VULNERABLE

VULNERABLE
The Law, Policy and Ethics of COVID-19

Edited by Colleen M. Flood, Vanessa MacDonnell,
Jane Philpott, Sophie Thériault,
and Sridhar Venkatapuram

University of Ottawa Press
2020

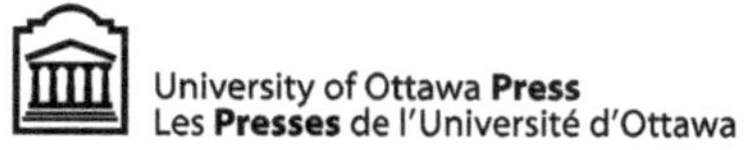

The University of Ottawa Press (UOP) is proud to be the oldest of the francophone university presses in Canada as well as the oldest bilingual university publisher in North America. Since 1936, UOP has been enriching intellectual and cultural discourse by producing peer-reviewed and award-winning books in the humanities and social sciences, in French and in English.
www.press.uOttawa.ca

Library and Archives Canada Cataloguing in Publication
Title: Vulnerable : the law, policy & ethics of COVID-19 / edited by Colleen M. Flood, Vanessa MacDonnell, Sophie Thériault, Sridhar Venkatapuram, Jane Philpott.
Other titles: Vulnerable (Ottawa, Ont.)
Names: Flood, Colleen M., editor. | MacDonnell, Vanessa, editor. | Thériault, Sophie, 1976- editor. | Venkatapuram, Sridhar, editor. | Philpott, Jane, 1960- editor.
Description: Some essays in French. | Includes bibliographical references and index.
Identifiers: Canadiana (print) 20200262610 | Canadiana (ebook) 20200262815 | ISBN 9780776636412 (hardcover) | ISBN 9780776636405 (softcover) | ISBN 9780776636429 (PDF) | ISBN 9780776636443 (Kindle) | ISBN 9780776636436 (EPUB)
Subjects: LCSH: COVID-19 (Disease)—Social aspects.
Classification: LCC RA644.C67 V85 2020 | DDC 362.1962/414—dc23

Legal Deposit: Third Quarter 2020
Library and Archives Canada

Production Team

Copy editing	James Warren Susan James Heather Lang Maryse Tremblay
Proofreading	France Beauregard James Warren Susan James Michael Waldin
Typesetting	Édiscript enr.
Cover design	Édiscript enr.

Cover image

Design by Clémence Labasse.
Images: Coronavirus copy space by BlackJack3D iStockPhoto.
Earth Eastern Hemisphere by NASA.

The University of Ottawa Press gratefully acknowledges the support extended to its publishing list by the Government of Canada, the Canada Council for the Arts, the Ontario Arts Council, the Social Sciences and Humanities Research Council and the Canadian Federation for the Humanities and Social Sciences through the Awards to Scholarly Publications Program, and by the University of Ottawa.

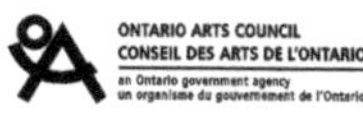

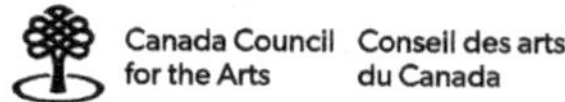

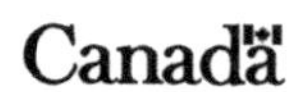

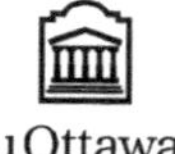

Table of Contents

SECTION E
THIS JOB IS GONNA KILL ME: WORKING AND COVID-19

SECTION F
GLOBAL HEALTH AND GOVERNANCE

Acknowledgments

Delivering a book in less than eight weeks from start to finish, particularly during and in response to a global pandemic, cannot be achieved without the support and generosity of many people.

First and foremost, we thank our stellar roster of contributors, who without exception willingly gave of their time and expertise and graciously accepted strict deadlines at a time of serious personal and professional challenges. We and our readers are indebted to you.

Thanks also to our research assistants from the University of Ottawa Centre for Health Law, Policy and Ethics and the University of Ottawa Public Law Centre for their superb support: Arianne Kent, Émilie Hogue, and Amber Miller. We are also very thankful to JD candidate Kelli White, Adjunct Professor Bryan Thomas, and Visiting Fellow Stephen Bindman for their insights, edits, and deft management of the many moving parts needed to make this expedited book a reality.

We are grateful for the support of the University of Ottawa's Associate Vice-President, Research, Promotion and Development Martine Lagacé, and for financial assistance from the Office of the Vice-President, Research, and Faculty of Law Deans Adam Dodek (Common Law Section) and Marie-Eve Sylvestre (Civil Law Section). Their financial support made it possible for this book to be accessible to all. And many thanks to the terrific staff at the University of Ottawa Press, led by Lara Mainville, especially Maryse Cloutier and Clémence Labasse, who agreed to move heaven and earth to publish this book in record time.

We would also like to express our appreciation to Associated Medical Services (AMS) for its generous financial support enabling the publication of this book and for recognizing the importance of this work at such a critical juncture in Canadian history.

And very special thanks to our peer reviewers: Professor Jocelyn Downie (Dalhousie University), Professor Greg Marchildon (University of Toronto), Professor Judy Fudge (McMaster University), Professor Alana Klein (McGill University), Professor Jean Leclair (Université de Montréal), Professor Catherine Régis (Université de Montréal), Professor Maxime St-Hilaire (Université de Sherbrooke), Professor Signa Daum Shanks (Osgoode Hall Law School, York University), and Professor Emma Cunliffe (University of British Columbia). Each took many hours at an extremely busy time for academics to provide reviews for the book and help us improve our analysis.

Finally, we dedicate this book to the hundreds of thousands whose lives were and will be lost prematurely to COVID-19; to the health care workers, caregivers, and front line responders who have accepted increased risk to their own health and life to care for others; and to all those harmed by COVID-19 and the responses. The destiny of humanity is interconnected and precarious. In that context, we have sought to shine a light on a new vulnerability and how some are much more vulnerable than others.

Reviews

No book could be more timely and important than *Vulnerable: The Law, Policy and Ethics of COVID-19*. This book explores the unconscionable health, social, and economic inequities revealed by COVID-19. It probes the profound weaknesses in many national responses, the deficiencies in global institutions, and the affronts to human rights and the rule of law. Above all, this marvellous book makes a compelling case for transparency, accountability, and justice. The book is a tour de force on the human, social, economic, and legal impacts of a once in a lifetime pandemic.

Lawrence O. Gostin
University Professor and Founding O'Neill Chair in Global Health Law, Georgetown University

Through *Vulnerable*, we are confronted with the failures and fissures in Canadian society exposed by the COVID-19 pandemic. This collection unmasks the extreme vulnerability to the ravages of inequality based on race, disability, age, and immigration status, and other sites of discrimination. By reflecting upon power, responsibility, and accountability, *Vulnerable* provides the reader with tools to use and paths to follow, to immediately begin to build our better normal.

Jocelyn Downie
James S. Palmer Chair in Public Policy and Law, Dalhousie University

In the wake of COVID-19, many of us are asking, "What just happened?" This book provides the answer. Leading scholars from across disciplines address the pandemic's impact, with vulnerability as the underlying theme. Why were some neighbourhoods hit harder than others? Do lessons learned equip us to better manage a "second wave?" Did Canadian federalism impede more effective responses? And what if a vaccine is delayed, or proves impossible? This book is an indispensable source of insight and advice, helping us understand not only what happened, but how to diminish the chances of it happening again.

Allan Rock
Former Minister of Health (Canada)
and Former President of the University of Ottawa

Pandemics and contagion bring out the best and worst in individuals and societies. They put into stark relief the strengths, weaknesses, gaps, and inequities in society, government policies, and institutional practices. Lessons from past events are often forgotten. This book presents crucial perspectives, to deal with the current pandemic and prepare for the future.

David Butler-Jones
First Chief Public Health Officer of Canada

What will our society look like now? *Vulnerable: The Law, Policy and Ethics of Covid-19* tackles this question head on, exposing the deadly health, social and economic failures of our past choices and proposing new and fairer frameworks for the tough decisions of the post-pandemic world.

Maureen McTeer
Canadian author and lawyer

Assembled in the midst of an unprecedented epidemic, this collection of 43 short essays examines vulnerabilities in Canada's defences against COVID-19, and the resultant consequences for vulnerable populations at home and abroad. It should be required reading for anyone who cares about Canadian public health policy, law, and ethics.

David Naylor
Co-Chair of the Federal COVID-19
Immunity Task Force

This important compilation comes at a time in Canada when we are looking back on the first months of a global pandemic and strengthening our foundation for future work. The authors' in-depth questioning and proposing of just and innovative approaches should inform how COVID-19 is addressed by public health and elected representatives.

Dr. Monika Dutt
Public Health and Preventive Medicine Specialist,
Sydney, Nova Scotia

INTRODUCTION

Overview of COVID-19: Old and New Vulnerabilities*

Colleen M. Flood, Vanessa MacDonnell,
Jane Philpott, Sophie Thériault, and Sridhar Venkatapuram

Within the span of a few months, a new virus named SARS-CoV-2 (which causes the disease COVID-19) has altered the course of nations and the world. Indeed, it is difficult to process all the rapid and sweeping changes to our lives, social interactions, government functioning, and global relations that the COVID-19 pandemic has caused. But the devastation it has and is producing, and the unequal distribution of harms within and across countries, demands global responses to pandemic control that prioritize equity. It is for this reason that in April 2020 we embarked on a collaborative effort with 69 authors to better understand the impact the pandemic is having on Canada and the world. This edited collection is the result of that collaboration. More than anything, this volume documents the vulnerabilities and interconnectedness made visible by the pandemic and the legal, ethical, and policy responses to it. These include vulnerabilities for people who have been harmed or will be harmed by the virus directly and those neglected or harmed by measures taken to slow its relentless march; vulnerabilities exposed in our institutions, governance, and legal structures; and vulnerabilities in other countries and at the global level where persistent injustices harm us all.

* We are grateful to Bryan Thomas, Stephen Bindman, and the peer reviewers for excellent comments on this introduction. We also thank Kelli White and Arianne Kent for their superb research assistance.

The book, comprising 43 short chapters, is divided into 6 subthemes: federalism and governance, accountability, civil liberties, equity, labour, and global health. Our approach is one primarily grounded in law, because of the critical nature of law in defining responsibilities, accountability, rights, distribution of wealth, and, indeed, health. We have included other important disciplines, including ethics, public policy, public health, and medicine. We begin this overview chapter by providing context for the pandemic with facts and figures (including what we do not know), before turning to discuss in more detail how we employ a lens of vulnerability throughout our analysis. Subsequently, for each of our subthemes, we highlight insights emerging from the chapters. We conclude by claiming that the COVID-19 pandemic forces us to reflect deeply on how we are governed and on our policy priorities in order to ensure pandemic preparedness, response, and recovery policies include all of us, not just some or the most privileged of us.

Context for a Modern-Day Plague

The Emergence of COVID-19

At the time of writing, the novel coronavirus SARS-CoV-2[1] has infected people in 213 countries and territories and on every continent except Antarctica.[2] As of June 27, 2020, over 495,781 people worldwide[3] have died, including the 8,504 people who have died in Canada.[4] The true death toll is certainly higher and will continue to rise.

The respiratory illness caused by SARS-CoV-2 was initially identified by regional health authorities in China after dozens of people with similar symptoms were treated in Wuhan, Hubei Province, in December 2019. This made headlines when the World Health

1. "COVID-19 Coronavirus Pandemic", online: *Worldometer* <https://www.worldometers.info/coronavirus/>.
2. "COVID-19 Has Infected Every Continent Except Antarctica", *The Times of India* (27 February 2020), online: <https://timesofindia.indiatimes.com/world/china/COVID-19-has-infected-every-continent-except-antarctica/articleshow/74327535.cms>.
3. "COVID-19 Dashboard" (27 June 2020), online: *Centre for Systems Science and Engineering at Johns Hopkins University* <https://www.arcgis.com/apps/opsdashboard/index.html#/bda7594740fd40299423467b48e9ecf6>.
4. See dashboard from the Canada Open Data Working Group, "COVID-19 in Canada", online: *Canada Open Data Working Group* <https://art-bd.shinyapps.io/covid19canada/>.

Organization (WHO) tweeted on January 4, 2020, that it was investigating a cluster of pneumonia-like cases in China.[5] A week later, the genetic sequence of the novel coronavirus was shared publicly.[6] Then, on January 13, Thailand reported the first case outside of China. On January 30, amid thousands of new cases in China, and infections spreading across countries, the WHO declared a "public health emergency of international concern," as required by International Health Regulations.[7]

By January 31, Italy was reporting its first cases as being two Chinese tourists who travelled to Rome from Wuhan and fell ill.[8] Italy was the first European country to report cases and its subsequent experience—hospitals filled beyond capacity, and a mounting death toll—was a cautionary tale for other countries.

At the beginning of February, reports emerged of an outbreak on the Diamond Princess cruise ship—then the largest cluster of cases—more than 200—outside of China.[9] By the third week of February, Iran reported a large outbreak; as an international travel hub, this raised further alarm among public health experts.[10]

As lockdowns were initiated across Latin America and Europe, infections spiked in all jurisdictions, followed soon after by a nationwide lockdown for India's 1.3 billion inhabitants. The WHO described the spread of the novel coronavirus as a "pandemic" on March 11. On March 26, the United States earned the unenviable distinction of leading the world in confirmed infections and deaths. Soon after, despite

---

5. "WHO Timeline—COVID-19" (27 April 2020), online: *World Health Organization* <https://www.who.int/news-room/detail/27-04-2020-who-timeline---COVID-19>; Hilary Brueck, "The WHO Made a Thinly Veiled Dig at Sweden's Loose Coronavirus Lockdown, Saying 'Humans Are Not Herds' and Old People are Not Disposable", *Business Insider* (11 May 2020), online: <https://www.businessinsider.com/herd-immunity-few-people-have-had-the-coronavirus-who-2020-5?fbclid=IwAR3ZcQ_3F7vdWCB-lDshXHzEifBobek_AFRgKI5JenRXfQQqWixw-W5d7I4>.
6. "Novel Coronavirus—China" (12 January 2020), online: *World Health Organization* <https://www.who.int/csr/don/12-january-2020-novel-coronavirus-china/en/>.
7. Derrick Bryson Taylor, "How the Coronavirus Pandemic Unfolded: A Timeline", *The New York Times* (12 May 2020), online: <https://www.nytimes.com/article/coronavirus-timeline.html>.
8. Iris Bosa, "Italy's Response to the Coronavirus Pandemic" (16 April 2020), online (blog): *Cambridge Core - Health Economics, Policy and Law (HEPL) Blog Series* <https://www.cambridge.org/core/blog/2020/04/16/italys-response-to-the-coronavirus-pandemic/>.
9. *Ibid.*
10. *Ibid.*

initial speculation that Africa might escape unscathed, infections and deaths began to be recorded there. At the time of writing, there are more than 130,000 confirmed cases on that continent.[11]

SARS-CoV-2: The Epidemiology

SARS-CoV-2 is a new virus. It is part of a family of coronaviruses that may be transmitted from animals to people. It is thought to have originated in a bat but was transmitted to humans via another vector or animal species. For decades, it has been recognized that with ever-increasing interactions between people and undomesticated animals and increasing globalization, novel coronaviruses will from time to time spread among human populations.[12] Previous examples include Severe Acute Respiratory Syndrome (SARS), which has caused 774 deaths worldwide to date,[13] and Middle East Respiratory Syndrome (MERS), which has caused 858 fatalities around the world to date.[14] With a reported 503,000 deaths in a few short months, the harm of the COVID-19 pandemic dwarfs that of the other outbreaks. Unfortunately, infectious disease experts agree that even more harmful viruses could emerge in the future.

As of June 27, 2020, there have been over 10 million cases of COVID-19 reported worldwide,[15] but the number is likely much higher, as many cases are asymptomatic and testing availability and infrastructure, use, and criteria vary significantly across jurisdictions, and there is no standardized approach to reporting.[16]

---

11. Jason Burke & Nyasha Chingoyo, "African Nations Fail to Find Coronavirus Quarantine Escapees", *The Guardian* (31 May 2020), online: <www.theguardian.com/world/2020/may/31/african-nations-fail-to-find-coronavirus-quarantine-escapees>.
12. Hongying Li et al, "Human-Animal Interactions and Bat Coronavirus Spillover Potential Among Rural Residents in Southern China" (2019) 1:2 J Biosafety & Health 84.
13. "SARS Basics Fact Sheet" (6 December 2017), online: *Centre for Disease Control and Prevention* <https://www.cdc.gov/sars/about/fs-sars.html>.
14. "Middle East Respiratory Syndrome Coronavirus (MERS-CoV)" (November 2019), online: *World Health Organization* <https://www.who.int/emergencies/mers-cov/en/>.
15. Worldometer, *supra* note 1.
16. Sometimes the claim is that labs were overwhelmed so that testing was not possible. See Kelly Crowe, "Why Isn't Canada Testing Everyone for Coronavirus?", *CBC News* (13 April 2020), online: <https://www.cbc.ca/news/health/coronavirus-covid19-testing-canada-1.5527219>. But, on the other hand, we see resistance on the part of some medical officers of health to increasing

Our epidemiological understanding of COVID-19 is greatly hindered by the quality and availability of data. Still, available data show some emerging patterns. Globally, it seems more men die than women: 69% of all coronavirus deaths reported across Western Europe have been male.[17] However, in Canada this trend is reversed, as the vast majority of deaths have occurred in long-term care homes, where the majority of residents and workers are women.[18] There are also significant differences in rates of death by age groups, with older people dying most.[19] A large sample in Italy found that 80% of deaths were among people aged 70 and older.[20] Nursing home residents and care workers in many high-income countries (HICs) have died in staggering numbers. At least one-third of COVID-19 deaths in the U.S. have been in nursing homes (whether residents or caregivers). Similarly, WHO figures indicate that almost half of all people who have died in Europe were residents of care facilities.[21] Canada has the highest proportion of deaths in long-term care settings among 14 countries in a study by the International Long-Term Care Policy Network, an incredible 82%.[22]

Initially, little data was collected on the socio-economic, racial, and ethnic backgrounds of victims. Once data began to be collected,

testing rates. See "Hamilton's Associate Medical Officer of Health Apologizes to Premier Doug Ford", *CBC News* (24 April 2020), online: <https://www.cbc.ca/news/canada/hamilton/bart-harvey-apology-doug-ford-1.5543557>.

17. Martha Henriques, "Why Covid-19 is Different for Men and Women", *BBC News* (12 April 2020), online: <https://www.bbc.com/future/article/20200409-why-covid-19-is-different-for-men-and-women>.

18. As of May 15, 55% of confirmed cases of COVID-19 are women, and women made up 53% of the total deaths in Canada. See Olivia Bowden, "More Canadian Women Have COVID-19 and are Dying as a Result. Here's Some Possible Reasons Why", *Global News* (17 May 2020), online: <https://globalnews.ca/news/6920505/more-women-have-coronavirus/>.

19. Anuja Vaidya, "6 Insights into COVID-19 Patient Care Patterns Worldwide" (12 May 2020), online: *Becker's Hospital Review* <https://www.beckershospitalreview.com/patient-safety-outcomes/6-insights-into-covid-19-patient-care-patterns-worldwide.html>.

20. David Wallace-Wells, "COVID-19 Targets the Elderly. Why Don't Our Prevention Efforts?", *New York Magazine* (13 May 2020), online: <https://nymag.com/intelligencer/2020/05/covid-targets-the-elderly-why-dont-our-prevention-efforts.html>.

21. Eimear Flanagan, "Coronavirus: Almost Half of Irish Covid-19 Deaths in Care Homes", *BBC News* (23 April 2020), online: <https://www.bbc.com/news/world-europe-52399869>.

22. International Long-term Care Policy Network & Care Policy and Evaluation Centre, "Country Reports: COVID-19 and Long-Term Care" (19 April 2020), online: *Resources to Support Community and Institutional Long-Term Care Responses to COVID-19* <https://ltccovid.org/country-reports-on-covid-19-and-long-term-care/>.

particularly in the United Kingdom and the United States, clear distribution patterns began to emerge. For example, people living in the poorest Scottish neighbourhoods were twice as likely to die as their wealthier neighbours.[23] The death rate was 86.5 per 100,000 in the poorest fifth of Scottish neighbourhoods, compared to 38.2 in the richest fifth. Socio-economic disadvantage is strongly correlated with vulnerability to infection and death from COVID-19.

In Canada, Quebec has the highest COVID-19 death rate per capita in the country (reportedly the seventh deadliest place in the world), propelled by very lethal outbreaks in the low-income neighbourhoods of Montréal.[24] Some have attributed this to the province's early spring break (i.e., Quebeckers travelled abroad and returned infected before provinces began taking strict measures).[25] It is clear, however, that hot spots of the outbreak in Montréal are in poorer areas, particularly among recent immigrants living in overcrowded housing,[26] some of whom work in long-term care facilities, placed there by temporary employment agencies.[27] The working hypothesis is that care workers bring the illness back to neighbourhoods, where it spreads rapidly because of poverty and crowding. The extent to which Montréal differs from other major cities in Canada is not yet known. Data suggest that within Toronto, poor neighbourhoods also have vastly higher reported cases than neighbouring wealthy suburbs.[28]

The socio-economic dimensions of COVID-19 transmissions and deaths in HICs is raising alarm regarding how the disease will impact low-to-middle income countries (LMICs). Lockdowns, which seem to

---

23. Tom Gordon, "Poorest Scots Twice as Likely to Die from Coronavirus", *The Herald* (13 May 2020), online: <https://www.heraldscotland.com/news/18445900.poorest-scots-twice-likely-die-coronavirus/>.
24. Tracey Lindeman, "Why Are so Many People Getting Sick and Dying in Montreal from Covid-19?", *The Guardian* (13 May 2020), online: <https://www.theguardian.com/world/2020/may/13/coronavirus-montreal-canada-hit-hard>.
25. Leyland Cecco, "Canada's Bid to Beat Back Coronavirus Exposes Stark Gaps Between Provinces", *The Guardian* (15 April 2020), online: <https://www.theguardian.com/world/2020/apr/15/canada-coronavirus-covid-19-provinces-trudeau>.
26. *Ibid.*
27. For a discussion of temporary employment agencies and long-term care, see Katherine Lippel, this volume, Chapter E-3.
28. Kelly Grant & Carly Weeks, "Examining Hot Spots for Community Spread Across Ontario", *The Globe and Mail* (29 May 2020), online: <https://www.theglobeandmail.com/canada/article-examining-hot-spots-for-community-spread-across-ontario/?utm_medium=Referrer:+Social+Network+/+Media&utm_campaign=Shared+Web+Article+Links>.

be the primary intervention, are often challenging in LMICs, if not impossible, due to poverty and population density.

The Policy Response to COVID-19

There have been very different political responses to COVID-19 across countries. At one end of the spectrum are countries that have implemented very restrictive measures. China set a global precedent, instituting what was then the largest quarantine in world history of the Wuhan region's sixty million people. This has since been eclipsed as other countries have locked down to a greater or lesser degree. Neighbouring countries such as Vietnam, South Korea, and Taiwan, perhaps enlightened by their earlier experience of SARS and H1N1, responded quickly to the Wuhan outbreak by shutting down borders and implementing aggressive testing and contact tracing, relying heavily on digital surveillance. They seem to have largely contained the virus; however, it is hard to predict what will happen as physical distancing restrictions are lifted.

At the other end of the spectrum, among Western countries, Sweden stands out for its embrace of a less restrictive approach that some media have dubbed "anti-lockdown." Sweden's chief epidemiologist pursued a strategy of mitigation: allow the virus to spread slowly without overwhelming the health system, without recourse to harsh social isolation restrictions, and attempt to shield the most vulnerable. Earlier in the pandemic, countries such as the U.K. and the U.S. also toyed with policies aimed at establishing "herd immunity"; namely that they would permit the virus to spread so that at a certain point enough people in the population would acquire immunity that the disease would significantly dissipate. However, both countries implemented lockdowns of varying degrees after enormous expert and popular outcry.

Canada's path through COVID-19 is perhaps best described as a middle ground. This approach has seen neither the federal nor provincial governments impose strict lockdowns (i.e., unlike in New Zealand, Canadian governments have not mandated that people stay in their homes, although they have encouraged it). Provinces have, however, imposed various restrictions on large and small gatherings, closed schools, universities, and nonessential businesses, locked down jails and long-term care institutions, and issued physical distancing guidelines. Both federal and provincial governments have provided significant funding to support affected businesses and employees.

Canadians have largely accepted this middle-way approach, and to date, the hospital system has not been overrun. There have been, however, significant provincial variations in infection rates. British Columbia, which acted the fastest amongst Canadian provinces in response to the outbreak, has for the moment succeeded in stemming what appeared initially to be a rather aggressive spread of the virus, using measures assessed as relatively "stringent" by the Oxford Stringency Index, developed to monitor country policies in response to the pandemic.[29] By contrast, infection and death rates in Quebec and Ontario remain high for reasons not yet fully understood although, as discussed earlier, outbreaks have been strongly correlated with socio-economic deprivation.

Across Canada, the vast preponderance of deaths (82%) have been associated with overrun long-term care institutions, with accounts of personal support workers forced to abandon their jobs for fear of the disease and for the health of their own families, sometimes leaving the frail elderly dehydrated, hungry, covered in feces, and in rare cases, left for dead. The military was called in to assist in Quebec and Ontario,[30] and in both cases, has issued devastating reports on the conditions they found.[31] Thus, while the Canadian approach has been successful to date in fending off an unmanageable surge in hospitals, a myopic focus on hospitals left long-term care homes and similar institutions exposed.

As infection rates have begun to drop, some countries are beginning to lift these measures, some gradually and others more quickly.

---

29. Brandon Tang, Sara Allin & Greg Marchidon, "British Columbia's Response to the Coronavirus Pandemic" (25 April 2020), online (blog): *Cambridge Core - HEPL Blog Series* <https://www.cambridge.org/core/blog/2020/04/25/british-columbias-response-to-the-coronavirus-pandemic>; Natalie Obiko Pearson, "Behind North America's Lowest Death Rate: A Doctor Who Fought Ebola", *Bloomberg News* (16 May 2020), online: <https://www.bloomberg.com/news/articles/2020-05-16/a-virus-epicenter-that-wasn-t-how-one-region-stemmed-the-deaths>. For the stringency index, see Oxford University, "Coronavirus Government Response Tracker" (last visited 13 May 2020), online: *Blavatnik School of Government* <https://www.bsg.ox.ac.uk/research/research-projects/coronavirus-government-response-tracker>.
30. "Long-Term Care COVID-19 Tracker" (last visited 13 May 2020), online: *National Institute on Ageing* <https://ltc-covid19-tracker.ca/>.
31. For Quebec, letter from Colonel T M Arsenault, and for Ontario, letter from Brigadier General C J A Mialkowski, both letters dated 19 May 2020 and on file with the authors.

The impact of COVID-19 on the economy has generated a great deal of concern in all countries. In some, the economic necessity to reopen is accompanied by a strong culture of personal freedom and resistance to government interventions. The epidemiological data is clearly just one consideration in deciding when and how to lift lockdowns.

It is already evident that every approach carries its own risk of unforeseen consequences. For instance, while the early shutdown of borders and lockdowns seems to have propelled some countries toward success (New Zealand, Taiwan, South Korea), other democracies that locked down quickly, such as India, Italy, Spain, and Greece, saw thousands of people moving between areas on the announcement of an impending lockdown.

Around the world, the priority now seems to be preventing transmission, protecting the vulnerable, and restarting work, commerce, and education. To do this, the focus is on known places and settings of vulnerability, alongside public health measures of hygiene, physical distancing, masking, testing, and tracing. Canada has not been a strong performer on testing and tracing, falling far below testing targets,[32] and there are significant disparities in testing rates across provinces.

The Unknowns

Many crucial factors remain unknown. First, while a vaccine is seen by many as the magic bullet, it is unknown when or even whether one will be developed; policies contingent on this hope may have to be recalibrated. Nor do we know whether, once a vaccine is developed, there will be a sufficient supply at a price that is affordable for all who need it. Second, the extent and duration of natural immunity produced from SARS-CoV-2 infection is another unknown. Third, we do not know the extent of the harmful consequences of all the policy measures taken to combat COVID-19. For example, an estimated 1.2 million children worldwide could die in the next six months due to the disruption of health services and food supplies caused by the coronavirus pandemic.[33] Lockdowns and physical isolation have led to severe

32. Omar Sachedina & Ben Cousins, "As Canadians Struggle to Receive COVID-19 Testing, Health Officials Recommend Expansion", *CTV News* (12 May 2020), online: <https://www.ctvnews.ca/health/coronavirus/as-canadians-struggle-to-receive-covid-19-testing-health-officials-recommend-expansion-1.4936998>.

33. Kate Hodal, "UNICEF: 6,000 Children Could Die Day Due to Impact of Coronavirus", *The Guardian* (13 May 2020), online: <https://www.theguardian.com/

job losses, economic recession, increased mental health issues, and rising domestic violence. In the longer run, we will have to account for both sides of the ledger, namely the people who were saved because of precautionary measures and the people who were lost or harmed. Fourth, we do not yet know which of the various approaches taken by governments to combat COVID-19 are most effective. This will be important to know when responding to further waves of infection. Some claim that Japan has been relatively successful because people commonly and willingly wear masks. Others suggest that the strict separation of suspected COVID-19 patients into separate hospitals or treatment facilities is key. Many analyses refer to the importance of testing and tracing, or the importance of acting early and closing borders. Others promote a strong focus on high-risk populations in long-term care settings, prisons, factories, and other sites. We need detailed scientific research into the range of approaches taken and the factors that determine their efficacy in order to understand the impact of different approaches on different vulnerable groups.

Vulnerability as an Organizing Theme

We employ a lens of vulnerability throughout our analysis. COVID-19 has exposed and created vulnerabilities that follow the fault lines of pre-existing structural inequities. COVID-19 has flourished in settings where people were already vulnerable because of government policies and corporate bottom lines. Many of the virus's hot spots in high-income countries (HICs)—long-term care homes, prisons, immigration detention centres, and slaughterhouses, among others—are spaces of acute vulnerability because they are sites of long-standing structural inequalities.

Governments have long tolerated substandard quality of care in long-term care homes, caused by, among other things, understaffing and low wages.[34] Oversight of public and private long-term care facilities varies between jurisdictions, but is often inadequate. In Ontario, for example, annual inspections have essentially evaporated in the

global-development/2020/may/13/unicef-6000-children-could-die-every-day-due-to-impact-of-coronavirus>.

34. Martine Lagacé, Linda Garcia & Louise Bélanger-Hardy, this volume, Chapter D-2; Matthew Kupfer, "'Something Is Bound to Break': More Long-Term Care Staff Needed, Families Say", *CBC News* (23 April 2020), online: <https://www.cbc.ca/news/canada/ottawa/madonna-care-community-orleans-staff-recruit-1.5541610>.

past two years: CBC News reports that in 2019, less than 1.5% of long-term care homes received annual inspections.[35]

Overcrowding is a well-documented feature of prisons and immigration detention centres around the world, caused by a combination of punitive criminal laws and policies around bail, inadequate community mental health services, harsh sentences for convicted offenders, and other factors.[36] Access to healthy food, hygiene products, and health care—the most basic obligations owed by the state to individuals in its care—are persistent problems.[37] The response to COVID-19 in federal and provincial prisons has been to increase lockdowns and/or segregation.[38] While jail staff in most Canadian prisons now appear to have access to personal protective equipment (PPE), prisoners in many facilities remain without access to masks and gloves.[39] With the majority of trials adjourned indefinitely, prisoners on remand face periods of pre-trial detention of uncertain length in conditions of great stress and exposure.[40]

Slaughterhouses have long been considered sites of insecurity and risk for workers.[41] In recent decades, government regulation has

35. Katie Pedersen, Melissa Mancini & David Common, "Ontario Scaled Back Comprehensive, Annual Inspections of Nursing Homes to Only a Handful Last Year", *CBC News* (15 April 2020), online: <https://www.cbc.ca/news/canada/seniors-homes-inspections-1.5532585>.
36. "Reasonable Bail?" (September 2013), online (pdf): *John Howard Society of Ontario* <https://johnhoward.on.ca/wp-content/uploads/2014/07/JHSO-Reasonable-Bail-report-final.pdf>.
37. Adelina Iftene, this volume, Chapter D-5; Deepan Budlakoti, "The Ottawa Jail Is No Vacation – Especially During COVID-19", *Ottawa Citizen* (22 May 2020), online: <https://ottawacitizen.com/opinion/budlakoti-the-ottawa-jail-is-no-vacation-especially-during-covid-19>.
38. Iftene, this volume, Chapter D-5; Criminalization and Punishment Education Project, News Release, "Government of Ontario Needs to Take Additional Steps to Reduce the Use and Harms of Imprisonment at the Ottawa-Carleton Detention Centre During the COVID-19 Crisis" (6 April 2020), online: *Criminalization and Punishment Education Project* <https://cp-ep.org/new-press-release-via-cpep/>; Office of the Correctional Investigator, *COVID-19 Status Update* (Ottawa: Office of the Correctional Investigator, 23 April 2020), online (pdf): *Office of the Correctional Investigator* <https://perma.cc/DT46-PADV>; Stephen Hoff, "Jail Guards Want COVID-19 Screening at Ottawa-Carleton Detention Centre", *CBC News* (1 April 2020), online: <https://www.cbc.ca/news/canada/ottawa/active-monitoring-ocdc-covid19-1.5516645>.
39. Iftene, this volume, Chapter D-5; Budlakoti, *supra* note 37; J.A.I.L. Accountability and Information Line, "People at the Ottawa Jail Echo This Demand!" (8 May 2020 at 15:34), online: *Twitter* <https://twitter.com/jail_line/status/1258842842916626433>.
40. Budlakoti, *ibid.*
41. Sarah Berger Richardson, "COVID-19 Disruption Reveals Challenges in our Meat Supply", *The Province* (16 April 2020), online: <https://theprovince.com/

led to the closure of small slaughterhouses and the emergence of supersized corporate abattoirs that employ large numbers of workers.[42] Two of the largest outbreaks of COVID-19 in Canada have been at Cargill slaughterhouses in Alberta and Quebec.[43] These plants rely heavily on the labour of immigrants and temporary foreign workers.[44] Temporary foreign workers often live in shared accommodation and share transportation to work because of low wages. Unionization has not prevented such workers from being forced back to work following large outbreaks.[45] Recent outbreaks amoungs migrant farmworkers in Ontario raise similar issues.

Indigenous Peoples, including First Nations on reserves, face unique challenges in dealing with COVID-19.[46] Colonialism and systemic discrimination, which are manifest in the chronic underfunding of essential services and infrastructure, heighten indigenous people's vulnerability. For instance, at the time of writing, 61 First Nations communities are under long-term drinking water advisories, making it very difficult to implement the basic hygiene measures to prevent the spread of the virus.[47] Moreover, the well-documented overcrowding and substandard housing on reserves

---

opinion/sarah-berger-richardson-covid-19-disruption-reveals-challenges-in-our-meat-supply>.

42. Sarah Berger Richardson, this volume, Chapter E-5.
43. Berger Richardson, this volume, Chapter E-5; Jennifer A Quaid, this volume, Chapter B-8. See also Kathryn Blaze Baum, Carrie Tait & Tavia Grant, "How Cargill Became the Site of Canada's Largest Single Outbreak of COVID-19", *The Globe and Mail* (2 May 2020), online: <https://www.theglobeandmail.com/business/article-how-cargill-became-the-site-of-canadas-largest-single-outbreak-of/>; Colin Harris, "Cargill Meat-Processing Plant to Shut Down After COVID-19 Outbreak", *CBC News* (10 May 2020), online: <https://www.cbc.ca/news/canada/montreal/cargill-chambly-covid-19-shut-down-1.5563539>.
44. Y Y Brandon Chen, this volume, Chapter D-8; Stephanie Babych, "Filipino Workers Face Backlash in Towns over COVID-19 Outbreaks at Packing Plants", *Calgary Herald* (29 April 2020), online: <https://calgaryherald.com/news/filipino-employees-not-to-blame-for-meat-packing-plant-outbreaks-that-have-surpassed-1000-cases>.
45. "Workers Return to Alberta Meat Plant Despite Union's Effort to Block Reopening Amid COVID-19", *CBC News* (4 May 2020), online: <https://www.cbc.ca/news/canada/calgary/cargill-plant-meat-union-reopen-high-river-1.5554298>.
46. Aimée Craft, Deborah McGregor & Jeffery G Hewitt, this volume, Chapter A-2; Anne Levesque & Sophie Thériault, this volume, Chapter D-6.
47. Indigenous Services Canada, "Indigenous Services Canada" (21 May 2020), online: *Government of Canada* <https://www.canada.ca/en/indigenous-services-canada.html>; Indigenous Services Canada, "Short-Term Drinking Water Advisories" (11 July 2019), online: *Government of Canada* <https://www.sac-isc.gc.ca/eng/1562856509704/1562856530304>.

prevent First Nations families from complying with physical distancing.[48]

It would be a mistake to speak of these as discrete phenomena, however. To do so would risk obscuring how the current situation is the predictable outcome of policy choices made by governments. The pandemic is not a natural disaster or an "act of God." The effects of COVID-19 are the result of choices: to tax and spend in ways that benefit some and disadvantage others;[49] to intervene or not intervene in the economy when market forces prevent individuals from meeting basic needs; to regulate in particular ways; to view health as the product of a combination of luck and personal choices rather than the product of colliding social, economic, and political factors; and to adopt particular foreign policies toward international cooperation, including foreign aid.

The theme of vulnerability also touches domestic and international institutions. The pandemic is a stark reminder of the fragility of democratic governance, the rule of law, and fundamental rights.[50] Governments in both new and established democracies have quickly dispensed with normal procedures to respond to the pandemic. While there is no doubt that governments must respond quickly in a public health crisis, some balance must be found between the need for dispatch and the need for considered and accountable policy responses. The closure of courts for a period of months for all but urgent matters is unprecedented and demonstrates the degree to which the judicial system has until now continued to be reliant on in-person hearings and paper filings.[51]

48. Craft, McGregor & Hewitt, this volume, Chapter A-2; Levesque & Thériault, this volume, Chapter D-6.

49. See generally Attiya Waris, *Tax and Development: Solving Kenya's Fiscal Crisis Through Human Rights* (Nairobi: Law Africa, 2013).

50. Vanessa MacDonnell, this volume, Chapter B-1; Gerald Daly, "Democracy and the Global Emergency – Shared Experiences, Starkly Uneven Impacts" (15 May 2020), online (blog): *Verfassungsblog* <https://verfassungsblog.de/democracy-and-the-global-emergency-shared-experiences-starkly-uneven-impacts/>; Steve Paikin, "Liberty vs Security in a Pandemic" (2 April 2020), online (video): *Facebook* <https://www.facebook.com/TheAgenda/videos/liberty-vs-security-in-a-pandemic/2691840667581128/>.

51. Aedan Helmer, "'There Is No Going Back': How COVID-19 Forced Courts into the Digital Age", *Ottawa Citizen* (17 May 2020), online: <https://ottawacitizen.com/news/local-news/there-is-no-going-back-how-covid-19-forced-courts-into-the-digital-age>; Paola Loriggio & Liam Casey, "COVID-19 Pandemic Forces Ontario Justice System 'Stuck in the 1970s' to Modernize", *CP24* (29 April 2020),

The pandemic has been used by some governments as a pretext for seizing further control over the levers of government.[52] Scholars of the democratic decline in Hungary have identified the coronavirus outbreak as an important "constitutional moment" in President Viktor Orban's quest for supremacy, a "coronavirus coup."[53] Weak systems of government are vulnerable along multiple axes—prone to further hollowing out when the opportunity presents itself and also unable to coordinate an effective response to the pandemic owing to unresponsive governance and corruption.[54] In the United States, for example, state governments have resorted to covertly importing PPE to avoid its being confiscated by the federal government for redistribution to political allies.[55]

The Edited Collection

To illustrate the different ways COVID-19 reveals existing vulnerabilities and creates new ones, our discussion is grouped into six sections: federalism, accountability, civil liberties, equity, labour, and global health. While many of the chapters have a Canadian focus, they contain insights that will also be of interest to an international audience. In some cases, there is significant disagreement between our contributors. We do not attempt to resolve these differences, but illuminate them to help us better design the best legal and policy responses to COVID-19. In what follows, we discuss in reverse order the themes as they appear in this book, in order to emphasize the interconnectedness of global and local issues.

---

online: <https://www.cp24.com/news/covid-19-pandemic-forces-ontario-justice-system-stuck-in-the-1970s-to-modernize-1.4917915>.

52. Dan Baer, "The Shocking 'Coronavirus Coup' in Hungary Was a Wake-Up Call" (31 March 2020), online: *Carnegie Endowment for International Peace* <https://carnegieendowment.org/2020/03/31/shocking-coronavirus-coup-in-hungary-was-wake-up-call-pub-81431>.
53. Renáta Uitz, "Pandemic as Constitutional Moment" (24 March 2020), online (blog): *Verfassungsblog* <https://verfassungsblog.de/pandemic-as-constitutional-moment/>.
54. See generally Ebrahim Afsah, "Dysfunctional Resilience in the Afghan Civil Service" J World Comparative L (forthcoming 2020).
55. Ross Ketschke, "'You Can Get Past This' Man Wins Battle with COVID-19", *WCVB* (last modified 17 May 2020), online: <https://www.wcvb.com/article/you-can-get-past-this-man-wins-month-long-battle-with-covid-19/32556120#>.

Global Health and Governance

This pandemic has reinforced truths that global health academics have espoused for a decade or more. First, it is now patently clear that health is not just a matter of domestic circumstances, but is also global.[56] Our health is interconnected, and some of us are more vulnerable than others as a result. Second, for well over two decades, expert observers of global governance for health have highlighted how power and politics at the supranational level significantly shape health and health inequities within countries.[57] And third, there are large global threats to health, such as climate change, antimicrobial resistance, and new and re-emerging infectious diseases. What is new or unexpected about COVID-19 is how quickly this health crisis has become a global political crisis, with the WHO at its epicentre.[58] As infections began to spread in various countries, China and the WHO became targets of ferocious criticism, accused of colluding in their failure to control the pandemic early on.[59]

The WHO presents itself as a scientific organization governed by member countries and providing technical assistance. When the WHO began providing clear messaging in January that countries should test, isolate, trace, and treat, countries worldwide began shutting down their borders. Moreover, following China's and Italy's examples, most countries began self-quarantining or implementing lockdowns by mid-March.[60] How and why that became the primary policy of government leaders is still unclear, nor is it clear that lockdowns were the most effective options, at least for all countries. In Low and Middle-Income Countries (LMICs), lockdowns produced staggering hardships for hundreds of millions of people. In India, millions of rural to urban migrants who survive on daily wages were

56. Paul Farmer, *Reimagining Global Health: An Introduction* (Berkeley: University of California Press, 2013).
57. Julio Frenk & Suerie Moon, "Governance Challenges in Global Health" (2013) 368:10 New England J Medicine 936.
58. Stephen Buranyi, "The WHO v Coronavirus: Why it Can't Handle the Pandemic", *The Guardian* (10 April 2020), online: <https://www.theguardian.com/news/2020/apr/10/world-health-organization-who-v-coronavirus-why-it-cant-handle-pandemic>.
59. Shawn Yuan, "Inside the Early Days of China's Coronavirus Coverup", *Wired* (1 May 2020), online: <https://www.wired.com/story/inside-the-early-days-of-chinas-coronavirus-coverup/>.
60. "Global COVID-19 Lockdown Tracker" (last updated 19 May 2020), online: *Global COVID-19 Lockdown Tracker* <https://covid19-lockdown-tracker.netlify.app/image.png>.

suddenly left with no work.[61] Millions took to the roads, returning to their villages and towns. In many LMICs, where millions live in densely populated slums, the basic prerequisites for lockdown survival—such as clean water, toilets, space, money to buy food, and refrigerators—do not exist. Those venturing out to find work or food were sometimes brutally beaten by police for breaking lockdown restrictions.[62] The implausibility of following physical distancing, combined with the inability of many LMICs to provide a safety net for their citizens during lockdown, brought resistance to the generic or "one size fits all" pandemic response.[63]

As High-Income Countries (HICs) transformed their hospitals to handle the pandemic, they also began transforming their foreign aid funding into COVID-19 support. In preparing their own national responses, LMICs found themselves competing in the global market against HICs for testing kits, ventilators, and protective gear. LMICs generally had inadequate supplies and health care workers to deal with the pandemic. Moreover, there has been an "eviction effect," where the pandemic response has diverted attention from other health care needs and infectious disease control programs.[64] The devastation from the lockdowns and shutdown of most health care and public health programs is expected to erase years of progress.[65]

As with the global competition for limited personal protective equipment (PPE)—masks, gloves, and so forth—and ventilators, there is a race to find a vaccine. Who will discover the vaccine first, who will get it first, and will LMICs get the vaccine? These are all open

61. "The Impact of COVID-19 on Informal and Migrant Workers in India" (13 May 2020), online: *International Growth Centre* <https://www.theigc.org/event/the-impact-of-covid-19-on-informal-and-migrant-workers-in-india/>.
62. Isaac Mugabi, "COVID-19: Security Forces in Africa Brutalizing Civilians Under Lockdown" (20 April 2020), online: *DW* <https://www.dw.com/en/covid-19-security-forces-in-africa-brutalizing-civilians-under-lockdown/a-53192163>.
63. Alex Broadbent & Benjamin T H Smart, "Why a One-Size-Fits-All Approach to COVID-19 Could Have Lethal Consequences", *The Conversation* (23 March 2020), online: <http://theconversation.com/why-a-one-size-fits-all-approach-to-covid-19-could-have-lethal-consequences-134252>.
64. Timothy Robertson et al, "Early Estimates of the Indirect Effects of the COVID-19 Pandemic on Maternal and Child Mortality in Low-Income and Middle-Income Countries: A Modelling Study" [2020] Lancet Global Health, online: *The Lancet* <https://www.thelancet.com/journals/langlo/article/PIIS2214-109X(20)30229-1/abstract>.
65. "Covid-19 is Undoing Years of Progress in Curbing Global Poverty", *The Economist* (23 May 2020), online: <https://www.economist.com/international/2020/05/23/covid-19-is-undoing-years-of-progress-in-curbing-global-poverty>.

questions. On May 4, the G-20 countries, except the U.S. and Russia, joined major philanthropists to raise nearly €8 billion (approximately C$12.3 billion) for research and development of diagnostics, therapies, and vaccines, promising these would all be public goods, and fairly distributed.[66] Meanwhile, private sector companies, most based in the U.S., are also racing to develop vaccines, which will not be public goods.[67] It will soon become clear whether global cooperation and solidarity are rhetoric or reality.

This Job Is Gonna Kill Me: Working and COVID-19

The health and safety of workers is a critical theme of the COVID-19 pandemic. In Canada and around the world, the implementation of lockdowns required the designation of "essential workers." The list varies by jurisdiction but generally includes health care, food services, transportation, utilities, communication, and some government employees.[68] These workers have been spared some of the economic hardships of their neighbours who have lost jobs. However, they and their families have taken on significant risks to their own physical and mental health.[69]

In the health sector, early public discourse focused on preparing hospitals, ensuring an adequate supply of test kits, ventilators, and PPE. It quickly became clear that the most vulnerable commodity could be the workers themselves.[70] This has been evident in Canada since the 2006 SARS Commission Report, led by the Honourable Justice Archie Campbell, which determined that "the health system

66. Giuseppe Conte et al, "As EU Leaders, We Want to Unite the World Against Coronavirus and End the Global Crisis", *The Independent* (2 May 2020), online: <https://www.independent.co.uk/voices/coronavirus-eu-response-leaders-fight-covid-19-vaccine-a9495716.html>.
67. Tom McCarthy, "The Race for a Vaccine: How Trump's 'America First' Approach Hinders the Global Search", *The Guardian* (12 May 2020), online: <https://www.theguardian.com/world/2020/may/12/the-race-for-a-vaccine-how-trumps-america-first-approach-slows-the-global-search>.
68. Public Safety Canada, "Guidance on Essential Services and Functions in Canada During the COVID-19 Pandemic" (2 April 2020), online: *Government of Canada* <https://www.publicsafety.gc.ca/cnt/ntnl-scrt/crtcl-nfrstrctr/esf-sfe-en.aspx>.
69. See Pat Armstrong, Hugh Armstrong & Ivy Bourgeault, this volume, Chapter E-1; Lippel, this volume, Chapter E-3.
70. Jane Philpott, "'Public Officials Should be Obsessed with Protecting the Health Workers Who Will Keep People Alive'", *Maclean's* (31 March 2020), online: <https://www.macleans.ca/opinion/public-officials-should-be-obsessed-with-protecting-the-health-workers-who-will-keep-people-alive/>.

generally did not understand its obligations under worker safety laws and regulations. There was a lack of understanding of occupational safety as a discipline separate from infection control."[71] Nurses, doctors, and other health workers constituted the largest single group of SARS cases, unlike with COVID-19. Therefore, training in safety protocols and provision of PPE in the health sector was a focus of the Campbell Report, emphasizing the precautionary principle "that safety comes first, that reasonable efforts to reduce risk need not await scientific proof."[72] COVID-19 has put a spotlight on the workforce in different ways. The largest outbreaks have been linked to crowded workplaces; inadequate infection control; shortages of PPE; and economic, political, and emotional incentives to continue working despite illness.[73] Long-term care homes have been a major site of outbreaks, as low wages force workers to take shifts at multiple facilities, risking spread of the disease.

The essays in this section of the book explore a range of intersections between the workforce and COVID-19, including privatization of health care, occupational health and safety, and the duties owed to and by health workers.[74] We also include a chapter about a COVID-19 outbreak in a group home for adults with disabilities to illustrate the reality of the day-to-day fight against COVID disease.

The section also provides an international perspective on labour issues, using the framework of the global food supply chain.

Equity and COVID-19

While COVID-19 has had widespread health, economic, and social impacts, some groups have been disproportionately affected both by the disease and by the measures taken to contain its spread.[75] The increased vulnerability of certain populations to COVID-19, such as people with disabilities, the elderly, women, people living in poverty or experiencing homelessness, and racialized and Indigenous

71. The SARS Commission, *Spring of Fear*, vol 1 (Toronto: The SARS Commission, December 2006) (The Honourable Justice Archie Campbell) at 22, online: *The Archives of Ontario* <http://www.archives.gov.on.ca/en/e_records/sars/report/index.html>.
72. *Ibid*, at 14, volume 2.
73. For a discussion of the causes of outbreaks in the workplace, see Lippel, this volume, Chapter E-3; Berger Richardson, this volume, Chapter E-5.
74. Vanessa Gruben & Louise Bélanger-Hardy, this volume, Chapter E-4.
75. Sridhar Venkatapuram, this volume, Chapter D-1.

peoples, should be attributed not to their inherent characteristics or their choices, but to pre-existing structural inequities.

This pandemic has exposed the systemic factors that lead to marginalization and vulnerability, including classism, ageism, ableism, racism, and colonialism. For instance, concerns have been raised that medical triaging policies and decisions, notably the distribution of ventilators, could discriminate against persons with disabilities.[76] Elderly people, especially in long-term care homes, have been disproportionately impacted by the disease.[77] Vulnerability to COVID-19 has also followed the fault line of race. The disease is reportedly disproportionately affecting racialized minorities, while also perpetuating racist discourses, for example against Asian Canadians, who are widely stigmatized as being responsible for the pandemic and vectors for its spread.[78] Racialized people, including migrants and temporary foreign workers, are also overrepresented in prisons, meat processing plants, and long-term care homes.[79] Furthermore, colonialism and the systemic discrimination in government laws, policies, and practices regarding First Nations, Inuit, and Métis communities, including those related to access to clean water, adequate housing, and health care, pose unique challenges in the context of COVID-19.[80]

Measures taken to contain the pandemic have exacerbated the vulnerability of marginalized groups and individuals. For example, persons with disabilities have been affected by the temporary closure or reduction of essential services and programs, including public transportation and programs funding mobility and other assistive devices.[81] Persons experiencing homelessness have suffered service reduction or outright closure of homeless shelters and drop-ins.[82] Confinement and quarantine measures also have a disproportionate impact for children and women living in violent homes, especially in Indigenous communities where access to safe houses is limited or

76. Jennifer A Chandler et al, this volume, Chapter D-10; Tess Sheldon & Ravi Malhotra, this volume, Chapter D-9.
77. Martha Jackman, this volume, Chapter D-3; Lagacé, Garcia & Bélanger-Hardy, this volume, Chapter D-2.
78. Jamie Chai Yun Liew, this volume, Chapter D-7.
79. Chen, this volume, Chapter D-8; Liew, this volume, Chapter D-7.
80. Craft, McGregor & Hewitt, this volume, Chapter A-2; Levesque & Thériault, this volume, Chapter D-6.
81. Sheldon & Malhotra, this volume, Chapter D-9.
82. Leilani Farha & Kaitlin Schwan, this volume, Chapter D-4.

non-existent.[83] Moreover, certain populations, including people living with mental illness and those experiencing homelessness, face unique challenges in respecting public health directives on the use of public spaces and physical distancing. They are therefore disproportionately subjected to sanctions and enforcement procedures under public health laws.[84]

COVID-19 is both a public health crisis and "profound human rights crisis,"[85] but it can also be an opportunity for transformative policy and law reforms. While emergency measures that are compliant with human rights are required to alleviate the immediate impacts of COVID-19 on persons and groups made vulnerable by structural inequities, confronting present and future health crises requires deep structural changes to promote more just and equitable societies.

Civil Liberties vs. Ideas of Public Health

Significant precautionary measures have been taken across all countries to control the pandemic. Some of these may conflict with civil liberties, such as freedom of association, freedom of religion, and mobility rights[86] (quarantine orders, closure of borders, lockdowns, and stay-at-home orders), as well as privacy rights (contact tracing, both traditional and digital).[87]

A public health perspective may at first blush seem to conflict with civil liberties, given its emphasis on preventing or curbing a pandemic that could cause death and suffering to many millions. However, as the various contributors in this section discuss, a clear focus on civil liberties is needed, not only so that the actions of public health officials are lawful (in the Canadian context, in compliance with the *Canadian Charter of Rights and Freedoms*), but also because maintaining respect for civil liberties may well produce sound public health policy. Public health measures, tailored to civil liberties, will likely achieve more buy-in from the public, particularly when precautionary measures are required for many months and possibly years.

---

83. Farha & Schwan, this volume, Chapter D-4; Levesque & Thériault, this volume, Chapter D-6.
84. Chandler et al, this volume, Chapter D-10.
85. Sheldon & Malhotra, this volume, Chapter D-9.
86. Delphine Nakache & Yves Le Bouthillier, this volume, Chapter C-5.
87. Teresa Scassa, Jason Millar & Kelly Bronson, this volume, Chapter C-2.

Governments may justify intrusion into civil liberties as being proportionate to the need to respond to a public health crisis on the scale of COVID-19, and we stress that courts are likely to be deferential to governmental choices in such a situation.[88] Civil rights are, of course, fundamental to our democracy, but no one wishes to "die with their rights on," which could occur if needed governmental measures to curb a disease outbreak or pandemic are sacrificed on a right's altar. However, as better evidence emerges on potential options to respond to the pandemic, courts may well hold governments to a more stringent standard and be more exacting in their review of whether measures taken are as respectful of civil liberties as possible while still achieving the objective of curbing the virus.

An important aspect of the analysis in this section is the acknowledgment that the *Charter*, particularly in health care, serves largely to protect civil rights (sometimes described as "negative" rights—being "free" from governmental intrusion). But it is presently not interpreted to protect "positive" socio-economic rights (requiring governmental expenditures), at least not without being tied to another *Charter* right, such as the right to equality under s. 15. Different contributors across this volume argue this is an impoverished view of rights and COVID-19 helps to illuminate that.[89]

Accountability

In any emergency, mechanisms for holding governments to account tend to be weakened, but COVID-19 has created unique accountability challenges.[90] The pandemic has disrupted sittings of legislatures and courts in many jurisdictions. U.K. Prime Minister Boris Johnson's hospitalization after contracting the virus exposed a disturbing lack of clarity around lines of succession should he be required to give up his functions.[91] Canadian Prime Minister Justin Trudeau self-isolated after his spouse tested positive, and spent the first two weeks of the nationwide lockdown working from home while Cabinet met on Parliament Hill.

---

88. Colleen M Flood, Bryan Thomas & Kumanan Wilson, this volume, Chapter C-1.
89. See particularly Jackman, this volume, Chapter D-3.
90. MacDonnell, this volume, Chapter B-1.
91. Thomson Reuters, "U.K. PM Boris Johnson Moved to Intensive Care as COVID-19 Symptoms Worsen", *CBC News* (6 April 2020), online: <https://www.cbc.ca/news/world/coronavirus-johnson-hospital-1.5522983>.

Some progress has been made toward resuming operation in Canadian institutions using videoconferencing and other technologies. But even when institutions are open, accountability is not guaranteed. Since mid-March, governments at the local, provincial, and federal levels have promulgated a flurry of emergency orders and regulations to respond to the pandemic, many sweeping in their scope. Ensuring meaningful review of these orders and regulations is an enormous challenge.[92] Legislative review of emergency legislation has generally been perfunctory. While courts are hearing urgent matters, and some non-urgent ones, it is difficult to be optimistic about their ability to serve as meaningful checks on executive or legislative overreach, both because of the limits of their jurisdiction and the limits of litigation as a tool for challenging a complex and networked government response to the pandemic.[93]

In the face of these challenges, the authors in this section suggest it is important to look beyond formal sources of accountability. This includes invisible sources of accountability within the executive and the legislature that shape the content of policy decisions and legislation in important ways, such as public servants and informal "off-stage" negotiations between political parties.[94] The media also plays a crucial accountability role. In today's media environment, "trusted and true" traditional news sources continue to be influential, but they compete for space with sources of information on social media.

In the context of a pandemic, where accurate data matters greatly, the cost of an informational vacuum or, alternatively, of misinformation, is terribly high. Governments have an obligation to be transparent about the data they are relying on in making policy, and about the trade-offs they are making. A lack of transparency jeopardizes public trust in government. In an information vacuum, misinformation can more easily take hold and spread.

One significant dimension of the COVID-19 response has been governments' willingness to partner with private corporations to ensure stable supply chains for PPE and other essential supplies. This section considers the accountability gap that can emerge when governments rely on private companies in this way.[95]

92. We are grateful for a conversation with Gabrielle Appleby on this point.
93. Paul Daly, this volume, Chapter B-6.
94. MacDonnell, this volume, Chapter B-1.
95. Yee-Fui Ng, "Political Constitutionalism: Individual Responsibility and Collective Restraint" (2020) Federal LR (forthcoming).

Who Does What? Challenges and Demands of Canadian Federalism

Good governance is needed to prepare for and respond to a pandemic, both in the initial stages and as evidence grows on the efficacy of different preventative measures. Simply put, good governance requires clear lines of responsibility about which orders of government and other institutions or actors will do what and when. Particularly in the early part of a pandemic, there is little time for the usual rhythm of democracy and thus clear lines of responsibility are even more essential.

In Canada, good governance is complicated by our disaggregated federation and the politicization of jurisdictional issues. For example, health is often portrayed as being solely a matter of provincial jurisdiction. But the Supreme Court of Canada has declared on multiple occasions that health is in fact a matter of *shared* jurisdiction.[96] Which order of government has jurisdiction depends on the context. In this section, we explore how dysfunctionality in federal-provincial relations was laid bare during the SARS outbreak in 2003: the federal government could not report key data about the outbreak to the WHO because Ontario's provincial government either could not or would not supply this data, resulting in the WHO issuing a travel ban.

SARS turned out to be a mere warm-up for COVID-19 in both scale and scope. Post-SARS, several significant changes were made to public health governance, notably the creation of the Public Health Agency of Canada (PHAC), and pan-Canadian committees supporting better coordination and sharing of data.[97] As COVID-19 has unfolded, Canada's performance was strengthened by these reforms; yet serious vulnerabilities remain.

First, the federal government in Canada—unlike other countries—has not declared COVID-19 a national emergency. Some see this decision as appropriately respectful of provincial jurisdiction. However, a failure to declare a national emergency also reveals a vulnerability in governance at the federal level. The *Emergencies Act*[98] is

96. *RJR-MacDonald Inc v Canada (AG)*, 1995 3 SCR 199 at para 32, 127 DLR (4th) 1; *Eldridge v British Columbia (AG)*, 1997 3 SCR 624 at para 24-25, 151 DLR (4th) 677; *Reference re Assisted Human Reproduction Act*, 2010 SCC 61 at para 57; *Canada (AG) v PHS Community Services Society*, 2011 SCC 44 at paras 67-70. For a full discussion, see Colleen M Flood, William Lahey & Bryan Thomas, "Federalism and Health Care in Canada: A Troubled Romance?" in Peter Oliver, Patrick Macklem & Nathalie Des Rosiers, eds, *The Oxford Handbook of the Canadian Constitution* (New York: Oxford University Press, 2017).
97. Mel Cappe, this volume, Chapter B-2.
98. *Emergencies Act*, RSC 1985, c 22 (4th Supp.)

very limited in when it can be invoked and the powers it contains, making it largely inadequate in the context of COVID-19. There is a possibility the federal government could declare an emergency with special legislation passed under the Peace Order and Good Government power of the Canadian Constitution, but our contributors differ in their views on the necessity of this.[99] One option to be considered going forward is an amendment to the *Public Health Agency of Canada Act*[100] that could provide a mechanism to declare a Public Health Emergency of National Concern.

Second, harkening back to SARS, the federal government still does not receive the public health data from the provinces required for epidemiological modelling to forecast the optimal containment and recovery strategies. PHAC has no authority to compel data from provincial, territorial, and private sector partners, even where national public health is compromised. Its ability to produce timely national surveillance on the health status of Canadians is severely limited by the lack of strong federal public health legislation.[101]

Third, there is both strength and vulnerability in the various approaches taken by governments across Canada. Variation can be a strength, as it may allow governments to respond to differences in needs and contexts. So, for example, our contributors discuss the quite different risks for Indigenous Peoples, and how Indigenous governments are taking greater precautionary measures than other governments. However, we also need to ask whether vastly different death rates per capita across the country can be attributed to factors beyond the immediate control of decision makers or instead to poor policy choices or policy implementation. For example, as of June 28, 2020, COVID-19 death rates per 100,000 population are 63.9 in Quebec, 18.4 in Ontario, and 3.4 in British Columbia.[102] One, of course, must account for differences in risk factors such as age and obesity, or factors such as the early spring break in Quebec (and the return of infected travellers), but we do not yet know whether these factors explain a more than 18-fold differences in per capita deaths as between, for example,

99. See Colleen M Flood & Bryan Thomas, this volume, Chapter A-6; Carissima Mathen, this volume, Chapter A-7.
100. *Public Health Agency of Canada Act*, SC 2006, c 5.
101. On the problems of not having the means to collect country-wide public health data, see Amir Attaran & Adam R Houston, this volume, Chapter A-5.
102. As of June 28, 2020, the number of deaths reported from COVID-19 were 5,448 in Quebec, 2,701 in Ontario, and 174 in British Columbia. See Canada Open Data Working Group, *supra* note 4. See also Pearson, *supra* note 29.

British Columbia and Quebec. Great differences in death rates are seen too in the U.S., with states that implemented strong physical distancing measures recording a death rate 35 times lower than those who did not.[103]

It is often said in the Canadian context that provincial variations provide a natural experiment where we can learn as much from our successes as from our mistakes, but in the context of COVID-19 these differences could represent needless loss of life. For example, at the time of writing there are concerns that Ontario, Canada's most populous province, is not sufficiently slowing the spread of infection, with the number of new cases per day at the end of June 2020 remaining near the highest levels since the beginning of the pandemic.[104] This is *not* to say that if there was but one governmental decision maker at the federal level that results would have been better, but at a minimum there needs to be a central conduit for clear information on the kinds of precautionary measures that all orders of government *should* be taking and the costs and consequences of not doing so.

Finally, variation in measures taken by various orders of government across Canada can provide significant challenges in managing a pandemic in terms of communication with the public. We discuss the myriad approaches taken by municipal governments to COVID-19, as well as differences across provinces. Although these many differences may well be justified by different contexts, the end result is a cacophony of different legal requirements, making it hard for people to understand what is required of them and perhaps contributing to compliance fatigue in the longer run.

Conclusion: Moving Forward

In the months and years to come, there will be important choices to be made as we adapt to a "new normal," prepare for what is said to be an inevitable second wave of the infection, and implement plans to rebuild our societies and the international order.

---

103. Charles Courtemanche et al, "Strong Social Distancing Measures in the United States Reduced The COVID-19 Growth Rate" (2020) 39:7 Health Aff 1.
104. Ed Tubb & Kenyon Wallace, "Far More Ontarians are Catching COVID-19 in Community Settings than Previously Known, Star Analysis Finds", *The Star* (23 May 2020), online: <https://www.thestar.com/news/canada/2020/05/23/far-more-ontarians-are-catching-covid-19-in-community-settings-than-previously-known-star-analysis-finds.html>.

At the domestic level, countries will develop a range of recovery plans. Some of these plans will tilt toward austerity, tacitly accepting that some will be left behind.[105] While health care budgets are unlikely to see significant cuts, other crucial public goods, such as education, could see their funding slashed.

Other countries will spend their way out of the economic downturn. These governments will invest significant funds to support their populations and build new infrastructure in the hope of stimulating the economy.[106] While temporary income support programs will eventually be phased out, some may become permanent. In Canada, for example, there will be pressure to convert the Canadian Emergency Response Benefit, a $500 weekly payment to individuals who became unemployed as a result of the pandemic, into a universal basic income program.[107] Economists have argued that recovery plans must be attentive to the gendered impacts of COVID-19 on the economy. Jobs held predominantly by women have been more significantly impacted than jobs held primarily by men, and access to childcare will be crucial to ensuring the return to the workforce of women.[108] In Canada, too, there will be pressure to significantly invest in and reform long-term care.

In short, states will be faced with choices. The weaknesses of some choices that countries have made to date have been exposed by COVID-19. Will countries now choose another path? Rather than ignoring our vulnerabilities and disregarding questions of human dignity, respect, and equity, we contend these values should shape the response going forward. Profound global inequities have created the preconditions

---

105. See generally Rory O'Connell et al, *Applying an International Human Rights Framework to State Budgetary Allocations: Rights and Resources* (Oxford: Routledge, 2014).
106. See Bob Rae & Mel Cappe, "We Can't Just Pick up the Pieces after the Pandemic Subsides – We Need to Keep Them Together", *The Globe and Mail* (30 March 2020), online: <https://www.theglobeandmail.com/opinion/article-we-cant-just-pick-up-the-pieces-after-the-pandemic-subsides-we-need>.
107. "Will This Pandemic's Legacy be a Universal Basic Income?", *Maclean's* (19 May 2020), online: <https://www.macleans.ca/opinion/will-this-pandemics-legacy-be-a-universal-basic-income>.
108. Jessica Smith Cross, "Women's Job Losses Require Strategies for an Economic 'She-covery'" (5 May 2020), online: *QP Briefing* <https://www.qpbriefing.com/2020/05/05/womens-job-losses-require-strategies-for-an-economic-she-covery>; Jordan Press & Teresa Wright, "Ottawa Quietly Probes Expanded Role for Child Care in Post-Pandemic Recovery", *The Globe and Mail* (17 May 2020), online: <https://www.theglobeandmail.com/politics/article-feds-quietly-probe-expanded-role-for-child-care-in-post-pandemic>.

for a pandemic. The solution to the health, economic, and social crises COVID-19 has precipitated is not to become more insular. Rather, it is to recognize that our future is co-determined with others, and to seize the benefits of our interconnectedness within and across countries. We hope this book, focused on vulnerability, will motivate responses and recovery plans with social justice as a central concern in addition to controlling infections and restarting the economy.

SECTION A

WHO DOES WHAT? CHALLENGES AND DEMANDS OF CANADIAN FEDERALISM

CHAPTER A-1

Have the Post-SARS Reforms Prepared Us for COVID-19? Mapping the Institutional Landscape

Katherine Fierlbeck* and Lorian Hardcastle**

Abstract

Effective pandemic management requires a clear and straightforward structure of communication and accountability. Yet the political realities of Canadian federalism preclude this. The fundamental theme of pandemic management in Canada is thus the tension between the need to make clear, coherent, and timely decisions, on the one hand, and the need to involve an exceptionally large array of political actors across different levels of government, on the other. The sudden outbreak of SARS in 2003 exposed several problems in coordinating the public health system. This led to a major restructuring of public health institutions in Canada. The 2009 H1N1 pandemic tested these reforms and identified new issues underlying the coordination of governmental actors. This chapter presents the legal and institutional context within which COVID-19 has emerged, and identifies both lessons learned from the past and the challenges that remain.

* McCulloch Professor of Political Science, Dalhousie University.

** Associate Professor, Faculty of Law and Cumming School of Medicine, University of Calgary.

Résumé
Les réformes intervenues après le SRAS nous ont-elles préparés à la COVID-19 ? Cartographie du paysage institutionnel

Pour gérer efficacement une pandémie, il faut une structure de communication et de reddition de comptes claire et simple. Or, les réalités politiques du fédéralisme canadien rendent la chose impossible. Le thème fondamental de la gestion des pandémies au Canada repose donc sur la tension entre la nécessité de prendre des décisions éclairées, cohérentes et opportunes, d'une part, et celle de faire intervenir un éventail exceptionnellement vaste d'acteurs politiques à différents paliers de gouvernement, d'autre part. L'épidémie soudaine de SRAS en 2003 a mis en évidence plusieurs problèmes de coordination du système de santé publique. Il s'en est suivi une restructuration majeure des institutions de santé publique au Canada. La pandémie de grippe H1N1 en 2009 a mis ces réformes à l'épreuve et a révélé de nouveaux problèmes sous-jacents à la coordination des différents intervenants gouvernementaux. Ce chapitre présente le contexte juridique et institutionnel dans lequel la COVID-19 a fait son apparition, et expose à la fois les leçons tirées du passé et les défis qui restent à relever.

A fundamental aspect of pandemic management is effective coordination between key units of governance within a state. Pandemic planning in all states involves horizontal coordination (between ministries or departments at the same level of government) and vertical coordination (communicating and implementing government directives to activity on the front line). But in a federal system, where the capacity to engage politically is constitutionally defined, the ability to coordinate pandemic responses becomes more difficult. In Canada, where the health care system is arguably more decentralized than in any other federal state in the OECD,[1] the problems of coordination are even more pronounced. In the first part of this chapter, we set out the formal distribution of decision-making authority in Canada with reference to pandemic planning. The second and third sections discuss how the responses to SARS and H1N1 shaped pandemic response

1. Ferran Requejo, "Federalism and Democracy: The Case of Minority Nations" in Michael Burgess & Alain-G Gagnon, eds, *Federal Democracies* (London and New York: Routledge, 2010) 175.

capacity within Canada's formal legal framework. We conclude by identifying both the lessons learned from Canada's legacy from past pandemics and some of the issues that remain.

Power to Regulate in Relation to a Pandemic

The Constitution[2] does not assign "health" to either the provinces or the federal government. Instead, both levels of government have responsibilities in this area. According to the Supreme Court of Canada, health is not "subject to specific constitutional assignment but instead is an amorphous topic which can be addressed by valid federal or provincial legislation, depending in the circumstances of each case on the nature or scope of the health problem in question."[3]

Several provincial heads of power are relevant to health, including the power to regulate hospitals,[4] property and civil rights, and matters of a merely local or private nature. These powers have resulted in provinces assuming many responsibilities in the health sector, including health insurance, the regulation of health professionals, the delivery of health care services, and the regulation of public health. Provincial public health laws cover a variety of topics, including the abatement of health hazards, inspection and closure of infected premises, reporting of communicable diseases, and examination and isolation of infected persons, all of which are generally enforced by medical officers of health. Most provincial public health laws establish a Chief Medical Officer of Health, who often has sweeping powers to implement public health orders they deem necessary to contain the spread of a communicable disease. Provinces also have emergencies legislation that allows them to take exceptional measures such as seizing goods and real property, closing premises, or limiting travel to or within the province.

The Constitution assigns the power to regulate "municipal institutions" to the provinces. There are several provincial approaches to the delegation of powers to municipalities.[5] However, generally speaking, they may take various actions in response to a pandemic,

2. *Constitution Act, 1982*, ss 91-92, being Schedule B to the *Canada Act 1982* (UK), 1982, c 11.
3. *Schneider v The Queen*, [1982] 2 SCR 112 at 142, 139 DLR (3d) 417. See also Martha Jackman, "Constitutional Jurisdiction Over Health" (2000) 8 Health LJ 95.
4. An exception to this is "marine hospitals," which are a federal head of power.
5. For a detailed discussion of municipal powers, see Alexandra Flynn, this volume, Chapter A-8.

such as closing or passing restrictions in relation to local businesses and municipal services (like playgrounds, libraries, and public transit), declaring a local state of emergency, and imposing fines for those who do not adhere to public health restrictions. Although there is considerable interprovincial variation, the delivery of public health services often occurs at the local or regional level. Throughout the 1990s, most provinces shifted responsibility for the planning and delivery of health services, including public health, to regional entities. The purpose of this reform was to improve integration of health services. Although some provinces have recently moved away from regional governance and toward a single provincial health authority, public health services are sometimes still delivered on a regional basis. Under another model, municipalities appoint public health units, which are tasked with the delivery of public health services.[6]

The Constitution assigns the federal government several powers that are relevant to public health, including quarantine and the criminal law. The latter has been interpreted broadly to include public health matters like drug regulation, tobacco control, and supervised consumption sites.[7] The federal government also has the power to "make laws for the peace, order and good government of Canada" (the POGG clause). According to the Supreme Court of Canada, the POGG clause is available in response to an emergency or a matter of "national concern,"[8] which could include a pandemic. The federal *Emergencies Act* sets out exceptional powers the government can exercise upon the declaration of an emergency.[9]

Indigenous-governmental relations are another important aspect of Canadian federalism,[10] both in terms of which level of government

6. Raisa B Deber et al, "A Cautionary Tale of Downloading Public Health in Ontario: What Does it Say about the Need for National Standards for More than Doctors and Hospitals?" (2006) 2:3 Healthcare Policy 60.
7. In *RJR MacDonald v Canada (Attorney General)*, Justice LaForest stated that "[t]he scope of the federal power to create criminal legislation with respect to health matters is broad, and is circumscribed only by the requirements that the legislation must contain a prohibition accompanied by a penal sanction and must be directed at a legitimate public health evil." [1995] 3 SCR 199 at 246, 127 DLR (4th) 1.
8. *Toronto Electric Com'rs v Snider et al*, [1925] 2 DLR 5, 1 WWR 785 (PC); *R v Crown Zellerbach Canada Ltd*, [1988] 1 SCR 401, 49 DLR (4th) 161.
9. *Emergencies Act*, RSC 1985, c 22 (4th Supp). For a discussion of the POGG clause and federal emergencies legislation, see Colleen M Flood & Bryan Thomas, Chapter A-6 and Carissima Mathen, Chapter A-7 in this volume.
10. For a detailed discussion of this issue, see Aimee Craft, Deborah McGregor & Jeffery Hewitt, Chapter A-2 of this volume. See also Robert Hamilton, "Indigenous Peoples and Interstitial Federalism in Canada" (2019) 24:1 Rev Const Stud 43.

is responsible for providing public health services to Indigenous communities, and in terms of First Nations' own jurisdiction to regulate public health matters. With respect to the former, the poor health status of Indigenous people living in Canada is well documented, as is the federal-provincial wrangling that causes or exacerbates health inequities.[11] Indigenous communities also have their own jurisdiction to pass regulations in response to a pandemic, either through bylaw-making powers assigned under the *Indian Act*,[12] a self-government agreement, or an asserted inherent constitutional right to self-government.

In sum, the reason Canadian federalism involves so many actors and institutions stems from the constitutional division of power. The key lessons learned from recent pandemic experiences generally revolve around the question of how to facilitate the intergovernmental coordination required to contain disease spread. As noted below, SARS taught us that we needed a more sophisticated institutional armature to facilitate coordination between jurisdictions; H1N1 brought home the realization that too many intermediate organizations in this framework could lead to confusion in determining roles and responsibilities. Some lessons—such as the need to share data as quickly and as comprehensively as possible—seem to have been poorly learned; other lessons (most painfully, that all pandemics are different) highlight the need to build agility and flexibility into decision-making. That long-term care homes rather than hospitals would be the epicentre of many of the biggest outbreaks, for example, was not appreciated soon enough by many jurisdictions: SARS had been limited to hospitals and, as those most vulnerable to H1N1 were younger rather than older cohorts, H1N1 did not force our attention to long-term care homes. But lessons are not just for governments; they are for all those involved in pandemic responses. And, as political decision makers have learned that they must listen and respond to front line workers, so too must those at the front line understand that pandemics are not simply a moment in time, but rather exist within a specific political context, one that constrains the political choices available to those at the helm.

11. See generally, Constance MacIntosh, "The Intersection of Aboriginal Public Health with Canadian Health Law and Policy" in Tracey Bailey, Timothy Caulfield & Nola Riles, eds, *Public Health Law and Policy in Canada*, 3rd ed (Toronto: Butterworths, 2013); Yvonne Boyer, *Moving Aboriginal Health Forward: Discarding Canada's Legal Barriers* (Vancouver: UBC Press, 2015).
12. *Indian Act*, RSC 1985, c I-5.

SARS

On March 7, 2003, a man was admitted to the Scarborough Grace Hospital in Ontario with symptoms of a respiratory illness. He waited in a crowded emergency department for over 16 hours, setting into motion a chain of infection that would eventually lead to 44 deaths. By March 23, SARS was officially declared a "reportable, communicable, and virulent" disease under provincial public health legislation. The outbreak lasted four months. Health care workers comprised a large proportion of the SARS deaths in Ontario and, while the virus was transmitted within families, there was little community spread.[13]

When analyzing the outbreak for the province three years later, the Honourable Archie Campbell stated that "[t]he surprise is not that Ontario's response to SARS worked so badly, but that it worked at all, given the lack of preparation and systems and infrastructure."[14] The Campbell Report, commissioned by the Government of Ontario, also highlighted the "profound lack of awareness" regarding best practices for, and commitment to, worker safety.[15] The National Advisory Committee on SARS and Public Health (the Naylor Report), with a national mandate, focused both on limitations in response capacity (training, resources, equipment, institutions) and on the need for greater coordination and communication.[16] This report noted that the epidemiological information necessary to respond to the outbreak was simply not available in a timely or systematic manner. The disease-tracking platform was a relic from the 1980s; data handling protocols were unclear or non-existent; and there was no central database. The Naylor Report looked closely at the need for collaboration between key players. It identified localized problems, such as turf wars between institutions and different practices across public health units (such as the determination of thresholds for quarantine).

---

13. There was likely little to no asymptomatic spread of SARS, and the incubation time for the virus was much shorter than for COVID-19.
14. The SARS Commission, *Spring of Fear*, vol 1 (Toronto: The SARS Commission, 2006) at 10, online: *Archives of Ontario* <http://www.archives.gov.on.ca/en/e_records/sars/report/index.html>.
15. This prompted both constitutional litigation and tort claims by health care practitioners: *Abarquez v Ontario*, 2009 ONCA 374; Lorian Hardcastle, "Governmental Tort Liability for Negligence in the Health Sector" (2004) 30:1 Queen's LJ 156.
16. National Advisory Committee on SARS and Public Health, *Learning from SARS: Renewal of Public Health in Canada* (Ottawa: Health Canada, 2003), online (pdf): *Government of Canada* <https://www.canada.ca/content/dam/phac-aspc/migration/phac-aspc/publicat/sars-sras/pdf/sars-e.pdf>.

But "the single largest impediment" to addressing SARS was "the lack of a collaborative framework and ethos among different levels of govt."[17] Patient confidentiality requirements made it difficult to release critical patient information to Health Canada (while a memorandum of understanding on data sharing between Ontario and Ottawa had been discussed, it was never finalized). Because roles for each government were not clearly spelled out, expertise was not optimally utilized. The Naylor Report catalyzed a major restructuring of public health institutions in Canada. During SARS, public health units both within provincial governments and Health Canada (as the Population and Public Health Branch) were poorly coordinated. Because of this, Canada lacked the kind of integrated and comprehensive health objectives and strategies that characterized other federal states. What was needed, suggested the report, was a new Canadian agency for public health led by a Chief Public Health Officer (CPHO).[18] The report argued that this federal government body should be answerable to Health Canada, in order to keep the chain of accountability clear, but be arm's length and thus not directly under the control of Health Canada.

At the same time, however, the political realities of Canadian federalism meant that it was also essential to bring the provincial governments on as equal partners in the development of a comprehensive national public health strategy. While the report discussed the possibility of a more hierarchical approach grounded in Ottawa's constitutional authority, the final blueprint was for a more collaborative system of horizontal governance sitting athwart the basic structure of vertical hierarchical accountability. Not only would the new organization have regional bodies geographically situated in each province, but at the heart of the agency would be a national "advisory board" with representative voices from each region of Canada. This horizontal integration would be reinforced by the secondment of federal public health officials to provincial public health units (and vice versa) to foster greater understanding of how public health policies

17. *Ibid* at 212.
18. Similarly, the Standing Senate Committee on Social Affairs, Science and Technology called for an arm's-length "Health Protection and Promotion Agency" that was national in scope and mandated to address public health emergencies. *Reforming Health Protection and Promotion in Canada: Time to Act* (Ottawa: Senate of Canada, 2003), online: *Senate of Canada* <https://sencanada.ca/content/sen/committee/372/soci/rep/repfinnov03-e.htm>.

and procedures functioned across jurisdictions. Finally, this culture of collaboration would need to be supported by an earmarked funding allocation of $300 million for joint public health activities.

The Naylor Report also identified problems in coordination between Canada and international actors, particularly around a lack of clarity about which level of government was to be in contact with the World Health Organization (WHO). WHO's unanticipated travel advisory for Toronto in April 2003 was at least partly due to the lack of clear and effective communication between levels of government, and thus the need for some form of vertical accountability was a priority. The Naylor Report found that the federal government's "uncertain authority in the face of a multi-provincial outbreak" was especially problematic, given that WHO moved to establish expectations with regard to surveillance, reporting, and disease outbreak management through its *International Health Regulations*.[19] These regulations, which are binding on WHO member states, are designed to "prevent, protect against, control and provide a public health response to the international spread of disease."[20] The need to implement these regulations informed the Naylor Report recommendations and helped to catalyze post-SARS changes to public health in Canada.

The Naylor Report's vision for a new public health system was close to what was finally established by the *Public Health Agency of Canada Act* in 2006.[21] The Public Health Agency of Canada (PHAC) is a federal agency of the Government of Canada, but the beating heart of the agency is the Pan-Canadian Public Health Network, comprising representatives from each province (generally Chief Medical Officers of Health or Assistant Deputy Ministers), and co-chaired by federal and provincial representatives. The governance model of the new body was ambitious and well received, but not without challenges. One key issue, for example, emerged from the development of electronic health data, and the need to amend privacy laws and to address sharing (as discussed in Amir Attaran & Adam R Houston, this volume, Chapter A-5).

While the mandate of the new public health agency went well beyond infectious disease control, the scar left by SARS meant that

19. *Supra* note 16 at 7.
20. World Health Organization, *International Health Regulations*, 3rd ed (Geneva: World Health Organization, 2005), article 2.
21. *Public Health Agency of Canada Act*, SC 2006, c 5. See also Katherine Fierlbeck, *Health Care in Canada: A Citizen's Guide to Policy and Politics* (Toronto: University of Toronto Press, 2011) at ch 5.

emergency preparedness and response was a major aspect of the new agency's directive. This focused on the integration of federal and provincial public health actors, including "a mechanism for dealing with health emergencies which would be activated in lockstep with provincial emergency acts in the event of a pan-Canadian health emergency."[22] Also important was the development of a common set of principles, the clarification of roles and responsibilities, the development of protocols for major disease outbreaks, the designation of lead F/P/T public health officials for crisis management (including local roles and responsibilities), the assessment of surge capacity in hospitals and laboratories, the assessment of the National Emergency Stockpile System, the creation of national epidemic response teams, and the clarification of the legal and regulatory context underlying public health management (especially pandemic response) in Canada.

When SARS struck, the federal government was already in the midst of reviewing its public health laws, most importantly the *Quarantine Act*.[23] This legislation was amended in June 2003 to add SARS to the list of contagious diseases to which the *Act* applied, although limited use was made of these legislative powers during the SARS outbreak. Although no federal quarantine officer issued a quarantine order against an individual, they detained one flight at the Vancouver International airport for decontamination.[24] In 2006, significant amendments to the *Quarantine Act*, which was largely unchanged since 1872, came into force. The legislation was modernized by, for example, focusing on air travel and authorizing the use of screening technology. The amendments also broadened the powers of quarantine officers to conduct medical assessments and detain travellers, and authorized the Governor in Council to make orders excluding classes of travellers who had been in foreign countries where there were communicable diseases. The federal government has made extensive use of the power to exclude travellers during COVID-19. To facilitate coordination, these amendments required quarantine officers to provide information to a province's public health authority regarding matters such as travellers being required to undergo medical examinations, detention orders, or flights diverted due to communicable

22. Naylor, *supra* note 16 at 216.
23. *Quarantine Act*, SC 2005, c 20.
24. Nola M Ries, "Quarantine and the Law: The 2003 SARS Experience in Canada (A New Disease Calls on Old Public Health Tools)" (2005) 43:2 Alta L Rev 529 at 534.

disease. The 2006 and subsequent minor amendments also facilitated coordination with international actors by bringing the *Quarantine Act* into line with the *International Health Regulations*.

The provincial response to SARS has been variable, with various amendments to provincial public health laws coming into force in the years following the SARS outbreak. When the disease hit Ontario, the government amended its *Health Protection and Promotion Act* to include SARS as a disease to which the legislation applied,[25] which meant that individuals such as health professionals had to report cases of the disease to public health officials and public health officials were empowered to require infected individuals to submit to examinations or isolate. The most significant amendment to provincial public health laws has been to clarify that public health orders, such as those compelling isolation, could be directed not only toward individuals, but to groups of persons.[26] These powers have been used extensively during COVID-19, for example, with respect to returning travellers and symptomatic individuals. Some provinces also made post-SARS changes to their emergencies laws to make them more responsive to disease outbreaks. For example, Ontario amended its *Emergency Management and Civil Protection Act* (as it is now called) to define "emergency" as including a situation caused by "a disease or other health risk."[27]

H1N1

H1N1 was the first real test of post-SARS public health reforms. The pandemic manifested itself in two waves in Canada, with the first peaking in May 2009, and the second, more severe wave, cresting in November 2009. Unlike SARS, the victims tended to be younger, with

25. *Health Protection and Promotion Act*, RSO 1990, c H 7.
26. *Ibid*, s 22(5.0.1). Toronto's Medical Officer of Health at the time of SARS explained the rationale for this amendment: "There was an instance wherein we had an entire group of people who needed to be put into quarantine on a weekend. It was physically and logistically impossible to issue orders person to person on a Saturday afternoon for 350 people who happened to live in three or four different health units all at once..." (The SARS Commission, *SARS and Public Health Legislation: Second Interim Report*, vol 5 [Toronto: The SARS Commission, 2006] at 320, online [pdf]: *Archives of Ontario* <http://www.archives.gov.on.ca/en/e_records/sars/report/v5.html>). See also *Public Health Act*, SBC 2008, c 28, s 39(3).
27. *Emergency Management and Civil Protection Act*, RSO 1990, c E 9, s 1.

three-quarters of the cases presenting in those under 30.[28] While the public health community had anticipated that a major influenza pandemic would be a form of avian influenza, with a potential mortality exceeding 50% in humans,[29] H1N1 turned out to be a much less virulent strain. Nonetheless, it challenged the response capacity of Canada's federal system in two ways: first, it was present throughout all provinces and territories; second, it was the first pandemic that involved the development and distribution of both an adjuvanted vaccine and an antiviral.[30]

H1N1 containment required three discrete forms of coordination: between federal institutions; between federal, provincial, and territorial jurisdictions; and across regional and municipal bodies within each province and territory. Collectively, these institutions comprised a sprawling fascia providing a comprehensive and responsive network linking vital information-gathering, analytical, and decision-making bodies throughout the country in real time. Key federal departments included not only Health Canada but also the Privy Council Office (representing the Prime Minister), Public Safety Canada (emergency management), the Canadian Food Inspection Agency (food safety), the Department of Foreign Affairs and International Trade (coordinating international communication), RCMP (domestic security), and the Canada Border Services Agency and Immigration Canada (to monitor cross-border movement), among others. These bodies were largely coordinated through the Federal Healthcare Partnership—Pandemic Planning Working Group and were guided by the Avian and Pandemic Influenza Preparedness Program.

Intergovernmental coordination occurred through the Conference of Deputy Ministers of Health and the young PHAC. Central to PHAC's organization was the Pan-Canadian Public Health Network, including the Council of Chief Medical Officers of Health embedded within it. These units had created the Pandemic Preparedness Oversight Committee in 2007 to streamline pandemic management. Existing public health network groups provided expert advice when needed. New task groups were set up to support the Pandemic Coordination

28. Donald E Low & Allison McGeer, "Pandemic (H1N1) 2009: Assessing the Response" (2010) 182:17 CMAJ 1874.

29. Harvey V Fineberg. "Pandemic Preparedness and Response: Lessons from the H1N1 Influenza of 2009" (2014) 370:14 New England J Medicine 1339.

30. An adjuvant is an ingredient added to a vaccine that helps promote a better immune response (and can thus reduce the amount of virus needed).

Committee for the duration of the pandemic. Facilitating communication between these groups was a web-based system called the Canadian Network for Public Health Intelligence. In a sense, however, the lessons of SARS were *too* well learned. The proliferation of bodies set up to support and coordinate government bodies itself led to delays in decision-making and a duplication of efforts; and the PHAC analysis following the H1N1 outbreaks called for greater clarity concerning the roles and responsibilities of all of the groups involved.[31]

Provincial and territorial jurisdictions also had serious organizational issues. Most provinces had regional governance structures in health care delivery, which made a centralized response to pandemic planning difficult. For example, Nova Scotia's nine district health authorities were given the responsibility of managing responses to potential pandemics, with the province becoming involved only when a district health authority (DHA) "could no longer adequately respond to the situation."[32] Yet there was no central review of district health authority plans, nor a clear sense of whether these plans existed at all. Further, information on the available stockpiles of supplies held by DHAs was not readily available, and the province was uncertain whether they could "legally require the DHAs to provide details of their supplies on hand and costs for those supplies."[33] Similar supply-related coordination problems have arisen during COVID-19, including a dispute between Ottawa and Alberta over the approval of testing technology[34] and problems with the distribution of personal protective equipment and testing supplies across the health sector. For example, while many hospitals were well stocked, long-term care homes often reported not having access to adequate supplies.

31. Public Health Agency of Canada and Health Canada, *Lessons Learned Review: Public Health Agency of Canada and Health Canada Response to the 2009 H1N1 Pandemic* (Ottawa: Public Health Agency of Canada, 2010), online (pdf): *Government of Canada* <https://www.canada.ca/content/dam/phac-aspc/migration/phac-aspc/about_apropos/evaluation/reports-rapports/2010-2011/h1n1/pdf/h1n1-eng.pdf>.

32. Nova Scotia Office of the Auditor General, *Pandemic Preparedness* (Halifax: Office of the Auditor General, 2010) at 12, online (pdf): *Office of the Auditor General* <https://oag-ns.ca/sites/default/files/publications/2009%20-%20Special%20Report%20-%20Pandemic%20Preparedness.pdf>.

33. *Ibid* at 20.

34. Ubaka Ogbogu & Lorian Hardcastle, "Crisis or Not, Alberta Must Not Do an End-Run Around Health Canada", *The Globe and Mail* (20 April 2020), online: <https://www.theglobeandmail.com/opinion/article-crisis-or-not-alberta-must-not-do-an-end-run-around-health-canada/>.

These concerns with decentralization are also illustrated by post-H1N1 changes to Ontario's *Health Protection and Promotion Act*, which gave the Chief Medical Officer of Heath (CMOH) more authority to respond to diseases in a coordinated manner. For example, these amendments empowered the CMOH to direct boards of health and local medical officers of health to adopt measures "if he or she feels that Ontarians would be better protected by a coordinated response to an outbreak...."[35] However, the tension between Ontario's Premier and the public health authorities regarding responsibility for COVID-19 testing illustrates that there is still lack of clarity regarding key roles and responsibilities within the province.

In most provinces, the deployment of health care workers across health regions was another concern. The nature of decentralized health authorities meant that it was difficult to move health care personnel where they would be needed. While collective bargaining provisions could generally be suspended in the event of a pandemic, unions were concerned about provisions that might require their members to drive long distances to report to work. These same challenges arose during COVID-19, with Ontario's Premier issuing an emergency order that allowed health service providers to redeploy staff to different locations, change the assignment of work (including assigning non-bargaining unit employees bargaining unit work), change scheduling, and defer vacations, among other measures.[36]

But if the decentralization of health authorities had led to difficulties in pandemic management in 2009, the more recent recentralization of health authorities in many provinces led to other kinds of issues. One was the effect on public health systems within these provinces. While the organization of public health varies considerably across provinces, most provinces had embedded public health at the municipal level, where it could most effectively provide guidance and assistance to local offices. With the centralization of health authorities, public health offices were increasingly amalgamated and expected to cover larger catchment areas. The concern here, as the Canadian

35. Ontario, Legislative Assembly, Standing Committee on Social Policy, "Health Protection and Promotion Amendment Act, 2011", *Official Report of Debates (Hansard), No SP-17* (22 March 2011), online (pdf): *Ontario Legislative Assembly* <https://www.ola.org/sites/default/files/node-files/hansard/document/pdf/2011/2011-03/committee-transcript-2-EN-22-MAR-2011_SP017.pdf>.

36. *Order Made Under Subsection 7.0.2(4) of the Emergency Management Act*, O Reg 74/20; *Order Made Under Subsection 7.0.2(4) of the Emergency Management Act* O Reg 77/20.

Public Health Association noted, was whether these reorganizations "have compromised the core functions of public health."[37]

COVID-19

The first Canadian case of COVID-19 was detected on January 25, 2020. Unlike SARS, which was largely confined to a few hospitals, COVID-19 presented more widely, with outbreaks in long-term care homes, meat processing factories, prisons, and Indigenous communities. The mortality rate of COVID-19 is considerable compared to recent pandemics, and, because it is a coronavirus rather than a strain of influenza, the development of a vaccine will be more protracted. Given important differences in transmission, mortality, and treatment, the public health actions taken in response to COVID-19 have been more sweeping and restrictive than with previous outbreaks. Although there is interprovincial variation, governments have limited gatherings, closed non-essential businesses, issued directions to health facilities, and declared states of emergency. This required tremendous horizontal coordination across government departments well beyond the health sector.[38]

As the only country outside of Asia with a significant experience of SARS, Canada had the advantage compared to other western states of being able to use the crisis to develop an institutional protocol for pandemic management. The legal framework following SARS, however, was not itself changed substantially after H1N1. Discussions in the wake of H1N1 did reference the Naylor Report's recommendations to harmonize legislative frameworks "to permit a determination of the legal status of the measures found to be necessary to meet the public health goal that is in the interests of all Canadians," including clarification on the use of POGG during pandemics.[39] Despite noting the need for greater collaboration, the Senate Report on H1N1

37. Canadian Public Health Association, *Public Health in the Context of Health System Renewal in Canada* (Ottawa: Canadian Public Health Association, 2019), online (pdf): *Canadian Public Health Association* <https://www.cpha.ca/sites/default/files/uploads/policy/positionstatements/phhsr-backgrounddocument-e.pdf>.

38. For example, this includes efforts undertaken by Ministries of Justice to move essential court proceedings online and provide law enforcement support for new offences linked to the violation of public health orders, implementing benefit plans to support Canadians who are out of work and coordinating with the United States government over the closure of the border, among other actions.

39. *Supra* note 16 at 24.

recommended that this be accomplished through federal/provincial/territorial (F/P/T) discussions and memoranda of understanding rather than legislation.[40] COVID-19 shows the need for further intergovernmental collaboration in areas such as national standards for testing and tracing and the distribution of medical supplies, perhaps including a future vaccine.

But the coordination of institutions and processes between jurisdictions is not simple merely because it is supralegal. While Canada was able to sublimate most regional differences (however temporarily) rather than use pandemic planning to political advantage, the structure of health care in Canada is by nature unwieldy and fragmented. The rapid collection and exchange of critical data is still beset with issues, one of which is simply the comparability of data collected in real time. The existence of key pandemic protocol means that governments, if not working "in lockstep," are able to coordinate fundamental policies and do not work at cross-purposes (such as bidding against each other for equipment or drugs). But pandemics vary considerably, and the details—especially in an uncertain and data-poor environment—can be more difficult to work out. With H1N1, a significant source of confusion for the public was the sequencing of vaccination, which varied across provinces. With COVID-19, conflicting messages arose over whether and how far one could travel within one's province, the acceptable size of social groups, and the use of face masks. These conflicting messages have been amplified through the widespread use of social media.

The formal roadmaps for pandemic management focus primarily on two sets of actors—federal and provincial/territorial governments—but the effective execution of public health policies often depends on the collaboration of four levels of government (including regional and municipal) with other jurisdictions (such as First Nation and Inuit) sitting crosswise on several of these concurrently. Pandemics also require government to coordinate with non-governmental entities, such as drug and device companies, private businesses such as the transportation and manufacturing sectors, and the unions representing health care workers.

Another lesson from both SARS and H1N1 that is easy to understand but difficult to operationalize has been the need for decision makers to comprehend the demands of those working on the front

40. *Supra* note 18 at 45.

lines, and to respond in a timely manner to their concerns.[41] The 2006 Campbell Report noted that "[w]hat we learned from SARS is that what is needed is a process to bring together the various partners—union, management, government, ministries, associations—to address these very complex systemic and legal issues, but we need to do that long before the crisis hits."[42] As the experiences with SARS, H1N1, and COVID-19 all illustrate, seemingly small issues for governmental decision makers (the adequacy of personal protective equipment or the clinical guidelines pulled together to guide health care professionals) had tremendous importance for health care workers. It is clear that further work on this is needed, not only within hospitals but within other parts of the health sector (namely, long-term care) and other essential parts of the economy (such as workers in the food supply chain who also suffered from high infection rates).

What have been the lessons of COVID-19 itself? These will only be identified with confidence once the dust has settled. But some observations are readily apparent now. All jurisdictions have realized the importance of communicating not only with each other but with their citizens to provide clear, consistent, and ongoing information regarding what is happening, what is expected of everyone, and what to anticipate. Chief medical officers of health across Canada have presented themselves as the public face of pandemic messaging. These same individuals have not mistaken consistency with rigidity and have, given the lack of key data and shifting scientific understanding of the virus, been willing to change their messaging when empirical information suggests new insights. We have a better understanding of how social structures (long-term care homes, food processing plants, penal institutions) can exacerbate and amplify the spread of disease. We have learned that we have *not* learned the importance of effective data sharing across jurisdictions. And we are also learning that large-scale pandemics are not phenomena that are isolated in time or space: they affect countless social and economic relationships, and must be understood as an ecosystem in themselves. That is why a major pandemic cannot simply be managed by appealing to a central authority. An understanding of intergovernmental relations throughout Canada's history shows clearly that any intemperate exercise of federal emergency powers would be seen as intrusive,

41. See Part E of this volume for an examination of these issues.
42. *Supra* note 26 at 271.

pernicious, illegitimate, and fundamentally destructive of intergovernmental relations in Canada. Faster containment of a pandemic would be won only at the cost of decades of provincial acrimony and bitterness, affecting intergovernmental relations across a wide swathe of programs and policies.

The hardest lesson may be the requirement that we invest in public health even (or especially) in periods where threats to public health are not on the horizon (and thus not on the political agenda). Faced with short electoral cycles and the competing financial demands of primary and acute care, public health across jurisdictions has a history of marginal funding. "The pattern," noted the Naylor Report, "is now familiar. Public health is taken for granted until disease outbreaks occur, whereupon a brief flurry of lip service leads to minimal investments and little real change in public health infrastructure or priorities."[43]

Conclusion

There is some speculation that disaggregated government exacerbated the spread of the pandemic in Italy.[44] To what extent has Canada's highly decentralized framework of health care governance affected our ability to address pandemic management? There are two responses to this question. The first simply says that, for better or worse, we have a constitutional structure that does not permit a national command-and-control model of health care governance (Italy, which is essentially a unitary state divided into organizational regions, can more usefully ask this kind of question). The second response is grounded in democratic theory. If there is regional variation across Canada, should we not be concerned if some regions seem to be performing more poorly? In the classical understanding of representational federalism, we should not: where a multitude of variables coalesce in political decision-making, the particular constellation of choices and values will have different outcomes in different jurisdictions. Who is to determine whether the choices made are legitimate? If regional governments are responsible for decisions taken, then their electorates will hold them answerable.

---

43. *Supra* note 16 at 64.
44. See e.g. Iris Bosa, "Italy's Response to the Coronavirus Pandemic" (16 April 2020), online (blog): *Cambridge Core* <https://www.cambridge.org/core/blog/2020/04/16/italys-response-to-the-coronavirus-pandemic/>.

The natural advantage of a federal system rests not only in its receptiveness to local interests, but also in the flexibility it affords some jurisdictions to see opportunities and take risks that others are unwilling to countenance. The multi-stage process of re-opening provincial economies, for example, is a natural experiment that will afford a much deeper understanding of policy effectiveness.[45] Pandemic conditions involve tremendous uncertainty; yet political decisions must be made. On the one hand, serious measures involving the curtailment of civil rights or the diminution of one's livelihood require the application of proportionality: are the potential outcomes so extreme that these measures are merited? The empirical information we have on this is limited and often in flux. On the other hand, the precautionary principle suggests that, when facing uncertainty, a more cautious strategy is preferable. Canadians will take different positions regarding the levels of relative risk they are willing to accept, and the particular balance between public health, civil liberties, and economic prosperity they prefer. Canada's federal structure, despite the complications and frustrations of coordinating activity between jurisdictions, will permit these political discussions to play themselves out in a manner that is receptive to diverse perspectives.

---

45. Quebec, despite having the highest number of cases, reopened various businesses and services between May 4 and 19, including elementary schools, daycares, stores, and the construction and manufacturing sectors. The sequencing of re-opening was quite different across regions as well, with businesses such as personal services (for example, hair salons) enjoying early opening in Alberta, but late-phase opening in Nova Scotia.

CHAPTER A-2

COVID-19 and First Nations' Responses

Aimée Craft,* Deborah McGregor,** and Jeffery Hewitt***

Abstract

This chapter considers the federal government's fettering of jurisdiction through inaction in the areas of clean water and housing. We consider a small sample of First Nations' responses, taken on the basis of their assertions of jurisdiction and responses to the particular needs and circumstances of their communities. We conclude that First Nations are best positioned to make policy and law in response to COVID-19, and that the federal government can and must work with First Nations communities on resourcing their plans for wellness and emergency preparedness in relation to the pandemic, in accordance with a *sui generis* application of the constitutional principle of subsidiarity in conjunction with other constitutional obligations such as the fiduciary duty of the Crown and its duty to act honourably. This chapter is contextualized by the theme of self-determination in Indigenous health, s. 35 of the *Constitution Act*, and the *United Nations Declaration on the Rights of Indigenous Peoples*.

* Associate Professor at the Faculty of Common Law, University of Ottawa and an Indigenous (Anishinaabe-Métis) lawyer from Treaty 1 territory in Manitoba.

** Canada Research Chair in Indigenous Environmental Justice, cross-appointed with Osgoode Hall Law School and the Faculty of Environmental Studies, York University.

*** Assistant Professor at Osgoode Hall Law School, former President of the Indigenous Bar Association of Canada, and currently director of the National Theatre School.

Résumé
La COVID-19 et les interventions des Premières Nations

Ce chapitre examine comment l'inaction du gouvernement fédéral dans les dossiers de l'eau potable et du logement constitue une entrave à sa compétence. Nous nous intéressons à un modeste échantillon d'interventions des Premières Nations, choisies sur la base de l'affirmation de leur compétence et de leurs réponses aux circonstances et aux besoins particuliers de leurs communautés. Nous concluons que les Premières Nations sont les mieux placées pour concevoir des politiques et des lois en réaction à la COVID-19 et que le gouvernement fédéral peut et doit travailler avec elles et financer leurs plans en matière de mieux-être et de préparation aux situations d'urgence en rapport avec la pandémie, selon une application *sui generis* du principe constitutionnel de subsidiarité en conjonction avec d'autres obligations constitutionnelles telles que l'obligation fiduciaire de la Couronne et son devoir d'agir honorablement. Ce chapitre est mis en contexte à travers le thème de l'autodétermination en matière de santé autochtone, conformément à l'article 35 de la *Loi constitutionnelle de 1982* et à la *Déclaration des Nations Unies sur les droits des peuples autochtones*.

"The great aim of our legislation has been to do away with the tribal system and assimilate the Indian people in all respects with the other inhabitants of the Dominion as speedily as they are fit to change."

– *Prime Minister John A. Macdonald,* 1887

"We need to make sure that all different orders of government, including Indigenous governments, are working together with the same goal, which we all share, which is keeping Canadians as safe as possible, recognizing that certain communities and certain individuals are more vulnerable."

– *Prime Minister Justin Trudeau,* 2020

It is no small task to discuss Indigenous responses to COVID-19. In large part, this subject is so daunting due to constitutional obscurities and legal fictions that frame the relationship between Indigenous people and the Crown. Indigenous vulnerability to pandemics must be understood within a broader context of historical and ongoing colonialism, which has disrupted and undermined the health and well-being of Indigenous people. In sum, the relationship is primarily governed through the Crown's unilateral creation of laws and policies, formed and deformed over centuries, and which aim to position Crown interests above those of Indigenous people, especially in relation to lands and resources. The Supreme Court of Canada refers to this relationship structure as the *reconciliation* of asserted/affirmed Crown sovereignty with the "prior occupation by Aboriginal people."[1]

Both prior to and since confederation, Canada adopted a federal project to assimilate Indigenous people into the citizenry, which continues today in a variety of forms, including chronic underfunding of essential services, leaving Indigenous people vulnerable to the COVID-19 pandemic. Indigenous people score far worse on virtually all indicators of health than the general public,[2] a situation that has been directly attributed to historical and ongoing processes of colonization.[3] Further, Indigenous communities currently face multiple health crises and have already experienced devastating pandemics with disastrous and ongoing impacts. The broader context for Indigenous people is characterized by increased risk and vulnerability, yet a capacity for resilience.

This chapter is not the place to recount the long, hostile, and violent history of Indigenous/Crown relations in Canada, but it is a place for attempting to offer a contemporary picture of some of the ways in which the long-standing federal approach has impacted COVID-19 responses for Indigenous people. We have scaled down our discussion to consider only federal COVID-19 responses in a First Nations context and the assertion of jurisdiction by First Nations in relation to their own people and territories. We have not captured Métis or Inuit responses, nor have we canvassed provincial responses. If we had taken on each of

1. *R v Van der Peet*, [1996] 2 SCR 507, 137 DLR (4th) 289.
2. Truth and Reconciliation Commission of Canada, *Canada's Residential Schools: The Legacy (The Final Report)*, vol 5 (Winnipeg: Truth and Reconciliation Commission of Canada, 2015). See also First Nations Child and Family Caring Society of Canada, "Victory for First Nations Children: Canadian Human Rights Tribunal Finds Discrimination Against First Nations Children Living On-Reserve" (26 January 2016), online (pdf): *First Nations Child and Family Caring Society of Canada* <https://fncaringsociety.com/sites/default/files/Information%20Sheet%20re%20CHRT%20Decision.pdf>.
3. James Anaya, "Report of the Special Rapporteur on the Rights of Indigenous Peoples" (2014), online: *United Nations* <https://undocs.org/A/HRC/27/52/AdFREEd.2>.

these dimensions, we would have only scratched the surface, especially given that the legal and policy context that applies to each First Nations, Inuit, Métis, and non-status people has different implications (what the federal government calls a "distinctions-based approach"). Instead, we have dived more deeply into the affirmations of jurisdiction and corresponding acts of First Nations governments (and their collaborations based on their exercise of jurisdiction). The achievement of Indigenous well-being and resilience must be understood within the context of self-determination, as outlined in the *United Nations Declaration on the Rights of Indigenous Peoples* (UNDRIP), in conjunction with the ongoing failures by the federal government to address basic human rights issues, such as housing and clean water on reserves, both of which have a direct impact on the ability to ensure the health and safety of First Nations.

> Self-determination holds the key to better Aboriginal health by allowing communities to develop programs that are suited to their own needs, and to do so in a holistic way, avoiding the jurisdictional disputes that have plagued progress in health and so many other areas where the residential schools still cast a large shadow.[4]

We have chosen a handful of First Nations examples that reflect First Nations self-determination in the area of health, aimed at mitigating the spread of COVID-19 and maintaining the health and wellness of First Nations people and communities. We suggest that First Nations, as the most proximate government, are best positioned to make policy and law in response to COVID-19 and that they should be supported financially in that endeavour by the federal government—in the form of a *sui generis* application of the constitutional principle of subsidiarity (where authority rests with the government that is closest to the context and the people). Our comments are shared in light of the continued efforts of Indigenous people to maintain and restore good relations and to live in wellness—key pillars of Treaties and Indigenous legal orders in Canada.[5]

---

4. Truth and Reconciliation Commission of Canada, *Canada's Residential Schools: The Legacy (The Final Report)*, vol 5 (Winnipeg: Truth and Reconciliation Commission, 2015).
5. Aimée Craft, "Ki'inaakonigewin: Reclaiming Space for Indigenous Laws" (Paper delivered at the Canadian Administration of Justice Conference, *Aboriginal Peoples and Law: "We Are All Here to Stay"*, Saskatoon, 14 October 2015).

Federal Government's Failure and the Argument for Enhanced First Nations Jurisdiction

Today, there are 634 First Nations in Canada, with more than 50 distinct languages; their financial, geographic, political, cultural, and social circumstances vary considerably.[6] There is no homogeneous way to refer to an Indigenous experience of COVID-19, other than increased vulnerabilities and risk. Furthermore, within each community there will be a range of opinions and perspectives depending on capacity, geography, and access to resources. Some communities have recent experience with pandemics, including those that were significantly affected by H1N1 and SARS.[7] Some now have emergency preparedness plans. Others have developed COVID-specific strategies.

As noted above, Indigenous people are confronted with disparities and disadvantages in every conceivable indicator of well-being.[8] Anne Levesque and Sophie Thériault, in the Equity section of this volume (see Chapter D-6), cover some of these issues, including the lack of responsiveness by governments and the wholly inadequate funding of existing responsibilities, in violation of human rights. Many First Nations communities across Canada are in a continual state of crisis and have declared states of emergency in their communities in the following areas: health (suicide crisis); infrastructure, including inadequate and over-crowded housing and unsafe drinking water; child welfare; and the climate crisis (fires, droughts, and floods). Governmental attempts to address these crises have been inadequate and have left Indigenous people more susceptible to COVID-19. These inequalities will only be exacerbated by the COVID-19 pandemic "largely due to the pre-existing and ongoing impacts of colonialism and racism."[9]

In our view, the federal government has fettered its jurisdiction by being non-responsive to ongoing human rights violations and by

6. René R Gadacz, "First Nations" in *The Canadian Encyclopedia*, (Toronto: Historica Canada, 2020), online: *The Canadian Encyclopedia* <https://www.thecanadianencyclopedia.ca/en/article/first-nations>.
7. Shanifa Nasser, "Early Signs Suggest Race Matters When it Comes to COVID-19. So Why Isn't Canada Collecting Race-Based Data?", *CBC News* (17 April 2020), online: <https://www.cbc.ca/news/canada/toronto/race-coronavirus-canada-1.5536168>.
8. *Supra* note 4.
9. Ontario Human Rights Commission, "Policy Statement on a Human Rights-Based Approach to Managing the COVID-19 Pandemic", online: *Ontario Human Rights Commission* <http://www.ohrc.on.ca/en/policy-statement-human-rights-based-approach-managing-covid-19-pandemic>.

failing to provide adequate resources to First Nations people (especially those living on reserve). As a result, applying the constitutional principle of subsidiarity in conjunction with other constitutional obligations such as the fiduciary duty of the Crown and its duty to act honourably, we focus our discussion on the actions taken as a result of Indigenous assertions of jurisdiction. Clearly, there is a need for coordination and transparency across jurisdictions in order to recognize and give effect to the distinct COVID-19 responses of First Nations.

Water and housing are two areas of federal *irresponsibility* that significantly increase the COVID-19 risk for First Nations. One of the cornerstones of COVID-19 prevention is frequent hand washing, which poses a particular challenge for First Nations due to lack of access to clean water: currently, 27 First Nations are under short-term water advisories.[10] The inadequacy of the government's response to this problem is illustrated by Indigenous Services Canada (ISC) advising (on its website) those communities on a "do not use" water advisory "... your water is not safe for any use. Use bottled water with soap or hand sanitizer with at least 60% alcohol to wash your hands. If you do not have access to running water, wash your hands in a large bowl and then throw out the water from the hand-washing bowl after each individual use."[11] This "hand-washing" advice ignores the overarching chronic water insecurity already existing in a number of First Nations communities, including the lack of access to bottled water in remote communities. Thus the "solutions" offered are wholly inadequate.

While there are opportunities for emergency responses from federal and provincial governments, both Ontario's *Emergency Management and Civil Protection Act*[12] and the federal *Emergencies Act*[13] do not specifically allocate federal financial aid for First Nations communities when declaring a state of emergency. In other words, even in the context of a pandemic or similar scale of emergency, Canadian law does not expressly include Indigenous jurisdictional capacity, despite the constitutional requirement to do so based on treaties and the *Constitution Acts, 1867* and *1982*. Thus, it is left to First Nations

10. Note that ISC data do not include B.C. First Nations or those that are part of the Saskatoon Tribal Council.
11. Indigenous Services Canada, *Coronavirus (COVID-19) and Indigenous Communities: Confirmed Cases of COVID-19* (Ottawa: Indigenous Services Canada, 2020), online: *Indigenous Services Canada* <https://www.sac-isc.gc.ca/eng/1581964230816/1581964277298#chap0>.
12. *Emergency Management and Civil Protection Act*, RSO 1990, c E 9.
13. *Emergencies Act*, RSC, 1985, c 22.

to provide leadership without full constitutionally recognized jurisdictional authority, given the occupation of the legislative field by the federal and provincial governments and their control over First Nations' financial and other resources.

The Ontario Human Rights Commission, as well as Thériault and Lévesque, argue for a human rights-based approach to managing COVID-19, with independent oversight and additional funding to protect Indigenous people's health and human rights, and the application of Jordan's Principle when jurisdictional disputes arise.[14] This failure to remedy water and housing insecurity puts First Nations citizens in more precarious positions in relation to COVID-19 than other citizens. In sustaining the precariousness, the federal government has abdicated responsibility, breached the Honour of the Crown and its fiduciary duty, and fettered its jurisdiction. In response, many First Nations have expressly (re)asserted their jurisdiction and continued with their responsibilities, examples of which are illustrated below.

The Federal COVID-19 Response

Despite all efforts, there are some cases of COVID-19 in First Nations. As of June 9, according to ISC there were 234 confirmed cases of COVID-19, 22 hospitalizations, 206 recovered cases and 6 deaths in First Nations communities (reserves) in Canada.[15] Some of the ISC data differs from First Nations' reporting,[16] although in some regions,

14. Levesque & Thériault, this volume, Chapter D-6. See also Ontario Human Rights Commission, "Policy Statement on a Human Rights-Based Approach to Managing the COVID-19 Pandemic", online: *Ontario Human Rights Commission* <http://www.ohrc.on.ca/en/policy-statement-human-rights-based-approach-managing-covid-19-pandemic>. See also TRC Call to Action 3; Canadian Human Rights Commission "Statement–Inequality Amplified by COVID-19 Crisis", online: *Canadian Human Rights Commission* <https://www.chrc-ccdp.gc.ca/eng/content/statement-inequality-amplified-covid-19-crisis>.
15. *Supra* note 12. ISC updates the numbers daily. Indigenous Services Canada, *Coronavirus (COVID-19) and Indigenous Communities: Confirmed Cases of COVID-19*, (2020). Online: <https://www.sac-isc.gc.ca/eng/1581964230816/1581964277298#chap0>. However, as commentators have noted (see <https://www.cbc.ca/news/indigenous/coronavirus-indigenous-data-gap-1.5556676>), community reporting is outpacing ISC data. The ISCs data do not include the number of recovered cases, the number, or names of First Nations communities affected, or account for First Nations members living off reserve. Further, the ISC only tracks cases of COVID in First Nations and Inuit communities.
16. Courtney Skye, "Colonialism of the Curve: Indigenous Communities & Bad COVID Data", Yellowhead Institute (12 May 2020), online: *Yellowhead*

the numbers are likely to be significantly under-reported because of a lack of testing. Health Canada is said to be mobilizing testing capacity, shipping personal protective equipment (PPE), and sending bottled water, hand sanitizer, isolation tents, and additional health professionals to communities. However, no concrete plan of action has been made publicly available, nor have the unique challenges of dealing with an outbreak on reserve been acknowledged, including issues with limited health infrastructure and services and those relating to the ability to self-isolate, quarantine, and physically distance.[17]

ISC's general COVID-19 strategy (see Figure A2.1 at the end of the chapter) has reported that the federal government will pay what it costs to respond to possible outbreaks in Indigenous communities. The media reports that, as of April 24, the government has allocated $145.6 billion in direct support for COVID-19 responses.[18] While Indigenous people make up roughly 4.5% of the Canadian population[19] as a whole, Indigenous-specific funding only accounts for 0.56% of the federal government's COVID-19 funding allocation. This has been widely criticized as insufficient and lacking an understanding of the issues that First Nations communities are facing.[20]

On March 18, 2020, the Minister for ISC announced the Indigenous Community Support Fund,[21] which includes $305 million for Indigenous people in Canada, with funds set aside to support regional, urban, and off-reserve Indigenous organizations. The allocation between First Nations ($215 million), Inuit ($45 million),

---

Institute <https://yellowheadinstitute.org/2020/05/12/colonialism-of-the-curve-indigenous-communities-and-bad-covid-data/>.

17. Teresa Wright, "COVID-19 Outbreaks in 23 First Nations Prompt Worries", *CTV News* (1 May 2020), online: <https://www.ctvnews.ca/canada/covid-19-outbreaks-in-23-first-nations-prompt-worries-1.4920181>.

18. Karina Roman, "By the Numbers: Federal Projected Spending on Direct Supports Due to COVID-19 Hits $145B", *CBC* (24 April 2020), online: <https://www.cbc.ca/news/politics/covid-19-economic-programs-1.5543092>.

19. Statistics Canada, *Aboriginal Peoples Highlight Tables*, 2016 Census (Ottawa: Statistics Canada, 2016), online: *Statistics Canada* <https://www12.statcan.gc.ca/census-recensement/2016/dp-pd/hlt-fst/abo-aut/Table.cfm?Lang=Eng&T=101&S=99&O=A>.

20. Teresa Wright, "Ottawa Response for COVID-19 Outbreak in Indigenous Communities Troubling", *National Observer* (15 March 2020), online: <https://www.nationalobserver.com/2020/03/15/news/ottawa-response-covid-19-outbreak-indigenous-communities-troubling>.

21. Indigenous Services Canada, *Indigenous Community Support Fund* (Ottawa: Indigenous Services Canada, 2020), online: *Indigenous Services Canada* <https://www.sac-isc.gc.ca/eng/1585189335380/1585189357198>.

and Métis ($30 million) is based on population (2016 census), remoteness, and community well-being. For a breakdown by province/territory, see Figure A2.2 at the end of the chapter.[22] According to the Minister, "these new funds will provide Indigenous leadership with the flexibility needed to design and implement community-based solutions to prepare for and react to the spread of COVID-19 within their communities."[23] Indigenous organizations providing services to Indigenous people in urban centres/off reserve received $15 million. The adequacy of the funding provided is contested: the Congress of Aboriginal Peoples filed an application in Federal Court claiming inadequate and discriminatory funding for off-reserve and urban Indigenous people.[24] Following this application, on May 21, 2020, the federal government announced an additional $75 million in COVID-19 funding for Indigenous individuals living off-reserve.[25] Other pockets of funds have been allocated by ISC to Indigenous communities for: a) public health short-term needs (implement pandemic plans, and for public health and primary care related to a COVID outbreak) ($100 million); b) short-term, interest-free loans and non-repayable contributions for businesses (up to $306.8 million); c) increased subsidies for the Nutrition North program ($25 million); d) "distinctions-based" support for post-secondary students ($75.2 million); and e) funds to support families in the Northwest Territories to move onto the land as a physical distancing measure ($2.6 million).[26]

22. *Ibid.*
23. *Ibid.*
24. Kristy Kirkup, "Congress of Aboriginal Peoples File Court Application Over Federal Funding Levels During COVID-19", *The Globe and Mail* (May 14 2020), online: <https://www.theglobeandmail.com/politics/article-congress-of-aboriginal-peoples-file-court-application-over-federal/?utm_source=First+Peoples+Law+Blog&utm_campaign=3cocf73dd4-EMAIL_CAMPAIGN_2019_07_10_09_19_COPY_01&utm_medium=email&utm_term=0_84105b31a3-3cocf73dd4-196448785>.
25. Rachel Aiello, "PM Offering $75 Million More in COVID-19 Aid to Indigenous People Living Off-Reserve", *CTV News* (21 May 2020), online: <https://www.ctvnews.ca/canada/pm-offering-75-million-more-in-covid-19-aid-to-indigenous-people-living-off-reserve-1.4947961>.
26. *Supra* note 22; Indigenous Services Canada, *COVID-19 Specific Funding Announced by Government of Canada to Support First Nations Public Health Response* (Ottawa: Indigenous Services Canada, 2020), online: *Indigenous Services Canada* <https://www.sac-isc.gc.ca/eng/1584819394157/1584819418553#b>; Indigenous Services Canada, News Release, "Indigenous, Territorial and Federal Leaders Mobilize Funding to Support Unique Northern Physical Distancing Initiative" (30 March 2020), online: *Indigenous Services Canada* <https://www.canada.ca/en/indigenous-services-canada/news/2020/03/

The federal government's Indigenous COVID-19 response continues to evolve as First Nations advocate for increased funding to address their distinct challenges and needs. Many First Nations are vulnerable to COVID-19, both the disease itself and the adverse consequences of measures taken in response, due to existing and longstanding economic, social, and health disparities. Recently, Grand Chief Perry Bellegarde of the Assembly of First Nations expressed concerns to the Standing Committee on Indigenous and Northern Affairs regarding the government's removal of pandemic restrictions that would impact First Nations. He stated that some "provincial governments are refusing to accept lawful decisions by First Nations to restrict traffic flow and gatherings among people" as part of First Nations exercising their inherent jurisdiction in their response to COVID-19.[27]

Indigenous Responses Relating to COVID-19

First Nations governments are the best placed and most proximate government to respond to needs, and to act in accordance within a variety of jurisdictional fields, including the management of health emergencies on their reserve. However, this must be understood in conjunction with the ongoing treaty and constitutional obligations of the federal government to fund the operation of this First Nations authority in response to COVID-19.

---

indigenous-territorial-and-federal-leaders-mobilize-funding-to-support-unique-northern-physical-distancing-initiative.html>; Indigenous Services Canada, *Relief Measures for Indigenous Businesses* (Ottawa: Indigenous Services Canada, 2020), online: *Indigenous Services Canada* <https://www.sac-isc.gc.ca/eng/1588079295625/1588079326171>; Health Canada, *Canada's COVID-19 Economic Response Plan: Indigenous Peoples (Making Personal Hygiene Products and Nutritious Food More Affordable)* (Ottawa: Health Canada, 2020), online: *Health Canada* <https://www.canada.ca/en/department-finance/economic-response-plan.html#individuals>; Health Canada, *Canada's COVID-19 Economic Response Plan: Indigenous Peoples (Providing Support to Indigenous Post-Secondary Students)* (Ottawa: Health Canada, 2020), online: *Health Canada* <https://www.canada.ca/en/department-finance/economic-response-plan.html#individuals>.

27. Teresa Wright, "Canada's Indigenous Leaders Say More Help Is Needed as COVID-19 Outbreaks Rise", *Global News* (8 May 2020), online: <https://globalnews.ca/news/6923971/coronavirus-canada-indigenous-concerns/>. See also House of Commons, "Standing Committee on Indigenous and Northern Affairs, INAN Meeting, No 7" (8 May 2020), online (video): *House of Commons*, <https://parlvu.parl.gc.ca/Harmony/en/PowerBrowser/PowerBrowserV2/20200508/-1/33202?Language=English&Stream=Video> [House of Commons].

Indigenous responses to the COVID-19 pandemic have been multiple and varied across Canada. However, they all build on multiple sources of authority for assuming the jurisdiction needed to protect citizens of First Nations. Some Nations have chosen to enact bylaws (a power granted to band councils under subsection 86(1) and (4) of the *Indian Act*) or have claimed their authority and rights under treaties. Others have affirmed their ongoing and inherent jurisdiction, recognized in the unceded title to their traditional territories, or have anchored their responses in their Indigenous legal orders, both in the exercise of customary laws and modern codified and legislated authority. Many have invoked their sovereign rights of self-determination, as provided for in UNDRIP and which is grounded in multiple sources of authority. Many First Nations have decided to continue with measures stricter than those of the provinces and adjoining municipalities, in the face of eventual multiple waves and spikes of infection. First Nations communities are not typically located near large urban centres and, therefore have increased vulnerability to infectious diseases such as COVID-19. By virtue of being Indigenous, there is also less health care infrastructure.

An increasing number of First Nations have declared a pandemic and a state of emergency, and have implemented COVID-19 responses, including restrictions consistent with federal and provincial jurisdictions. Some First Nations have implemented lockdowns, travel restrictions, curfews, 24-hour surveillance, checkpoints, as well as failure-to-comply fines. First Nations have limited options to enforce their pandemic responses through *Indian Act* bylaw provisions. It should be noted that First Nation responses vary and change over time as new information and cases emerge in their communities.

The following examples illustrate the affirmations of jurisdiction by many First Nations in Canada in core areas relating to the overall wellness and protection of citizens of those Nations, for example, in areas of: transport; trade and commerce; health; education; matters of a local and private nature; property and civil rights; and emergency law-making powers. By regulating the "who, what, and where," First Nations have taken positive and preventive measures to ensure the health and wellness of their community members; have created emergency responses and regulated trade; and have also limited travel to, from, and within their territories (both reserves and traditional territories). They have collaborated among themselves and with other governments to ensure these orders are respected. They have also called upon others to account for their actions, including municipal, provincial, and federal governments, particularly where there has been conflict in the application and implementation of their orders. This is illustrative of the extent to which First Nations' governmental responsibilities are impacted by municipalities, provinces, and the federal government, yet most First Nations operate without the benefit of a taxable base, the security of multi-year funding, or the ability to incur debt. In sum, the current funding for First Nation communities is one that relies on agreement between the federal and provincial Crowns. The lack of specific inclusion of Indigenous people in emergency legislation along with a disregard by the settler population (access to tobacco, cottages) of the interests and needs of Indigenous people is demonstrative of the ongoing asymmetrical Indigenous/Crown relationship that places the existence of Indigenous people at risk in favour of the settler population.

Trade, Land Leases, and Mobility

To contain COVID-19, by early April a number of communities in Ontario, such as Six Nations,[28] Rama First Nation,[29] and Wahta First Nation,[30] temporarily closed their communities to varying degrees, including their tobacco retailers.[31] Councils issued these orders through their inherent rights jurisdiction and via *Indian Act* powers. Restrictions on gatherings (no more than five people) and requests to stay at home were already in place for the general population in Ontario.[32] However, the response of many non-residents to Six Nations and Rama's notices of temporary closure was to ignore the stay-in-place protocol and

28. Jennifer K Baker, "Chief Calls for Closure of Smoke Shops After Two COVID-19 Cases Reported in Six Nations", *CTV News* (29 March 2020), online: <https://kitchener.ctvnews.ca/chief-calls-for-closure-of-smoke-shops-after-two-covid-19-cases-reported-in-six-nations-1.4873315>.
29. Justin Rydell, "Wahta First Nation Also Closes Non-Essential Business, Ending Tobacco Sales", *CTV News* (8 April 2020), online: <https://barrie.ctvnews.ca/wahta-first-nation-also-closes-non-essential-business-ending-tobacco-sales-1.4888729>.
30. *Ibid.*
31. Lindsay Richardson, "Influx of Non-Residents Chasing Gas, Smokes and Pot Putting First Nation Communities at Risk" *APTN News* (7 April 2020), online: <https://www.aptnnews.ca/national-news/influx-of-non-residents-chasing-gas-smokes-and-pot-putting-first-nation-communities-at-risk/>.
32. Ontario Ministry of Health, "Statement from the Chief Medical Officer of Health" (30 March 2020), online: *Ontario Ministry of Health* <https>//news.ontario.ca/mohltc/en/2020/03/statement-from-the-chief-medical-officer-of-health.html>.

travel to these First Nations communities to stock up on cigarettes. Simultaneously, there was an increase in online racism against First Nations communities that issued temporary closures.[33]

To mitigate against the risk of infection within the Nation, some First Nations communities are limiting access to the reserve to residents only (and in some cases excluding non-resident citizens of the nation). This is in step with, for example, a province closing its borders to others (as Quebec has done, for example) or Canada closing the border to the United States to slow the spread of COVID-19. As we write, warmer weather approaches and many First Nations in Ontario are discouraging non-resident cottagers from travelling to their communities due to the increased potential for the spread of COVID-19. Another unique constitutional question arises in this context: can non-resident mobility rights under section 6 of the *Charter* be restricted by the application of First Nations jurisdiction and the protection of "rights or freedoms that pertain to the aboriginal peoples of Canada" against charter claims?[34]

There have been tensions between First Nations that have exercised their jurisdictional assertion to protect the health of their people and non-resident cottagers. Cottage leases located on reserves are subject to various laws, including the *Indian Act*[35] and the *First Nation Lands Management Act*.[36] Generally, reserve lands cannot be privately owned, though they can be leased to non-residents and are often used for non-resident cottagers. First Nations retain the right as to whether or not to renew a cottage lease by way of statute[37] or inherent right.[38] A different question arises when First Nations communities wish to exercise public health authorities to prevent a non-resident cottager from entering their community, where to do so would put the community at risk.

33. Kim Uyede-Kai, "COIVD-19 and the Racism Pandemic We Need to Talk About" (April 2020), online: *Shining Waters Regional Council* <https://shiningwatersregionalcouncil.ca/wp-content/uploads/2020/04/COVID-19-and-Racism-Pandemic-SWRC-revised.pdf>; Roberta K Timothy, "Coronavirus Is Not the 'Great Equalizer'—Race Matters: U of T Expert", *U of T News* (8 April 2020), online: <https://www.utoronto.ca/news/coronavirus-not-great-equalizer-race-matters-u-t-expert>.
34. *Canadian Charter of Rights and Freedoms*, s 25, Part I of the *Constitution Act, 1982*, being Schedule B to the *Canada Act 1982* (UK), 1982, c 11.
35. *Indian Act*, RSC, 1985, c I-5, ss 38 and 53.
36. *First Nation Land Management Act*, SC 1999, c 24, s 18(1)(b).
37. *Williston v Canada (Minister of Indian Affairs and Northern Development)*, 2005 FC 829.
38. *Devil's Gap Cottagers (1982) Ltd v Rat Portage Band No 38B*, 2008 FC 812.

For example, Walpole First Nation, located at the Michigan border, has advised non-residents and cottagers not to come to the community.[39] Whitefish River First Nation (WRFN) commenced a phased approach to pandemic planning and implemented travel restrictions, which have become increasingly restrictive over time as COVID-19 cases increase. Currently, only "residents" are permitted access to the community (and can leave for essential services). Chief Shining Turtle pointed out "that phase one of the response was signage, phase two was a letter informing cottagers that they could not access their seasonal dwellings and phase three was bringing in concrete barriers" in case they were required to physically prevent people from entering the reserve. "I get it," he said. "People don't want to be in Sudbury, Toronto, or Hamilton while this is going on. But the question you have to ask yourself, 'is this essential?'" Some cottagers with leased shoreline property in WRFN seem to be startled with the First Nation asserting their inherent jurisdiction during a pandemic, complaining about their restricted access to the reserve, stating that their seasonal cottages are their only "residences" and that they therefore meet the residency requirement. The cottage leases clearly indicate the cottagers are seasonal residents only. However, First Nations' jurisdiction was challenged by settler seasonal cottagers, despite the fact that similar measures were being suggested in adjoining municipalities in Ontario. It was observed that a "number of summer residents were flocking to their properties, many returning from COVID hot spots such as Florida and Toronto."[40] The WRFN updated their trespass by-law to address emergency measures and support the community pandemic plan.

First Nations communities will continue to face challenges from those who do not respect their inherent jurisdiction, particularly if their pandemic and recovery plans are not coordinated across jurisdictions. The Assembly of First Nations has stated that First Nations must be at any table dealing with the health crisis, and arguably should be the ultimate decision-making authority with respect to the wellness and safety of their communities.[41]

---

39. "Walpole Island First Nation Restricts Access to Non-Residents Due to COVID-19", *CBC* (2 April 2020), online: <https://www.cbc.ca/news/canada/windsor/walpole-island-first-nation-restricts-access-covid19-1.5518628>.

40. Michael Erskine, "Birch Island Denies Access to Cottagers with Leased Lots", *Manitoulin Expositor* (15 April 2020), online: <https://www.manitoulin.ca/birch-island-denies-access-to-cottagers-with-leased-lots/>.

41. House of Commons, *supra* note 28.

Wellness and Cultural Appropriateness

The Truth and Reconciliation Commission of Canada (TRC) called on the federal government to close the gap in health outcomes between Indigenous and non-Indigenous communities and for the recognition of Indigenous healing practices.[42] First Nations have stepped into this jurisdictional sphere in response to COVID-19, often with limited resources and funding. Combining the authority to act with respect to both wellness and emergency, some First Nations have enacted and implemented their own "disease emergency" by-laws under the *Indian Act*.[43] The by-laws range from mandating self-isolation or quarantine; mandating physical-distancing; restricting travel; restricting access to public spaces or businesses; and establishing emergency shelters for citizens who are homeless or living in precarious housing situations. Orders have been enforced through fines (and in some cases provide for imprisonment).

Proactive and culturally appropriate efforts relating to wellness, including the harvesting and distribution of traditional medicines, is supported through formal and informal networks that build on the jurisdiction of Nations, and is given effect through various forms of leadership, including those who have the responsibility to harvest, make, share, and look after medicines (including traditional foods). In addition, some of the formal COVID-19 preparedness plans include instructions for traditional methods of cleaning, harvesting, and preparing traditional medicines and guidance on ceremonies.[44] Some indicate that Elders and healers should be involved in incorporating traditional medicines and wisdom pertaining to contagious illnesses like COVID-19.[45] Many have also included information on sustaining well-being and mental health during physical distancing.

An important component of cultural appropriateness includes methods of communication of information, including in Indigenous

42. Truth and Reconciliation Commission of Canada, *Calls to Action* (Winnipeg: Truth and Reconciliation Commission, 2015).
43. Heiltsuk Nation, "By-Law No 21, Heiltsuk Disease Emergency By-Law"(2020), online (pdf): *Heiltsuk Nation* <http://www.heiltsuknation.ca/wp-content/uploads/2020/04/2020-03-31-Disease-Emergency-By-law.pdf>.
44. Six Nations of Grand River, "Coronavirus (COVID-19) Preparedness" (2020), online (pdf): *Six Nations of Grand River* <http://www.sixnations.ca/hpnsCovid19PreparednessImportantInformation.pdf>.
45. Nishnawbe Aski Nation, "COVID-19 Pandemic Plan" (2020), online (pdf): *Nishnawbe Aski Nation* <http://www.nan.on.ca/upload/documents/community-covid-19-pandemic-plan-templat.pdf>.

languages; see, for example, the Protecting Our Home Fires initiative from the Morning Star Lodge in five Indigenous languages.[46] Other examples include collaborations relating to the release of information in culturally and linguistically appropriate ways, including using humour, health care workers, and Elders to engage in online platforms like Kahkakiw, a Cree-speaking Raven puppet.[47]

Conclusion

Many First Nations have decided to continue with measures stricter than those of the provinces, in the face of eventual multiple waves and spikes of infection. Further, the positive reclamation of jurisdiction, wellness, language, and culture by Indigenous communities, as well as the continued practices rooted in a holistic approach derived from a connection with land, water, and other parts of creation will affirm the continued and ongoing wellness of Indigenous Nations in the face of the COVID-19 pandemic and beyond. By most accounts, First Nations approaches seem to be working. The difficult decisions made by many First Nations communities have contributed directly to the well-being of those communities.

In an unprecedented data-sharing agreement between First Nations and the Province of Manitoba, Indigenous rates of COVID infection are being tracked. As of June 5, there were no cases on First Nations reserves in Manitoba (only 16 cases off reserve).[48] First Nations in Northern Manitoba had set strict rules as to who can enter into their communities. Against the wishes of local First Nations, Manitoba Hydro was planning for a massive 1000+-person shift change, the third week in May, including workers from other jurisdictions in Canada and other countries, a business decision that would put the local First Nations citizens' health and well-being at risk. Citizens of the Tataskweyak Cree Nation turned vehicles away from their territory, specifically from going up to the Keeyask Dam construction

46. Morning Star Lodge, "Protecting Our Home Fires" (last visited 26 May 2020), online: *Indigenous Health Lab* <http://www.indigenoushealthlab.com/protecting-our-home-fires>.
47. Kitatipithitamak Mithwayawin, "Indigenous-led Countermeasures to Coronavirus (COVID-19) and Other Pandemics Then, Now and Into the Future" (2020), online: *Kitatipithitamak Mithwayawin* <https://covid19indigenous.ca/>.
48. Manitoba First Nations COVID-19 Pandemic Response Coordination Team PRCT BULLETIN, <https://d5d8ad59-8391-4802-9f0a-f5f5d600d7e9.filesusr.com/ugd/38252a_861c0280bab14bfab61cceaee7121320.pdf?index=true>.

camp. Manitoba Hydro then filed an injunction against the respective First Nations to end the "protests". Leaders of the four Keeyask Cree Nations (who are partners in the Keeyask project) have called for First Nations' participation in a new plan to resume construction and manage the movement of workers. Examples like this illustrate the need for First Nations' forward jurisdiction, with coordinated support from the provinces and the federal government to put the health and safety of First Nations ahead of the non-essential construction of hydroelectric infrastructure.

The TRC has stated that UNDRIP is the framework for reconciliation in Canada. UNDRIP finds its root in the recognition of Indigenous self-determination. Although Canada has committed to implementing UNDRIP, only the British Columbia government has passed legislation to that effect. In light of the COVID-19 pandemic, the United Nations has asked governments to consider the application of UNDRIP and, as a first recommendation, the recognition of "Indigenous peoples' representative institutions, authorities, and governments as the legitimate representatives of Indigenous peoples."[49]

We have argued in this chapter that Indigenous-led responses, as affirmations of First Nations' jurisdiction and self-determination, are supported by one of the basic tenets of federalism, namely the principle of subsidiarity, as well as by s. 35 of the *Constitution Act* and all corresponding obligations, together with commitments in international law pursuant to UNDRIP. In this light, the federal government can and must work with First Nations on resourcing their plans for wellness and emergency preparedness in relation to the COVID-19 pandemic.

---

49. UN Department of Economic and Social Affairs, "Indigenous Peoples & the COVID-19 Pandemic: Considerations", online (pdf): *United Nations* <https://www.un.org/development/desa/indigenouspeoples/wp-content/uploads/sites/19/2020/04/COVID19_IP_considerations.pdf>.

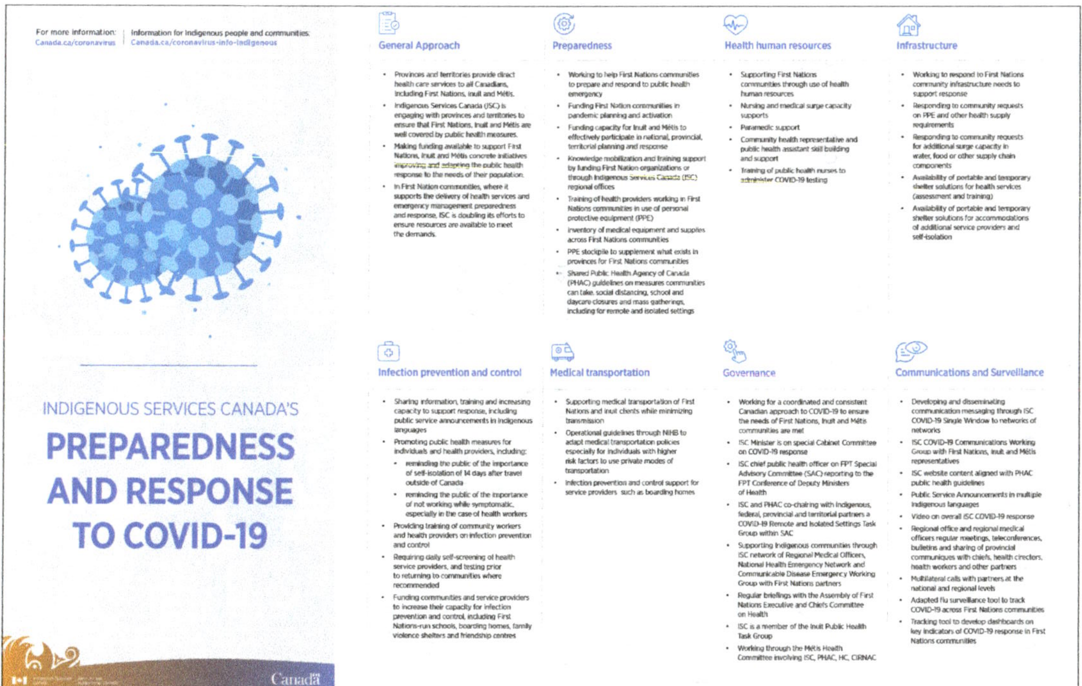

Figure A2.1 Information for Indigenous People and Communities

Source: Indigenous Services Canada, *Preparedness and Response to COVID-19* (Ottawa: Indigenous Services Canada, 2020), online: *Indigenous Services Canada* https://www.sac-isc.gc.ca/DAM/DAM-ISC-SAC/DAM-HLTH/STAGING/texte-text/preparedness_response_COVID-19_1584463875030_eng.pdf.

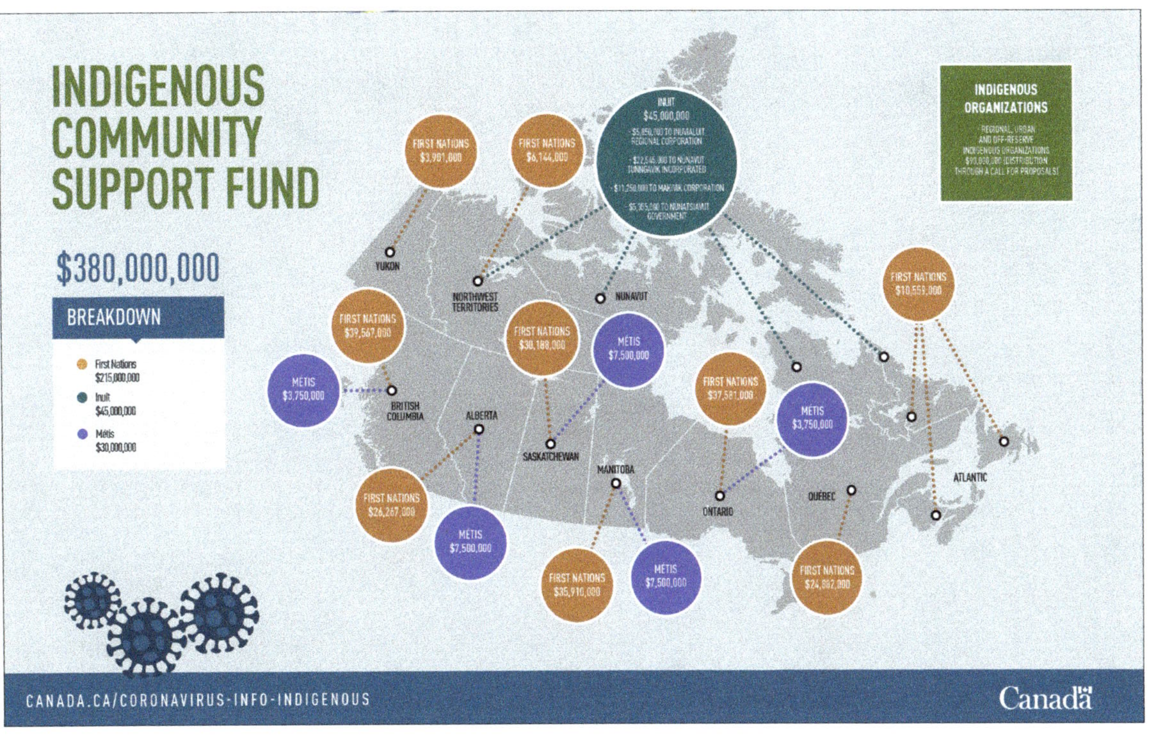

Figure A2.2 Indigenous Community Support Fund

Source: Indigenous Services Canada, *Indigenous Community Support Fund* (Ottawa: Indigenous Services Canada, 2020), online: *Indigenous Services Canada* https://www.sac-isc.gc.ca/eng/1585189335380/1585189357198.

CHAPITRE A-3

Réflexions sur la mise en œuvre de la *Loi sur la santé publique* au Québec dans le contexte de la pandémie de COVID-19*

Michelle Giroux**

Résumé

L'état d'urgence sanitaire a été décrété au Québec le 13 mars 2020 en raison de la pandémie de COVID-19. Une première depuis l'adoption, en 2002, de la *Loi sur la santé publique* (LSP) du Québec. Ce texte présente d'abord le contexte québécois en matière de santé publique, puis entame une réflexion sur la mise en œuvre de la LSP dans le contexte de la pandémie actuelle. Le Programme national de santé publique du Québec insiste sur les déterminants sociaux de la santé, et précise très clairement que les populations les plus vulnérables doivent être au centre des préoccupations. Pourtant, ce sont quand même ces populations qui sont les plus particulièrement affectées par la présente crise sanitaire. Les problèmes qui prévalaient avant la COVID-19 dans le réseau de la santé et des services sociaux sont exacerbés par la pandémie, et la situation dans les centres d'hébergement et de soins de longue durée (CHSLD) en est un triste exemple. Aurait-on pu éviter la dégradation des soins prodigués dans ces établissements et permettre aux personnes en établissement psychiatrique d'être soignées avec

---

* Merci à mes chères collègues Audrey Ferron-Parayre, Marie-France Fortin et Sophie Thériault pour leurs précieux conseils lors de la relecture de versions antérieures de ce texte.

** Professeure titulaire, Faculté de droit, Section de droit civil de l'Université d'Ottawa.

plus de dignité, pour ne mentionner que ceux-là, malgré la COVID-19 ? Si la santé publique avait été une priorité et qu'elle n'avait pas été confrontée aux lacunes du réseau de la santé et des services sociaux et au financement défaillant pour mener à bien sa mission, en serait-on arrivé là ? Au-delà du droit, la prise en considération de ces enjeux relève de l'éthique et du politique. Souhaitons que cette pandémie et ses victimes n'aient pas été vaines, et qu'elles permettent l'émergence d'une société plus juste.

Abstract

Discussion on the Implementation of the Quebec *Public Health Act* in the Context of the COVID-19 Pandemic

On March 13, 2020, Quebec declared a public health emergency in response to the COVID-19 pandemic, a first since Quebec adopted the *Public Health Act* in 2002. This chapter first provides background on public health in Quebec, then discusses the implementation of the *Public Health Act* in the context of the current pandemic. Quebec's *Programme national de santé publique* (Public Health Program) focuses on the social determinants of health and clearly outlines how the most vulnerable populations should be at the centre of these concerns. Yet, the current crisis has affected these populations the most. The pandemic has exacerbated problems that prevailed in the health and social services system prior to COVID-19, and the situation in residential and long-term care centres (CHSLD) is an unfortunate example. Could we have avoided the deterioration of care in these facilities? And could patients in psychiatric institutions, to name just a few, have been treated with more dignity despite COVID-19? If public health had been a priority and had not been faced with the failings of the health and social service system and the lack of funding to properly carry out its mission, would the situation have been the same? Beyond the law, these issues must be discussed in the context of ethics and politics. Let us hope that this pandemic and its victims have not been in vain, and that they will lead to the emergence of a more just society.

À Eric, Julien et Paul
pour avoir testé la signification
de « famille » en période de pandémie.

« Il y a dans l'homme plus de choses à admirer qu'à mépriser. »
Albert Camus, *La peste*

En accueillant l'année 2020, qui aurait pu prédire qu'un virus, même si on l'avait déjà identifié en Chine, la rendrait à ce point historique ? Dès le 30 janvier 2020, l'Organisation mondiale de la santé (OMS) déclarait l'état d'urgence sanitaire international conformément au pouvoir que lui donne le *Règlement sanitaire international* (RSI)[1]. Au Québec, plusieurs lois s'intéressent à la santé de la population, mais c'est en vertu de la *Loi sur la santé publique* (LSP)[2], adoptée en 2001, que l'état d'urgence sanitaire (ÉUS) a été décrété le 13 mars 2020[3]. Les dispositions de la LSP concernant l'ÉUS sont ici testées pour la première fois. Ce texte s'attardera d'abord à la définition, aux fonctions et à l'organisation de la santé publique en sol québécois pour expliquer le fondement des décisions prises par les autorités depuis la déclaration de l'ÉUS (partie I). Puis, une réflexion sur la mise en œuvre de la LSP en période de COVID-19 sera entamée (partie II).

La santé publique au Québec en période de COVID-19 : définition, fonctions et organisation

Comment définir la santé publique ? « S'agit-il d'une notion davantage associée aux situations d'urgence constituant une menace pour la santé de la population ou s'agit-il d'un concept qui résulte de la somme des états de santé individuels[4] […] » ? La LSP adoptée en 2001 préconise

1. Organisation mondiale de la santé, *Règlement sanitaire international* (2005), en ligne : *Organisation mondiale de la Santé* <https://www.who.int/ihr/publications/9789241580496/fr/>.
2. La *Loi sur la santé publique*, RLRQ, c S-2.2 [LSP] constituera le principal point de mire de notre analyse.
3. *Concernant une déclaration d'urgence sanitaire conformément à l'article 118 de la Loi sur la santé publique*, 177-2020, (13 mars 2020), en ligne : *gouvernement du Québec* <https://cdn-contenu.quebec.ca/cdn-contenu/adm/min/sante-services-sociaux/publications-adm/lois-reglements/decret-177-2020.pdf?1584224223>.
4. Louise Lussier, « Protection de la santé publique, éthique et droit : pour une définition des concepts » (1995) 2:1 Ruptures, revue transdisciplinaire en santé 18

une définition large et contemporaine de la santé publique. Non seulement elle s'intéresse à la « menace à la santé », mais également aux « situations comportant des risques pour la santé[5] ». D'ailleurs, le Programme national de santé publique du Québec insiste sur les déterminants sociaux de la santé et précise très clairement que les populations les plus vulnérables doivent être au centre des préoccupations[6]. La présente crise sanitaire ne démontre-t-elle pas qu'il faudrait en faire davantage pour assurer la mission plus large de la santé publique ?

Les fonctions ou les stratégies essentielles associées à la santé publique sont : la *surveillance*, la *prévention*, la *promotion* et la *protection* de l'état de santé de la population[7]. La déclaration d'urgence sanitaire découle de la fonction liée à la *protection*. C'est la mesure la plus coercitive permise dans la LSP lorsqu'il existe une menace à la santé de la collectivité. Bien que le terme « menace » ne soit pas défini dans la LSP ni ailleurs, l'article 118 de la LSP précise qu'une déclaration d'état d'urgence sanitaire ne sera possible que « lorsqu'une *menace grave* à la santé de la population, *réelle ou imminente*, exige *l'application immédiate de certaines mesures* [...] pour protéger la santé de la population » (je souligne). La pandémie de COVID-19 répond clairement à ces critères.

Quant à l'organisation de la santé publique dans la province de Québec, elle est plutôt centralisée, à l'instar de l'organisation générale du système de santé québécois et tel qu'il découle de l'application de la *Loi sur les services de santé et services sociaux* (LSSSS)[8]. D'ailleurs, contrairement à ce qui prévaut dans les autres provinces canadiennes et sur le plan national, le directeur national de la santé publique du Québec (DNSPQ) relève du ministre de la Santé et des Services sociaux, auprès duquel il occupe un poste de sous-ministre adjoint « pour conseiller et assister le ministre et le sous-ministre dans l'exercice de leurs responsabilités en santé publique[9] ». On note également

---

aux p 18-19. Voir aussi Christelle Colin, « La santé publique au Québec à l'aube du XXIe siècle » (2004) 16:2 Santé publique aux p 185-195.

5. LSP, *supra* note 2, art 1, 118, 53.
6. Voir Québec, ministère de la Santé et des Services sociaux, *Programme national de santé publique 2015-2025 : pour améliorer la santé de la population du Québec*, (Québec, gouvernement du Québec, 2015) à la p 65.
7. Voir LSP, *supra* note 2, art 8.
8. *Loi sur les services de santé et les services sociaux*, RLRQ, c S-4.2 ; Marie-Ève Couture-Ménard, « La santé publique au Québec : organisation et fonctions essentielles » dans Mélanie Bourassa Forcier et Anne-Marie Savard, dir, *Droit et politiques de la santé*, 2e éd, (Montréal : LexisNexis, 2018), aux p 569-571.
9. *Loi sur le ministère de la Santé et des Services sociaux*, RLRQ, c M-19.2, art 5.1 ; LSP, *supra* note 3, art 2.

qu'en cas d'ÉUS, les directives du DNSPQ ont la même force exécutoire que celles du ministre[10]. Certains ont soulevé des questions quant à l'indépendance du DNSPQ : étant sous-ministre, n'est-il pas un subalterne du ministre ? D'autres voient plutôt l'intégration de son poste à l'intérieur du Ministère comme une façon d'assurer une meilleure coordination des orientations et des décisions[11].

En période d'ÉUS, les mesures prévues à l'article 123 de la LSP permettent au gouvernement ou au ministre habilité en ce sens d'agir « sans délai et sans formalité », et permettent notamment d'« ordonner la vaccination obligatoire », « la fermeture d'établissement d'enseignement ou tout autre lieu de rassemblement », d'« interdire l'accès à tout ou partie du territoire ou n'en permettre l'accès qu'à certaines personnes et qu'à certaines conditions, ou ordonner, lorsqu'il n'y a pas d'autre moyen de protection, pour le temps nécessaire, l'évacuation des personnes de tout ou partie du territoire ou leur confinement […] ». Alors que la première mesure n'a pas été utilisée dans la présente pandémie, et n'est de toute façon pas possible étant donné l'absence de vaccin pour contrer le virus SARS-CoV-2 à ce jour, les deux dernières mesures ont quant à elles été mises en pratique[12]. Les pouvoirs sont encore plus vastes que ceux expressément énumérés à l'article 123 de la LSP, le paragraphe 8 précisant qu'on peut également « ordonner toute autre mesure nécessaire pour protéger la santé de la population ». Ces pouvoirs sont-ils trop larges[13] ou ne sont-ils pas justifiés généralement en période de pandémie[14] ?

10. LSP, *supra* note 2, art 124.

11. Mireille Lacroix, « The Quebec Public Health System: A Modern Model » dans Tracey M Bailey, Timothy Caulfield et Nola M Ries, dir, *Public Health Law & Policy in Canada*, (Markham: Lexis/Nexis Butterworths, 2005), aux p 497-504.

12. À noter que le gouvernement fédéral a aussi le pouvoir d'ordonner la vaccination de la population, *Loi sur les mesures d'urgence*, LRC 1985, c 22 (4e suppl).

13. Martine Valois, « Droit et urgence ne font pas bon ménage », *La Presse* (14 avril 2020), en ligne : <https://plus.lapresse.ca/screens/d38c4dc8-1860-41d9-9c80-eda6bbfb8b24__7C___0.html?utm_medium=Facebook&utm_campaign=Internal+Share&utm_content=Screen&fbclid=IwAR0UNcIu6BmabZuV8nFuSDuOPsk4BnOk6qXYK> ; Maxime St-Hilaire, « Urgence et droit n'ont jamais fait bon ménage, mais la Loi sur la santé publique compte certes d'importants défauts (réponse à Martine Valois) » (15 avril 2020), en ligne : À qui de droit <https://blogueaquidedroit.ca/2020/04/15/urgence-et-droit-nont-jamais-fait-bon-menage-mais-la-loi-sur-la-sante-publique-compte-certes-dimportants-defauts-reponse-a-martine-valois/>.

14. Marie-Eve Couture Ménard et Marie-Claude Prémont, « L'équilibre vital entre droits individuels et intérêt collectif en temps de pandémie » (22 avril 2020), en ligne : À qui de droit <https://blogueaquidedroit.ca/2020/04/22/lequilibre-vital-entre-droits-individuels-et-interet-collectif-en-temps-de-pandemie/>.

Les actions en matière de santé publique visent la population en général et constituent *a priori* une exception justifiée à la violation de droits individuels[15], en particulier des droits à la liberté, à l'inviolabilité et à la sécurité de la personne[16]. Cependant, les mesures prises pour protéger la collectivité doivent être proportionnelles à la menace qui la guette, respecter les principes de justice fondamentale et les limites raisonnables dans une société libre et démocratique[17].

Les mesures concernant la distanciation physique, le confinement ou le port du masque, pour ne nommer que celles-ci, ont changé au fur et à mesure de l'évolution des connaissances sur le virus SARS-CoV-2[18]. Force est de constater que celui-ci était encore parfaitement inconnu il y a quelques mois seulement, que celui-ci est parfois même « asymptomatique » et que cela rend plus ardu le déploiement des règles de santé publique pour éviter la contagion. Si on ajoute à cela les problèmes d'approvisionnement en matériel sanitaire, tel que les masques ou les gants, comme on l'a vu, on comprend que les autorités doivent considérer ce facteur dans leurs décisions. Par contre, elles doivent s'assurer de bien justifier les décisions prises, de façon à démontrer leur caractère essentiel et la légitimité de l'atteinte aux libertés individuelles. À la lumière de ces quelques règles, on comprend mieux les hésitations du DNSPQ d'imposer ou non le masque, étant donné la situation de pénurie et par souci d'équité envers tous les citoyens qui n'ont peut-être pas tous accès à un masque. Sans compter que des amendes élevées, allant de 1 000 $ à 6 000 $, accompagnent le non-respect d'une ordonnance. Ces amendes sont certes utiles pour convaincre la population de l'importance de respecter les mesures, mais elles peuvent être inappropriées pour certains groupes

15. Voir notamment, LSP, *supra* note 2, art 5.
16. Sur le droit à l'inviolabilité en droit des personnes, voir *Code civil du Québec*, SQ 1991, c 64, art 10 ; Dominique Goubau avec la collaboration d'Anne-Marie Savard, *Le droit des personnes physiques*, 6e éd, (Montréal : Éditions Yvon Blais, 2019), au para 103. Quant à la liberté et à la sécurité, voir *Charte canadienne des droits et libertés, Loi constitutionnelle de 1982* (R-U), constituant l'annexe B de la *Loi de 1982 sur le Canada* (R-U), 1982, c 11, art 7.
17. *R* c *Oakes*, [1986] 1 RCS 103, 26 DLR (4th) 200. Voir l'article suivant pour une réflexion à ce sujet : Catherine Régis, Jean-Louis Denis et Jean-François Gaudreau-DesBiens, « La pandémie nous montre qu'il faut consolider la capacité d'agir de l'État et mettre à profit l'innovation née dans l'urgence », Options politiques (11 mai 2020), en ligne : <https://policyoptions.irpp.org/magazines/may-2020/reflechir-a-lapres-crise-en-politique-et-en-sante/>.
18. Sur ces questions et sur la collaboration essentielle, mais pas toujours facile entre les différents niveaux de gouvernement, voir Fierlbeck et Hardcastle, chapitre 1, section A ; Robitaille, chapitre 2, section A ; ainsi que Flood et Thomas, chapitre 6, section A.

dans la population[19]. Cependant, on comprend moins bien lorsque le même DNSPQ invoque la violation des droits individuels pour expliquer qu'il ne peut imposer le port du masque, les règles en matière de santé publique justifiant toutes mesures essentielles pour contrer le virus SARS-CoV-2.

Réflexions sur la *Loi sur la santé publique* au Québec en période de COVID-19

Alors que la pandémie actuelle s'étire et qu'une solution vaccinale n'est pas envisageable à court terme, des drames de toutes sortes s'accumulent : familiaux, psychosociaux, médicaux, etc. On constate notamment des problèmes d'accès aux soins en matière de santé mentale[20], de même qu'en établissements de soins de longue durée. Des chirurgies oncologiques sont reportées[21]. Les problèmes qui existaient avant la COVID-19 sont exacerbés par la pandémie et la situation dans les centres d'hébergement et de soins de longue durée (CHSLD) en est un triste exemple. Après la COVID-19, aurons-nous à faire face à une autre crise, associée à une « épidémie de problèmes sociaux » portant tout autant atteinte à la dignité humaine ?

Depuis la déclaration de l'ÉUS, on a vu l'application de plusieurs décrets et directives ministériels concernant notamment les CHSLD du Québec[22]. Dans ce contexte, il n'est pas étonnant de constater le dépôt de nouvelles actions collectives pour dénoncer le traitement des personnes âgées pendant la pandémie de la COVID-19[23], ou la modifi-

19. LSP, *supra* note 2 : les sanctions pénales sont prévues aux articles 138-142. Pour l'inadéquation de ces peines sur la population des sans-abri, voir Skolnik, chapitre 4, section C. Voir aussi le Communiqué de la Commission des droits de la personne et des droits de la jeunesse, « Contraventions des jeunes en situation d'itinérance : comment s'isoler quand on vit dans la rue » (15 avril 2020), en ligne : *La commission des droits de la personne et des droits de la jeunesse* <http://www.cdpdj.qc.ca/fr/medias/Pages/Communique.aspx?showItem=910>.
20. Texte collectif, « D'autres oubliés de la COVID-19 », *Le Devoir* (13 avril 2020), en ligne : <https://www.ledevoir.com/opinion/idees/577959/d-autres-oublies-de-la-covid-19>.
21. SA, « Report de chirurgies oncologiques : des victimes collatérales de la covid-19 » (8 avril 2020), en ligne : *Medlegal Avocats* <https://medlegal.ca/report-de-chirurgies-oncologiques-des-victimes-collaterales-du-covid-19/>.
22. Pour plus de détails sur la situation en établissement de soins de longue durée, voir Jackman, chapitre 3, section D ; et Lagacé, Garcia et Bélanger-Hardy, chapitre 2, section D.
23. Mentionnons la demande d'autorisation d'une action collective contre le CHSLD Sainte-Dorothée, *Jean-Pierre Daubois* c *Centre d'hébergement et de soins de longue*

cation à d'autres demandes déjà autorisées, car la crise actuelle a exacerbé les problèmes déjà présents avant la COVID-19[24]. Néanmoins, il est important de noter que la LSP prévoit, à l'article 123 *in fine*, que « [l]e gouvernement, le ministre ou toute autre personne ne peut être poursuivi en justice pour un acte accompli de *bonne foi* dans l'exercice ou l'exécution de ces pouvoirs[25] ». Quel est l'impact de cette immunité étatique ? De prime abord, elle semble essentielle en période de pandémie lorsque les actions sont dictées par la bonne foi. Cependant, « une imputabilité juridique accentuée de l'État permettrait[-t-elle] une gestion plus efficace des crises sanitaires ou [...] le litige judiciaire collectif en responsabilité contre l'État a[-t-il] le pouvoir d'engendrer des changements sociaux positifs dans le domaine de la santé publique[26] » ?

À une époque où d'autres pandémies se sont déroulées, comme celle de la peste noire au Moyen-Âge, ou bien celles subséquentes de variole ou de grippe espagnole, les mesures sanitaires et d'hygiène, de même que la médecine, n'étaient pas ce qu'elles sont aujourd'hui. Il semblait donc naturel et vital que les mesures de santé publique priorisent la salubrité et l'hygiène, tout en combattant les maladies infectieuses, « dans la foulée du courant hygiéniste de la fin du XIXe siècle, correspondant à l'urbanisation massive opérée avec le début de la société industrielle[27] ». Une fois les grandes maladies contagieuses contrôlées, le domaine de la santé publique a été délaissé et moins financé[28] ; le curatif tourné sur la santé individuelle allait prédominer jusqu'à l'éclosion de la prochaine crise. À l'heure où la gestion des égouts, aqueducs et déchets n'est plus à organiser (quoiqu'elle nécessite sans cesse une vigilance), les mesures de santé publique ne devraient-elles pas inclure les préoccupations sociales dont certaines ont déjà notamment été identifiées par la recherche en sciences sociales ou en psychologie, au-delà des données scientifiques sur le virus ?

---

durée Sainte-Dorothée et Centre intégré de services de santé et de services sociaux de Laval, Cour supérieure, district de Montréal, dossier no 500-600-001062-203.

24. Voir Améli Pineda, « La crise amplifierait une action collective contre les CHSLD », *Le Devoir* (9 mai 2020), en ligne : <https://www.ledevoir.com/societe/sante/578623/action-collective-la-crise-amplifierait-une-action-collective-contre-les-chsld>.
25. Ces immunités statutaires, souvent conditionnelles à la bonne foi, s'ajoutent aux immunités de droit public, voir Fortin, chapitre 7, section B.
26. Lara Khoury, « Crises sanitaires et responsabilité étatique envers la collectivité » (2016) 46 RDUS aux p 261-288.
27. Louise Lussier, *supra* note 4 à la p 21.
28. *Ibid* à la p 22.

Cela permettrait de protéger la vie lorsqu'une menace grave est imminente, comme c'est assurément le cas de la COVID-19 (mission de protection de santé publique), mais également d'éviter de provoquer des épidémies de phénomènes sociaux, comme celles qui risquent d'émaner, par ricochet, étant donné la durée de la présente pandémie. Par exemple, le fait de ne pas pouvoir être accompagné correctement en CHSLD ou de ne pas pouvoir accéder à des soins de santé mentale appropriés, quand il y a risques pour la santé (mission de promotion et de prévention)[29]. Mais comment trouver un meilleur équilibre pendant et après la pandémie de COVID-19 ? Ce n'est pas simple.

La pandémie de la COVID-19 illustre d'une part la fragilité ou la difficulté d'assurer les acquis, comme les règles d'hygiène par exemple. La crise sanitaire ramène aux besoins de base et de sécurité, les deux premiers niveaux dans la pyramide de Maslow, si tant est qu'elle tienne toujours, vu les nombreuses critiques formulées à son égard[30]. Faut-il ajouter que pour pouvoir se préoccuper des besoins de base, encore faut-il être en vie. Cela tend à justifier l'accent actuellement mis sur la menace par la Santé publique.

Mais d'autre part, la durée de la pandémie de COVID-19 démontre que si l'accent est seulement posé sur la menace grave, sans prise en considération des autres risques pour la santé pour éviter des épidémies de problèmes sociaux, la Santé publique n'aura peut-être pas assuré le mandat attendu d'elle au 21e siècle.

La LSP adoptée en 2001 inclut les nouvelles règles en matière de protection de la santé publique, dont font partie celles concernant la déclaration de l'ÉUS, mais comprend également des règles qui témoignent d'une vision plus large de la santé publique, incluant des actions concrètes pour surveiller certains problèmes de santé individuels, mais qui sont largement présents dans la population. On a ainsi adopté des mesures pour limiter les effets dévastateurs du cancer. Pour contrer ce fléau, la surveillance s'est accrue et on a insisté sur la promotion des saines habitudes de vie. Un certain financement a suivi, mais on n'a jamais réussi à intégrer parfaitement ces enjeux aux priorités du réseau. Le sous-financement et « la dévalorisation du statut de

---

29. LSP, *supra* note 2, art 53 ; Marie-Ève Couture-Ménard, *supra* note 8 à la p 594.
30. Philippe Mouillot, « Comment le coronavirus réhabilite les besoins de la pyramide de Maslow », The Conversation (4 mars 2020), en ligne : <https://theconversation.com/comment-le-coronavirus-rehabilite-la-pyramide-des-besoins-de-maslow-132779>.

la santé publique » sont rappelés à maintes reprises[31]. Les soins curatifs s'imposant toujours, « certains pouvoirs [de la LSP] demeurent pour le moment inexploités ou seulement faiblement exploités[32] ».

Aurait-on pu éviter la dégradation complète des soins en CHSLD, ou permettre aux personnes en établissement psychiatrique d'être soignées avec dignité, malgré la COVID-19, si la santé publique avait été une priorité et qu'elle n'avait pas été confrontée aux lacunes des réseaux de santé et au financement défaillant pour mener à bien sa mission ? Au-delà du droit, la prise en considération de ces enjeux relève de l'éthique et du politique[33].

Conclusion

La définition et le rôle de la santé publique évoluent avec les crises sanitaires et aussi, par conséquent, les législations qui les encadrent. La pandémie de COVID-19 pose des défis accrus si on la compare avec le SRAS ou encore avec la grippe A (H1N1) et justifie d'ailleurs l'utilisation inédite de l'état d'urgence sanitaire. Elle s'étire et ses effets sont souvent invisibles. En matière de pandémie, comme c'est le cas à la suite d'un accident, il est toujours plus facile de comprendre après coup ce qui aurait pu être fait autrement pour éviter le pire. De la même manière, l'approche de la santé publique varie dans l'histoire et son financement dépend de l'importance qu'on y accorde[34]. Souhaitons que cette pandémie et ses victimes n'aient pas été vaines et qu'elles permettent de mieux prioriser les enjeux de santé publique ainsi que leur gestion et par conséquent, l'émergence d'une société encore plus égalitaire[35].

31. Voir notamment Trevor Hancock et Art Eggleton, « La santé publique doit devenir une priorité », Options politiques (20 septembre 2018), en ligne : <https://policyoptions.irpp.org/magazines/september-2018/la-sante-publique-doit-devenir-une-priorite/>.
32. Sur l'impact des politiques publiques sur la santé de la population, voir Marie-Ève Couture-Ménard, *supra* note 8 aux p 590-596.
33. Louise Lussier, *supra* note 4 à la p 34.
34. *Ibid* à la p 22.
35. Voir Laureen Laboret, « Ce que l'on peut apprendre de l'épidémie de peste noire du Moyen-Âge » (11 avril 2020), en ligne : <https://ici.radio-canada.ca/nouvelle/1692333/peste-noire-pandemie-lecons-histoire>.

CHAPITRE A-4

La COVID-19 au Canada : le fédéralisme coopératif à pied d'œuvre

David Robitaille*

Résumé

Outre ses impacts sur la santé des populations, une crise sanitaire comme celle de la COVID-19 comporte d'importants défis de gouvernance multiniveaux dans une fédération comme le Canada. La Constitution attribue des pouvoirs exclusifs à chacun des paliers fédéral et provincial, dans des perspectives nationale et régionale, tandis que les municipalités exercent des compétences locales déléguées. De nouvelles matières, comme les contrôles interprovinciaux de personnes, non expressément attribuées au Parlement ou aux provinces, ont aussi fait surface. Dans ce contexte, nous avançons que si la coordination et la collaboration intergouvernementales ne sont pas toujours acquises, la crise de la COVID-19 a montré que le fédéralisme canadien et sa décentralisation relativement équilibrée ne constituent pas nécessairement des obstacles à l'endiguement d'une urgence nationale, un enjeu qui comporte en réalité de nombreuses variables locales.

* Professeur titulaire et codirecteur du Centre de droit public, Faculté de droit, Université d'Ottawa.

Abstract
COVID-19 in Canada: Cooperative Federalism at Work

Aside from its impact on the health of populations, a health crisis such as the COVID-19 one involves substantial multilevel governance challenges in a federation such as Canada. The Constitution grants exclusive powers to both the federal and provincial governments at the national and regional level, while municipalities exercise delegated local power. New matters such as the interprovincial control of people, not expressly attributed to Parliament or the provinces, have also arisen. In this context, we would argue that if intergovernmental coordination and collaboration are not always achieved, the COVID-19 crisis has shown that Canadian federalism and its relatively balanced decentralization does not necessarily impede the management of a national emergency, an issue that, in reality, is comprised of numerous local variables.

Ce n'est pas le fruit du hasard si les provinces ont pu intervenir rapidement pour prendre des mesures visant à limiter la pandémie de la COVID-19. Ce n'est pas non plus parce qu'il aurait sous-estimé l'importance de cette dernière ou fait preuve de laxisme que le gouvernement fédéral n'est pas intervenu aussi promptement, sauf sur le plan politico-fiscal, par son pouvoir de dépenser, qu'il a tôt fait d'utiliser pour annoncer une aide financière massive, notamment aux agriculteurs, aux aînés, aux entreprises, aux étudiants, aux associations sportives et aux travailleurs[1]. C'est plutôt en raison de la structure même de notre régime constitutionnel. En effet, les provinces disposent de compétences de proximité leur permettant d'intervenir dans l'intérêt des collectivités locales. En revanche, ont plutôt été attribuées au Parlement et au gouvernement du Canada des compétences sur des matières dont l'appréhension efficace nécessite une approche uniforme et une perspective nationale. Nous avançons dans ce texte qu'une centralisation poussée n'est pas nécessaire ni souhaitable, en

1. Si cette aide a été saluée par plusieurs, elle pourrait à long terme avoir d'importants impacts sur l'autonomie provinciale et les champs de compétences des provinces, surtout si le gouvernement fédéral impose des conditions en retour. Voir : Daniel Béland *et al*, « A Critical Juncture in Fiscal Federalism? Canada's Response to COVID-19 » [2020] Revue canadienne de science politique 1, DOI : <https://doi.org/10.1017/S0008423920000323>.

ce qui concerne la lutte contre une pandémie dans une fédération comme le Canada. De multiples réalités culturelles, démographiques, économiques, politiques, sanitaires et sociales différentes, sur le terrain, favorisent au contraire une répartition équilibrée des compétences. La Constitution canadienne répond bien à ce besoin, tandis que le gouvernement fédéral s'est montré respectueux des différentes réalités canadiennes et de l'autonomie provinciale, tout en exerçant un nécessaire leadership de coordination.

Les compétences fédérales : une perspective nationale

Pour contribuer à limiter les conséquences d'une crise sanitaire, le Parlement et le gouvernement fédéral disposent de nombreuses compétences aux dimensions interprovinciales et internationales. C'est le cas du commerce interprovincial et d'intérêt national en général, du service militaire, de la navigation, des entreprises de transports interprovinciaux et internationaux, de la « quarantaine et l'établissement et maintien des hôpitaux de marine », du droit criminel et de la compétence concurrente sur l'agriculture et l'immigration[2]. Le gouvernement a donc, par exemple, limité et aménagé les transports par avion et par train à l'intérieur du Canada[3], collaboré avec le gouvernement du Québec en envoyant des soldats en renfort dans les établissements pour personnes âgées[4], pris des mesures à l'égard des ressortissants et travailleurs étrangers[5], fermé les frontières internationales et pris des mesures de quarantaine à l'égard des citoyens canadiens de retour au pays après des séjours à l'étranger[6].

2. *Loi constitutionnelle de 1867* (R-U), 30 et 31 Vict, c 3, art 91, reproduit dans LRC 1985, annexe II, n°5, art 91 (2), (7), (10), (11), (27), et art 92(10)(a), 95.
3. Transports Canada, *Arrêté d'urgence n° 2 imposant certaines restrictions aux bâtiments à passagers en raison de la maladie à coronavirus 2019 (COVID-19)*, Ottawa, Transports Canada, 20 avril 2020 ; Transports Canada, *Arrêté en vertu de l'article 32.01 de la Loi sur la sécurité ferroviaire en raison de la COVID-19 (MO 20-04)*, Ottawa, Transports Canada, 27 mars 2020 ; Transports Canada, *Arrêté d'urgence visant à interdire à certaines personnes d'embarquer sur les vols au Canada en raison de la COVID-19*, Ottawa, Transports Canada, 27 mars 2020.
4. Marie Vastel, « Bientôt 1350 soldats à Montréal », *Le Devoir* (7 mai 2020), en ligne : <https://www.ledevoir.com/politique/canada/578512/bientot-1350-soldats-a-montreal>.
5. *Règlement modifiant le Règlement sur l'immigration et la protection des réfugiés (Loi sur les mesures d'urgence et Loi sur la mise en quarantaine)*, DORS/2020-91.
6. Gouvernement du Canada, *Décret visant la réduction du risque d'exposition à la COVID-19 au Canada (obligation de s'isoler)*, CP 2020-0175, en ligne : *Gouvernement du Canada* <https://decrets.canada.ca/attachment.php?attach=38989&lang=fr>;

Si la compétence sur la quarantaine n'a fait l'objet d'aucune interprétation approfondie par nos tribunaux, elle permet certainement au gouvernement fédéral de prévoir l'isolement temporaire obligatoire des citoyens de retour au pays et d'imposer des dépistages, examens ou vérifications aux voyageurs, sous réserve bien entendu de respecter la *Charte canadienne des droits et libertés*[7].

Certains préconisent une interprétation très vaste des compétences fédérales pour lutter efficacement contre une pandémie, similaires à celles sur l'aéronautique ou l'énergie nucléaire, de manière à ce que le gouvernement fédéral soit en mesure d'imposer ses vues et sa gestion de crise aux provinces[8]. Pour cette même raison, d'autres ont souhaité que le gouvernement fédéral ait recours à la *Loi sur les mesures d'urgence*[9]. Mis à part le pouvoir d'urgence sur lequel nous reviendrons en conclusion, nous sommes plutôt d'avis que les compétences fédérales doivent se limiter aux aspects internationaux et interprovinciaux d'une pandémie[10], si tant est que l'on accorde de l'importance à l'équilibre entre l'autonomie locale et l'intérêt national en tant que principe fondateur du Canada[11]. Une interprétation évolutive de la Constitution ne saurait aller plus loin, puisque cet « arbre vivant » ne peut pousser au-delà de « ses limites naturelles[12] ». C'était

---

Transports Canada, *Arrêté d'urgence n° 3 visant à interdire à certaines personnes d'embarquer sur les vols à destination du Canada en raison de la COVID-19*, Ottawa, Transports Canada, 24 mars 2020.

7. À ce sujet, voir les chapitres de nos collègues dans ce volume. Voir également Catherine Régis, Jean-François Gaudreault-Desbiens et Jean-Louis Denis, « Gouverner dans l'ombre de l'État de droit en temps de pandémie », Options politiques (5 mai 2020), en ligne : <https://policyoptions.irpp.org/fr/magazines/may-2020/gouverner-dans-lombre-de-letat-de-droit-en-temps-de-pandemie/>.
8. Amir Attaran et Kumanan Wilson, « A Legal and Epidemiological Justification for Federal Authority in Public Health Emergencies » (2007) 52 RD McGill 381 aux p 386-392 et 399-402.
9. *Loi sur les mesures d'urgence*, LRC (1985), c 22 (4e suppl). À ce sujet, voir Carissima Mathen, chapitre A-7, de ce volume.
10. Kerri Gammon, « Pandemics and Pandemonium: Constitutional Jurisdiction Over Public Health » (2006) 15 Dal LJ 1 aux p 29-30 ; Nola M Ries, « Quarantine and the Law: The 2003 SARS Experience in Canada (A New Disease Calls on Old Public Health Tools) » (2005) 43 Alta L Rev 529 à la p 533.
11. *Renvoi relatif à la Loi sur les valeurs mobilières*, 2011 CSC 66, [2011] 3 RCS 837; *Consolidated Fastfrate Inc c Western Canada Council of Teamsters*, 2009 CSC 53 aux para 29-39, [2009] 3 RCS 407; Hugo Cyr, « Autonomy, Subsidiarity, Solidarity: Foundation of Cooperative Federalism » (2014) 23:4 Forum constitutionnel 20; Bruce Ryder, « Equal Autonomy in Canadian Federalism: The Continuing Search for Balance in the Interpretation of the Division of Powers » (2011) 54 SCLR 565.
12. *Edwards c Attorney General for Canada*, [1930] AC 124 à la p 136, 1929 UKPC 86.

d'ailleurs avec ce contexte à l'esprit que la compétence sur la quarantaine a été attribuée au Parlement[13]. C'est aussi l'intention qu'a eue ce dernier en adoptant la *Loi sur la mise en quarantaine* qui ne vise que le contexte des voyages internationaux, ce qui n'est pas sans importance dans l'interprétation constitutionnelle[14].

Cela ne signifie pas que l'intervention fédérale n'est pas nécessaire; au contraire, comme nous l'avons souligné, le gouvernement fédéral est intervenu, avec raison, par des mesures à l'intérieur de ses champs de compétences et par son « pouvoir » de dépenser. L'endiguement d'une pandémie requiert nécessairement une approche concertée, sauf que concertation n'est pas forcément synonyme de centralisation constitutionnelle ou législative, mais de leadership politique municipal, provincial et fédéral coordonné[15]. La gestion de la crise de la COVID-19 au Canada a d'ailleurs été marquée par une étroite collaboration entre les provinces et le fédéral :

> Ottawa is heeding the calls of the provinces and territories to respect their jurisdiction and use the *Emergencies Act* powers only as a last resort. We have never seen our premiers and prime minister getting along so well. [...] In short, the operational, front-line response is being led at the provincial-territorial level, but it is being backed by a national approach of sharing information and coordinating action through high-level venues like first ministers' meetings and institutions such as the Public Health Agency of Canada[16].

---

13. *La Municipalité du village de Saint-Louis du Mile End v La Cité de Montréal* (1886), 2 MLR SC 218 à la p 224, cité par Andrée Lajoie et Patrick A Molinari, « Partage constitutionnel des compétences en matière de santé au Canada » (1978) 56 R du B can 579 à la p 585; Ries, *supra* note 10 à la p 532; *Canada, Commission royale des relations entre le Dominion et les provinces*, à la p 33, cité dans *Schneider c La Reine*, [1982] 2 RCS 112 à la p 136, 139 DLR (3d) 417.
14. *Banque canadienne de l'Ouest c Alberta*, 2007 CSC 22 au para 91, [2007] 2 RCS 3.
15. Gammon, *supra* note 10 à la p 35; Mathen, chapitre A-7 ; Robert Schertzer et Mireille Paquet, « How Well is Canada's Intergovernmental System Handling the Crisis? », Options politiques (8 avril 2020), en ligne : <https://policyoptions.irpp.org/magazines/april-2020/how-well-is-canadas-intergovernmental-system-handling-the-crisis/>.
16. Schertzer et Paquet, *ibid*. Voir aussi Stéphanie Chouinard, « COVID-19 Crisis Sheds Light on Blind Spot of Canadian Federalism: Interprovincial Collaboration », *i*Politics (9 avril 2020), en ligne : <https://ipolitics.ca/2020/04/09/covid-19-crisis-sheds-light-on-blind-spot-of-canadian-federalism-interprovincial-collaboration/> ; Mathen, chapitre A-7.

Une compétence fédérale sur la quarantaine aussi vaste que celle sur l'aéronautique donnerait par ailleurs à Ottawa une compétence exclusive, indivisible et prépondérante, ce qui laisserait peu de place aux provinces[17]. Cela ne nous semble pas souhaitable compte tenu de tous les aspects différents que comporte une pandémie qui constitue, en réalité, un agrégat de plusieurs compétences différentes[18]. En effet, comme l'a montré la crise de la COVID-19, les moyens pour enrayer ou contrôler cet enjeu sanitaire sont très variés, notamment : fermeture des écoles, des commerces non essentiels, des salles à manger de restaurants, des tribunaux et des lieux publics municipaux; confinement forcé de certains groupes de personnes; interdiction des rassemblements; limites aux déplacements interrégionaux dans une même province; limite aux déplacements internationaux et interprovinciaux; interventions dans les foyers pour personnes âgées; gestion des pénitenciers et des hôpitaux; intervention de l'armée; soutien économique massif; développement d'un vaccin ou de médicaments; et fermeture de voies de circulation locales aux automobiles pour laisser plus d'espace à la distanciation physique des piétons. Nous voyons mal comment ces mesures pourraient être centralisées entre les mains du gouvernement fédéral qui ne dispose pas toujours de la proximité et des connaissances suffisantes pour agir efficacement sur le plan microterritorial, d'où l'importance d'institutions provinciales et locales fortes. Pour cette même raison, bien que la jurisprudence du Conseil privé comporte des passages suggérant qu'une épidémie soit d'intérêt national[19], la perspective d'une compétence fédérale exclusive et indivisible pour lutter contre un tel fléau serait plutôt difficile à défendre aujourd'hui.

Par ailleurs, l'échec de la collaboration entre les gouvernements provinciaux nous semble tout aussi périlleux que de reconnaître une compétence exclusive très vaste à un État central qui l'exercerait de manière inefficace sans égard aux réalités locales que les gouvernements provinciaux et municipaux sont en mesure de mieux comprendre dans toutes leurs subtilités en raison de leur proximité

17. *Québec (Procureur général) c Canadian Owners and Pilots Association*, 2010 CSC 39, [2010] 2 RCS 536 ; *R. c Crown Zellerbach Canada ltd*, [1988] 1 RCS 401 aux p 432-434, 49 DLR (4e) 161 ; *Renvoi : Loi anti-inflation*, [1976] 2 RCS 373 aux p 444-453, (1976) 68 DLR (3d) 452.

18. Gammon, *supra* note 10 aux p 14-21.

19. Gammon, *supra* note 10 aux p 14-15.

inhérente avec leurs citoyens[20]. À cet égard, des auteurs soulignent que si des variations ont été observées entre les interventions municipales, « [i]*n general,* [...] *Canadian municipalities have responded to the pandemic in remarkably consistent ways*[21] ». D'autres concluaient que « [s]*o far, governments in Canada have been doing a remarkably good job at working together to protect the safety and lives of Canadians*[22] ». Cela ne veut pas dire que les approches provinciales sont sans failles[23] ni qu'une coordination efficace est chose facile à concrétiser[24], au contraire. Sur ce point, nos collègues Attaran et Houston se désolent du manque d'approche unifiée en ce qui concerne le partage d'informations entre les gouvernements provinciaux et fédéral relativement à la COVID-19[25]. Si c'était le cas, il s'agirait effectivement d'une lacune importante. Mais l'adoption d'une loi obligeant les provinces à colliger de l'information adéquate sur la pandémie et à la partager, comme le suggèrent nos collègues, serait sans doute considérée inconstitutionnelle; ni le Parlement ni les provinces ne peuvent normalement forcer l'autre palier à agir dans ses champs de compétences[26], d'où l'importance d'une approche concertée. Par ailleurs, une démonstration claire de l'inefficacité du fédéralisme en temps de pandémie ne nous semble pas avoir été faite et paraît liée davantage à une conception politique différente sur le Canada que sur une base empiriquement neutre. Il faut toutefois souligner la pertinence de la suggestion faite par Da Silva et St-Hilaire qui privilégient la négociation d'une

20. Alain-G Gagnon, « Penser l'après-COVID-19 : pandémie, fédéralisme et concertation », *La Presse* (28 avril 2020), en ligne : <https://www.lapresse.ca/debats/opinions/202004/27/01-5271147-penser-lapres-covid-19-pandemie-federalisme-et-concertation.php> ; Gammon, *supra* note 10 à la p 36 ; Mathen, chapitre A7. Voir aussi : *Catalyst Paper Corp c North Cowichan (District)*, 2012 CSC 2, [2012] 1 RCS 5 ; *114957 Canada Ltée (Spraytech, Société d'arrosage) c Hudson (Ville)*, 2001 CSC 40, [2001], RCS 241 ; *Nanaimo (City) c Rascal Trucking ltd.*, 2000 CSC 13, [2000] 1 RCS 342 ; *Produits Shell Canada Ltée c Vancouver (Ville)*, [1994] 1 RCS 231, 110 DLR (4e) 1 (j. McLachlin).

21. David A Armstrong et Jack Lucas, « Measuring and Comparing Municipal Policy Responses to COVID-19 » (2020) R Can science politique 1, DOI : <https://doi.org/10.1017/S000842392000044X>. Pour de plus amples développements sur cette question, voir Alexandra Flynn, chapitre A8.

22. Schertzer et Paquet, *supra* note 16.

23. Voir Colleen M Flood et Bryan Thomas, chapitre A6.

24. Pour de plus amples développements, voir Katherine Fierlbeck et Lorain Hardcastle, chapitre A1.

25. Voir Amir Attaran et Adam R Houston, chapitre A5.

26. *Québec (Procureur général) c Canada (Procureur général)*, 2015 CSC 14, [2015] 1 RCS 693.

entente de coordination entre les provinces et le gouvernement fédéral, ce qui assurerait sans doute une plus grande prévisibilité et une cohésion des mesures prises en temps de pandémie[27].

Les compétences provinciales : une perspective locale

Si le Parlement peut intervenir en matière de santé à partir de compétences plus spécifiques comme celles relatives au droit criminel[28] et à la quarantaine, il est de jurisprudence constante que la santé, matière non attribuée par le constituant de 1867, soit un domaine de compétence partagé[29] qui relève toutefois principalement des compétences provinciales quant aux hôpitaux, à la propriété et aux droits civils et aux questions de nature purement locale[30]. Il s'agit de la plus importante compétence provinciale dérivée en contexte pandémique. Comme le souligne la professeure Mathen, cette attribution de pouvoir a permis aux provinces de développer, au cours du dernier siècle, leur expertise en ce domaine[31].

Bien que la Constitution reconnaisse au Parlement une compétence spécifique sur la quarantaine en contexte international et qu'elle ne prévoit pas l'équivalent intraprovincial, les provinces disposent certainement du pouvoir d'imposer l'isolement de leurs populations en temps de crise sanitaire. Il est d'ailleurs révélateur que les premières décisions dans lesquelles les tribunaux ont reconnu la vaste compétence des provinces en santé aient été rendues dans des contextes de pandémies[32]. En ce qui concerne la mise en quarantaine de citoyens déjà présents en sol canadien, qui ne reviennent pas d'un voyage international, il appartient

27. Micheal Da Silva et Maxime St-Hilaire, « Pandemic Preparedness and Responsiveness in Canada: Exploring the Case for an Intergovernmental Agreement », blogue du Centre d'études constitutionnelles, en ligne : <https://ualawccsprod.srv.ualberta.ca/2020/06/pandemic-preparedness-and-responsiveness-in-canada-exploring-the-case-for-an-intergovernmental-agreement/>.
28. *RJRMacDonald Inc c Canada (Procureur général)*, [1995] 3 RCS 199 aux para 28-44, 127 DLR (4e) 1.
29. *Canada (Procureur général) c PHS Community Services Society*, 2011 CSC 44 au para 68, [2011] 3 RCS 134.
30. *Loi constitutionnelle 1867*, *supra* note 2, arts 92(7), 92(13) et 92(16) ; *Bell Canada c Québec (CSST)*, [1988] 1 RCS 749 à la p 761, 51 DLR (4e) 161 ; *Association québécoise des vapoteries c Procureure générale du Québec*, 2019 QCCS 1644 au para 235 ; Martha Jackman, « Constitutional Jurisdiction Over Health in Canada » (2000) 8 Health L J à la p 110 ; Ries, *supra* note 10 à la p 533.
31. Mathen, chapitre A7
32. Lajoie et Molinari, *supra* note 13 aux p 584-585.

conséquemment aux provinces de prendre des mesures de confinement ou d'isolement physique et social qui découlent non seulement de leur compétence sur la santé, mais aussi de celle sur les transports et les commerces locaux[33].

Durant la pandémie de la COVID-19, plusieurs provinces ont toutefois décidé, unilatéralement, d'aller plus loin et d'effectuer différents types de contrôles à leurs frontières interprovinciales, en limitant les entrées de citoyens canadiens habitant d'autres provinces, ce qui nous a paru, à première vue, douteux sur le plan du partage des compétences. Ce fut le cas du Nouveau-Brunswick, de la Nouvelle-Écosse, de l'Île-du-Prince-Édouard et du Québec[34], dont les policiers demandaient aux voyageurs les raisons de leur entrée dans la province et n'acceptaient généralement que les passages jugés essentiels ou les travailleurs des domaines de la santé, du commerce et des transports commerciaux ne présentant aucun symptôme. Si ces mesures ont certainement été prises dans l'objectif de protéger la santé publique dans les provinces, leurs impacts interprovinciaux les rendraient peut-être inconstitutionnelles, selon la gravité de leurs effets. Nul doute, d'ailleurs, que le Parlement dispose d'une compétence sur le sujet en raison de ses nombreuses implications interprovinciales et des compétences dont il bénéficie déjà, comme les ouvrages de transport interprovinciaux.

Il faut toutefois reconnaître que le contrôle des passages de citoyens à une frontière interprovinciale en contexte de pandémie fait également entrer en jeu plusieurs compétences provinciales. Les impacts d'une pandémie peuvent considérablement varier d'une province à l'autre en fonction d'un nombre important de facteurs, notamment l'âge et la santé de la population, le type, l'efficacité et la solidité du système de soins de santé, les mesures d'assistance socioéconomiques, etc. Vu les nombreuses variables nationales, régionales et locales qu'implique cette question, celle-ci n'est sans doute pas suffisamment distincte des enjeux de compétences provinciales pour justifier une compétence fédérale indivisible. Son attribution exclusive au Parlement et au gouvernement du Canada pourrait aussi entraîner un déséquilibre du fédéralisme canadien en empêchant des provinces, en

33. *Loi constitutionnelle 1867*, *supra* note 2, art 92(10).
34. Voir : La Presse Canadienne, « COVID-19 : Des régions du pays ferment la porte aux autres Canadiens », *Acadie Nouvelle* (21 mars 2020), en ligne : <https://www.acadienouvelle.com/actualites/2020/03/21/covid-19-des-regions-du-pays-ferment-la-porte-aux-autres-canadiens/>.

temps de crise, de prendre des mesures rapides et essentielles afin de protéger leurs populations[35].

Compte tenu de la jurisprudence récente favorisant généralement le fédéralisme coopératif[36], il est tout à fait possible que les provinces bénéficient d'une compétence accessoire sur les mouvements interprovinciaux de citoyens, liée à leur compétence sur la santé, et peut-être même d'une compétence partagée avec le fédéral étant donné les nombreux aspects locaux de cet enjeu non expressément attribué par la Constitution. On pourrait ainsi avancer que des contrôles limités et temporaires, permettant les déplacements interprovinciaux essentiels, constituent des mesures valides nécessaires à l'application des lois provinciales sur la santé et la sécurité publiques. Si de telles mesures avaient des effets jugés trop importants sur l'équilibre constitutionnel, des mesures plus modestes pourraient plus aisément être validées par un tribunal, par exemple l'imposition de tests de dépistage et d'un isolement forcé aux citoyens entrant dans une province, mais sans que l'accès leur soit refusé. S'il fallait en plus que le gouvernement fédéral appuie ces mesures comme ce semble avoir été le cas, un juge hésiterait d'autant plus à les juger inconstitutionnelles[37] : « On recommande aux gens de rester chez eux, de ne pas aller chez les voisins. Ça s'applique aux États-Unis, mais ça s'applique aussi aux provinces avoisinantes », a répondu M. Trudeau[38].

Par ailleurs, en cas de conflit clair entre des décisions fédérales et provinciales, les premières auraient prépondérance[39]; il pourrait y avoir conflit, par exemple, si une province faisait fi de la fermeture obligatoire des frontières canadiennes imposées par le gouvernement

35. « Je n'ai pas à attendre après le fédéral pour faire ce que je perçois nécessaire pour le bien-être de notre province. [...] Je veux plutôt m'assurer que l'on prenne les mesures efficaces entre les frontières », affirmait le premier ministre du Nouveau-Brunswick. Voir : Jean-François Boisvert, « Pas de fermeture des frontières du N.-B. pour le moment, mais... », *Acadie Nouvelle* (23 mars 2020), en ligne : <https://www.acadienouvelle.com/actualites/2020/03/23/pas-de-fermeture-des-frontieres-du-n-b-pour-le-moment-mais/>.

36. *Orphan Well Association c Grant Thornton Ltd*, 2019 CSC 5, [2019] 1 RCS 150; *R c Comeau*, 2018 CSC 15, [2018] 1 RCS 342 ; *Saskatchewan (PG) c Lemare Lake Logging Ltd*, 2015 CSC 53, [2015] 3 RCS 419 ; *Renvoi relatif à la Loi sur les valeurs mobilières*, *supra* note 11 ; *Consolidated Fastfrate Inc c Western Canada Council of Teamsters*, *supra* note 11 ; *Banque canadienne de l'Ouest c Alberta*, *supra* note 14.

37. *Goodwin c Colombie-Britannique (Superintendent of Motor Vehicles)*, 2015 CSC 46 au para 33, [2015] 3 RCS 250.

38. La Presse Canadienne, *supra* note 34.

39. *Saskatchewan (PG) c Lemare Lake Logging Ltd*, 2015 CSC 53 aux para 15 à 23, [2015] 3 SCR 419.

fédéral. Il va toutefois sans dire, sur ce point, que l'idéal politico-pratique est que le gouvernement fédéral exerce un leadership de concertation interprovinciale et fédérale-provinciale[40].

Conclusion

Tout ce qui précède pourrait cependant être écarté en temps de crise sanitaire si le Parlement décidait d'exercer son pouvoir constitutionnel en matière d'urgence[41]. La prudence est toutefois de mise à cet égard puisque cette compétence extraordinaire permet de suspendre temporairement le partage des compétences et peut avoir des impacts importants sur les droits et libertés fondamentaux. Au moment d'écrire ces lignes, le Canada était d'ailleurs, depuis trois mois, plongé en pleine crise de la COVID-19 et le gouvernement fédéral n'avait toujours pas eu recours à ce pouvoir. Cela montre, en partie du moins, la prudence du gouvernement par rapport à cette compétence[42], dont l'utilisation pourrait créer plus de tort que de bien au sein de la fédération[43].

La *Loi sur les mesures d'urgence*[44] exprime elle aussi cette prudence. En effet, non seulement son préambule prévoit que les mesures prises doivent respecter la *Charte canadienne*, mais la loi montre un souci marqué pour la démocratie parlementaire et pour le respect des compétences provinciales[45]. Ces balises strictes et les pouvoirs, peut-être trop limités compte tenu de l'urgence[46], que la loi accorde

40. « Je parlerai avec les premiers ministres des provinces ce soir des mesures que nous pouvons prendre en tant que pays », a déclaré Justin Trudeau […]. « Nous devons continuer d'être coordonnés […] ». Voir : Lina Dib, « Les premiers ministres discuteront de la fermeture des frontières entre les provinces », *La Presse* (23 mars 2020), en ligne : <https://www.lapresse.ca/covid-19/202003/23/01-5266002-les-premiers-ministres-discuteront-de-la-fermeture-des-frontieres-entre-les-provinces.php>.

41. *Toronto Electric Commissioners v Snider*, [1925] 2 DLR 5 à la p 16, 55 OLR 454 ; Jackman, *supra* note 30 aux p 102-103.

42. Hélène Buzzetti et Marie Vastel, « Toujours pas de Loi sur les mesures d'urgence à Ottawa », *Le Devoir* (10 avril 2020), en ligne : <https://www.ledevoir.com/politique/canada/576834/point-de-presse-trudeau-10-avril>.

43. Mathen, chapitre A7.

44. *Ibid.*

45. *Ibid*, 3e attendu du préambule, art 6(1), 10, 14 et 58-3. Sur cette question, voir aussi : Maxime St-Hilaire, « Urgence et droit n'ont jamais fait bon ménage, mais la *Loi sur la santé publique* compte certes d'importants défauts (réponse à Martine Valois) » 15 avril 2020, en ligne (blogue) : À qui de droit <https://blogueaquidedroit.ca/2020/04/15/urgence-et-droit-nont-jamais-fait-bon-menage-mais-la-loi-sur-la-sante-publique-compte-certes-dimportants-defauts-reponse-a-martine-valois/>.

46. Flood et Thomas, chapitre A-6.

au gouvernement sont aussi susceptibles d'expliquer pourquoi ce dernier n'y a pas encore eu recours[47].

Si la décentralisation qui découle du partage des compétences implique en partie ce que certains considèrent comme une approche fragmentée, il n'en demeure pas moins que les provinces et municipalités canadiennes sont intervenues face à la COVID-19 par des mesures tout de même assez similaires bien que non identiques dans les détails; exception faite, peut-être, de l'ouverture généralisée des écoles primaires au Québec, la province faisant sur ce point bande à part en Amérique du Nord. L'amélioration des conditions de vie des personnes marginalisées nécessite aussi des mesures à long terme qui se prêtent mal à l'exercice temporaire du pouvoir fédéral d'urgence[48]. Face à un enjeu qui comporte de nombreuses ramifications locales, il nous semble, en effet, que la Constitution canadienne exprime un bon équilibre entre une approche fondée strictement sur les résultats, mais moins respectueuse de la diversité, et une approche fondée sur la coordination intergouvernementale et le respect des collectivités canadiennes[49].

47. *Ibid.*
48. Mathen, chapitre A-7.
49. Voir Fierlbeck et Hardcastle, chapitre A-1.

CHAPTER A-5

Pandemic Data Sharing: How the Canadian Constitution Has Turned into a Suicide Pact

Amir Attaran* and Adam R. Houston**

Abstract

For decades, public health professionals, scholars, and on multiple occasions, the Auditor General of Canada have raised warnings about Canada's dysfunctional system of public health data sharing. Current, timely, and complete epidemiological data are an absolutely necessary, but not sufficient, precursor to developing an effective response to the pandemic. Nonetheless, it remains true that nearly two decades after data sharing proved a catastrophic failure in the 2003 SARS epidemic, epidemiological data still are not shared between the provinces and the federal government. This is largely due to a baseless and erroneous belief that health falls purely within the jurisdiction of the provinces, despite the Supreme Court of Canada's clear conclusions to the contrary, which has misled Canada to rely on voluntary data sharing agreements with the provinces that are not merely ineffective, but actually inhibit data sharing. As outlined in this chapter, there is no reason for this to be the case, since Canada already possesses statutory powers, under the *Statistics Act* and the *Public Health Agency of Canada Act*, to oblige provinces to share critical epidemiological data in a timely manner. It must exercise those powers, both in response to

* Professor, School of Epidemiology and Public Health, Faculty of Law, University of Ottawa.

** PhD Candidate (Law), Faculty of Law, University of Ottawa.

COVID-19 and against the foreseeable certainty of even more serious public health emergencies in the future.

Résumé

Partage de données en temps de pandémie : comment la Constitution canadienne s'est transformée en un pacte de suicide

Depuis des décennies, les professionnels de la santé publique, les universitaires et, à maintes reprises, le vérificateur général du Canada, ont lancé des avertissements quant au dysfonctionnement du système canadien de partage des données en santé publique. Des données épidémiologiques fiables, à jour et complètes, sont un précurseur absolument nécessaire, mais non suffisant, pour préparer une réponse efficace à la pandémie. Néanmoins, force est de constater que près de deux décennies après l'échec catastrophique de la mise en commun des données lors de l'épidémie de SRAS en 2003, il n'y a toujours aucun partage des données épidémiologiques entre les provinces et le gouvernement fédéral. Cela est essentiellement attribuable à une perception erronée et sans fondement selon laquelle la santé relève uniquement de la compétence des provinces, en dépit des conclusions contraires sans équivoque de la Cour suprême du Canada. Cette perception trompeuse s'est traduite par des accords volontaires de partage de données entre le fédéral et les provinces, accords non seulement inefficaces, mais qui entravent en fait ce partage. Comme mentionné dans ce chapitre, il n'y a aucune raison que ce soit le cas, puisque le Canada possède déjà des pouvoirs statutaires, en vertu de la *Loi sur la statistique* et de la *Loi sur l'Agence de la santé publique du Canada*, pour obliger les provinces à fournir des données épidémiologiques indispensables en temps utile. Il doit exercer ces pouvoirs, à la fois en réponse à la COVID-19 et dans la perspective prévisible d'urgences de santé publique encore plus graves à l'avenir.

> *The choice is not between order and liberty. It is between liberty with order and anarchy without either. There is danger that, if the court does not temper its doctrinaire logic with a little practical wisdom, it will convert the constitutional Bill of Rights into a suicide pact.*[1]

For decades, public health professionals, scholars, and on multiple occasions the Auditor General of Canada have raised warnings about Canada's dysfunctional system of public health data sharing. These warnings have been reiterated in the wake of repeated outbreaks—most prominently SARS in 2003, but also food-borne listeriosis in 2008 and H1N1 influenza in 2009. Every single time, the warnings have been clear that unless Canada better prepares itself for a pandemic, many thousands could die, as when the Spanish Flu killed an estimated 55,000 Canadians between 1918 and 1920.

Almost exactly a century later, COVID-19 arrived. While SARS killed 44 people in total in Canada, as of mid-May of 2020, COVID-19 is killing several times that many *every day*. Nor is satisfactory progress being made, for unlike some countries, including those far more seriously affected such as Spain and Switzerland, which sharply reversed and crushed the epidemic's growth, in Canada there is only minimal reversal after over two months of moderate lockdown. (See Figure A5.1.)

Why? The most fundamental problem is that epidemic responses are handicapped by a mythological, schismatic, self-destructive view of federalism, which endures despite being flagrantly wrong. Who among us has not heard it emptily parroted that "health is provincial," rather than the shared jurisdiction the Supreme Court of Canada has said it is?[2]

Nowhere is federal-provincial dysfunction more apparent than in the realm of epidemiological data. When provinces collect detailed "microdata" on each COVID-19 case—the *absolutely indispensable* raw

1. Justice Robert Jackson in *Terminiello v City of Chicago*, 337 US 1 (1949) at para 107.
2. *RJR-MacDonald Inc v Canada (AG)*, [1995] 3 SCR 199 at para 32, 127 DLR (4th) 1; *Eldridge v British Columbia (AG)*, [1997] 3 SCR 624 at paras 24–25, 151 DLR (4th) 577; *Reference re Assisted Human Reproduction Act*, 2010 SCC 61 at para 57; *Canada (AG) v PHS Community Services Society*, 2011 SCC 44 at paras 67–70.

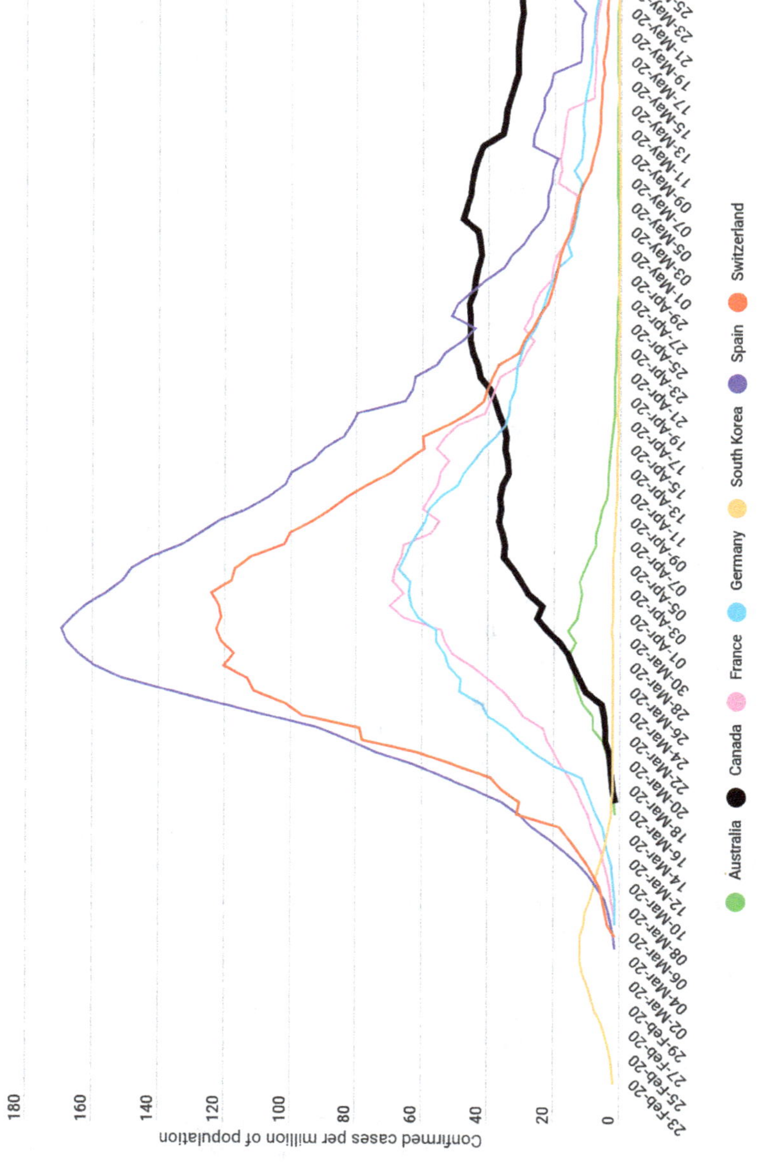

Figure A5.1 Confirmed COVID-19 Cases (per million of population, 7-day rolling average).

Source: European CDC.

data that epidemiologists require to analyze a pandemic and model strategies to vanquish it—the provinces insist that the data belong to them, to share or not with the federal government as they please. Worse, the Public Health Agency of Canada (PHAC) does not challenge this view.

Our thesis is that between them, the federal and provincial governments have failed to exchange the data which are the *sine qua non* for Canada battling COVID-19 scientifically and effectively. Just as farmers need accurate weather information from Environment Canada to plant, and businesses need precise economic information from Statistics Canada to thrive, public health planners need timely and complete epidemiological information to battle emerging pandemics. Without complete, timely epidemiological data from all parts of the country, it is *impossible* to navigate scientifically, and Canada must instead cross this maelstrom blindfolded, at an intolerable cost of wasted lives and money.

In this chapter, we discuss the history of how Canada reached this situation, and what can be done to fix it, while reminding readers of previous warnings foretelling the very crisis of epidemiological data sharing and avoidable death that Canada now faces.[3]

The History of Canada's Pandemic Governance

Canada has a sorry history of reactively legislating for public health only after being clobbered by a crisis.

Parliament created the first federal Department of Health in 1919, while the failures in Canada's response to the Spanish Flu pandemic were on full display.[4] It did so *in terrorem*, following a massive second wave of the influenza in fall 1918 that claimed nearly as many as died in the First World War.[5] While the *agent* of the pandemic was a new influenza virus, the *cause* of much excess death was Canada's

3. Amir Attaran & Kumanan Wilson, "A Legal and Epidemiological Justification for Federal Authority in Health Emergencies" (2007) 52 McGill LJ 381; Amir Attaran, "A Legislative Failure of Epidemic Proportions" (2008) 179 Can Medical Assoc J 9; Amir Attaran & Elvina Chow, "Why Canada Is Dangerously Unprepared for Epidemic Diseases: A Legal and Constitutional Diagnosis" (2011) 5 JPPL 287.
4. *An Act Respecting the Department of Health*, SA 1919, c 16. See (1919) Canada 8-9 George V, Parliament of the United Kingdom; (1919) Canada 9-10 George V, 13th Parl, 2nd Sess, 1919, 87–90.
5. Mark Humphries, *The Last Plague: Spanish Influenza and the Politics of Public Health in Canada* (Toronto: University of Toronto Press, 2012).

dysfunctional federation: despite measures the federal government imposed at national borders, the provinces proved unable to coordinate competently on basic measures within Canada, such as identifying the ill and ensuring they were isolated. All this was grimly admitted in a report completed for Cabinet amid the second wave by Vincent Massey, the future Governor General, which read: "A federal department of public health is justified now that it is clear that Provincial Governments are no longer competent to deal with Public Health in its new and wider application, and that their efforts require correlation and amplification."[6]

Yet the same incoordination and provincial inability of a century ago is now repeating with COVID-19. There is no uniformity in the quarantine or physical distancing rules of provinces; even on the seemingly uncontroversial matter of screening who has the disease, no two provinces agree.[7] Often the disunity is tragic farce: in mid-March as Quebec's premier called to isolate returning travellers, Ontario's premier encouraged families to "go away, have a good time, enjoy yourself" for spring break,[8] and the prime minister dithered, perhaps because of his health minister's scientifically wrong opinion that shutting borders to disease was "not effective at all."[9]

While not the only element underpinning an effective, coordinated response across Canada, proper data sharing is an indispensable component. Canada should be better coordinated than this, because between the Spanish Flu and COVID-19 was the Severe Acute Respiratory Syndrome (SARS) epidemic of 2003, which hit Canada worse than any other country outside Asia, and which furnished federal and provincial governments impetus to prepare effectively for the future.

They did not.

---

6. *The Report to the Vice-Chairman of the War Committee*, File 10-3-1, vol 2, vol 19, RG 29 (Ottawa: Library and Archives Canada).
7. Brieanne Olibris & Amir Attaran, "Lack of Coordination and Medical Disinformation in Canadian Self-Assessment Tools for COVID-19" [2020] medRxiv, DOI: https://doi.org/10.1101/2020.04.14.20065631.
8. Global News, "Coronavirus Outbreak: Doug Ford Tells Families to 'Have Fun' and 'Go Away' During March Break", *Global News* (2020), online: <https://globalnews.ca/video/6668414/coronavirus-outbreak-doug-ford-tells-families-to-have-fun-and-travel-during-march-break>.
9. Global News, "Coronavirus Outbreak: Hajdu Stresses Shutting Down Borders Over Illness 'Not Effective at All'", *Global News* (2020), online: <https://globalnews.ca/video/6560512/coronavirus-outbreak-hajdu-stresses-shutting-down-borders-over-illness-not-effective-at-all>.

SARS presented different challenges than the Spanish Flu. Not only was it extremely dangerous, with a case fatality rate over 10%, but this time the World Health Organization (WHO) demanded epidemiological data from Canada about the scope of the epidemic, particularly in Toronto.

Canada had no way to fulfil this demand, because a jurisdictional fight broke out and Ontario refused to share its epidemiological data with Health Canada. So little sharing occurred that Health Canada had to glean data from Ontario's press conferences![10] This left Health Canada in no position to answer WHO, which grew afraid that Canada was concealing epidemiological data—which it was, via immature federal-provincial squabbling. WHO therefore recommended against travelling to Toronto, making Canada one of only two countries ever to face that sanction (the other was notoriously secretive China).[11]

Later, Ontario established a SARS commission of inquiry to probe the causes of WHO's sanction.[12] In a blistering report, Justice Archie Campbell found that a jurisdictional battle between Ontario and Ottawa got in the way, and exhibited little judicial restraint in warning about the consequences:

> If a greater spirit of federal-provincial cooperation is not forthcoming in respect of public health protection, Ontario and the rest of Canada will be at greater risk from infectious disease and will look like fools in the international community.[13]

Justice Campbell also reviewed three other federal and provincial investigations into SARS—it was a cottage industry—and concluded that "one thing [is] crystal clear: the greatest benefit from new public

---

10. National Advisory Committee on SARS and Public Health, "Learning from SARS: Renewal of Public Health in Canada" (2003) at 202, online (pdf): *Health Canada* <https://www.canada.ca/content/dam/phac-aspc/migration/phac-aspc/publicat/sars-sras/pdf/sars-e.pdf>.
11. World Health Organization, "WHO Extends its SARS-Related Travel Advice to Beijing and Shanxi Province in China and to Toronto, Canada" (23 April 2003), online: *World Health Organization* <https://www.who.int/mediacentre/news/notes/2003/np7/en/>.
12. Government of Ontario, The SARS Commission, *The SARS Commission Report*, vol 1 (Toronto: The SARS Commission, December 2006) (The Honourable Justice Archie Campbell), online (pdf): *The Archives of Ontario* <http://www.archives.gov.on.ca/en/e_records/sars/report/index.html>.
13. *Ibid* at 193, vol 4.

health arrangements can be a new federal presence in support of provincial delivery of public health."[14]

SARS led to the creation of a new branch of the federal government, the Public Health Agency of Canada, but as we discuss in the next section, PHAC has utterly failed to solve the federal-provincial data schism, which places Canada in violation of international law. According to WHO's *International Health Regulations* passed after SARS, Canada must share epidemiological information with WHO, including:

> ... clinical descriptions, laboratory results, sources and type of risk, numbers of human cases and deaths, conditions affecting the spread of the disease and the health measures employed.[15]

Not one of these things is now being exchanged reliably between the provinces and PHAC, to say nothing of Canada being able to supply it to WHO. Simply put, Canada failed to learn the lessons of SARS.

The Public Health Agency of Canada

PHAC was originally created under the Liberal government in 2004, although the legislation formalizing its creation was left to the incoming Conservative government.[16] As the Parliamentary Secretary to the Minister of Health explained:

> First, the Public Health Agency of Canada must have specific regulatory authorities for the collection, management, and protection of public health information to ensure that the agency can receive the information it needs. As the SARS outbreak clearly showed, it is important for the government to have the ability and the means to assess accurate information... This is of particular importance because of the growing threat of an influenza pandemic or other public health emergencies... The bill provides that authority.[17]

14. *Ibid.*
15. World Health Organization, "International Health Regulations" (2005) art 5, annex 1, online: *World Health Organization* <https://www.who.int/ihr/publications/9789241580496/en/>.
16. C-5, *An Act Respecting the Establishment of the Public Health Agency of Canada and Amending Certain Acts*, 1st Sess, 39th Parl, 2006 (assented to 12 December 2006).
17. *House of Commons Debates*, 39-1, Vol 141, No 039 (13 June 2006) at line 1605, online: *House Publications* <https://www.ourcommons.ca/DocumentViewer/en/39-1/house/sitting-39/hansard>.

Presciently, the New Democratic Party complained at the time that although the legislation gave Cabinet the power to make regulations to collect epidemiological information, it placed *no corresponding duty on provinces* to share information.[18] This omission is echoed in WHO's 2018 review of Canada's compliance with the obligations set out in the *International Health Regulations*:

> While existing legislation does not specify terms for interjurisdictional sharing—which remains voluntary between provinces and territories and the federal levels—informal collegial relationships with provincial and territorial health authorities have been essential for public health surveillance and response to acute public health events across Canada.[19]

WHO went on to caution that the failure to ensure information sharing might "negatively affect [Canada's] ability to efficiently and effectively implement public health actions in response to an acute public health event."[20]

A decade before WHO's evaluation, in 2008, the Auditor General of Canada similarly warned:

> To obtain routine surveillance information, [PHAC] relies on the goodwill of the provinces and territories. However, due to gaps in its information-sharing agreements with them, it is not assured of receiving timely, accurate, and complete information. A data-sharing agreement recently signed with Ontario re-established the regular flow of information about individual cases after two years when this flow was limited. However, the Agency has not reached similar data-sharing agreements with the remaining provinces and territories.[21]

18. *Ibid* at line 1725.
19. World Health Organization, "Joint External Evaluation of IHR Core Capacities of Canada" (2019) at 27, online (pdf): *World Health Organization* <https://www.who.int/ihr/publications/who-whe-cpi-2019.62/en/>.
20. *Ibid* at 2.
21. House of Commons, *Surveillance of Infectious Diseases—Public Health Agency of* Canada (Ottawa: Office of the Auditor General of Canada, May 2008) at 2, online: *Office of the Auditor General of Canada* <https://www.oag-bvg.gc.ca/internet/English/parl_oag_200805_05_e_30701.html>.

This was hardly the Auditor General's first warning: her 2008 report complains that "fundamental weaknesses noted in our 1999 and 2002 reports remain."[22]

With over 7,000 Canadians dead at the time of this writing and no ceiling in sight, COVID-19 bears out the consequences of these ignored warnings, and the unalloyed failure of voluntary agreements with the provinces. On any given day, a comparison of the total number of cases in Canada known to PHAC with PHAC's available epidemiological "microdata" (containing details of sex, age, hospitalization or intensive care status, means of infection, deaths, and so forth) demonstrates that PHAC lacks particulars on *half* of the cases that exist. Such a giant omission essentially makes accurate epidemiological modelling and forecasting—basically scientific planning to manage the pandemic—entirely impossible.

Indeed, Canada is so primitive that the provinces and PHAC often exchange COVID-19 epidemiological data by fax machine! Fax rules because a federal-provincial project to establish modern "national surveillance and reporting systems" through the Canada Health Infoway never bore fruit.[23]

So too with two failed intergovernmental agreements since SARS. The first, a Memorandum of Understanding (MOU) for public health emergencies, is so jejune as to be self-parodying:

> This MOU is an expression of intent by the parties to explore, review, and undertake the measures set out in this MOU with a view to making appropriate administrative, policy and legislative changes considered advisable by each party to give effect to the intentions expressed in this MOU.[24]

Although the federal, provincial, and territorial health ministers all agreed in principle to this MOU in 2008, only in the case of Ontario is

22. *Ibid.*

23. Canada Health Infoway, "Public Health Surveillance: Developing a Pan-Canadian Solution to Protect Canadians" (last visited 26 May 2020), online: *Canada Health Infoway* <https://www.infoway-inforoute.ca/en/174-what-we-do/digital-health-and-you/stories/clinician-stories/380-public-health-surveillance-developing-a-pan-canadian-solution-to-protect-canadians>.

24. Pan-Canadian Public Health Network, "Federal/Provincial/Territorial Memorandum of Understanding (MOU) on the Sharing of Information During a Public Health Emergency" (last modified 9 July 2012), online: *Pan-Canadian Public Health Network* <http://www.phn-rsp.ca/pubs/mou-is-pe-pr/index-eng.php>.

it clear that the intended follow-up of an information-sharing agreement between PHAC and each province and territory was completed.[25]

Not until 2014, over a decade after SARS and following the listeriosis and H1N1 influenza outbreaks, was this MOU superseded by another intergovernmental pact, the *Multi-Lateral Information Sharing Agreement* (MLISA).[26] The language of MLISA sounds legalistic—Ottawa and the provinces are "Parties" in the style of a treaty—but it is misleading, because MLISA's so-called "mandatory obligations" to share information lack any legislated foundation and are non-binding. The trickery is not surprising: MLISA was drafted by Alberta, notoriously opposed to federal powers. Whether it has been signed by other provinces is unknown; PHAC refuses to say.

Yet foolishly, PHAC behaves as if MLISA were binding anyway, including certain "mandatory" provisions intended to neuter PHAC's ability to publish timely, important analyses such as disease models and forecasts. Clause 20(f) stipulates that before publishing any analysis of data sourced from a province, PHAC must first give the province "thirty (30) calendar days from receipt of the notice and Analysis to provide its comments." Worse, if the analysis makes use of subprovincial data—by region, city, or postal code, for example—then PHAC must "obtain the written permission of the Originating Party before it may Publish the Analysis," which is tantamount to a veto.

MLISA has thus made the sharing of timely epidemiological information *worse* since SARS. No competent public health planner wishes to confront a rapidly shifting pandemic using an epidemiological analysis that is a month obsolete—assuming that provinces grant permission for the analysis at all—just as no sane captain would set sail using last month's weather forecast. Yet the bromide that "health is provincial" is such a strong dogma that, although constitutionally wrong, PHAC thinks this natural.

Thanks to MLISA, several months into the pandemic, PHAC has failed to publish an epidemiological model of the COVID-19 crises unfolding in the country, provinces, or cities, though it unveils crude,

25. Canada, Standing Committee on Public Accounts, "Government Response to the Report of the Standing Committee on Public Accounts Chapter 5, Surveillance of Infectious Diseases—Public Health Agency of Canada of the May 2008 Report of the Auditor General of Canada (18 September 2009), online: <https://www.ourcommons.ca/DocumentViewer/en/40-2/PACP/report-12/response-8512-402-83>.

26. Pan-Canadian Public Health Network, "Multi-Lateral Information Sharing Agreement (MLISA)" (2014), online (pdf): *Pan-Canadian Public Health Network* <http://www.phn-rsp.ca/pubs/mlisa-eng.pdf>.

non-scientific forecasts for show. The Western democracies that have turned the course of COVID-19 most effectively, such as Germany, Norway, and Switzerland, have proper scientific models, in some cases *published daily*.

How and Why to Fix This

We believe there must be mandatory federal law—not just failing, voluntary agreements—that obliges provinces to share epidemiological data, in a timely, transparent, accessible, and auditable manner. It is inarguable that a law of this kind can be constitutional, even if it affects provincial health institutions.[27]

But some—including David Robitaille in this volume (see Chapter A-4)—think federal legislation of this kind undesirable, and prefer federal-provincial cooperation. We strongly disagree. Speaking not merely as lawyers, but with the backing of advanced training in immunology and years of experience with infectious disease, COVID-19 is neither history's last pandemic, nor "severe" in the spectrum of what scientists can foresee. Natural evolution can generate nightmare viruses combining the high transmissibility of COVID-19 with much higher case fatality rates (for example, 30% for the Middle Eastern Respiratory Syndrome), and virologists are even engineering such chimeras experimentally in laboratories today.[28] The jurisprudential notion that bare federal-provincial cooperation, demonstrably failing for "mild" COVID-19, could suffice for a far more terrifying biological reality such as this is simply too naïve to credit.

Currently, there are two federal statutes that could be used, but aren't. As with all laws of Parliament, both benefit from the Supreme Court of Canada's presumption of constitutionality, and both are *intra vires* the "statistics," "quarantine," or "criminal law" powers in s. 91 of the *Constitution Act, 1867*.[29]

S. 15 of the *Public Health Agency of Canada Act* permits the Governor in Council to make regulations respecting "the collection, analysis, interpretation, publication and distribution of information relating to public health," subject to parts of the *Department of Health Act*, and in turn the *Statistics Act*. It would be simple for Cabinet to

27. *Canada (AG) v PHS Community Services Society*, 2011 SCC 44 at para 50.
28. Talha Burki, "Ban on Gain-of-Function Studies Ends" (2018) 18:2 Lancet Infectious Diseases 148.
29. *Desgagnés Transport Inc v Wärtsilä Canada Inc*, 2019 SCC 58.

issue a regulation requiring provinces to share designated epidemiological data, and to do so in a prescribed, secure electronic form, which experts like Statistics Canada could build. S. 15 also helpfully empowers Cabinet to craft bespoke protections for confidential or personal health information, which is indispensable for critical life-saving interventions such as cellphone-based contact tracing of persons exposed to the COVID-19 virus, and in doing so Cabinet may deviate from the *Privacy Act* and the *Personal Information Protection and Electronic Documents Act*.[30]

Alternatively, s. 13 of the *Statistics Act* permits the Chief Statistician of Canada to issue a mandatory request for epidemiological data to any "person having the custody or charge of any documents or records that are maintained in any department [including in a province] or in any municipal office, corporation, business or organization." While easier to use than s. 15 of the *Public Health Agency of Canada Act*, this mechanism has the disadvantage that it only allows *existing* data to be collected.

We recommend using both these statutory powers at once for COVID-19. We further recommend for COVID-19 specifically that: (i) any Cabinet regulation under s. 15 of the *Public Health Agency of Canada Act* should concomitantly declare an emergency for the duration of the pandemic under the federal Peace, Order, and Good Government power (POGG) and the ratio in *Re: Anti-Inflation Act*;[31] and (ii) that a province's eligibility to receive billions of dollars of emergency federal relief should be conditioned on furnishing epidemiological data per the ratio in *Re: Canada Assistance Plan (B.C.)*.[32] Supreme Court precedent leaves no doubt that both the POGG emergency and federal spending power may be used to enforce compliance with data sharing.

Taken together, these two statutory powers, reinforced by other laws as we have just described, can:

- oblige provinces to hew to a single COVID-19 case definition established by PHAC for statistical comparability;
- oblige provinces to report epidemiological data according to a single method established by Statistics Canada;

30. See the derogations in the *Personal Information Protection and Electronic Documents Act*, SC 2000, c 5, ss 7(3)(c1)(iii), 7(3)(e); *Privacy Act* RSC 1985, c P-21, s 8(2).
31. [1976] 2 SCR 373, 68 DLR (3d) 452.
32. [1991] 2 SCR 525 at 567, 83 DLR (4th) 297.

- oblige telecommunications and Big Data companies to furnish cellphone-based data for tracing COVID-19 case contacts;
- implement bespoke privacy and confidentiality rules which are precisely tailored to the COVID-19 pandemic; and
- create both a precedent and a template for future pandemics.

We understand that others dislike these proposals, and that provinces will object. So what? Timely, effective epidemiological information is the *sine qua non* of saving lives from COVID-19—probably many thousands of them—and being ready for future pandemics. Epidemiological information alone does not ensure a successful pandemic response of course, but its continued absence *always* guarantees failure. The choice is either to use legal tools already existing in statute and Supreme Court precedent, courageously, or to fashion Canada's Constitution into the scaffold of our own demise.

CHAPTER A-6

The Federal *Emergencies Act*: A Hollow Promise in the Face of COVID-19?

Colleen M. Flood* and Bryan Thomas**

Abstract

Throughout March and April 2020, as the COVID-19 pandemic unfolded in Canada, Prime Minister Trudeau was repeatedly asked in his daily news conferences whether or not he would invoke the *Emergencies Act*. His response was that health care is a provincial matter, and the federal government would play a support role to the provinces. Rightly, the Act can only be triggered when a province has not been able to respond appropriately to a public health emergency, jeopardizing not only the health of people within a province but also other Canadians. However, there are other significant limitations within the Act such that even when a matter has risen to a level requiring a federal response, the Act may prevent the federal government from intervening or at least leave its powers unclear. We test three case-scenarios in the context of COVID-19 where arguably provincial steps have been insufficient, thus triggering the need for a national response. In so doing, we demonstrate the limitations of the *Emergencies Act* and suggest, post-COVID-19, there must be a discussion on whether the Act is fit for purpose.

* University Research Chair and Director of the Centre for Health Law, Policy and Ethics, University of Ottawa.

** Senior Research Associate and Adjunct Professor, Centre for Health Law, Policy and Ethics, University of Ottawa.

Résumé

La *Loi sur les mesures d'urgence* fédérale : une promesse vide de sens dans le contexte de la COVID-19 ?

En mars et avril 2020, alors que la pandémie de COVID-19 s'installait au Canada, le premier ministre Trudeau s'est fait questionner à maintes reprises, lors de ses conférences de presse quotidiennes, sur son intention de recourir ou non à la *Loi sur les mesures d'urgence*. Il répondait que les soins de santé sont de compétence provinciale et que le gouvernement fédéral allait soutenir les provinces. À juste titre, la *Loi* ne peut être invoquée que lorsqu'une province n'a pas été en mesure de réagir de manière appropriée à une urgence de santé publique, mettant en péril non seulement la santé de sa population, mais aussi celle d'autres Canadiens. Cependant, la *Loi* comporte d'autres restrictions importantes. Ainsi, même lorsqu'une situation exige une intervention du gouvernement fédéral, la *Loi* peut l'empêcher d'intervenir ou ne précise pas s'il a le pouvoir de le faire. Nous testons trois cas de figure dans le contexte de la COVID-19, dans lesquels les mesures provinciales ont sans doute été insuffisantes, ce qui aurait justifié une réponse nationale. Ce faisant, nous démontrons les limites de la *Loi sur les mesures d'urgence* et suggérons de discuter, une fois la pandémie passée, de l'adéquation de la *Loi* à ses objectifs.

Health is frequently described as primarily a matter of provincial jurisdiction,[1] and provinces have issued significant public health orders in response to the COVID-19 pandemic.[2] Despite some commonalities across provinces (for example, the closure of elementary and secondary schools and non-essential businesses), the overall response is best described as a patchwork. For example, at the time of writing, size restrictions on public gatherings vary from 50 people (British Columbia) to gatherings of 5 (Ontario) to *any* size (Quebec, Nunavut,

1. For more nuance on the division of powers vis-à-vis health, see Colleen M. Flood, William Lahey & Bryan Thomas, "Federalism and Health Care in Canada: A Troubled Romance?", in Peter Oliver, Patrick Macklem & Nathalie Des Rosiers, eds, *The Oxford Handbook of the Canadian Constitution* (New York: OUP 2017).
2. For a review of various orders, see Craig Forcese, "Repository of Canadian COVID-19 Emergency Orders" (2020), online (blog): *Intrepid* <https://www.intrepidpodcast.com/blog/2020/3/19/repository-of-canadian-covid-19-emergency-orders>.

and Northwest Territories). Likewise, provinces have varied in their approach to interprovincial travel, with Quebec turning away recreational travellers from Ottawa to Gatineau, several provinces requiring incoming travellers to self-isolate for 14 days (for example, Manitoba and Nova Scotia), and other provinces imposing no restrictions (Ontario, Alberta, British Columbia).[3] Provinces vary as well in their approaches to testing—methods for accessing a test (central hotlines, GP referrals), speed of receiving results, overall volume, and efforts at directing testing toward "hot spots."[4] Some provinces have demonstrably failed to adequately manage the terrible outbreak of COVID-19 in long-term care homes, with Ontario and Quebec calling upon assistance by the Canadian military, who have reported horrific conditions.[5]

Some critics of the patchwork approach argue that the federal government should invoke the *Emergencies Act*[6] to ensure a clear and unified response to COVID-19[7]—avoiding the confusion and skepticism arising from conflicting rules across jurisdictions. Internationally, the World Health Organization declared a "public health emergency of international concern" on January 30, 2020, and since that time many countries have declared national emergencies. Our review of international responses indicates that Canada stands alone among federated developed countries in not declaring an emergency or issuing a national lockdown.[8]

Those opposed to invoking the Act posit that the provinces have available to them all of the powers that the federal government might

---

3. Globe Staff and Wire Services, "What Is the Reopening Plan in My Province? A Guide", *The Globe and Mail* (1 April 2020), online: <https://www.theglobeandmail.com/canada/article-coronavirus-rules-by-province-physical-distancing-open-closed/#rulesque>.
4. Robert Jones, "Pace of COVID-19 Testing Picks Up, but N.B. Still Lags Behind Other Provinces", *CBC News* (26 March 2020), online: <https://www.cbc.ca/news/canada/new-brunswick/coronavirus-covid-19-testing-new-brunswick-1.5510396>.
5. Murray Brewster & Vassy Kapelos, "Military Reports Horrific Conditions, Abuse in Ontario Nursing Homes", *CBC News* (26 May 2020), online: <https://www.cbc.ca/news/politics/long-term-care-pandemic-covid-coronavirus-trudeau-1.5584960>.
6. *Emergencies Act*, RSC, 1985, c 22 (4th Supp), s 58 (1).
7. Peter Mazereeuw, "Ottawa Should Trigger Emergencies Act Amid COVID-19 Crisis, Says Retired General and Former Liberal Andrew Leslie", *The Hill Times* (26 March 2020), online: <https://www.hilltimes.com/2020/03/26/ottawa-should-trigger-emergencies-act-amid-covid-19-crisis-says-retired-general-and-former-liberal-andrew-leslie/241166>.
8. Deutsche Welle, "Coronavirus: What Are the Lockdown Measures Across Europe?", *DW* (14 April 2020), online: <https://www.dw.com/en/coronavirus-what-are-the-lockdown-measures-across-europe/a-52905137>.

employ under a national lockdown, even if they have not used them uniformly.[9] Skeptics also note that any rules set by the federal government may require provincial cooperation for their implementation.[10] Whether such cooperation would be forthcoming is an open question. Also, of course, it is not clear that the federal government would do a better job than any particular province.

Invoking the *Emergencies Act* would constitute an exercise of executive power (an order of the Governor in Council), and as such the legislation contains several important checks and balances, including the requirement of consultation with affected provinces and a review by Parliament with seven sitting days.[11] Reflecting the importance of division of powers in the Canadian federation, the Act empowers the federal government to respond to urgent and critical yet *temporary* situations that endanger Canadians at a scale and scope that exceeds the capacity or authority of the provinces to deal with, and that cannot be dealt with under any other law of Canada.[12] We contemplate three situations that arguably fall within these parameters:

1) *A Canada-wide lockdown*. Following the example of over 100 other jurisdictions, such as Italy, the U.K., and New Zealand, the federal government may wish to enforce lockdown orders for all of Canada (or for a province or provinces that have not been able to sufficiently control the outbreak), mandating that people stay in their homes except for essential travel (groceries, hospital visits, essential work).
2) *Increased testing and tracing*. Most commentators agree that a massive expansion of testing and contact tracing is needed before physical distancing restrictions can be lifted. We explore whether the federal government could declare a national emergency to attend to this problem.[13]

9. John Paul Tasker, "The 'Measure of Last Resort': What Is the *Emergencies Act* and What Does it Do?", *CBC News* (23 March 2020), online: <https://www.cbc.ca/news/politics/trudeau-emergencies-act-premier-1.5507205>.
10. Hanna Jackson, "Coronavirus: Should Canada Restrict Travel Between Provinces, Territories?", *Global News* (March 23, 2020), online: <https://globalnews.ca/news/6717323/coroanvirus-travel-between-provinces/>.
11. *Emergencies Act*, *supra* note 6 at s 58(1).
12. *Emergencies Act*, *supra* note 6 at s 3.
13. World Health Organization, "WHO Director-General's Opening Remarks at the Media Briefing on COVID-19", *World Health Organization* (16 March 2020), online: <https://www.who.int/dg/speeches/detail/who-director-general-s-opening-remarks-at-the-media-briefing-on-covid-19---16-march-2020>.

3) *Protecting long-term care homes*. Some provinces—particularly in Ontario and Quebec—appear to have failed to sufficiently test workers and residents in long-term care homes or to provide workers with protective gear. We explore the potential for the federal government to invoke the *Emergencies Act* to ensure Canada-wide standards.

Scenario 1: Can the Federal Government Establish and Enforce a Lockdown?

Although it is possible to implement lockdowns on a province-by-province basis, using provincial emergency measures laws, a key advantage of a national lockdown order is that it would avoid the confusion of conflicting messages from the municipal, provincial, and federal governments. Such benefits must be weighed against the costs of bold federal action—notably the intrusion into provincial jurisdiction—and the possibility a province-by-province approach may be more agile and responsive to local needs than a blanket national response.

Having declared a public welfare emergency, the federal government can issue one or more specific orders enumerated under the section 8 of the *Emergencies Act*, which empowers it to issue orders with respect to "the regulation or prohibition of travel to, from or within any specified area, where necessary for the protection of the health or safety of individuals." *Prima facie,* this would seem to enable a lockdown.

The next step is to gauge whether such a lockdown order could survive application of the Act's limitation clause:

> 4. Nothing in this Act shall be construed or applied so as to confer on the Governor in Council the power to make orders or regulations… **(b)** providing for the detention, imprisonment or internment of Canadian citizens or permanent residents within the meaning of subsection 2(1) of the *Immigration and Refugee Protection Act* on the basis of race, national or ethnic origin, colour, religion, sex, age or mental or *physical disability* (emphasis added)

This strict limitation clause reflects that the *Emergencies Act* replaced the *War Measures Act*—legislation that gained infamy when used to forcibly intern Japanese Canadians during the Second World War and again with Pierre Elliot Trudeau's heavy-handed response to the October Crisis. This limitation clause is more categorical than, for example, the guarantee of equality before the law granted under section 15 of the *Canadian Charter of Rights and Freedoms*.[14] First, the *Emergencies Act* forbids any and all detention on the basis of enumerated traits, whereas section 15 of the *Charter* is limited to *discriminatory* treatment of enumerated and analogous classes. Second, protections offered by section 15 are subject to the section 1 "reasonable limits" clause. The Act does not create the possibility for the federal government to "detain" individuals on the basis of enumerated traits (for example, require a lockdown of individuals exposed to COVID-19) and justify this measure as "demonstrably justified in a free and democratic society."[15]

Assuming that being infected with SARS-CoV-2 (or being at high risk of same) does constitute a physical disability, a further question is whether a national lockdown could be construed as targeting individuals "on the basis of" disability. This seems unlikely: such an order would apply to *all* residents, after all—the aim of physical distancing is to limit channels of transmission between the infected and non-infected. Perhaps there are scenarios where the federal government, having invoked the *Emergencies Act*, would seek to enforce isolation orders specifically targeting those infected with SARS-CoV-2 or at-risk populations, and this would seem to potentially run afoul of that Act's categorical limitations clause, as an *ultra vires* form of "detention"[16] on the basis of physical disability.

Declaring a federal lockdown is one thing, but enforcing it is another. Section 9 of the *Emergencies Act* bars the federal government from commandeering provincial and municipal police forces. With RCMP officers accounting for approximately 30% of all police personnel in the country, a switch to a federally controlled lockdown could see a drastic *reduction* in enforcement powers. It is possible that provinces and municipalities would cooperate and join their police forces with the RCMP for a Canada-wide lockdown. But if federal-provincial-territorial cooperation were to be forthcoming, this raises the question of why a federally controlled

14. *Canadian Charter of Rights and Freedoms*, Part I of the *Constitution Act, 1982*, being Schedule B to the *Canada Act 1982* (U.K.), 1982, c 11, s 15.
15. *Ibid*, s.1.
16. Physical force is not required under the criminal law definition of "detention"; "psychological detention" is established where the individual has a legal obligation to comply with a restrictive request or demand. *R v Grant*, 2009 SCC 32.

lockdown is necessary, as opposed to continued reliance on cooperative federalism.[17]

Scenario 2: Can the *Emergencies Act* Support the Ramping Up of Testing and Contact Tracing?

The *Emergencies Act* might also be invoked to ensure there is appropriate testing and contact tracing of cases across Canada.[18] At the time of writing this chapter, provincial efforts at testing and contact tracing have been mixed. In several large provinces (Ontario, Alberta, and British Columbia), officials have been instructing patients with mild symptoms to self-isolate rather than seek testing. Testing has been seriously backlogged in some provinces, while others have been testing *below* their available capacity.[19] The Act has no provision explicitly authorizing the federal government to establish minimum levels of testing and tracing for the provinces. However, section 8 does provide for the establishment of "emergency shelters and hospitals,"[20] and as such may be interpreted to permit the federal government to establish testing sites.

If (and this is a *big* if) testing was ramped up, the Act might also be employed to enhance Canada's lacklustre efforts at contact tracing, at least in some provinces.[21] South Korea's highly praised response to the outbreak (at least prior to a second wave) has been supported, in part, by the use of GPS data from cellphones and cars.[22] Retracing infected

17. This is not to deny that there are good reasons to be concerned *generally* about the efficacy and accountability of cooperative federalism within the public health sphere; see The SARS Commission, *The SARS Commission Interim Report: SARS and Public Health in Ontario* (Toronto: The SARS Commission, 15 April 2004) (Commissioner: The Honourable Justice Archie Campbell) at 66, online: *Archives of Ontario* <http://www.archives.gov.on.ca/en/e_records/sars/report/Interim_Report.pdf>. See also Amir Attaran & Adam R Houston, this volume, Chapter A-5.
18. Colleen M Flood, Teresa Scassa & David Robertson, "How Invoking the *Emergencies Act* Could Help Canada Better Track, Contain COVID-19", *CBC News* (27 March 2020), online: <https://www.cbc.ca/news/opinion/opinion-covid-coronavirus-emergency-measures-act-tracking-1.5510999>.
19. Andrew Russel, "Ontario Conducting Fewer than 3,000 COVID-19 Tests Despite Daily Capacity of 13,000", *Global News* (April 8, 2020), online: <https://globalnews.ca/news/6793481/coronavirus-covid-19-tests-ontario-capacity/>.
20. *Emergencies Act, supra* note 6, s 8(g).
21. Michael Wolfson, "Who Should We Really be Testing for COVID-19", *Toronto Star* (28 April 2020), online: <https://www.thestar.com/opinion/contributors/2020/04/28/who-should-we-really-be-testing-for-covid-19.html>.
22. Editorial, "Show Evidence that Apps for COVID-19 Contact Tracing Are Secure and Effective", *Nature* (29 April 2020), online: *Nature* <https://www.nature.com/articles/d41586-020-01264-1>.

patients' movements in this way, health officials have been able to notify individuals who had crossed paths with the virus.[23] In Canada, the federal government could utilize section 8(1) of the *Emergencies Act* (power over use and disposal of "property") to access data held by telecommunications companies. There are obvious privacy concerns here as the *Personal Information Protection and Electronic Documents Act* (PIPEDA) bars commercial entities from sharing personal information without consent.[24] To navigate these restrictions, new bespoke legislation[25] is likely needed that specifically, and temporarily, circumvents PIPEDA for contact tracing.

Scenario 3: Can the *Emergencies Act* Support Improved Protections in Long-term Care Homes?

At the time of writing this chapter, most COVID-19 deaths in Canada have occurred in long-term care homes. Provincial responses—particularly in Quebec and Ontario—have been too little, too late. For example, the Ontario government only recently (April 10, 2020) issued directives that all staff and visitors must wear surgical masks.[26] An addendum notes that, pursuant to the *Retirement Homes Act*, "retirement homes must take all *reasonable steps* to follow the required precautions and procedures outlined in this directive" (emphasis added). Moreover, within Ontario, we see that some municipalities have taken more extensive steps to control outbreaks in long-term care homes, raising the question of why this has not become a provincial or Canadian standard.[27] In response to devastating accounts

23. Max Fisher & Choe Sang-Hun, "How South Korea Flattened the Curve" *New York Times* (23 March 2020), online: <https://www.nytimes.com/2020/03/23/world/asia/coronavirus-south-korea-flatten-curve.html>.
24. PIPEDA contains some provisions allowing for disclosure without consent. For example, s 3(e) allows non-consensual disclosure in emergencies that impact "the life, health, or security of an individual." On our understanding, this provision is intended to protect specific individuals, and not to be used for collective, public health purposes. For a discussion of privacy concerns, both ethical and legal, see Teresa Scassa, Jason Millar & Kelly Bronson, this volume, Chapter C-2.
25. Passed pursuant to the peace, order, and good government power, for a critique see Carissima Mathen, this volume, Chapter A-7.
26. Ontario Ministry of Health and Long-Term Care, "Directive #5 for Hospitals within the Meaning of the *Public Hospitals Act* and Long-Term Care Homes within the Meaning of the *Long-Term Care Homes Act*, 2007", online (pdf): *Ontario Retirement Communities Association* <https://www.orcaretirement.com/wp-content/uploads/CMOH-Directive-5-Revised-2020-04-10.pdf>.
27. Karen Howlett, "With an Early Focus on Seniors' Residences, Kingston Has so far Avoided the Brunt of COVID-19", *The Globe and Mail* (28 April 2020), online:

of long-term care workers abandoning their roles, leaving patients dehydrated, hungry, and laying in squalor, the federal government has issued *guidelines* for COVID-19 infection control recommending (*inter alia*) that long-term care homes limit visitors and staff wear face masks and don robust personal protective equipment when assisting symptomatic residents.[28] Besides guidelines, the federal government has offered financial support to boost the incomes of workers so they don't need to work in multiple facilities.

We contend there is a public health case for more robust federal measures beyond "guidance" and offers of funding. The *Emergencies Act* could and should be used to (temporarily through the pandemic) require that optimal personal protective equipment is available and mandatory where appropriate, in long-term care homes and other facilities.[29] This would allow the federal government to temporarily upgrade its guidelines to enforceable national rules. But we note again the limitations of the Act, which does not empower the federal government, even if it has declared an emergency, to mandate uniform testing of long-term care workers.

Conclusion

As the pandemic outbreak evolves, it is possible other usages of the *Emergencies Act* beyond the three-case scenarios presented here (protecting residents and workers in long-term care homes, lockdown, and contact tracing) will emerge. Our aim has been to identify areas where the Act might arguably be used to address matters that have eclipsed the ability or the willingness of provinces to respond, as well as identify legal barriers and pragmatic limitations.

Much of the media discussion seems to assume that use of the *Emergencies Act* will necessarily be draconian. In fact, the Act could

<https://www.theglobeandmail.com/canada/article-with-an-early-focus-on-seniors-residences-kingston-has-so-far/>.

28. Government of Canada, *Infection Prevention and Control for COVID-19: Interim Guidance for Long Term Care Homes* (Ottawa: Government of Canada, 8 April 2020), online: *Government of Canada* <https://www.canada.ca/en/public-health/services/diseases/2019-novel-coronavirus-infection/prevent-control-covid-19-long-term-care-homes.html#a6.3.1>.

29. Canadian Federation of Nurses Unions, Press Release, "Canada Must Act Urgently to Protect all Health Care Workers, Before it's too Late", Silas Tells Federal Health Committee" (7 April 2020), online: *Canadian Federation of Nurses* Unions <https://nursesunions.ca/canada-must-act-urgently-to-protect-all-health-care-workers-before-its-too-late/>.

be used for a more regulatory purpose; a federal order mandating clear and consistent rules of personal protective equipment across the continuum of care, for the COVID-19 pandemic period, hardly represents a return to the darkest moments of the *War Measures Act*. Overall, we argue that in a number of important respects, the Act is too restrictive. As we have outlined, the internal limitations clause would appear to prohibit the selective detainment of individuals "disabled" by COVID-19. The Act also doesn't appear to enable national requirements for testing, for example, in long-term care homes. In fact, the Act sounds a hollow promise: it does not sufficiently enable a time-limited federal response to an *actual* public health emergency, COVID-19, in cases where provincial action has been insufficient.

CHAPTER A-7

Resisting the Siren's Call: Emergency Powers, Federalism, and Public Policy

Carissima Mathen*

Abstract

Virtually everyone in Canada would describe the COVID-19 pandemic as an emergency. The federal government's decisions—to close borders and order Canadians into quarantine—suggest that it shares this view. Yet it has neither declared an emergency nor triggered the federal *Emergencies Act*. The lack of such action has been criticized. At the same time, there has been less focus on the emergency powers available to Parliament under the "peace, order and good government" clause in s. 91 of the *Constitution Act 1867*. In this chapter, I explore three demands that would require emergency branch legislation: regulating long-term care; providing relief to persons under residential and commercial tenancies; and instituting nation-wide testing. Examining the emergency branch's benefits and drawbacks, I argue that emergency powers must be approached with continual caution, with due appreciation for the operational and political complexities inherent in a federal state. While a national, "top-down" approach may be effective in some situations, in others it is preferable to encourage regional responses and inter-governmental cooperation.

* Professor, Faculty of Law, University of Ottawa.

Résumé
Résister au chant des sirènes : pouvoirs d'urgence, fédéralisme et politiques publiques

Presque tout le monde au Canada décrirait la pandémie de COVID-19 comme une urgence. Les décisions du gouvernement fédéral – fermer les frontières et ordonner la mise en quarantaine de la population – suggèrent qu'il est du même avis. Pourtant, il n'a pas déclaré l'état d'urgence ni eu recours à la *Loi fédérale sur les mesures d'urgence*. On le lui a d'ailleurs reproché. En même temps, moins d'attention a été accordée aux pouvoirs d'urgence que détient le Parlement en vertu de la disposition relative à « la paix, l'ordre et le bon gouvernement » prévue à l'article 91 de la *Loi constitutionnelle de 1867*. Dans ce chapitre, j'explore trois demandes qui nécessiteraient des dispositions législatives s'appliquant aux situations d'urgence : la réglementation des soins de longue durée, l'aide aux personnes sous bail résidentiel et commercial, et le dépistage à l'échelle nationale. En examinant les avantages et les inconvénients de telles mesures législatives, je soutiens que les pouvoirs en cas d'urgence doivent être abordés avec une prudence constante, en tenant compte des complexités opérationnelles et politiques inhérentes à un État fédéral. Si une approche nationale peut être efficace dans certaines situations, dans d'autres, il est préférable d'encourager les initiatives régionales et la coopération intergouvernementale.

Virtually everyone in Canada would describe the COVID-19 pandemic as an emergency. At the time of writing, there are almost 70,000 confirmed cases and 5,000 deaths. Unemployment is at record levels; schools, theatres, and shopping malls have closed; many people continue to stay at home; and there are whispers of a depression. Scores of people have been deprived of the joys of family and community life. Hugs and handshakes feel like relics of a lost civilization.

The federal government has made many decisions that would be inconceivable in ordinary times, including closing the Canadian border to non-nationals; requiring those returning to the country to quarantine for 14 days; instructing international air carriers to refuse to board anyone displaying symptoms of the virus; and mandating masks on domestic flights. In a matter of weeks, Parliament enacted new social programs at a cost of hundreds of billions of dollars.[1] And yet, unlike the provinces, the federal government has not declared a national emergency. Nor has it triggered the federal *Emergencies Act*.[2]

To some, including Colleen M. Flood and Bryan Thomas in Chapter A-6 of this volume, that suggests fundamental flaws in the *Emergencies Act*.[3] Others have called out the government for shirking its duty.[4] There are demands for it to do more.

In this chapter, I take a somewhat different approach, focusing on the specific ability to enact laws under the emergency branch of the "peace, order, and good government" power (POGG).[5] Examining three policy areas, I examine the benefits and drawbacks of possible emergency legislation. While such laws might provide a measure of assistance, they come with certain risks—risks that are heightened during a health pandemic requiring extensive inter-governmental cooperation.[6]

The POGG Emergency Power

The *Constitution Act, 1867* enumerates federal and provincial powers. Traditionally, provinces have jealously guarded their powers against federal encroachment. Early cases circumscribed federal authority, under s. 91, to "make laws for the peace, order and good government of Canada."[7] For years, national emergencies were thought to be the

1. Government of Canada, *Canada's Economic Response to COVID-19* (Ottawa: Government of Canada, 2020), online: *Government of Canada* <https://www.canada.ca/en/department-finance/economic-response-plan.html>.
2. *Emergencies Act*, RSC, 1985, c 22 (4th Supp).
3. See Colleen M Flood & Bryan Thomas, this volume, Chapter A-6; and "Liberty v. Security in a Pandemic", *TVO The Agenda* (2 April 2020), online: <https://www.tvo.org/video/liberty-vs-security-in-a-pandemic?utm_source=TVO&utm_campaign=2031b263c3-EMAIL_CAMPAIGN_1_17_2019_10_56_COPY_01&utm_medium=email&utm_term=0_eadf6a4c78-2031b263c3-24183137>.
4. Christopher Guly, "Is it Time to Invoke the Federal Emergencies Act?", *The Tyee* (27 March 2020), online: <https://thetyee.ca/News/2020/03/27/Time-For-Emergencies-Act/>.
5. *Constitution Act, 1867* (UK), 30 & 31 Vict, c 3, s 91, reprinted in RSC 1985, Appendix II, No 5 [*Constitution Act, 1867*]. The POGG power has three "branches": new matters, national concern, and emergencies. While both national concern and emergency involve incursions into provincial jurisdiction, the emergency branch has the greatest relevance to a global health pandemic.
6. See David Robitaille, this volume, Chapter A-4.
7. *Constitution Act, 1867*, *supra* note 5.

only circumstance in which POGG could be used.[8] Even as that position softened, the judicial approach remained cautious.[9]

The emergency power is legislative. Parliament, not the Prime Minister or Cabinet, decides whether an emergency exists and what the response should be. Obviously, legislation requires more time than executive action. The government must negotiate with different parties (especially when it is in a minority), and ensure passage through the Commons and the Senate.[10] A number of COVID-related laws have passed extraordinary swiftly,[11] but alacrity is hardly a given.

The emergency branch shelters laws that cannot be subsumed within other federal subjects. Because it subverts the ordinary division of powers, courts have long insisted that emergency branch use must be temporary.[12] While such laws can be maintained for a time following the crisis, they must have an endpoint. Ideally, Parliament should invoke the power expressly. At the very least, there should be evidence that Parliament apprehended an emergency when it passed the law.[13]

Emergency legislation is not shielded from judicial review.[14] Courts may be asked whether Parliament apprehended a particular situation as an emergency and whether the legislation was intended

8. *AGAC (Ont) v AG (Can)* (Local Prohibition) [1896] 348; 5 Cart BNA 295 (PC).
9. *Fort Frances Pulp & Power Co Ltd v Manitoba Free Press Co Ltd*, [1923] 3 DLR 629, [1923] AC 695.
10. For a discussion of the Senate of Canada's role during the pandemic, see Vanessa MacDonnell, this volume, Chapter B-1.
11. *COVID-19 Emergency Response Act, No 2*, SC 2020, c 6 (introduced and assented to 11 April 2020); *Canada Emergency Student Benefit Act*, SC 2020, c 7 (first reading 29 April 2020, assented to 1 May 2020).
12. *R v Crown Zellerbach Canada Ltd*, [1988] 1 SCR 401 at 431–432, 1 DLR (4th) 161; *Re: Anti-Inflation Act*, [1976] 2 SCR 373 at 378, 68 DLR (3d) 452 [*Re Anti-Inflation*].
13. While there have been occasional exceptions to the demand for express articulation, at the very least a reviewing court requires some evidence that Parliament apprehended an emergency at the time that it passed the relevant legislation: *Re Anti-Inflation*, *ibid*; Christopher Nardi, "Why Would He Pick a Fight with Us? COVID-19 Raises Tensions Between Trudeau Government and Quebec", *National Post* (8 May 2020), online: <https://nationalpost.com/news/politics/why-would-he-pick-a-fight-with-us-covid-19-raises-tensions-between-trudeau-government-and-quebec>.
14. For a provincial example, see *Sprague v Her Majesty the Queen in right of Ontario*, 2020 ONSC 2335. See, from New Zealand, *Christiansen v DG (Health)*, [2020] NZHC 887, online (pdf): *Courts of New Zealand* <https://courtsofnz.govt.nz/assets/cases/Christiansen-v-The-Director-General-of-Health-Reasons-NZHC-887.pdf>.

to respond to it.[15] Equally, such laws are subject to the *Canadian Charter of Rights and Freedoms*.[16]

Emergency Laws and COVID-19

The pandemic has profoundly affected all areas of social and economic life; and revealed cracks in the country's health and social welfare systems. Under the division of powers, provinces have exclusive authority over "property and civil rights" and "all matters of a merely local or private nature"[17]—in other words, over those aspects of life most at risk from the virus. But, spurred in part by the different levels of provincial success in combatting COVID-19,[18] the federal government has faced repeated calls to intervene.

Promoting Health and Well-being: Long-term Care Homes

One of the pandemic's cruellest features is its ravaging of long-term care homes, where hundreds of thousands of Canadians receive life-affirming care. Deaths in such homes have vastly outpaced the population at large. The premier of Quebec has described the province as fighting two pandemics—one in long-term care homes and one in the general population.[19]

Long-term care homes are not considered part of the primary health care system.[20] Many are privately owned and operated for

15. *Re Anti-Inflation Act*, *supra* note 12.
16. The Canadian Civil Liberties Association has launched a *Charter* challenge against provincial travel restrictions and prohibitions on travel: Brian Platt, "Civil Liberties Group Filing Charter Challenge over Newfoundland's Ban on Travel Into Province", *National Post* (21 May 2020), online: <https://nationalpost.com/news/politics/civil-liberties-group-filing-charter-challenge-over-newfoundlands-ban-on-travel-into-province>. Other constitutional provisions, such as those concerning Indigenous rights, must also be respected.
17. *Constitution Act, 1867*, *supra* note 5 s 92(7), (14), (16).
18. Justin McElroy, "Why B.C. is Flattening the COVID-19 Curve While Numbers in Central Canada Surge", *CBC News* (6 April 2020), online: <https://www.cbc.ca/news/canada/british-columbia/bc-ontario-quebec-covid-19-1.5524056>. B.C. has 3 deaths per 100,000 while Quebec has over 35 deaths per 100,000.
19. Colin Harris, "COVID-19 in Quebec: Virus Creates '2 Separate Worlds,' Says Premier—Long-Term Care Homes vs. Rest of Society", *CBC News* (24 April 2020), online: <https://www.cbc.ca/news/canada/montreal/covid-19-quebec-april-24-1.5543521>.
20. Dr Amit Arya, "COVID-19 Rips Bandage Off Open Wound that Is Our Nursing Home System", *CBC News* (26 April 2020), online: <https://www.cbc.ca/news/opinion/opinion-nursing-homes-conditions-1.5541155>.

profit.[21] Whether public or private, almost all feature chronic understaffing by poorly paid workers juggling multiple jobs.[22] This has contributed to "case clusters" of COVID-19 in homes in British Columbia, Ontario, and Quebec.[23] Workers complain of inadequate personal protective equipment, and in some especially notorious incidents, they have even walked off the job, leaving residents lying in soiled beds, unfed and ill, for days.[24]

Numerous provinces have struggled to contain the spread of the disease, going so far as to ask members of the Canadian Armed Forces to deploy to the homes. While some provinces and even cities have slowed the spread,[25] at the time of writing, the situation in long-term care homes was linked to over three-quarters of deaths nationwide.[26] The federal government has faced increasing pressure to step in. In cooperation with provinces, it has created guidelines for best practices, but many consider such tools useless without a centralized compliance mechanism.

Those raising the need for federal intervention tend to focus on prohibiting for-profit centres; setting minimum staffing requirements and rates of pay; preventing workers from moving between homes; mandating the use of personal protective equipment; and creating

---

21. Anne Leclair, "Coronavirus: Working Conditions at Residence Herron and Owner's Past Under Scrutiny", *Global News* (16 April 2020), online: <https://globalnews.ca/news/6824575/working-conditions-owner-residence-herron-scrutiny/>.
22. See Pat Armstrong, Hugh Armstrong & Ivy Bourgeault, this volume, Chapter E-1.
23. Colin Perkel, "New Nursing Home Cluster Amid COVID Case Rise and Economic Gloom", *The Canadian Press* (27 March 2020), online: <https://www.ctvnews.ca/health/coronavirus/new-nursing-home-cluster-amid-covid-case-rise-and-economic-gloom-1.4871210>.
24. Leclair, *supra* note 22. See also the horrendous situation that occurred at the Participation House facility in Markham, Ontario: Sean Davidson, "Fourth Resident of Participation House in Markham Dies of COVID-19", *CP24* (24 April 2020), online: <https://www.cp24.com/news/fourth-resident-of-participation-house-in-markham-dies-of-covid-19-1.4911362>.
25. B.C., in particular, acted quickly and effectively: Natalie Obiko Pearson, "COVID-19: B.C.—The Virus Epicentre that Wasn't", *The Province* (16 May 2020), online: <https://theprovince.com/news/local-news/covid-19-b-c-the-virus-epicentre-that-wasnt/wcm/cfc1a7d6-1f92-405e-8bb6-4bc8426404b6>. See also the striking success of the City of Kingston, Ontario: Kimberley Johnson, "Kingston Officially Clear of Positive COVID-19 Cases", *CTV News* (9 May 2020), online: <https://ottawa.ctvnews.ca/kingston-officially-clear-of-positive-covid-19-cases-1.4932364>.
26. Marieke Walsh and Ivan Semeniuk, "Long-Term Care Connected to 79 Per Cent of COVID-19 Deaths in Canada", *The Globe and Mail* (28 April 2020), online: <https://www.theglobeandmail.com/politics/article-long-term-care-connected-to-79-per-cent-of-covid-19-deaths-in-canada/>.

national education and certification standards. The federal government might be able to achieve some of that through its spending power coupled with conditions.[27] It is unclear, though, whether a mere "opt-in" system would satisfy demands that are both framed as universal and relate to specific operational conditions. The federal government has rarely sought to exert a similar level of control through health care transfers; and doing so might prompt *vires* concerns that it was trying to control the services themselves. To rapidly ensure national standards, emergency powers might be required.[28]

Protecting Against Economic Insecurity: Rent

COVID-19 has created acute economic need. Millions of Canadians have lost jobs, seen their businesses crumble, or watched investments dwindle. Parliament has expanded existing support programs and created others out of whole cloth, including the Canada Emergency Response Benefit (CERB) and Canada Emergency Wage Subsidy.[29] To date, federal actors have rejected implementing a universal basic income.[30]

Residential and commercial tenancies are a pressing concern. Given the vast difference in rents across the country, the CERB ($2,000 per month) does not provide equivalent relief.[31] And, despite a new federal commercial rent subsidy, many businesses report being asked to vacate their premises.[32]

---

27. *Re Canada Assistance Plan* [1991] 2 SCR 525, 83 DLR (4th) 297; *Winterhaven Stables Limited v Canada (Attorney General)*, 1988 ABCA 334, 53 DLR (4th) 413.
28. The federal government might argue that long-term care homes should be regulated under the "national concern" branch of POGG, but caselaw concerning that branch has tended not to favour the federal government: *Re Anti-Inflation Act*, *supra* note 13; *R v HydroQuébec*, [1997] 3 SCR 213, 151 DLR (4th) 32; *R v MalmoLevine*, 2003 SCC 74; *R v Caine*, 2003 SCC 74. *Ontario Hydro v Ontario (Labour Relations Board)*, [1993] 3 SCR 327, 107 DLR (4th) 457 is a rare exception.
29. Government of Canada, *Canada's COVID-19 Economic Response Plan* (Ottawa: Government of Canada, 2020), online: *Government of Canada* <https://www.canada.ca/en/department-finance/economic-response-plan.html>.
30. Teresa Wright, "Trudeau Rejects Turning CERB's $2,000 a Month Into a Universal Benefit for Canadians", *National Post* (23 April 2020), online: <https://nationalpost.com/news/universal-benefit-minimum-basic-income-justin-trudeau-cerb>.
31. Ricardo Tranjan, "The Rent Is Due Soon: Economic Insecurity and COVID-19" (2020), online: *Canadian Centre for Policy Alternatives* <https://www.policyalternatives.ca/publications/reports/rent-due-soon>.
32. Tanya Mok, "Toronto Pizza Joint Shuts Down After Not Getting Rent Relief from Landlord" (2 May 2020), online (blog): *Blog TO* <https://www.

Aside from instituting a moratorium on residential evictions and issuing the occasional small subsidy,[33] provinces have been unwilling or unable to do more. Parliament could, by emergency legislation, enact a moratorium on all residential and commercial evictions. It could institute a national regime of rent control, as it did during the Second World War (which the Supreme Court of Canada upheld).[34] Or, it could lift the obligation to pay rent for a period of time.[35]

The Struggle for Nationwide Testing

In the battle against the pandemic, a rallying cry is "testing, testing, testing." Epidemiologists are categorical in stating that testing is core to managing the spread of the virus, safeguarding the health care system, and, eventually, lifting the punishing restrictions on all of us.[36]

Compared to other countries, Canada has had only modest success in achieving the necessary levels of testing.[37] The federal government has tried to assist provinces in procuring supplies and ramping up lab capacity.[38] As with long-term care homes, the federal government could develop guidelines for testing criteria. To actually take over testing from the provinces, however, likely would require a new

---

blogto.com/eat_drink/2020/05/toronto-pizza-joint-shuts-down-after-not-getting-rent-relief-landlord/>.

33. British Columbia achieving the most generous to date, offering up to $500 a month to residential tenants: BC Housing, "Supporting Renters, Landlords During COVID-19" (25 March 2020), online: *BC Housing* <https://www.bchousing.org/news?newsId=1479155088004>. Some provinces have offered nothing.
34. *Reference re Wartime Leasehold Regulations*, [1950] SCR 124, [1950] 2 DLR 1.
35. New Democratic Party, "Ask Justin Trudeau to Stop Payments and Waive Fees" (2020), online: *New Democratic Party* <https://www.ndp.ca/rent-freeze>.
36. Leslie Young, "Social Distancing Is Crucial, but Canada also Needs More Coronavirus Testing: Experts", *Global News* (24 March 2020), online: <https://globalnews.ca/news/6726525/social-distancing-testing-coronavirus/>; Warren Bell, "Robust Testing for COVID-19 Is Critical Missing Link", *National Observer* (10 April 2020), online: <https://www.nationalobserver.com/2020/04/10/opinion/robust-testing-covid-19-critical-missing-link>.
37. Acknowledging that this is a moving target, Canada's performance thus far has not been in the top tier of countries worldwide: Tonda MacCharles, "Canada Must Triple its COVID-19 Testing Before Loosening Restrictions, Experts Say", *Toronto Star* (23 April 2020), online: <https://www.thestar.com/politics/federal/2020/04/22/canada-must-triple-its-covid-19-testing-before-loosening-restrictions-experts-say.html>.
38. Catherine Tunney, "Trudeau Offering Provinces, Territories Help to 'Scale Up' Testing, Contact Tracing", *CBC News* (21 May 2020), online: <https://www.cbc.ca/news/politics/trudeau-testing-contact-tracing-1.5578714>.

legislative framework. The authority to do that is murky. The *Canada Health Act* is primarily a funding and insurance mechanism; it does not enable the federal government to provide health services to the general public.[39] Asserting emergency powers is a straightforward way for Parliament to erect such a regime.

Assessing the Benefits and Drawbacks of Emergency Laws

Benefits: Consistency, Capacity, and Reassurance

There is no question that the COVID-19 pandemic represents a previously unimaginable threat to national well-being. It is not surprising that many would look to the federal government for leadership. To the extent that such leadership was expressed through emergency legislation, it could provide the following benefits.

First, federal emergency laws might bring a welcome measure of *consistency*. Instituting nationwide policies around COVID-19 testing, for example, would address confusion over the criteria by which persons are able to access it.[40] Such consistency might be especially prized when the need to track the course of a disease is constant among subnational units. The aim would be to scale up to the best practices available. The same can be said about economic security: vulnerable persons ought not to receive varying relief simply because of their province of residence.

Second, to the extent that the federal order has greater *capacity*, emergency legislation might be a logical tool to wield it. Current levels of need, especially economic, are far beyond the fiscal envelope of most provinces. The sheer cost of such things as reforming long-term care or

39. *Canada Health Act* RSC, 1985 c C-6. Note the following from the preamble: "WHEREAS the Parliament of Canada recognizes ... that it is not the intention of the Government of Canada that any of the powers, rights, privileges or authorities vested in Canada or the provinces under the provisions of the *Constitution Act, 1867*, or any amendments thereto, or otherwise, be by reason of this Act abrogated or derogated from or in any way impaired..."
40. There are stark differences in per capita testing across the country. Most troublingly, Ontario and Quebec have consistently failed to meet their own targets, and together account for 85% of cases nationwide: Ivan Semeniuk, "COVID-19 Testing Shortfall Spurs Quest for Radical Approaches as Provinces Look to Reopen", *The Globe and Mail* (14 May 2020), online: <https://www.theglobeandmail.com/canada/article-covid-19-testing-shortfall-spurs-quest-for-radical-approaches-as/>. But see Amanda Connoly, "National Coronavirus Testing Strategy Wouldn't Work for Canada, Trudeau Says", *Global News* (7 May 2020), online: <https://globalnews.ca/news/6916991/national-coronavirus-testing-strategy-canada/>.

protecting renters is likely to deter provincial action. While the federal government's resources are not unlimited, it is the country's largest repository of wealth, as well as the greatest generator of revenue.

At the same time, however, it might appear irresponsible for the government to simply transfer funds to the provinces to meet needs as they see fit. Recent programs have been delayed by federal-provincial negotiation over mechanics and details.[41] Passing emergency legislation would provide an immediate framework by which the necessary supports could be supplied.

Finally, an emergency law has an enormous signalling function. In rallying public sentiment or conveying a situation's gravity, such a law has few rivals. When examined closely, the calls for federal intervention can be understood as demands for *reassurance*. COVID-19 has dealt Canada a profound emotional shock. Emergency legislation could increase public confidence that national institutions are fully seized of the issue and are devoting all possible resources to dealing with it.

Drawbacks: Operational Obstacles and Push-Back

While emergency federal legislation can be beneficial, it does have drawbacks and risks. While they do not apply equally to the laws mooted above, they merit serious consideration.

Intuitively, a uniform response should be more coordinated and, therefore, effective. But the nature of a crisis can pose *operational obstacles,* at least two of which are relevant here. First, COVID-19 has not had the same effect across the country.[42] That cuts against the kind of top-down approach that the federal order is best suited to impose. Certainly, it would be counterproductive to roll out a public health response independent of provincial and municipal authorities. Arguably, the actors closest to the relevant populations are best able to both assess relevant needs and vulnerability, and deliver the necessary services.

A second obstacle is that the very nature of the division of powers spurs the different orders of government to develop specialized

41. Ryan Tumulty, "Trudeau Announces Wage Top-ups for Frontline Workers, but Details Unclear", *National Post* (8 May 2020), online: <https://nationalpost.com/news/canada/covid-19-front-line-workers-minimum-wage-top-up>.
42. Patrick Cain, "Coronavirus: How COVID-19 Is Spreading Across Canada", *Global News* (14 April 2020), online: <https://globalnews.ca/news/6700788/coronavirus-covid-19-canada-cases-data/>. Some of the variance may be due to the different levels of testing in the different provinces.

competencies.[43] For example, the ability of the Canada Revenue Agency to design and distribute the CERB to some seven million Canadians in just a few weeks is directly related to the expertise it has developed under the federal taxation power. Conversely, provinces have been delivering health care and ordering private relationships for over a century.[44] It would take considerable time for the federal government to create comparable systems.[45] Indeed, an ongoing emergency may be the worst time to attempt such a transformation.

The differential expertise is compounded by the fact that emergency powers are temporary. Sometimes, that will be sufficient, as with, say, a short-term scheme for rent relief or nationwide testing. Other problems require more durable solutions. The pandemic has highlighted long-standing issues of social inequality and political powerlessness. While seniors, for example, may have more *acute* needs because of COVID-19, those needs predate and will long outlast the virus. That does not, necessarily, argue against short-term relief. But Parliament cannot address such vulnerabilities on an ongoing basis. Absent a constitutional amendment, as was done for old age pensions,[46] Parliament cannot federalize long-term care homes or their workers. The fact that such control will eventually cede to the provinces is an important factor in assessing the utility of intervention. That factor is only heightened when one considers the second risk of emergency legislation.

That risk is the likelihood of provincial *push-back*. The federal-provincial relationship rarely runs smoothly.[47] The depth of current

43. *114957 Canada Ltée (Spraytech, Société d'arrosage) v Hudson (Town)*, 2001 SCC 40 at para 3; see also Alexandra Flynn, this volume, Chapter A-8.
44. To be sure, the federal government does have some expertise in health care, including providing sevices to the military and Indigenous persons, as well as regulating drug and medical devices safety.
45. For a similar argument, see David Robitaille, this volume, Chapter A-4: "Nous voyons mal comment ces mesures pourraient être centralisées entre les mains du gouvernement fédéral qui ne dispose pas toujours de la proximité et des connaissances suffisantes pour agir efficacement sur le plan micro-territorial, d'où l'importance d'institutions provinciales et locales fortes."
46. *Constitution Act, 1867*, *supra* note 5, s 94A.
47. Several provinces have launched constitutional references about the validity of the 2018 *Greenhouse Gas Pollution Pricing Act*, which mandates a national fuel charge and enacts performance standards for large industrial facilities. There have also been difficult disagreements over the Trans Mountain Pipeline expansion and the United Nations Declaration on the Rights of Indigenous Peoples. Carissima Mathen, "Carbon Tax Court References a Chapter in Fed-Prov Power Struggle" (23 May 2019), online: *Policy Options* <https://policyoptions.irpp.org/magazines/may-2019/carbon-tax-court-references-chapter-fed-prov-power-struggle/>;

regional divisions is evident in the makeup of the current Parliament—the governing Liberal caucus has no elected MPs from Saskatchewan or Alberta.

The emergency branch could inflame existing tensions and create new ones. The early days of the pandemic were marked by striking levels of federal-provincial cooperation.[48] But politics inevitably returns. COVID-19 demands a high degree of collaboration among federal, provincial, and municipal actors.[49] The federal government bears a particular responsibility to ensure a functional relationship with provinces. To be sure, when provincial failures imperil the country, or certain of its citizens, the federal government should intervene.[50] But it cannot afford to appear dismissive or cavalier about provincial jurisdiction. It is no accident that the current *Emergencies Act* requires extensive consultation with provincial governments.[51] While not a constitutional imperative, it creates a political expectation of cooperation, around which the federal order must tread carefully.

The title of this chapter invokes the siren: a mythological creature with powerful, ceaseless attraction. In *The Odyssey*, Ulysses bound himself to the mast of his ship to resist her call, even as he was forced to navigate close to it.[52] Even when they must be contemplated, emergency powers demand similar restraint. In the current pandemic, the emergency branch may enable decisive action to mitigate staggering social and personal costs.[53] But absent provincial buy-in, such action risks significant national friction that could threaten the cooperation required to vanquish COVID-19.

Carissima Mathen, *Courts Without Cases: The Law and Politics of Advisory Opinions* (Oxford: Hart, 2019) at chapter 5; *Reference re Greenhouse Gas Pollution Pricing Act*, 2019 SKCA 40; *Reference re Environmental Management Act*, 2020 SCC 1.

48. Éric Grenier, "The Pandemic Is Breaking Down Political Barriers Between Provincial and Federal Governments", *CBC News* (5 April 2020), online: <https://www.cbc.ca/news/politics/grenier-provincial-federal-cooperation-1.5521531>. But see Christopher Nardi, "'Why Would He Pick a Fight with Us?' COVID-19 Raises Tensions Between Trudeau Government and Quebec", *National Post* (8 May 2020), online: <https://nationalpost.com/news/politics/why-would-he-pick-a-fight-with-us-covid-19-raises-tensions-between-trudeau-government-and-quebec>.
49. On the exercise of municipal powers, see Flynn, this volume, Chapter A-8.
50. Arguably, the lack of a coordinated scheme to collect data on COVID-19 qualifies. See Amir Attaran & Adam R Houston, this volume, Chapter A-5.
51. See Flood & Thomas, this volume, Chapter A-6.
52. Homer, *The Odyssey*. See also Jon Elster, *Ulysses and the Sirens: Studies in Rationality and Irrationality* (Cambridge, UK: Cambridge University Press, 1984).
53. See Flood & Thomas, this volume, Chapter A-6.

CHAPTER A-8

Municipal Power and Democratic Legitimacy in the Time of COVID-19*

Alexandra Flynn**

Abstract

As COVID-19 swept through Canada, cities were at the front lines in curbing its spread. From March 2020, municipalities introduced such measures as restricting park access, ticketing those lingering in public places, and enforcing physical distancing requirements. Local governments have also supplemented housing for the vulnerable and given support to local "main street" businesses. Citizens expected their local governments to respond to the pandemic, but few people know how constrained the powers of municipalities are in Canadian law. Municipalities are a curious legal construct in Canadian federalism. Under the Constitution, they are considered to be nothing more than "creatures of the province." However, courts have decided in many cases that local decisions are often considered governmental and given deference. This chapter focuses on the tensions in this contradictory role when it comes to municipal responses to COVID-19, particularly when those responses take the form of closure of public spaces, increased policing by by-law officers, and fines. I conclude that municipalities serve an important role in pandemic responses,

* Many thanks to Mariana Valverde, Colleen M. Flood, and an anonymous peer reviewer for their thoughtful comments and suggestions. All errors and omissions are my own.

** Assistant Professor, Allard School of Law, UBC.

alongside provincial and federal governments. Provincial law should be amended to capture the important role of municipalities in Canadian federalism, especially in the area of municipal finance.

Résumé
Pouvoirs municipaux et légitimité démocratique à l'ère de la COVID-19

Lorsque la COVID-19 a traversé le Canada, les municipalités ont été en première ligne pour freiner sa propagation. À compter de mars 2020, elles ont adopté certaines mesures, comme la restriction de l'accès aux parcs, l'émission de contraventions en cas de regroupements dans les lieux publics et l'application des règles de distanciation physique. Les administrations municipales ont également mis un plus grand nombre de logements à la disposition des personnes vulnérables et ont soutenu les entreprises locales. Les citoyens attendaient de leurs gouvernements locaux qu'ils réagissent à la pandémie, mais peu d'entre eux savent à quel point les pouvoirs des municipalités sont limités dans la loi canadienne. Les municipalités sont une étrange construction juridique au sein du fédéralisme canadien. En vertu de la Constitution, elles sont considérées comme de simples « créatures des provinces ». Cependant, à plusieurs occasions, les tribunaux ont jugé que les décisions prises par les autorités locales comptaient comme des décisions gouvernementales qui, à ce titre, doivent être respectées. Ce chapitre porte sur les tensions de ce rôle contradictoire lorsqu'il s'agit, pour les municipalités, de réagir à la COVID-19, en particulier quand ces réactions se traduisent par la fermeture de lieux publics, l'intensification des interventions par les agents chargés d'appliquer les règlements et l'imposition d'amendes. Je conclus que les municipalités jouent un rôle important en temps de pandémie, aux côtés des gouvernements provinciaux et fédéral. Les lois provinciales devraient être modifiées pour tenir compte du rôle primordial des municipalités au sein du fédéralisme canadien, en particulier dans le domaine des finances municipales.

Municipal councils have a perplexing role within Canada's federal system, stemming from the constitution.[1] On the one hand, under s. 92 of the *Constitution Act*, "In each Province the Legislature may exclusively make Laws in relation to Matters coming within the Classes of Subjects next hereinafter enumerated," which includes "Municipal Institutions in the Province."[2] Provincial governments and some courts have interpreted this section to mean that provinces alone set the rules regarding what municipalities can and cannot do. On the other hand, much jurisprudence from the Supreme Court of Canada (SCC) has referenced municipalities as "governments," giving deference to municipal decision makers on the grounds that local governments are closest to the people and thus aware of the on-the-ground realities that residents face.

This chapter focuses on the conflicting legal position vis-à-vis municipal authorities and puts it in the context of the role municipalities have played in addressing COVID-19. First, I situate municipal authority within Canadian federalism based on jurisprudence and legislation. Next, I discuss how selected Canadian cities have responded to the crisis, focusing on the closure of public space, fines for violating physical distancing by-laws, and increased policing. I conclude that despite lacking proper authority and proper stable funding, municipalities are playing a governmental role in response to the pandemic within a complex intergovernmental landscape that includes federal and provincial governments, First Nations, and public bodies like health authorities. Moving forward, cities must be granted clear authority within provincial legislation, including powers to declare emergencies and secure revenue, in part to ensure that the needs of the most vulnerable are considered.

Municipal Authority in Canada

The *Constitution Act, 1867* provides that municipal institutions in a province are within that province's exclusive jurisdiction, which legally speaking makes them administrative bodies subject to judicial review.[3] Provinces set out municipal authority in legislation, often a

1. Ron Levi & Mariana Valverde, "Freedom of the City: Canadian Cities and the Quest for Governmental Status" (2006) 44 Osgoode Hall LJ 409.
2. *Constitution Act, 1867* (UK), 30 & 31 Vict, c 3, reprinted in RSC 1985, Appendix II, No 5, s 92(8).
3. See, e.g. *R v Greenbaum*, [1993] 1 SCR 674 at 688-689, 100 DLR (4th) 183; *Shell Canada Products Ltd v Vancouver (City)*, 1994 1 SCR 231, 110 DLR (4th) 1; *Nanaimo*

general act that applies to all municipalities, and retain the power to override local decisions. Many larger cities, such as Montréal, have been granted more expansive powers, including more options for raising revenue and greater oversight in such matters as infrastructure and housing.[4] In addition to municipal acts, numerous other pieces of legislation enable local governments.[5] Legislation may also empower such bodies as health authorities or school boards, which overlap with municipal power.

Municipalities must act within jurisdictional limits or courts will "quash municipal action as *ultra vires*, or beyond its legal competence."[6] The notion of cities as "creatures of the province" was articulated by the Ontario Superior Court in *East York v Ontario (AG)*, a challenge to the unilateral amalgamation of six municipalities into the "megacity" of Toronto, which set out four principles regarding the constitutional status of municipalities: (i) municipal institutions lack constitutional status; (ii) municipal institutions are creatures of the legislature and exist only if provincial legislation so provides; (iii) municipal institutions have no independent autonomy and their powers are subject to abolition or repeal by provincial legislation; and (iv) municipal institutions may exercise only those powers which are conferred upon them by statute.[7]

Despite these purportedly blunt lines of authority set out in the constitution, the SCC has acknowledged numerous times that municipalities are democratic governments that represent their residents.[8] The SCC has carved out a distinct role for local democracies, with municipal decisions almost always judicially reviewed on a standard

---

(City) v Rascal Trucking Ltd, 2000 SCC 13; *114957 Canada Ltée (Spraytech, Société d'arrosage) v Hudson (Town)*, 2001 SCC 40 [*Spraytech*].

4. See e.g. *Municipal Government Act*, RSO 1990, c M-26; *Charter of Ville de Montréal*, RSO 2000, c 56, Schedule I, c C-11.4; *City of Toronto Act, 2006*, SO 2006, c 11, Schedule A at s 1(1).
5. See e.g. *Planning Act*, RSO 1990, c P.13 and *Municipal Conflict of Interest Act*, RSO 1990, c M.50, which apply to all Ontario municipalities.
6. Stanley Makuch, Neil Craik & Signe B Leisk, *Canadian Municipal and Planning Law* (Toronto: Thomson Carswell, 2004) at 81.
7. *East York v Ontario (AG)* (1997), 34 OR (3d) 789, 76 ACWS (3d) 1020 (Gen Div); aff'd (1997), 36 OR (3d) 733, 153 DLR (4th) 299 (CA); leave to appeal to SCC refused ([1998] 1 SCR vii at 797-98), see Supreme Court of Canada, "Bulletin of April 9, 1998" (1998), online: *Supreme Court of Canada* <https://decisions.scc-csc.ca/scc-csc/bulletins/en/item/166/index.do?q=east+york+%28borough%29>.
8. See e.g. *Pacific National Investment Ltd v Victoria (City)*, 2000 SCC 64, reconsideration/rehearing refused.

of reasonableness.[9] In interpreting municipal action through a deferential lens, however, the SCC has applied the language of the constitution as a "living tree"[10] that must be "tailored to the changing political and cultural realities of Canadian society," and "continually be reassessed in light of the fundamental values it was designed to serve."[11]

The SCC has applied the principles of cooperative federalism and subsidiarity in order to characterize municipalities as stewards of the local community.[12] In *Canadian Western Bank v Alberta*, the SCC explained, "The fundamental objectives of federalism were, and still are, to reconcile unity with diversity, promote democratic participation by reserving meaningful powers to the local or regional level and to foster co-operation among governments and legislatures for the common good."[13] Courts are careful to state that an expansive view of municipal authority must not "invent municipal authority where none exists."[14] But once municipalities are created and empowered, constitutional principles imbue respect for their decisions.

The respect given to municipalities by the courts is rooted in the closeness of citizens to local governments and the democratic and representative nature of their decision-making. The SCC stated that subsidiarity operates as a principle affirming that "legislative action is to be taken by the government that is closest to the citizen and is thus considered to be in the best position to respond to the citizen's concerns."[15] However, the principle may not be used to override the division of powers in the constitution.[16] Even before COVID-19 came to cities across Canada, spatial poverty, discrepancies in racial diversity, and a lack of affordable housing across neighbourhoods and communities were evident in large urban areas.[17] The SCC's rationale

9. *Catalyst Paper Corp v North Cowichan (District)*, 2012 SCC 2, recently referenced by the SCC in *Canada (Minister of Citizenship and Immigration) v Vavilov*, 2019 SCC 65 at para 108.
10. *Edwards v Attorney-General for Canada*, [1930] 1 DLR 98, [1930] AC 124.
11. *Ibid.*
12. See e.g. *Canadian Western Bank v Alberta*, 2007 SCC 22 (CanLII) at paras 22-23.
13. *Ibid.*
14. *Spraytech*, *supra* note 4 at 366.
15. See *Reference re Assisted Human Reproduction Act*, 2010 SCC 61 at para 183.
16. *Ibid* at para 72.
17. See e.g. Alan Walks, *Income Inequality and Polarization in Canada's Cities: An Examination and New Form of Measurement* (Toronto: University of Toronto Cities Centre, 2013), online (pdf): <https://perma.cc/9J35-3VZJ>; and David Hulchanski, *The Three Cities Within Toronto: Income Polarization among Toronto's Neighbourhoods, 1970–2005* (Toronto: University of Toronto Cities Centre, 2010); and Roger Keil, Melissa Ollevier & Erica Tsang, "Why Is There No Environmental Justice in

for deference to municipalities is reflected in enhanced local aid for the most vulnerable during COVID-19.

Municipal Responses to COVID-19

Globally, COVID-19 was first felt in cities, which are home to over 50% of the world's population and have dense populations living in close proximity to one another. In Canada, municipalities swiftly introduced strict measures to curb COVID-19's expansion based on their spheres of authority, including closing playgrounds and increasing shelter beds. In contrast to the experience in the United States, Canadian cities have worked in partnership with federal and provincial governments, and with public health agencies, throughout the pandemic.[18] Table A8.1 (p. 138) summarizes selected measures introduced by eight large municipalities in the country.[19]

The following observations can be drawn regarding municipal responses to COVID-19. First, most municipalities declared states of emergency at a similar time to those introduced by federal and provincial governments.[20] States of emergency permit governments at all levels to "prevent, reduce or mitigate a danger of major proportions that could result in serious harm to people or property" without the usual checks and balances of the political process.[21] Municipalities must declare states of emergency within the limits prescribed by provincial limitations.[22] Almost all local Ontario governments, regardless of size, have made declarations. In contrast, the Province of British Columbia suspended municipal states of emergency other than in Vancouver,

---

Canada?" in Julian Agyeman et al, eds, *Speaking for Ourselves: Environmental Justice in Canada* (Vancouver: University of British Columbia Press, 2009) at 78.

18. Robert Schertzer & Mireille Paquet, "How Well Is Canada's Intergovernmental System Handling the Crisis?", *Policy Options* (8 April 2020), online: <https://policyoptions.irpp.org/magazines/april-2020/how-well-is-canadas-intergovernmental-system-handling-the-crisis/>; Gabriel Eidelman & Jack Lucas, "Municipal Leaders Happy with Team Canada Approach to COVID", *Policy Options* (1 May 2020), online: <https://policyoptions.irpp.org/magazines/may-2020/municipal-leaders-happy-with-team-canada-response-to-covid/>.
19. Canadian Urban Institute, "City Watch Canada" (last visited 1 May 2020), online: *City Watch Canada* <https://citywatchcanada.ca>.
20. Michael Watts, Susan Newell & Amanda Arella, "The Ontario State of Emergency–COVID-19" (3 April 2020), online: *Osler, Hoskin & Harcourt LLP* <https://www.osler.com/en/resources/critical-situations/2020/the-ontario-state-of-emergency-covid-19>.
21. *Ibid.*
22. *Emergency Management and Civil Protection Act*, RSO 1990, c E9, s 4(1).

which has its own charter, is a big city, and has highlighted vulnerable people living in the downtown eastside.[23] British Columbia's rationale was that the COVID-19 response required a consistent approach across communities, much to the chagrin of smaller municipalities who do not think provincial coordination is sufficiently responsive to local needs.[24]

Ensuring a uniform regulation across the province was critical in the early days of the pandemic, especially given the close proximity of municipalities to one another in denser areas. However, municipal states of emergency may provide enhanced protection for local residents not captured at the provincial scale. This is especially important as prohibitions are lifted and smaller communities experience a greater influx of visitors. Some municipalities fear an influx of tourists and visitors, a concern that does not apply uniformly across the province and that has the potential to overwhelm local services.[25] For example, over two dozen leaders of smaller coastal towns and First Nations urged the Province of British Columbia to limit outside travel "for fishing, hunting and other leisure activities" into their communities following COVID-19 infections in small towns elsewhere, a request that was not granted.[26] Local states of emergency enable municipalities to address the specific needs of local communities, which differ dramatically from one another in geographic size, population, density, levels of tourism, and socio-economic disparity.[27] Provinces may not be as aware of the needs of particular localities.

---

23. McCarthy Tetreault, "COVID-19: Emergency Measures Tracker" (last updated 11 May 2020), online: *McCarthy Tetrault* <https://www.mccarthy.ca/en/insights/articles/covid-19-emergency-measures-tracker>. See also Government of British Columbia, "COVID-19: Frequently Asked Questions related to Provincial Orders" (last updated 8 May 2020), online: *Government of British Columbia* <https://www2.gov.bc.ca/gov/content/safety/emergency-preparedness-response-recovery/local-emergency-programs/local-government-first-nations-faq/provincial-orders-faq>, citing *Emergency Program Act*, RSBC 1996, Ch 111, s 14.
24. Joel Ballard, "Coastal First Nations and Municipalities Vow Continued COVID-19 Enforcement, Potential Hwy 16 Checkpoint", *CBC News* (1 May 2020), online: <https://www.cbc.ca/news/canada/british-columbia/haida-nation-enforcement-hwy-16-1.5552247>.
25. See e.g. District of Tofino, "COVID-19 Updates" (29 March 2020), online: *District of Tofino* <http://tofino.ca/blog/view/covid-19-updates>.
26. Natalia Balcerzak, "'We Don't Understand': B.C. Coastal Communities Brace for Tourists as Province Opens Hunting, Fishing Season", *The Narwhal* (28 April 2020), online: <https://thenarwhal.ca/coronavirus-bc-coastal-communities-brace-tourists-province-hunting-fishing-season/>.
27. Nathaniel Basen, "COVID-19: The Week in Review with Epidemiologist David Fisman (May 17–22)", *TVO* (23 May 2020), online: <https://www.tvo.org/article/covid-19-the-week-in-review-with-epidemiologist-david-fisman-may-17-22>.

Second, enforcement of physical distancing by-laws or rules made under provincial emergency powers differs across the country.[28] Some local governments have focused on using "snitch lines," where residents are encouraged to report transgressive behaviour to local authorities. And while cities have limited public amenities like playgrounds, local governments differ on their approach to outdoor movement. For example, Vancouver residents have been given greater use of parks, sidewalks, and bike paths than those in Montréal, Toronto, and Ottawa.[29] Municipalities also differ in their focus on sanctions. In some cities, residents who violate physical distancing rules—like sitting on park benches—are issued heavy fines or threats of imprisonment.[30] In contrast, other municipalities focus on educating the public through signage and warnings rather than sanctions.

Third, Canada's large cities recognize that particular populations require proactive assistance, in particular those experiencing homelessness, who were identified as especially vulnerable in previous Canadian pandemics.[31] Each city has introduced specific aid in the form of shelter space or hotel rooms. Missing are services for the vast number of low-income seniors, young people, and precariously employed persons, who have been most affected by library and community centre closures that deprive many of Internet access and a warm place to spend their days.[32] Cities are not yet responding to the broad range of needs experienced by vulnerable people, due to a lack of secure funding. Canadian pandemics such as H1N1 revealed great disparity in their effects on vulnerable people, especially low-income and racialized people.[33] Researchers are tracking the policing

---

28. See e.g. City of Ottawa, "State of Emergency: COVID-19 in Ottawa" (last visited 21 May 2020), online: *City of Ottawa* <https://ottawa.ca/en/health-and-public-safety/covid-19-ottawa/rules-and-restrictions>.
29. Canadian Urban Institute, *supra* note 19. See also National Capital Commission, "Update: Queen Elizabeth Driveway Pilot Project", online: *National Capital Commission* <https://ncc-ccn.gc.ca/closures/pilot-project-temporary-closure-queen-elizabeth-driveway-motor-vehicle-traffic>.
30. McCarthy Tetreault, *supra* note 23.
31. Kristy E Buccieri & Rebecca Schiff, eds, *Pandemic Preparedness and Homelessness: Lessons from H1N1 in Canada* (Toronto: Canadian Observatory on Homelessness Press, 2016).
32. Rob Gillezeau, Lindsay Tedds & Gilliant Petit, "Here's How Municipalities Should Respond to COVID-19", *Policy Options* (23 April 2020), online: <https://policyoptions.irpp.org/magazines/april-2020/heres-how-municipalities-should-respond-to-covid-19/>.
33. Janet E Mosher, "Accessing Justice amid Threats of Contagion" (2014) 51:3 Osgoode Hall LJ 919.

of provincial public health and emergency laws related to COVID-19 in Canadian cities to see whether particular populations are disproportionately affected.[34]

Fourth, all of the canvassed municipalities cite significant financial impacts from the pandemics. Most notable is a reduction in property tax payments, which accounts for 70% of municipal budgets. Local governments are also obtaining less revenue through fees, as many cities stopped enforcement of parking fees, have cancelled fee-paying recreation programs, and halted permits. Many municipalities have introduced layoffs to reduce operating expenses.[35] While provincial and federal governments have also experienced a loss of revenue, they are able to run deficits. Municipalities cannot do so and are hence very limited in their ability to raise revenue. The financial impact of COVID-19 should be taken as a reason for provincial governments to change outmoded legislation that prevents even the largest cities from engaging in the same deficit financing practices that ordinary citizens with mortgages take for granted.

Democratic Legitimacy in the Time of COVID-19

Cities are one of many responders in a federal model that includes federal and provincial governments, First Nations, and administrative bodies such as boards of health and school boards. Emergency legislation exposes the tensions in the municipal responses to COVID-19. Local governments are entrusted to bypass usual processes to immediately address matters of public safety if the matter can be addressed at that scale. For example, Ontario's act provides that "A declaration

34. Alex Luscombe & Alexander McClelland, "Policing the Pandemic Enforcement Report, April 14, 2020 -May 1, 2020" (2020), online: *Policing the Pandemic Mapping Project* <www.policingthepandemic.ca>. "Snitch lines" refer to encouragement by municipalities to report alleged COVID-19 violations to a dedicated phone or online "snitch line", or to general municipal information lines. COVID-19 violations may be municipal or provincial.
35. See e.g. Josh Pringle "4,280 Part-Time City of Ottawa Employees Laid off Due to COVID-19 Pandemic", *CTV News* (6 April 2020), online: <https://ottawa.ctvnews.ca/4-280-part-time-city-of-ottawa-employees-laid-off-due-to-covid-19-pandemic-1.4884667>; Jeremy Thompson, "City of Edmonton Temporarily Lays off 900 More Staff as $163M Shortfall Looms", *CTV News* (27 April 2020), online: <https://edmonton.ctvnews.ca/city-of-edmonton-temporarily-lays-off-900-more-staff-as-163m-shortfall-looms-1.4913647>; and Sean Kavanagh, "Nearly 700 City of Winnipeg Workers Receive Layoff Notices", *CBC* (15 April 2020), online: <https://www.cbc.ca/news/canada/manitoba/city-winnipeg-layoff-staff-covid-finances-1.5533139>.

of emergency should be made at the lowest level of jurisdiction."[36] It is up to the province alone to decide if a municipal order is valid.[37] This leaves a great deal of discretion to provinces to override local expertise.[38]

In my view, municipalities should have greater protection in two ways in order to affirm their important role in Canadian federalism. First, the principle of cooperative federalism is not enshrined in legislation and thus stands on shaky ground. Certain matters require provincial or federal attention based on scale.[39] However, legislative design can affirm local expertise in matters delegated to municipal governments without contravening emergency responses at the provincial scale. For example, the Province of British Columbia upheld Vancouver's state of emergency based in part on the city's unique legislative basis, the *Vancouver Charter*, and because it respects the city's expertise in responding to the needs of particular populations.[40] Other Canadian provinces have upheld municipal states of emergency on matters that do not conflict with provincial or federal orders.

Second, municipalities, which all across Canada enjoy good credit ratings and thus low interest rates, are also limited in their power to raise revenue, which will constrain their ability to introduce the measures that they identify as necessary. Despite the size of their governments, large cities may not carry deficits and thus will require provincial bailouts. Canadian cities have long advocated for legislative reform with respect to municipal finance and COVID-19 may be the impetus to do so.[41] These reforms will enable municipalities to exercise their important role in pandemic response, particularly when it comes to the needs of the most vulnerable.

---

36. *Emergency Management and Civil Protection Act, supra* note 22.
37. *Ibid*, s 4(4).
38. Note an upcoming leave to appeal that may impact provincial override of municipal decisions: *City of Toronto v Attorney General of Ontario* (2020) leave accepted by the Supreme Court of Canada (38921).
39. See Carissima Mathen, Chapter A-7 this volume.
40. Government of British Columbia, *supra* note 23.
41. See e.g. Keith Gerein, "COVID-19 Has Exposed the Weaknesses in How We Treat Municipalities", *Edmonton Journal* (9 May 2020), online: <https://edmontonjournal.com/news/local-news/keith-gerein-covid-19-has-exposed-the-weaknesses-in-how-we-treat-municipalities/>; Enid Slack & Tomas Hachard, "COVID-19 Crisis Creates Chance to Re-Examine Provincial Funding of Cities", *The Toronto Star* (6 April 2020), online: <https://www.thestar.com/opinion/contributors/2020/04/06/covid-19-crisis-creates-chance-to-re-examine-provincial-funding-of-cities.html>.

Conclusion

In their responses to COVID-19, the role of municipalities in taking action to represent the interests of their local communities has never been so clear. Local governments are acting as stewards of local communities, including working cooperatively with other governments to provide support for the most vulnerable. In the early days of COVID-19, provinces have generally reflected provincial respect for the local role. However, gaps have been exposed. To ensure a protected role within Canadian federalism, including securing enhanced funding tools for municipalities, provincial legislation must be amended to secure their responses to local emergencies and to raise revenue, particularly for larger cities. Legislative design of emergency legislation can ensure that municipal responses are tailored to their local communities and do not conflict with provincial action.

Table A8.1 Municipal responses to COVID-19 (to May 11, 2020)

	Municipal state of emergency[42]	Physical distancing by-laws[43]	"Snitch" line[44]	Focus on fines and sanctions[45]	Assistance for the most vulnerable[46]	Projected deficit
Halifax	No	No	No	Yes	Yes	Yes[47]
Montréal	Yes	No	Yes	Yes	Yes	No[48]
Ottawa	Yes	No	Yes	Yes	Yes	Yes[49]
Toronto	Yes	Yes	Yes	Yes	Yes	Yes[50]
Winnipeg	Yes	Yes	No	No	Yes	Yes[51]
Calgary	Yes	Yes	No	No	Yes	Yes[52]
Edmonton	Yes	Yes	Yes	No	Yes	Yes[53]
Vancouver	Yes	Yes	Yes	No	Yes	Yes[54]

42. Canadian Urban Institute, "City Watch Canada" (last visited 1 May 2020), online: *City Watch Canada* <https://citywatchcanada.ca>.
43. *Ibid.*
44. Luscombe & McLellan, *supra* note 34.
45. *Ibid;* Canadian Urban Institute, *supra* note 19.
46. *Ibid.*
47. City of Halifax Budget Committee, *Proposed 2020/21 Budget Recast for COVID-19 Impacts* (Halifax: City of Halifax, 2020) at 8, online (pdf): Halifax <https://www.halifax.ca/sites/default/files/documents/city-hall/regional-council/200512bc3.pdf>.
48. Amy Luft, "Montreal Plans to Cut Spending to Make up for COVID-19 Revenue Losses", *CTV News* (23 April 2020), online: <https://montreal.ctvnews.ca/montreal-plans-to-cut-spending-to-make-up-for-covid-19-revenue-losses-1.4908984>.
49. Josh Pringle, "City of Ottawa Facing Multi-Million Dollar Budget Deficit Due to COVID-19", *CTV News* (22 April 2020), online: <https://ottawa.ctvnews.ca/city-of-ottawa-facing-multi-million-dollar-budget-deficit-due-to-covid-19-1.4906957>.
50. Oliver Moore, "Pandemic Could Push Toronto's Budget Shortfall to Nearly $2.8-billion, Mayor Says", *The Globe and Mail* (17 April 2020), online: <https://www.theglobeandmail.com/canada/article-pandemic-could-push-torontos-budget-shortfall-to-nearly-28-billion/>.
51. Sean Kavanagh, "Winnipeg City Council Report Shows Losses in Millions Because of COVID-19", CBC (2 April 2020), online: <https://www.cbc.ca/news/canada/manitoba/city-winnipeg-report-tax-deferral-lost-revenue-covid-1.5519266>.
52. Adam MacVicar, "City of Calgary Facing $235M Financial Gap if Pandemic Continues Through December", *Global News* (30 April 2020), online: <https://globalnews.ca/news/6889351/calgary-235m-financial-gap-covid-pandemic-december/>.
53. Jeremey Thompson, "City of Edmonton Temporarily Lays off 900 More Staff as $163M Shortfall Looms", *CTV News* (27 April 2020), online: <https://edmonton.ctvnews.ca/city-of-edmonton-temporarily-lays-off-900-more-staff-as-163m-shortfall-looms-1.4913647>.
54. City of Vancouver, News Release, "Council Approves Delay in Property Tax Payment Deadline to September 30" (29 April 2020), online: *City of Vancouver* <https://vancouver.ca/news-calendar/council-approves-delay-in-property-tax-payment-deadline-to-september-30.aspx>.

SECTION B

MAKING SURE SOMEONE IS ACCOUNTABLE: PUBLIC AND PRIVATE RESPONSIBILITIES

CHAPTER B-1

Ensuring Executive and Legislative Accountability in a Pandemic*

Vanessa MacDonnell**

Abstract

Holding the executive and the legislature to account is a perennial challenge in an emergency. Even by emergency standards, however, COVID-19 has presented serious accountability challenges. The current situation raises questions about how we ensure that the executive and Parliament are held accountable in a public health crisis like the one COVID-19 has precipitated. I explore some of these questions in this chapter. In doing so, I attempt a fair assessment of the challenges the executive and Parliament face in such a crisis, and suggest ways that nodes of accountability might be found both within and outside the political branches when they are not operating as usual.

* I am grateful to Amelia Calbry-Muzyka for her excellent research assistance, to Mel Cappe, Paul Daly, Jennifer A. Quaid, Stephen Bindman, and Charlie Feldman for their helpful comments, and to the peer reviewers for their suggestions for improvement. The facts in this chapter are current to May 23, 2020.

** Associate Professor, University of Ottawa Faculty of Law and Co-Director, uOttawa Public Law Centre.

Résumé
Tenir les pouvoirs exécutif et législatif responsables en situation de pandémie

Il s'agit d'un défi continu d'exiger que les pouvoirs exécutif et législatif soient tenus responsables de leurs décisions en situation d'urgence. La COVID-19 a posé de sérieux problèmes en matière de reddition de comptes. La situation actuelle soulève des questions sur la manière de garantir que les pouvoirs exécutif et législatif sont tenus responsables dans le contexte d'une crise de santé publique comme celle dans laquelle la COVID-19 nous a plongés. J'explore certaines de ces questions dans ce chapitre. Ce faisant, je tente d'évaluer de manière juste les défis auxquels ces pouvoirs sont confrontés lors d'une telle crise, et je suggère des moyens pour trouver des axes de responsabilité, tant au sein des pouvoirs politiques qu'ailleurs, lorsque les circonstances sont exceptionnelles.

Holding the executive and the legislature to account is a perennial challenge in an emergency.[1] The executive typically has a significant margin to respond to an unfolding crisis using authority already granted to it by the legislature.[2] Where additional authority (especially authority to spend) is required, the usual processes of pre-legislative and legislative scrutiny may be compressed or simply scuttled.[3] Bills are drafted hastily, reviewed by legislators quickly or not all, and enacted.[4] It then falls to the courts, and possibly keen

1. On the various meanings of accountability in a parliamentary system, see Carol Harlow, "Accountability and Constitutional Law" in Mark Bovens, Robert E Goodin & Thomas Schillemans, eds, *The Oxford Handbook of Public Accountability* (Oxford: Oxford University Press, 2014) 195.
2. I am grateful to Charlie Feldman for pointing this out to me.
3. On the "usual" processes, see Gabrielle Appleby, "An excellent @auspublaw-blog post by Andrew Edgar explaining how Cth & NSW have implemented emergency public health measures. An important call-out for public lawyers to scrutinise these measures as ordinary accountability mechanisms don't apply. https://auspublaw.org/2020/03/law-making-in-a-crisis-commonwealth-and-nsw-coronavirus-regulations/" (29 March 2020 at 20:26), online: *Twitter* <twitter.com/Gabrielle_J_A/status/1244420785462063105>.
4. See generally Stephen Gardbaum, "Comparative Political Process Theory" [2020] Intl J Constitutional L [forthcoming in 2020], online: *SSRN* <papers.ssrn.com/sol3/papers.cfm?abstract_id=3596328>; Thomas Kaplan, "Congressional Leaders Agree on $1.3 Trillion Spending Bill as Deadline Looms", *The New York*

parliamentary committees, to determine *post hoc* whether the political branches overreached.

All of these elements have been evident in the federal government's and Parliament's initial responses to COVID-19.[5] Even by emergency standards, however, the pandemic has presented serious accountability challenges. The public health crisis initially prompted the adjournment of the Senate and the House of Commons and the near-total closure of the courts.[6] Prime Minister Trudeau and some members of his Cabinet were forced to self-isolate after potential exposure to COVID-19. In the weeks that followed, the political parties engaged in protracted discussions about how they might meet safely to enact further legislation to deal with the social and economic fallout of the pandemic.[7]

At the time of writing, some two months after the initial lockdown, progress has been made toward resuming normal operations. The Senate and the House of Commons are sitting periodically, and some committee hearings have resumed, mostly online.[8] While a range of matters are proceeding in virtual courtrooms, the courts remain closed for in-person hearings.[9] But at a moment when the federal government is both exercising extraordinary powers and seeking new powers to respond to the pandemic, the principal means of accountability—parliamentary debate, scrutiny by a parliamentary committee, and judicial review[10]—remain hobbled.

The current situation raises questions about how we ensure that the executive and the legislature are held accountable in a public

---

Times (21 March 2018), online: <www.nytimes.com/2018/03/21/us/politics/congress-spending-deal-government-shutdown.html>; Ian Dunt, "'You Don't Even Know What You're Voting For': MP Paints Damning Portrait of Life in Westminster", *Politics* (16 June 2013), online: <politics.co.uk/news/2013/06/16/you-don-t-even-know-what-you-re-voting-for>.

5. See Paul Thomas, "Parliament Under Pressure: Evaluating Parliament's performance in Response to COVID-19" (3 April 2020), online: *Samara Canada* <www.samaracanada.com/democracy-monitor/parliament-under-pressure> [Thomas, "Parliament Under Pressure"].
6. *Ibid.*
7. *Ibid.*
8. *Ibid.*
9. See Amy Salyzyn, "'Trial by Zoom': What Virtual Hearings Might Mean for Open Courts, Participant Privacy and the Integrity of Court Proceedings", *Slaw* (17 April 2020), online: <www.slaw.ca/2020/04/17/trial-by-zoom-what-virtual-hearings-might-mean-for-open-courts-participant-privacy-and-the-integrity-of-court-proceedings>.
10. See generally Appleby, *supra* note 3.

health crisis like the one COVID-19 has precipitated. I explore some of these questions in this chapter. In doing so, I attempt a fair assessment of the challenges the executive and Parliament face in such a crisis, and suggest ways that nodes of accountability might be found both within and outside the political branches when they are not operating as usual. My discussion here is focused on accountability in the sense of ensuring the lawfulness of legislation and executive action.[11] It is important to note, however, that robust oversight also enhances the quality of executive action and legislation quite apart from any question of lawfulness. In an emergency, both forms of oversight are crucial, as there is a risk both of overreach and of errors made in haste.

At the same time, it is important to be realistic about how much oversight is possible in the initial stages of a pandemic.[12] In a national emergency, vigorous opposition by politicians or push-back from the courts may be perceived as unpatriotic. Since the beginning of the outbreak, governments at all levels have spoken of the importance of adopting a "Team Canada" approach to COVID-19. This has resulted in an unusual level of cooperation between and across orders of government.[13] This collaborative spirit has extended across the aisle in Parliament. While there are obvious benefits to such an approach, there are also drawbacks, the most significant of which is the risk of weaker oversight.[14] This can be detrimental to civil rights and to the separation of powers in both the short and long terms.[15]

---

11. See generally Yee-Fui Ng, "Political Constitutionalism: Individual Responsibility and Collective Restraint" Federal L Rev [forthcoming in 2020]; Paul Daly, this volume, Chapter B-6.
12. On the need to view these issues through a temporal lens, see Colleen M Flood, Bryan Thomas & Kumanan Wilson, this volume, Chapter C-1; Gabrielle Appleby, Vanessa MacDonnell & Ed Synot, "The Pervasive Constitution: The Constitution Outside the Courts", Federal L Rev [forthcoming in 2020].
13. See e.g. "Alberta to Send Personal Protective Equipment to Ontario, Quebec, B.C.", *CBC News* (11 April 2019), online: <www.cbc.ca/news/canada/edmonton/alberta-to-send-personal-protective-equipment-to-ontario-quebec-b-c-1.5529989>; Susan Delacourt, "'He's My Therapist': How Chrystia Freeland and Doug Ford Forged an Unlikely Friendship in the Fight Against COVID-19", *Toronto Star* (3 April 2020), online: <www.thestar.com/news/insight/2020/04/03/hes-my-therapist-how-chrystia-freeland-and-doug-ford-forged-an-unlikely-friendship-in-the-fight-against-covid-19.html>.
14. Oren Gross & Fionnuala Ní Aoláin, *Law in Times of Crisis: Emergency Powers in Theory and Practice* (Cambridge, UK: Cambridge University Press, 2006).
15. See generally Mark Tushnet, "Emergencies and the Idea of Constitutionalism" in Mark Tushnet, ed, *The Constitution in Wartime: Beyond Alarmism and Complacency* (Durham & London: Duke University Press, 2005) 39; Gross & Ní Aoláin, *ibid;* Harlow, *supra* note 1, at 200-01.

In examining how some measure of accountability might be achieved in these circumstances, I suggest we ought to pay attention to both the visible and less visible modes of accountability that exist within the political system. Discussions of accountability should include the expert advice provided by civil servants and the informal, "off-stage" negotiations within and between political parties that shape the content of legislation before it is introduced. There is evidence that these accountability mechanisms played an important role in tailoring the initial response to COVID-19.

The Senate of Canada has also emerged as an important source of accountability during the pandemic. While the Senate has always been characterized (if not viewed) as a chamber of "sober second thought," changes to the Senate appointments process in 2016 have increased its independence.[16] The vast majority of senators now sit either as unaffiliated senators or as members of recognized parliamentary groups that are not aligned with the federal political parties. While the Senate expedited the passage of the five pieces of pandemic-related legislation it has considered since March, its committees will play a significant role in scrutinizing the government's response to the pandemic. Two Senate committees have begun to examine issues related to COVID-19, while a third, special committee on "Lessons Learned from the COVID-19 Pandemic and Future Preparedness" will begin work "no earlier" than October 2020.[17]

A group of fifty senators recently penned an open letter advocating for the adoption of a universal basic income as part of the longer-term response to the pandemic.[18] In doing so, they seemed to seek an active role in shaping the government's response to COVID-19 rather than simply reacting to it. This discussion is likely to intensify as the government transitions from the early stages of its pandemic response to a period of active economic recovery.

16. Paul G Thomas, "Moving Toward a New and Improved Senate" (March 2019), online (pdf): *IRPP Study No 70* <irpp.org/wp-content/uploads/2019/03/Moving-Toward-a-New-and-Improved-Senate.pdf> [Thomas, "New and Improved Senate"].

17. Government Representative Office in the Senate of Canada, "3 Senate Committees to Study COVID-19 Pandemic" (15 April 2020), online: *Senate of Canada* <senate-gro.ca/news/senate-committees-study-pandemic> [Senate of Canada, "Committees"].

18. Kim Pate, "Open letter from Senators to @JustinTrudeau @cafreeland @ Bill_Morneau calls for further evolution of CERB to implement Minimum #BasicIncome #SenCA #cdnpoli" (21 April 2020 at 16:05), online: *Twitter* <twitter.com/KPateontheHill/status/1252690030595846147>.

Finally, while there is robust academic debate on the courts' relative effectiveness in an emergency, it is essential that they remain open to hear challenges to executive and legislative overreach and government inaction during the pandemic.[19] The current lockdown has imposed dramatic restrictions on individuals' liberties. It is becoming increasingly obvious that the burden of these restrictions is not borne equally.[20] There is no guarantee that majoritarian political processes will be effective in addressing the disparate impact of lockdown policies on vulnerable groups. In fact, history suggests that they are not effective in performing this function. Courts are uniquely suited to addressing these types of claims—it is a core component of their mandate under the *Canadian Charter of Rights and Freedoms*.[21] As the courts continue to figure out how to operate remotely, they ought to prioritize and expedite the hearing of challenges to executive overreach, the constitutionality of legislation, and government inaction.

I begin this chapter by examining Parliament's response to COVID-19 to date. I then turn to a discussion of accountability "behind the veil"—that is, nodes of accountability that might be invisible to the ordinary observer, but which can have an important effect on government decision-making and law-making. In the third section of this chapter, I outline the oversight role the Senate has assumed in the pandemic, and in the fourth section, I argue that, notwithstanding their limitations, the courts remain important accountability checks in a public health crisis.

---

19. Mark Tushnet refers to courts as "weak reads in a crisis": see Mark Tushnet, "The Political Constitution of Emergency Powers: Parliamentary and Separation-of-Powers Regulation" (2007) 3:4 Intl J Law in Context 275 at 277 (internal quotation marks removed). For a contrary view, see Kent Roach, "Comparative Constitutional Law and the Challenges of Terrorism Law" in Rosalind Dixon & Tom Ginsburg, eds, *Comparative Constitutional Law* (Northampton, MA: Edward Elgar Publishing, 2011) 532. On inaction, see "Legal Challenge Citing Canada's Failure to Protect Prisoners' Health During COVID-19: Notice of Application" (12 May 2020), online: *Canadian HIV/AIDS Legal Network* <www.aidslaw.ca/site/notice-of-application-prison-covid/?lang=en> [HIV/AIDS Legal Network Notice of Application].
20. See Section D: Equity and COVID-19, this volume.
21. *Reference Re Secession of Quebec*, [1998] 2 SCR 217, 161 DLR (4th) 385; *United States v Carolene Products Co*, 304 US 144 (1938); Ran Hirschl, *Towards Juristocracy: The Origins and Consequences of the New Constitutionalism* (Cambridge, MA: Harvard University Press, 2004) at 1-2.

Parliament as Accountability Check

Discussions of Parliament's role in holding the executive to account tend to begin with what happens in the Senate and House of Commons and in parliamentary committees. There is good reason for this: these are the primary fora for public scrutiny of legislation and executive action.[22] However, they are not the only sites of accountability in our political system. In the context of the current pandemic, it is important to look beyond these fora to consider what additional role less visible forms of oversight might be playing.

Before adjourning in mid-March at the beginning of the pandemic, the House of Commons expedited the passage of legislation authorizing the executive to spend without prior parliamentary approval for a period of three and a half months.[23] It did so by means of the "unanimous consent" procedure. This procedure permits the House "to depart from, vary or abridge the rules it has made for itself" where there is unanimous support for use of a different procedure.[24] The House of Commons used this procedure to adopt a motion deeming the bill to have been passed at each stage rather than going through the usual three-reading process for the adoption of legislation.[25] As Thomas explains, "[t]here was no debate on the merits of the motion, and the motion was adopted before the text of C-12 was presented to the House of Commons."[26] The legislation passed in the Senate on the same day.[27]

Parliament has since enacted four further pieces of COVID-19-related legislation. These bills were also passed with dispatch. The

22. See Jonathan Malloy, "The Adaptation of Parliament's Multiple Roles to COVID-19" Can J Political Science [forthcoming in 2020].

23. Bill C-12, *An Act to Amend the Financial Administration Act (special warrant)*, 1st Sess, 43rd Parl, 2020. See generally Thomas, "Parliament Under Pressure", *supra* note 5.

24. Marc Bosc & André Gagnon, eds, *House of Commons Procedure and Practice*, 3rd ed (Ottawa: House of Commons, 2017) at Chapter 12, online: *House of Commons Canada* <www.ourcommons.ca/About/ProcedureAndPractice3rdEdition/ch_12_5-e.html>; Thomas, "Parliament Under Pressure", *supra* note 5. Interestingly, some of the motions adopted by unanimous consent since the outset of the pandemic have signalled agreement on procedure but not on substance. For example, the March 24 unanimous consent motion in the House of Commons was adopted on division: see *House of Commons Debates*, 43-1, Vol 149, No 32 (24 March 2020) [Hansard 24 March 2020].

25. See Thomas, "Parliament Under Pressure", *supra* note 5.

26. For the precise details, see Thomas, "Parliament Under Pressure", *ibid*.

27. Senate of Canada, *Debates of the Senate*, 43-1, Vol 151, No 17 (13 March 2020).

House of Commons used the unanimous consent procedure to fast-track the adoption of each of the bills, though the procedure to which the parties agreed on each of these subsequent occasions included limited opportunities for debate.[28] *Charter* Statements for each of the bills were tabled on the same day the bills were considered. Study and debate of the bills in the Senate were similarly abbreviated. The Minister of Finance and a Department of Finance official appeared briefly before the Senate sitting as a Committee of the Whole to answer questions about Bills C-13 and C-14, two packages of primarily economic measures. The Minister of Employment, Workforce Development and Disability Inclusion attended with a departmental official to answer questions about Bill C-15, legislation designed to provide emergency relief to students, and the Minister of Agriculture and Agri-Food and two government officials appeared to discuss Bill C-16, which amended the *Canadian Dairy Commission Act*.[29] On each of these occasions, a number of senators then spoke in support of the Bill at third reading.

Things are somewhat more encouraging when we consider the role that parliamentary committees are playing in reviewing the government's response to the pandemic. The Senate and the House of Commons have variously authorized or mandated committees to provide ongoing oversight of the government's response to COVID-19. As noted above, three different Senate Committees have been or will be pressed into service to study the measures put in place to address the pandemic and the economic crisis it has precipitated. One of these committees is specifically tasked with thinking proactively about how Canada can be better prepared for future public health emergencies.[30]

On the House side, a motion passed by unanimous consent on April 20 established the Special Committee on the COVID-19 Pandemic to sit "while the House stands adjourned."[31] The Committee, which consists of all sitting members of the House of Commons, is currently meeting three times per week and has a broad mandate that includes "considering ministerial announcements," "allowing members to

28. Hansard 24 March 2020, *supra* note 24; *House of Commons Debates*, 43-1, Vol 149, No 34 (20 April 2020) [Hansard 20 April 2020]; *House of Commons Debates*, 43-1, Vol 149, No 35 (29 April 2020); *House of Commons Debates*, 43-1, Vol 149, No 36 (13 May 2020).
29. RSC 1985, c C-15.
30. Senate of Canada, "Committees", *supra* note 17.
31. Hansard 20 April 2020, *supra* note 28.

present petitions," and "questioning ministers of the Crown, including the Prime Minister, in respect of the COVID-19 pandemic."[32] A March 24 motion instructed the House of Commons Standing Committees on Health and Finance to "meet at least once per week … for the sole purpose of receiving evidence concerning matters related to the government's response to the COVID-19 pandemic."[33] As of May 21, these committees have met fourteen and sixteen times, respectively, and have heard from a wide range of witnesses from both within and outside government. Six other committees have also met to discuss the impact of COVID-19 on matters falling within their remit.[34]

The March 24 motion also requires the Minister of Finance to report in writing to the Finance Committee every two weeks on the implementation of aspects of the *COVID-19 Emergency Response Act*,[35] and to be available to the Committee to answer questions about the report. The motion creates a mechanism for reporting concerns about the government's implementation of the Act to the House of Commons, at which time the House must convene to debate the issues the Committee has identified. It also tasks the Finance Committee with a full review of the Act within six months of enactment. One of the most recent laws enacted in response to COVID-19, *An Act respecting Canada emergency student benefits (coronavirus disease 2019)*, provides for a review of the Act by a committee of the House of Commons and/or the Senate before the end of September 2021.[36]

To date, scrutiny of legislation in the Senate and House of Commons chambers has been minimal. However, work in committee has ramped up dramatically in a matter of weeks. These committees are hearing evidence from both government officials and from individuals, communities, institutions, businesses, and organizations. Their testimony is providing important information about how the

32. House of Commons, *Journals*, 43rd Parl, 1st Sess, No 34 (20 April 2020).
33. Hansard 24 March 2020, *supra* note 24.
34. The House of Commons Standing Committee on Government Operations and Estimates, the House of Commons Standing Committee on Human Resources, Skills and Social Development and the Status of Persons with Disabilities, the House of Commons Standing Committee on Indigenous and Northern Affairs, the House of Commons Standing Committee on Agriculture and Agri-Food, the House of Commons Standing Committee on Industry, Science and Technology, and the House of Commons Standing Committee on Procedure and House Affairs.
35. SC 2020, c 5.
36. SC 2020, c 7, s 16.

pandemic is affecting different sectors and how the measures the government has implemented are responding—or not—to those impacts.[37]

Off-Stage Accountability

The importance of what occurs off-stage in both the pre-legislative and legislative processes emerges very strongly from the research of British scholars Meg Russell and David Gover.[38] In an exhaustive study of the U.K. law-making process, Russell and Gover explain that parliamentarians have more "influence" on the policy process than is generally acknowledged.[39] This influence can take many forms. For example, the executive may propose legislation in a particular form because of the "anticipated reactions" of the opposition.[40] One research participant in Russell and Gover's study explained that "the sponsoring department will have a sense of what it thinks it can ask Parliament, where it might need to concede, and what it shouldn't even ask because it would be too unacceptable."[41] This sense of what is possible is obviously more critical in a minority government such as the current one, but it is always a factor.

The importance of anticipating reactions is magnified in an emergency because of the need to clear the way for the speedy passage of legislation. The general contours of emergency legislation are therefore more likely to be crafted against the backdrop of "anticipated reactions." The Government may go so far as to actively negotiate the contents of "the package" in advance with some or all opposition parties. Again, negotiation is more likely in a minority government situation.[42]

We have seen this type of negotiation occurring in response to COVID-19. The scrutiny of proposed legislation has taken place almost

37. I am grateful to Amelia Calbry-Muzyka for pointing this out to me.
38. Meg Russell & Daniel Gover, *Legislation at Westminster: Parliamentary Actors and Influence in the Making of British Law* (Oxford: Oxford University Press, 2017). In the Canadian context, see Paul G Thomas, "Parliament and Legislatures: Central to Canadian Democracy?" in John C Courtney & David E Smith, eds, *The Oxford Handbook of Canadian Politics* (Oxford: Oxford University Press, 2010) 153 [Thomas "Parliament and Legislatures"].
39. Russell & Gover, *ibid* at 7.
40. *Ibid* at 8.
41. *Ibid* at 269.
42. Thomas, "Parliament and Legislatures", *supra* note 38 at 160.

entirely behind the scenes before a bill is introduced in the House of Commons. Media reports suggest that the parties have engaged in protracted, sometimes heated, negotiations about the content of some of the bills enacted in response to the pandemic. For example, a March 24 sitting of the House convened to consider Bill C-13 (the *COVID-19 Emergency Response Act*) was adjourned temporarily to allow the parties to continue negotiating the content of the Bill.[43]

Significant concessions appear to have been secured through these negotiations.[44] The most publicized has been the removal of provisions that would have permitted the executive to authorize new expenditures without prior parliamentary approval into 2022.[45] But there are others. As I have noted, the bills passed and motions adopted by unanimous consent in recent weeks have empowered parliamentary committees to take an active role in monitoring the government's response to COVID-19.[46] In addition, one of the motions "call[s] upon the government to provide regular updates to representatives of opposition parties on its management of the COVID-19 pandemic, including a bi-weekly conference call between the finance critics of recognized parties and the Minister of Finance."[47] Another gives the Auditor General an important role in scrutinizing government expenditures related to the pandemic.[48] Some of these accountability measures were absent in the first draft of the legislation or motion and were negotiated subsequently.[49]

In ordinary times, we might expect off-stage bartering to be heavily interest-based or to involve the exchange of support for one initiative for support of another. However, there is reason to believe that this kind of bartering has been attenuated in the context of the

43. Robert Fife & Bill Curry, "Government, Opposition Reach Deal on Emergency Bill to Respond to Coronavirus Economic Fallout", *The Globe and Mail* (24 March 2020), online: <www.theglobeandmail.com/politics/article-liberals-pull-one-controversial-tax-and-spend-measure-from-emergency>; Thomas, "Parliament under Pressure", *supra* note 5; Rachel Emmanuel, "COVID-19 Aid Bill Could Have Passed Quickly if Liberals Dropped Demand for New Powers: CPC Source", *iPolitics* (25 March 2020), online: <ipolitics.ca/2020/03/25/covid-19-aid-bill-could-have-passed-quickly-if-liberals-dropped-demand-for-new-powers-cpc-source> [Emmanuel].
44. Thomas, "Parliament Under Pressure", *supra* note 5.
45. *Ibid*; Emmanuel, *supra* note 43.
46. Thomas, "Parliament Under Pressure", *ibid*; Emmanuel, *ibid*.
47. Hansard 24 March 2020, *supra* note 24.
48. *House of Commons Debates*, 43-1, Vol 149, No 33 (11 April 2020) [Hansard 11 April 2020]. See also Thomas, "Parliament Under Pressure", *supra* note 5.
49. Emmanuel, *supra* note 43; Thomas, "Parliament Under Pressure", *ibid*.

present emergency.[50] To be sure, the fact that negotiations take place off-stage means that interest-based bargaining does not carry the same repercussions as public politicization of the pandemic response would. But the evidence suggests that the early pandemic response in Canada has not, generally, been politicized.[51] This is not inevitable, however, as the situation in the United States makes clear.[52] In this depoliticized, more collaborative space, discussions and negotiations are more likely to focus on issues of accountability—how much authority does the executive require to respond to the pandemic? Would certain measures overreach? How should the government's spending be overseen by Parliament on an ongoing basis?

In short, off-stage accountability must be considered in evaluating how the legislature holds the executive to account in a pandemic. Of course, it is not a substitute for on-stage accountability, particularly as time goes on. As Thomas notes, off-stage negotiations do not tend to promote transparency or representation. He reports, for example, that a relatively exclusive group of MPs from each party were part of the negotiations that led to the development of the early pieces of coronavirus legislation.[53] At the same time, no MP ultimately objected to the agreements that were struck.[54] Moreover, it would be a mistake to ignore these levers in evaluating the overall accountability dynamics of the current situation, especially in light of their apparent effectiveness in securing more transparent and representative forms of oversight. It now falls to parliamentary committees to take advantage of their mandates.

Another node of off-stage accountability can be found within the executive itself. Civil servants in both the legal and policy spheres provide expert advice to politicians on how legislation and government programs should be structured.[55] This includes providing legal

---

50. Zack Beauchamp, "Canada Succeeded on Coronavirus Where America Failed. Why?", *Vox* (4 May 2020), online: <www.vox.com/2020/5/4/21242750/coronavirus-covid-19-united-states-canada-trump-trudeau>, citing Eric Merkley et al, "A Rare Moment of Cross-Partisan Consensus: Elite and Public Response to the COVID-19 Pandemic in Canada" Can J Political Science [forthcoming in 2020].

51. *Ibid.*

52. Beauchamp, *supra* note 50.

53. Thomas, "Parliament Under Pressure", *supra* note 5. See also Malloy, *supra* note 22.

54. I am grateful to Charlie Feldman for this point.

55. See generally Gillian E Metzger, "Foreword: 1930s Redux: The Administrative State Under Siege" (2017) 131 Harv L Rev 2 at 71-72: "The administrative state—with its bureaucracy, expert and professional personnel, and internal

advice on the limits of the state's authority.[56] Government lawyers have always played this role, though it is one that has grown in importance with the arrival of the *Canadian Charter of Rights and Freedoms*.[57] While government lawyers face a delicate balancing act in seeking to be perceived as both helpful and impartial,[58] they are duty-bound to "see that the administration of public affairs is in accordance with law."[59] Ministers are, of course, free to reject the advice of government lawyers, but they must nonetheless contend with it. When the lawyer's advice is that a proposed law is unlikely to survive scrutiny on judicial review, the risk of ignoring it is much higher.[60] In short, government lawyers can perform an important accountability function within government, even if they do so behind the veil.[61]

There are good reasons to think that civil servants are capable of being effective in a public health crisis, as former Clerk of the Privy Council Mel Cappe argues in his contribution to this volume.[62] For example, it is not unusual for government lawyers to be asked to provide legal advice or to draft legislation in a compressed time frame. Lines of accountability within the Department of Justice itself ensure that advice on important issues and draft legislation is thoroughly

institutional complexity—performs critical constitutional functions and is the key to an accountable, constrained, and effective executive branch."

56. See generally Vanessa MacDonnell, "The Civil Servant's Role in the Implementation of Constitutional Rights" (2015) 13:2 Intl J Constitutional L 383; Gabrielle Appleby, *The Role of the Solicitor-General: Negotiating Law, Politics and the Public Interest* (Oxford: Hart Publishing, 2016); Adam M Dodek, "Lawyering at the Intersection of Public Law and Legal Ethics: Government Lawyers as Custodians of the Rule of Law" (2010) 33:1 Dal LJ at 1.
57. Janet Hiebert, *Charter Conflicts: What Is Parliament's Role?* (Montréal: McGill-Queen's University Press, 2002); James B Kelly, *Governing with the Charter: Legislative and Judicial Politics and Framers' Intent* (Vancouver: University of British Columbia Press, 2005).
58. See Donald J Savoie, "First Ministers, Cabinet, and the Public Service" in John C Courtney & David E Smith, eds, *The Oxford Handbook of Canadian Politics* (Oxford: Oxford University Press, 2010) 172 at 180-82; M Deborah MacNair, "Government Lawyers and the Elusive Concept of the Public Interest: A Canadian Perspective" in Gabrielle Appleby, Patrick Keyzer & John M Williams, eds, *Public Sentinels: A Comparative Study of Australian Solicitors-General* (London: Routledge, 2014) 249 at 253.
59. *Department of Justice Act*, RSO 1985, c J-2, s 4(a). See also MacDonnell, *supra* note 56; Hiebert, *supra* note 57.
60. Hiebert, *supra* note 57.
61. John Mark Keyes, "Loyalty, Legality and Public Sector Lawyers" (2018) Ottawa Faculty of Law Working Paper No 2018-18, online: *SSRN* <papers.ssrn.com/sol3/papers.cfm?abstract_id=3200076>.
62. Mel Cappe, this volume, Chapter B-2.

vetted before it reaches the political executive, providing some assurance of their quality.

At the same time, the U.S. experience suggests that caution is needed before concluding that government lawyers will invariably give impartial advice in a pandemic. The "Torture Memos" written by Justice Department lawyer John Yoo justifying the mistreatment of Afghan detainees on the thinnest of legal grounds loom large in thinking through how government lawyers support the political executive in an emergency.[63] Like other actors who play a role in responding to the pandemic, government lawyers may feel a natural inclination to "support the team." As long as this prompts them to provide advice on how the government can achieve its objectives within the limits set down by the constitution and other laws, there is no issue.[64] Such advice is entirely consistent with the government lawyer's duties and fulfills an important accountability function at a moment when accountability checks may be weakened.

The Role of the Senate

Prior to the pandemic, the independent Senate had already emerged as an important body in holding the government to account.[65] In 2014, Justin Trudeau announced that he was removing all Liberal senators from the Liberal Caucus. Upon becoming Prime Minister, he implemented an independent Senate appointments process.[66] Since that process was created in 2016, Trudeau has appointed fifty-two Senators.[67] Paul J. Thomas explains that "[t]he Senate has not been completely transformed. However, enough change has occurred in the past five years that it is possible to contrast the "old, partisan,

63. "A Guide to the Memos on Torture", *The New York Times* (2005), online: <archive.nytimes.com/www.nytimes.com/ref/international/24MEMO-GUIDE.html?mcubz=3>.
64. Mary Dawson, "The Impact of the Charter on the Public Policy Process and the Department of Justice" (1992) 30:3 Osgoode Hall LJ 595 at 603.
65. On the role of upper chambers in ensuring accountability, see generally Russell & Gover, *supra* note 38 at 7-8.
66. Government of Canada, "Independent Advisory Board for Senate Appointments" (4 March 2020), online: *Government of Canada* <www.canada.ca/en/campaign/independent-advisory-board-for-senate-appointments.html>.
67. Office of the Prime Minister of Canada, News Release, "The Prime Minister Announces the Appointment of Two Senators" (31 January 2020), online: *Office of the Prime Minister of Canada* <pm.gc.ca/en/news/news-releases/2020/01/31/prime-minister-announces-appointment-two-senators>.

government-controlled" Senate with the "new, nonpartisan, independent Senate" that continues to take shape."[68] It is not uncommon for independent senators to seek amendments to or even vote against government legislation.[69] And while the Senate dutifully passed the emergency legislation rushed through in response to the pandemic, Senate Committees are poised to play a significant role in scrutinizing the government's response to COVID-19.

Given that debate in the Senate Chamber and in Senate committees has been limited to date, it is perhaps logical to begin by asking what accountability role senators might be playing off-stage. The picture that emerges is mixed. Thomas reports that senators were involved in the negotiations that preceded Bill C-12 but not those that preceded Bill C-13.[70] Regardless of whether senators are playing a role in these informal discussions, however, their "anticipated reactions" are an important consideration in any legislative response to COVID-19.[71] The tendency has been for senators to scrutinize but not ultimately impede the passage of government legislation.[72] However, it is conceivable that legislation which is perceived as being sufficiently problematic could be delayed in the Senate while amendments are proposed.[73] The political disincentives to delay COVID-19-related legislation are, of course, quite strong; however, it is a possibility to which government must be alert. Given the relative independence of individual senators, moreover, anticipated reactions cannot be expected to fall into predictable categories. In short, the Senate's newfound independence requires the federal government to anticipate and be responsive to a range of potential reactions from senators.[74]

Some senators have also been making use of spaces off-stage—specifically, the media and the public square—to make the case for

68. Thomas, "New and Improved Senate", *supra* note 16.
69. Government Representative Office in the Senate, "Towards an Independent Senate: A Progress Report to Canadians" (22 August 2019), online (pdf): *Senate GRO* <senate-gro.ca/wp-content/uploads/2019/08/Report-to-Canadians-English.pdf> [GRO, "Progress Report"]; Emmett Macfarlane, "The Renewed Canadian Senate: Organizational Challenges and Relations with the Government" (May 2019), online: *IRPP Study No 71* <irpp.org/wp-content/uploads/2019/05/The-Renewed-Canadian-Senate-Organizational-Challenges-and-Relations-with-the-Government.pdf>.
70. Thomas, "Parliament under Pressure", *supra* note 5.
71. See generally Russell & Gover, *supra* note 38 at 67.
72. GRO, "Progress Report", *supra* note 69.
73. Macfarlane, *supra* note 69.
74. Thomas, "New and Improved Senate", *supra* note 16; Macfarlane, *ibid.*

a universal basic income.[75] One of the centrepieces of the government's economic response to the pandemic has been the Canadian Emergency Response Benefit (CERB). The CERB provides Canadians who have lost their jobs as a result of the pandemic with a lump sum payment of $2,000 every four weeks.[76] This amount is considerably more than some recipients would receive under federal employment insurance or provincial social assistance schemes.[77] Observers have noted that it may be difficult for the federal government to revert to the pre-pandemic scheme once the economy re-opens. Many, including a significant number of senators, see this as an opportunity to institute a universal basic income at the federal level. It is noteworthy that these senators seem intent on leading on this issue rather than reacting, and that they are appealing directly to the people for support for their policy position.

Senate committees are currently organizing themselves to review the government's response to the pandemic and to consider the longer-term social and economic issues raised by COVID-19. Committee review has long been at the centre of the Senate's work, and some of its reports have proven to be highly influential.[78] The Senate's newfound independence may alter the dynamics of committee review by injecting a less partisan tone into committee deliberations. Senate committees thus have a distinct and important role to play in studying the government's response to COVID-19. The transition from the old to the new Senate has not been without its challenges.[79] Macfarlane reports, for example, that the combined effect of the Senate's recent independence and the relative "inexperience" of a large number of

75. Art Eggleton & Hugh Segal, "COVID-19 Presents Lessons in How a Guaranteed Basic Income Program Could Work", *Ottawa Citizen* (29 April 2020), online: <ottawacitizen.com/opinion/eggleton-and-segal-covid-19-presents-lessons-in-how-a-guaranteed-basic-income-program-could-work>.

76. "Canada Emergency Response Benefit", online: *Government of Canada* <www.canada.ca/en/services/benefits/ei/cerb-application.html>.

77. Andrew Coyne, "The CERB is Nothing Like a Basic Income, But it Might be the Platform We Use to Build One", *The Globe and Mail* (22 May 2020), online: <www.theglobeandmail.com/opinion/article-the-cerb-is-nothing-like-a-basic-income-but-it-might-be-the-platform>.

78. See generally CES Franks, "The Canadian Senate in Modern Times" in Serge Joyal, ed, *Protecting Canadian Democracy: The Senate You Never Knew* (Montréal & Kingston: McGill-Queen's University Press, 2003) 151; Andrea Lawlor & Erin Crandall, "Committee Performance in the Senate of Canada: Some Sobering Analysis for the Chamber of 'Sober Second Thought'" (2013) 51:4 Commonwealth & Comparative Politics 549.

79. Macfarlane, *supra* note 69.

new senators has sometimes impacted the institution's effectiveness.[80] Assuming these challenges can be overcome as senators begin to find their footing, however, committee review in the Senate is likely to provide an important measure of accountability.

In sum, the Senate is well positioned to hold the government to account for its response to COVID-19. This role is a natural one for the Senate, one that it draws on both its traditional expertise in studying national issues and its more recent status as an independent institution capable of scrutinizing and improving government legislation.[81] In fact, provided that the worst of its growing pains are now behind it, the Senate's response to the pandemic could prove to be a defining moment for the institution, when it finally emerges as an independent, effective body that contributes materially to enhancing the quality of our democracy.

Keeping Courts Open

Writing more than a decade ago, Mark Tushnet was candid in his pessimism about the courts' ability to serve as a check on executive and legislative excesses in an emergency. In particular, he worried that the concept of proportionality that is at the heart of constitutional rights analysis in so many jurisdictions is not up to the task of protecting civil rights in a crisis.[82] Many of the concerns he identified, including the courts' propensity to defer to legislatures where there is an informational gap between the courts and the political branches, are also live issues in the context of COVID-19.[83] By contrast, Kent Roach offers a somewhat different perspective. After evaluating the courts' response to the national security crisis precipitated by 9/11, he argued that they have *not* been particularly deferential to the executive and the legislature.[84]

80. *Ibid*.
81. Thomas, "New and Improved Senate", *supra* note 16; Macfarlane, *supra* note 69. On "improv[ing]" government legislation, see GRO, "Progress Report", *supra* note 69.
82. Tushnet, *supra* note 15. See also Sujit Choudhry, "So What Is the Real Legacy of *Oakes*? Two Decades of Proportionality Analysis under the Canadian Charter's Section 1" (2006) 34 SCLR (2d) at 501.
83. Colleen M Flood, Bryan Thomas & Kumanan Wilson, this volume, Chapter C-1.
84. Kent Roach, "Comparative Constitutional Law and the Challenges of Terrorism Law" in Rosalind Dixon & Tom Ginsburg, eds, *Comparative Constitutional Law* (Northampton, MA: Edward Elgar Publishing, 2011) 532.

While there are likely elements of truth to both accounts, there has never been any question that the courts would actually be *open* to hear cases. COVID-19 is testing this bedrock assumption about our system of government. In Ontario, for example, the Superior Court of Justice has assured Ontarians that the courts are open,[85] but they are currently operating at a fraction of their normal volume. The Superior Court has authorized "urgent matters" to proceed virtually. The list of cases deemed urgent has grown longer since the outset of the pandemic, and the Court has acknowledged that "[t]o promote access to justice, to minimize growing caseloads, and to maintain the effective administration of justice in Ontario, it is incumbent that the Court expand its operations beyond urgent matters."[86] The Superior Courts are currently treating certain child protection and family matters as urgent, as well as civil and commercial cases "where immediate and significant financial repercussions may result if there is no judicial hearing." It is also hearing COVID-related cases that arise under the provincial *Health Protection and Promotion Act*[87] and "urgent requests for injunctions related to COVID-19," plus "[a]ny other matter that the Court deems necessary and appropriate to hear on an urgent basis." Criminal trials are currently adjourned, though courts are still hearing bail reviews, guilty pleas and sentencing.[88] At the time of writing, some non-urgent civil and criminal matters are beginning to be heard in some judicial districts in Ontario, on a jurisdiction-by-jurisdiction basis.[89]

---

85. Ontario Superior Court of Justice, "Consolidated Notice to the Profession, Litigants, Accused Persons, Public and the Media" (13 May 2020), online: *Ontario Courts* <www.ontariocourts.ca/scj/notices-and-orders-covid-19/consolidated-notice> [Consolidated notice].
86. Ontario Superior Court of Justice, "Notice to the Profession, the Public and the Media Regarding Civil and Family Proceedings—Update" (2 April 2020), online: *Ontario Courts* <www.ontariocourts.ca/scj/notice-to-the-profession-the-public-and-the-media-regarding-civil-and-family-proceedings-update>; Consolidated notice, *ibid.*
87. RSO 1990, c H7.
88. Consolidated notice, *supra*; Ontario Court of Justice, "COVID-19: Notice to Counsel and the Public re: Criminal Matters in the Ontario Court of Justice" (11 May 2020), online: *Ontario Courts* <www.ontariocourts.ca/ocj/covid-19/covid-19-criminal-matters/>.
89. See, for example, Ontario Superior Court of Justice, "Notice to the Procession—Protocol for Civil Matters in the Superior Court of Justice, Central East Region (Effective May 19, 2020)" (19 May 2020), online: *Ontario Courts* <www.ontariocourts.ca/scj/notices-and-orders-covid-19/notice-ce-civil-matters/#Civil_Matters_Adjourned>.

The Federal Court of Canada initially agreed to hear "urgent" or "exceptional" matters, as well as other cases "by request of a party." It has since added any case that can be decided in writing, as well as matters "at the Court's initiative," noting that, "[t]he Court has identified a substantial number of matters that are ready to proceed, or are close to being ready to proceed."[90] The scope of the former category is potentially vast, given that the Court's most recent Practice Direction "encourages parties to consent to proceed in writing with respect to any matter that would have normally been determined in person, by teleconference or videoconference."

In many respects, courts at all levels have done a remarkable job of adapting to the new environment. A largely paper-based justice system has been moved online in a matter of weeks in the midst of a pandemic.[91] This has been easier for appeal courts than for trial courts, which still face significant challenges in figuring out how to hear matters involving live witnesses whose credibility must be assessed. But the Superior Court is no doubt also correct in suggesting that it is a matter of considerable urgency that the courts continue to increase their capacity to hear matters, whether online or in person. This is particularly true as it relates to challenges to executive overreach, unconstitutional legislation, and government inaction. This includes cases that challenge the lawfulness of the executive and the legislature's response to COVID-19 and cases that challenge overreach or inaction unrelated to the pandemic.[92] While the former cases arguably fall within the scope of the Superior Court's current Practice Direction, the latter may not unless the court exercises its discretion to allow such matters to proceed. The Federal Court's Practice Direction

---

90. "Updated Practice Direction and Order (COVID-19)" (4 April 2020), online (pdf): *Federal Court of Canada* <www.fct-cf.gc.ca/content/assets/pdf/base/FINAL%20-%20EN%20Covid-19%20Amended%20Practice%20Direction%20Order.pdf>; "Practice Direction and Order (COVID-19): Update #2 (29 April 2020)" (29 April 2020), online (pdf): *Federal Court of Canada* <www.fct-cf.gc.ca/Content/assets/pdf/base/Covid-19-Updated-Practice-Direction-Order-2-April-29-2020-FINAL-E.pdf>.

91. Aedan Helmer, "'There is no Going Back': How COVID-19 Forced Courts into the Digital Age", *Ottawa Citizen* (16 May 2020), online: <ottawacitizen.com/news/local-news/there-is-no-going-back-how-covid-19-forced-courts-into-the-digital-age>; Paola Loriggio & Liam Casey, "COVID-19 Pandemic Forces Ontario Justice System 'Stuck in the 1970s' to Modernize", *CP24* (29 April 2020), online: <www.cp24.com/news/covid-19-pandemic-forces-ontario-justice-system-stuck-in-the-1970s-to-modernize-1.4917915>.

92. See Daly, this volume, Chapter B-6.

is more agnostic, in that it refers to general urgency as the primary criterion for deciding whether to hear a matter.

To date, both the Federal Court and the Ontario Superior Court have heard and decided a number of COVID-related cases.[93] This is important for several reasons. As I have noted, the executive and the legislature are moving quickly. The margin of error is higher than it would normally be. Additionally, the scope of the potential impact on rights in this pandemic is vast. Governments at all levels have promulgated laws, regulations, and emergency orders that place significant constraints on individual rights and freedoms. Moreover, the enforcement of these laws and regulations is not neutral; rather, it tends to disproportionately limit the freedoms of some groups over others, as the chapters in the Equity section of this volume make plain. Courts have a special responsibility to address these types of issues.

Going forward, both the Federal Court and the provincial superior courts must continue to ensure that public law actions challenging state and legislative overreach are given priority, whether those challenges arise from the pandemic or not.[94] The same is true with challenges to government delay or inaction, which is now the subject of multiple actions in the Federal Court.[95]

Conclusion

Canadian institutions have been forced to adapt rapidly to the challenges posed by COVID-19. The challenges in this context are not limited to the public health crisis and its impact on the economy. Rather, they include ensuring basic access to, and functioning of, institutions. The executive, Parliament, and the courts have made a great deal of progress in a short time. Political parties that engage in highly partisan ways in normal times have thus far chosen the path of collaboration—though some cracks are beginning to show.[96] Courts are adapting to new ways of working and are doing what they can

93. See e.g. *McCulloch v Canada (Attorney General)*, 2020 FC 565 [*McCulloch*].
94. For a pessimistic view of the effectiveness of courts in providing accountability in the context of COVID-19, see Daly, this volume, Chapter B-6.
95. McCulloch, *supra* note 93; HIV/AIDS Legal Network Notice of Application, *supra* note 19.
96. Mike Blanchfield, "Tories want Parliament Declared 'Essential Service,' Regular House Sittings", *National Post* (22 May 2020), online: <nationalpost.com/pmn/news-pmn/canada-news-pmn/tories-want-parliament-declared-essential-service-regular-house-sittings>.

to ensure that courts are open. Real challenges remain, however. In thinking through these challenges, it is important to consider all available accountability mechanisms.

In this chapter, I have suggested that off-stage accountability mechanisms are playing an important role in structuring the government's response to the pandemic. These mechanisms include informal negotiations between the parties prior to legislation being proposed and the impartial advice of public servants, especially government lawyers. As time goes on, one would hope that some of the off-stage debate between the parties will move to a more public forum.

I have also suggested that the Senate is well placed to hold the executive to account for its response to COVID-19, through a combination of its traditional role as a chamber of sober second thought, its more recent independence, and its increasing willingness to actively take on the role of advocating for certain policy proposals. Finally, courts must be open to hear challenges to executive and legislative overreach and government inaction, particularly given the disparate impact of pandemic policies on the most vulnerable.

CHAPTER B-2

Good Governance: Institutions, Processes, and People

Mel Cappe*

Abstract

There are several determinants of success in managing a pandemic, but good governance is key. In this short chapter, I elaborate on why good governance matters in a pandemic. I underscore the key attributes of good governance, focusing on strong institutions, robust processes of decision-making, and the right people making those decisions. In this pandemic, Canadian institutions have displayed some of their weaknesses and inadequacies, but on the whole have performed relatively resiliently. Processes of decision-making have been adapted to improve performance, and the people in leadership jobs have largely risen to the challenges they faced. As to institutions, processes, and people, we have been relatively well served.

Résumé

Bonne gouvernance : institutions, processus et individus

Lorsqu'il s'agit d'évaluer le succès de la gestion d'une pandémie, il existe plusieurs facteurs déterminants, mais la bonne gouvernance est essentielle. Dans ce court chapitre, j'explique pourquoi la bonne gouvernance est importante en temps de pandémie. J'en souligne

* Professor in the Munk School of Global Affairs and Public Policy, University of Toronto.

les principales caractéristiques, en insistant sur la nécessité de pouvoir compter sur des institutions fortes, des processus décisionnels solides et des personnes compétentes pour prendre des décisions. Dans le contexte de la pandémie actuelle, les institutions canadiennes ont révélé certaines de leurs lacunes et de leurs insuffisances, mais dans l'ensemble, elles se sont montrées plutôt efficaces. Les processus décisionnels ont été adaptés pour améliorer leur rendement, et les personnes occupant des postes de direction ont été à la hauteur des défis qui se sont présentés. Ainsi, en ce qui concerne les institutions, les processus et les individus, nous avons été relativement bien servis.

There are several determinants of success in managing a pandemic, but good governance is key. In the next few years, we will look across states and sub-national governments to assess why some were more successful than others. However, at the moment, there seem to be several indicia of good performance. Democracies with high levels of social trust, strong institutions, science-based decision-making, and technocratic leaders seem to have done well, as have some autocratic states. However, unscientific, populist-led countries such as Brazil and the U.S. appear to have done less well.

In this short chapter, I elaborate on why good governance matters in a pandemic. I underscore the key attributes of good governance, focusing on strong institutions, robust processes of decision-making, and the right people making those decisions. Of course, there is an important interplay among these three factors.

Institutions

Institutions matter.[1] Acemaglu and Robinson have long held that the strength of political and economic institutions determines good governance, which in turn determines economic and social success.[2] Three types of institutions affect performance in the context of a pandemic like COVID-19: those charged with operations (for example, Chief

1. Daron Acemoglu & James A Robinson, *Why Nations Fail: The Origins of Power, Prosperity, and Poverty* (New York: Crown Publishers, 2012).
2. Daron Acemoglu & James A Robinson, *The Narrow Corridor: States, Societies and the Fate of Liberty* (New York: Penguin Press, 2019).

Medical Officers of Health [CMHOs]); those responsible for coordination (for example, Cabinet committees); and those that deliver accountability (for example, parliamentary committees). Of course, there is much overlap in function across these three.

Federations such as Canada, Belgium, the U.S., and Switzerland have the advantage of experimentation across provinces and cities but also experience the friction costs of collaboration.[3] While each jurisdiction may be sovereign in its own domain, complexity necessitates some measure of coordination. Inter-jurisdictional operations and sharing of information requires informal, relationship-based meta-institutions to facilitate exchange and joint delivery. Although the federal system may be fractured and fragmented, these institutions of collaboration and coordination provide mechanisms of exchanging ideas and delivering collective action in the form of initiatives such as physical distancing measures and income transfers.

Operational Organizations

There are several operational organizations that are delivering services like testing and tracing as part of the COVID-19 response. Such institutions include the Chief Medical Officers of Health, Ministers of Health and other portfolios and their Deputy Ministers, the public service at large, hospitals and their administrators, engineers, front line workers (for example, orderlies, nurses, and doctors), as well as Canadian Blood Services and HemaQuébec, and pan-Canadian health organizations such as the Canadian Institute for Health Information and the Canadian Agency for Drug and Technologies in Health.

These institutions are essential to ensuring success in fighting a pandemic. Prior to SARS, federal public health authorities were located in Health Canada and other departments such as Agriculture Canada. The SARS post-mortem identified the need to draw together public health functions from across government to form the relatively independent Public Health Agency of Canada (PHAC).[4] We have been

3. For a constructive view of federalism, see David Robitaille, this volume, Chapter A-4. For a more contrarian and cynical view, see Amir Attaran & Adam R Houston, this volume, Chapter A-5.
4. National Advisory Committee on SARS and Public Health, *Learning from SARS: Renewal of Public Health in Canada*, by David Naylor et al, Catalogue No H21-220/2003E (Ottawa, ON: Health Canada, October 2003).

relatively well served by having had PHAC coordinating, informing, and explaining to the public how to respond to COVID-19 as well as providing public health policy advice within government. For its part, Health Canada ultimately remains responsible for federal public health policy.

COVID-19 has taken a particular toll on individuals in long-term care homes.[5] Ontario now has a Minister of Long-Term Care supported by a department. Whereas in the past long-term care has been a small piece of the health care portfolio. It was only when Premier Ford last shuffled his Cabinet that he gave separate responsibility for long-term care to a junior minister. While the department has not performed particularly well since its creation, it has provided focused political attention to the issue.[6] Given the significant number of deaths in long-term care facilities, it is likely that we will see this model revamped in Ontario and possibly replicated in other jurisdictions.

The federal public service provides non-partisan, dispassionate, professional advice and service delivery. Some unheralded heroes have emerged in the response to COVID-19. Programmers and program delivery specialists at Employment and Social Development Canada (ESDC) and the Canada Revenue Agency (CRA), as well as policy people in those departments and at Finance Canada, have risen to the challenge of developing new policies and programs on an almost daily basis to fill gaps in existing programs—and in record time.[7] It became clear that the system for delivering employment insurance (EI), which was built in the 1970s using an outdated computer language, with complex qualification criteria, and usually processed fewer than 10,000 applications a week, would be ineffective at delivering employment insurance payments to the millions suddenly left unemployed by COVID-19. The government turned to the CRA to deliver the Canada Emergency Relief Benefit (CERB). Remarkably, those who qualified for EI or the CERB received their benefits from Service Canada within a few weeks. This achievement is all the more remarkable given that most public servants were working from home as part of an organization not structured to do so.

5. See Colleen M Flood, Bryan Thomas & Kumanan Wilson, this volume, Chapter C-1.
6. "Long-Term Care COVID-19 Tracker", online: *National Institute on Ageing* <ltc-covid19-tracker.ca/>.
7. Nick Taylor-Vaisey, "Pulling off a Bureaucratic Miracle: How the CERB Got Done", *Maclean's* (4 May 2020), online: <www.macleans.ca/politics/ottawa/pulling-off-a-bureaucratic-miracle-how-the-cerb-got-done/>.

For an institution known for its risk aversion and its plodding and deliberate nature, the public service has served Canadians well in this crisis to date. The creation, design, and delivery of a benefit like this could have taken months, but the public service rose to the occasion and met the challenge, going from conception to delivery in roughly three weeks. Ministers took the advice of the scientific establishment based in departments like Agriculture, Environment, and, of course, Health. But they came to a judgment on the policy choice by balancing that advice against the economic and social consequences of not doing so.

Comparisons internationally will be undertaken in the future. But overall, the professional, non-partisan public service has performed well.

Coordination and Collaboration

As noted, there are several institutions whose primary purpose is to exchange information and coordinate action.[8] These institutions allow government departments to coordinate activity, governments to collaborate in messaging and in action, and subject-matter specialist organizations to learn from each other. These include Federal/Provincial/Territorial First Ministers tables, the Council of Ministers of Health of Canada, and the Conference of Deputy Ministers of Health (a coordinating body with some executive functions), pan-Canadian health organizations such as the Canadian Partnership Against Cancer, the Canadian Patient Safety Institute, the Canadian Foundation for Healthcare Improvement, the Canadian Centre on Substance Use and Addiction, and the Canadian Mental Health Commission.

First Ministers have used executive federalism, meaning intergovernmental negotiations at the highest levels, to effectively coordinate action on COVID-19. Although First Ministers generally meet from time to time, the regular weekly telephone calls during this crisis have been important for First Ministers to share information and coordinate policy. The inauguration of a federally funded, provincially differentiated wage top-up for essential workers is the result of this kind of collaboration.[9] While these teleconferences and virtual meet-

8. For an elaboration of the need for coordination and collaboration, see Grégoire Webber, this volume, Chapter B-3.
9. Office of the Prime Minister, News Release, "Prime Minister Announces Agreements to Boost Wages for Essential Workers" (7 May 2020), online: *Office of*

ings take place in secret, it is precisely this secrecy that allows them to be effective. In these frank exchanges, ministers can discuss trade-offs across priorities and find common ground for action.

The Council of Chief Medical Officers of Health meets regularly to discuss population and public health issues. By meeting and working collaboratively over time on non-urgent issues, these public health officials develop familiarity and establish trust. This pays off when they are called on to quickly make decisions and exchange information in a crisis. In demonstrating that they can take science-based decisions collectively without political involvement on issues such as cannabis, tobacco, vaping, and substance abuse, the Chief Medical Officers of Health established a level of trust that has proven essential in responding to the pandemic. Confidence is easy to lose, but hard to build.

The institution of the Clerk of the Privy Council[10] plays a coordinating role[11] within the federal government. Although a creature of statute, the office of the most senior public servant is given no specific powers. The Clerk derives authority by speaking with the voice of the Prime Minister. The clerks use committees of Deputy Ministers to ensure coordination and concerted action, and they use the accountability that Deputy Ministers have to the Prime Minister to enforce that coordination.

The network of Canadian Cabinet Secretaries also builds relations among heads of public services before crises arrive, which, as with the Chief Medical Officers of Health, builds trust and confidence to solve problems during a crisis. Before 9/11, Canadian Cabinet Secretaries had built up personal relationships that allowed them to coordinate across governments even when there was tension among their First Ministers. This network is used to this day.

Public-Facing Institutions

There are also governance institutions that are public-facing or that act as instruments of accountability. Auditors General (AGs) will have an *ex post* role in holding government to account. The question for AGs will not be whether mistakes were made; it is inevitable that

the Prime Minister <pm.gc.ca/en/news/news-releases/2020/05/07/prime-minister-announces-agreements-boost-wages-essential-workers>.

10. *Public Service Employment Act*, SC 2003, c 22, s 126.
11. "Clerk and Deputy Clerk" (last modified 16 September 2019), online: *Privy Council Office* <www.canada.ca/en/privy-council/corporate/clerk/role.html#toco>.

there were. Rather, it is whether they were the right mistakes in light of imperfect information.[12]

Consider the role of daily press conferences. The Prime Minister and Premiers are expected to demonstrate leadership. Some have done much better than anyone might have expected. For instance, Premier Doug Ford of Ontario has used his simple, "man-of-the-people" communication style to great effect and been praised from all sides.[13] Alberta Premier Jason Kenney has for the moment put aside the inter-party rivalry of federal/provincial relations.[14] And Prime Minister Trudeau has played multiple roles, building confidence and calming the public all while delivering policy and programs to deal with the crisis.

The Chief Medical Officers of Health have also played a crucial role—with most doing very well. In several cases, political leaders have taken a back seat to let their respective Chief Medical Officer of Health play a leadership role. Similarly, although Tina Namieskowski is the President of the Public Health Agency of Canada, she is not playing a public role, leaving confidence-building to Canada's Chief Medical Officer of Health Dr. Theresa Tam. At the provincial and local levels, Chief Medical Officers of Health who have performed in stellar fashion include Dr. Eileen de Villa (Toronto), Dr. Deena Hinshaw (Alberta), and Dr. Bonnie Henry (British Columbia).[15] Conversely, Premier Ford has called out some local Chief Medical Officers of Health who have not taken the initiative to promote testing or deal with the long-term care facilities in their regions.[16] In some cases, provincial counterparts have been criticized for being off message and insensitive to the evident data.[17]

12. See Vanessa MacDonnell, this volume, Chapter B-1.
13. Marie Henein, "My Uncomfortable Reality: Doug Ford is the Leader Ontario Needs", *The Globe and Mail* (9 April 2020), online: <www.theglobeandmail.com/opinion/article-my-uncomfortable-reality-doug-ford-is-the-leader-ontario-needs>.
14. "Alberta to Send Personal Protective Equipment to Ontario, Quebec, B.C.", *CBC News* (11 April 2020), online: <www.cbc.ca/news/canada/edmonton/alberta-to-send-personal-protective-equipment-to-ontario-quebec-b-c-1.5529989>.
15. Meagan Fitzpatrick, "Chief Medical Officers Are Leading Canada through COVID-19 Crisis—And Many Are Women", *CBC News* (2 April 2020), online: <www.cbc.ca/news/health/women-chief-medical-officers-canada-1.5518974>.
16. Ryan Rocca, "'Pick Up the Pace': Doug Ford Says Some Local Medical Officers Falling Behind on COVID-19 Testing", *Global News* (5 May 2020), online: <globalnews.ca/news/6907247/coronavirus-doug-ford-local-medical-officers-testing>.
17. See David Fisman interviewed on "What Is Ontario Doing Wrong on COVID-19?" (22 April 2020), online (podcast): *The Big Story* <thebigstorypodcast.ca/2020/04/22/what-covid-19-can-teach-us-about-being-wrong/>.

Parliament and its committees have stepped up to play a crucial role in holding government to account. The federal government initially overreached in proposed legislation[18] by trying to appropriate to itself discretion to spend without parliamentary approval. The Opposition stopped that before it was tabled. Nevertheless, the legislation was approved in record time. It began in preparation on March 17, 2020, and was tabled on March 24, passed both houses, and given Royal Assent on March 25. The challenge function of Parliament worked, but not to the impairment of the approval function.[19] More broadly, Parliament has adapted to the need to continue to meet while doing so at distance: distance within the Chamber and distance from the Chamber. This ability to adapt is key in a crisis.

Processes of Decision-Making

Processes matter. Niall Ferguson argues that institutions degenerate and decline when their capacity for structured and rigorous decision-making is undermined. Adapting decision processes to the challenge of the moment ensures they can accomplish their ends while facing the challenge of COVID-19.[20]

Good governance requires inclusive, informed, and accountable processes, including administrative, Cabinet, parliamentary, intergovernmental, and international processes. What follows is a brief discussion of some of these processes.

In Westminster parliamentary democracies, Cabinet requires adherence to a few key principles, such as solidarity. But a pandemic requires that the adaptation of decision processes be effective. Speed and effectiveness require better use of Cabinet committees and deployment of talent in new ways. After 9/11, the Prime Minister created a Cabinet Committee that had long been advised, chaired by the Deputy Prime Minister, to deal with international security and intelligence issues. With the pandemic challenging Cabinet's capacity to respond well and fast, the PM created the Cabinet Committee on the Federal Response to the Coronavirus Disease (COVID-19), chaired by Deputy Prime Minister Chrystia Freeland. If spies and civil rights

18. *COVID-19 Emergency Response Act*, SC 2020, c 5.
19. See MacDonnell, this volume, Chapter B-1, discussing "off-stage" negotiations and accountability.
20. Niall Ferguson, *The Great Degeneration: How Institutions Decay and Economies Die* (London: Allen Lane, 2012).

protectors needed to be at the table for when security and intelligence decisions were made in 2001, then doctors and economists needed to be at the table in 2020 for COVID-19. Specialized Cabinet committees allow for deliberative consideration of interconnected issues to optimize decision-making where there are a multitude of objectives.

The quality of decision-making is always dependent on the quality and availability of the data and the evidence on which that data is based. The decision about whether to recommend the wearing of masks or force lockdowns has been the subject of much criticism. However, in the presence of imperfect information, policy leaders must make decisions based on the medical, scientific, economic, and social assessments available to them.[21] After the fact we assess their decisions with perfect hindsight. The adequacy and appropriateness of a decision should be evaluated based on the information available at the time the particular decision was taken. With inadequate information of the viral loads, immunities, testing, and transmission of SARS-CoV-2, medical and policy leaders did the best they could.[22] Optimal decisions *ex ante* look very different from perfect decisions *ex post*.[23]

Moreover, the judgment of ministers requires optimality in risk taking.[24] That means seeking adequate information, exercising due diligence in its assessment, understanding the consequences of decisions, and knowing what risks to take.[25] It also means being prepared to change the decision upon discovering or receiving new information. The recommendation to wear masks is an example of responding to the evolving base of evidence in this pandemic.

Some key decisions on mitigation and on health resource allocation may be judged to be wrong in the long term. However, they appear remarkably well taken based on the imperfect information available at the time.

---

21. See Flood, Thomas & Wilson, this volume, Chapter C-1, discussing information inadequacy and the precautionary principle as well as proportionality.
22. On weighing risks, see Gillian Tett, "Is it Safe to Go to the Shops, See a Friend or Get on a Plane?", *Financial Times* (8 May 2020), online: <www.ft.com/content/a69afc14-904a-11ea-9b25-c36e3584cda8>.
23. Marc Fleurbaey, "Welfare Economics, Risk and Uncertainty" (2018) 51:1 Can J of Economics 5.
24. See Michael Howlett, "Policy Analytical Capacity and Evidence-Based Policy-Making: Lessons from Canada" (2009) 52:2 Can Public Administration 153.
25. For a discussion of the duty of governments to seek adequate information see Jula Hughes & Vanessa MacDonnell, "Social Science Evidence in Constitutional Rights Cases in Germany and Canada: Some Comparative Observations" (2013) 32:1 NJCL 23.

People

People matter.[26] The elusive characteristics of leadership are dependent on the right people being in the right job and performing at or beyond their capacity to lead the public in crisis.[27]

Strong institutions and robust decision-making processes require competent people. Competence is partly determined by a person's background and training and partly by their character and judgment. The comments on the personalities of the Chief Medical Officers of Health above are instructive.

Health Minister Patty Hajdu has performed with competence and compassion. Having worked on homelessness in a mid-sized city, she is well placed to understand their vulnerability to COVID-19. Deputy Prime Minister Chrystia Freeland has used her experience dealing with the Americans and Europeans on trade to develop arrangements with the U.S. regarding borders. Jean-Yves Duclos, President of the Treasury Board, a former scholar of income security, played an important role in developing income supplements. And, Procurement Minister Anita Anand, a former law professor, contributed beyond her portfolio responsibilities, as did Finance Minister Bill Morneau. Internationally, Jacinda Ardern of New Zealand and Angela Merkel of Germany have shown strong leadership based on science.[28]

The principles of competence, character, and judgment also extend to senior members of the public service. The Clerk of the Privy Council, Ian Shugart, having been Deputy Minister of Health and of ESDC as well as Director of the Medical Research Council (the predecessor to the Canadian Institutes of Health Research), and Graham Flack, the Deputy Minister of ESDC, having been a senior official in social policy and at Finance Canada, were well positioned to gear up quickly to face the crisis. They had also built up trust over years of working together.

---

26. Ian Green & André Côté, *Leading by Example: 50 Prominent Canadians Talk to Us about the Federal Public Service and Why Leadership Matters* (Ottawa, ON: Public Policy Forum, 2007).
27. For U.S. presidential examples, see Doris Kearns Goodwin, *Leadership: In Turbulent Times* (New York: Simon and Schuster, 2018).
28. See "Coronavirus: How New Zealand Relied on Science and Empathy", *BBC* (20 April 2020), online: <www.bbc.com/news/world-asia-52344299>; Katrin Bennhold, "Relying on Science and Politics, Merkel Offers a Cautious Virus Re-entry Plan", *New York Times* (15 April 2020), online: <www.nytimes.com/2020/04/15/world/europe/coronavirus-germany-merkel.html>.

We turn to our political and public service leaders not only to provide government policy and program response, but also to provide that elusive sense of leadership that instills confidence and trust. Regardless of their political stripe, Canadian leaders have realized the public turns to them for decisiveness, calm, and fairness.[29] They have largely risen to the occasion, some excelling well beyond expectations. The comparison of Canadian political leaders with those in the U.S. and the U.K. has been rather stark in this regard.

You do not need the "great person" theory of history to recognize that the backgrounds, characters, and nature of people in leadership positions matter. Flexibility, adaptability, and professionalism have become watchwords for ministerial performance. Clearly, a Prime Minister must choose his Ministers and Deputy Ministers partially on their past performance, but more importantly on how he, she, or they judges they will perform in a crisis.

Conclusion

Good governance is often taken for granted. It is only when it is needed that it matters. Effective institutions, robust decision-making processes, and competent and compassionate people create effective governance. And they have to be adaptable. In this pandemic, Canadian institutions have displayed some of their weaknesses and inadequacies, but on the whole have performed resiliently. Processes of decision-making have been adapted to improve performance. And the people in the jobs of leadership have largely risen to the challenges. As to institutions, processes, and people, on balance, Canadians have been well served.

29. Not surprisingly, not all public health officers have performed in distinguished fashion. In the cut-and-thrust of immediate policy creation, non-taxed universal payments to seniors embodies unnecessary leakage to those who do not need it.

CHAPTER B-3

The Duty to Govern and the Rule of Law in an Emergency*

Grégoire Webber**

Abstract

Across the world, the legislative and judicial branches of government have retreated in part during the COVID-19 pandemic, while members of the executive branch have assumed greater responsibilities. Is such a shift in responsibilities justified by this emergency or exceptional situation? This chapter explores this question by reviewing the duty to govern, the duty to govern in compliance with the Rule of Law, the constrained nature of any emergency or exceptional powers, and the duty incumbent on those exercising extraordinary authority to return to the normal situation as much as circumstances allow.

Résumé

Le devoir de gouverner et la primauté du droit en situation d'urgence

Partout dans le monde, les pouvoirs législatif et judiciaire ont fléchi durant la pandémie de COVID-19, tandis que le fardeau du pouvoir

* For comments on a previous draft, thanks are owed to the editors, reviewers, and Victoria Carmichael, Jean Thomas, Owen Rees, and Stéphanie Vig.

** Canada Research Chair in Public Law and Philosophy of Law, Queen's University, and Visiting Fellow, London School of Economics and Political Science. Email: gregoire.webber@queensu.ca.

exécutif s'est alourdi. Une telle situation d'urgence ou exceptionnelle justifie-t-elle ce changement ? Ce chapitre explore cette question, en analysant le devoir de gouverner, le devoir de gouverner dans le respect de la primauté du droit, la nature contraignante de tout pouvoir d'urgence ou exceptionnel et le devoir qui incombe à ceux et celles qui exercent un pouvoir extraordinaire de revenir à la normale dans la mesure où les circonstances le permettent.

The Duty to Govern

The COVID-19 pandemic vividly captures the need for coordinated action in the community. Absent a pattern of coordination, the life and health of the community's members would be at radically increased risk. The candidate patterns of coordination all contemplate coordination between means and ends—how to flatten the curve, how to increase the maximum capacity of our hospitals, how to address economic losses—and between persons for whose good the ends are sought—who is to be classified as an essential worker, who is to be tested, who is to self-isolate. The range of possible patterns of coordination is highlighted by the different strategies pursued in different jurisdictions. Even if some fare better by the metrics of health, or the economy, or liberty of movement, or government support, no one pattern of coordination can be said to be superior to all the others in respect of every metric taken together. Yet, despite the absence of a single right answer to the question of which pattern of coordination should be adopted, the failure to settle on any one pattern would be unreasonable.

Any one member of the community can contemplate independently of the others which pattern of coordination should be the community's, with the more imaginative identifying a greater range of candidate patterns. But that independence cannot be maintained when one moves beyond contemplating different possibilities to determining which pattern of means-to-ends and which roles for which persons should be favoured, not only by oneself, but by everyone. The practical question confronting each member of a community is not best captured as "What should *I* do?" but rather as "What should *we* do?" What should we do about social gatherings, public schools, and our borders? Without settling on a pattern, the advantages of coordination will be frustrated or realized imperfectly or too late. What is more, coordination in the community will be desirable not only for each finite, episodic project, but also for projects carried on over time: maintaining emergency preparedness, addressing the mounting public debt, confronting the failings exposed by present circumstances. Here, too, the failure to settle upon a pattern of coordination will be, in many instances, unreasonable, even if reason identifies no one pattern as *the* pattern that should be selected.

How, then, is a community to settle upon a pattern of coordination? In the final analysis, there are only two reasonable ways to secure a pattern of coordination: *unanimity* or *authority*.[1] Both aim to bring all persons to the same view: the first directly on which pattern of coordination is to be selected; the second indirectly on how to settle which scheme is to be selected. There can be no denying that some measure of unanimity successfully resolves some coordination problems in a community. Yet, for a greater number of matters, only authority will be available to settle, *decisively*, which coordination pattern will be the community's. Authority secures what unanimity cannot: a way of settling, in the absence of unanimity, what is to be done by members of a community. Such need is all the more immediate when, as is the case in responding to a health pandemic, there is need to secure a pattern of coordination now, without delay.

On this understanding, authority is a relationship between persons in authority and the community's members. This relationship can aptly be labelled one of "service,"[2] captured by common references to persons in political authority as "public servants" exercising a "public service." The service in question is fulfilled in part by settling patterns of coordination. As illustrated by the challenges of the COVID-19 pandemic, persons in authority would fail to do their duty if they failed to settle on a pattern of coordination.[3] With this failure in mind, we come to see how authority *over* a community's members is synonymous with a responsibility *for*.

---

1. See Yves R Simon, *A General Theory of Authority* (Notre Dame: University of Notre Dame Press, 1980) at 40; John Finnis, *Natural Law and Natural Rights*, 2nd ed (Oxford: Oxford University Press, 2011) at 232. See further Leslie Green, "The Duty to Govern" (2007) 13:3/4 Legal Theory 165.
2. See e.g. Joseph Raz, *The Morality of Freedom* (Oxford: Oxford University Press, 1986) at chapter 3.
3. On whether, in a federation, such coordination should be achieved at the national level, see David Robitaille, this volume, Chapter A-4; Colleen M Flood & Bryan Thomas, this volume, Chapter A-6; Carissima Mathen, this volume, Chapter A-7.

Governing Through Law

The first responsibility of a government is to govern. The responsibility to govern is exercised in important measure by directing what is to be done by the members of a community. It is not the only way to govern or the whole of it. A government may also govern by guiding, nudging, recommending, and proposing.[4] But the direction associated with law has special status, for it renders non-optional certain conduct by community members. When reasonable, law is a reason for action. It seeks to provide direction to each community member by answering the question: What are we to do?

In well-formed legal systems, the duty to govern is widely shared. The principles of checks and balances and the separation of powers counsel the distribution of executive, legislative, judicial responsibilities to different persons and institutions. Such distribution of the duty to govern provides defence against tyranny and is in the service of liberty and the Rule of Law.[5] Good legal systems will not award all or near all authority to the same person or institution.

In such systems, the institution with primary law-making responsibility will be the legislature. The legislature will be designed to promote responsible law-making, recognizing that the duty to govern will be frustrated by incompetent, imprudent, or unwise directives. The law-making process will emphasize deliberation, so that the reasons for and against a legislative proposal will be freely debated.[6] Such a deliberative process will expand the time needed to make law, but it will help to ensure that the law conforms to the Rule of Law.

Among the many requirements associated with the Rule of Law[7] are that laws will be promulgated (published and made readily available), clear (understandable by one who reads them), coherent (so that one directive does not require an action that another directive prohibits), prospective (so that the directive governing conduct today is not decided tomorrow), not impossible to comply with (so that one is

4. On "the technique of suasion," see Paul Daly, this volume, Chapter B-6.
5. See Jeremy Waldron, *Political Political Theory* (Cambridge: Harvard University Press, 2016) at chapter 3.
6. See Vanessa MacDonnell, this volume, Chapter B-1.
7. On which, see Lon L Fuller, *The Morality of Law* (New Haven: Yale University Press, 1969); Joseph Raz, "The Rule of Law and its Virtue" (1977) 93 Law Quarterly Review 198; Joseph Raz, "The Law's Own Virtue" (2019) 39:1 Oxford J Leg Stud 1; Margaret Jane Radin, "Reconsidering the Rule of Law" (1989) 69:4 BUL Rev 781; Tom Bingham, *The Rule of Law* (London: Allen Lane, 2010).

inevitably in breach of the law), and generally stable *over* time (such that the laws governing conduct in a community are not changing too frequently). These requirements are associated with the idea of reciprocity between those in authority and those subject to law, so that voluntary collaboration is made possible by-laws apt to be followed.[8]

Though not without their blemishes, well-formed legal systems have a good record of complying with these Rule of Law requirements, in part because of the law-making process that favours due consideration and deliberation prior to enactment. But such commitment to consideration and deliberation is not always possible, as exceptional or emergency situations may arise.

A State of Exception

A well-formed legal system will anticipate exceptional or emergency situations. It may do so by enumerating such situations, such as war, invasion, insurrection, or a public health crisis, though there are reasons to resist too exhaustive a list.[9] A legal system may require that a number of different persons or institutions concur in the judgment that an emergency situation has emerged, for example by requiring a resolution of the legislature and requiring its renewal at regular intervals. Such requirement will temper the risk of abuse, but there is another order of risk in the event that debate over a resolution delays urgent action or in the event that the legislature is incapacitated due to the emergency.

The risk of abuse of power is nonetheless live because, in awarding extraordinary powers to a person or small set of persons, the legal system does precisely what the principles of checks and balances and the separation of powers warn against doing. In many established legal systems, it is to members of the executive branch that extraordinary powers are vested.[10] Across the world, the legislative and judicial

8. See Fuller, *supra* note 7, chapter II; see also Kristen Rundle, *Forms Liberate: Reclaiming the Jurisprudence of Lon L Fuller* (Oxford: Hart Publishing, 2012).
9. See Alexander Hamilton, *The Federalist Papers* (Ann Arbor: ProQuest, 2015) at no 23: "The circumstances that endanger the safety of nations are infinite; and for this reason no constitutional shackles can wisely be imposed on the power to which the care of it is committed." See now Council of Europe, European Commission for Democracy Through Law, *Compilation of Venice Commission Opinions and Reports on States of Emergency*, CDL-PI(2020)003, (2020).
10. See John Ferejohn & Pasquale Pasquino, "The Law of the Exception: A Typology of Emergency Powers" (2004) 2:2 Intl J of Constitutional L 210.

branches of government have retreated in part during the COVID-19 pandemic whereas members of the executive branch—understood to include public health officials—have assumed greater responsibilities.

Even when extraordinary powers are authorized by law, such powers are in some respects a departure from the law, since the law that governs during the normal situation is set aside in small or large ways. Some argue that where the law fails to vest extraordinary powers or does so in imperfect ways, an exception to the legal order may be decided upon so as to enable one to act in the face of an exceptional or emergency situation.[11] Is there justification for sure departures—be they large or small or complete—from the law that governs during the normal situation?

Any sound justification will draw on two reasons. The first relates to the need to settle patterns of coordination. An emergency situation may require rapid decisions on which direction to issue to members of a community. The quickly changing public health advice in the early days of the COVID-19 pandemic illustrates such need in the face of a fluid situation, with near-daily shifts in direction on the size of permissible gatherings, the merits of border closings, the duration of school closures, and the range of essential services. To such end, a single person or small group of persons will have greater capacity to respond to changing circumstances than would a large deliberative body.

The second reason affirms that the person or persons awarded extraordinary powers do so on commission: they are to exercise such powers with a view to ending the emergency situation. Their mandate is fundamentally conservative: it is to return to the normal situation.[12] Once the normal situation is re-established, the justification for extraordinary powers is spent and the commission is concluded. In acting on commission, those with extraordinary powers affirm the understanding that all authority, in both normal and emergency situations, is a service and a benefit not to the person or persons who rule, but to the members of the community.

Even when justified, the exercise of extraordinary powers may raise challenges for the Rule of Law.

---

11. See Carl Schmitt, *Political Theology* (Cambridge: MIT Press, 1986); Carl Schmitt, *Dictatorship. From the Origin of the Modern Concept of Sovereignty to the Proletarian Class Struggle* (Cambridge, UK: Polity Press, 2014).
12. See Ferejohn & Pasquino, *supra* note 10.

Challenges for the Rule of Law

Against the requirements of the Rule of Law, the directives issued further to extraordinary powers may leave much to be desired. Though such directives will be *published*, their promulgation and diffusion may not have the prominence of legislative enactments and so be less readily available and known to the community members. Some members may struggle to distinguish between directives that have the force of law and recommendations that have the force of advice. In turn, the needs of an exceptional or emergency situation may require a great number of directives in quick succession, thereby increasing the risk of *contradiction* between directives. These same needs may require those with responsibility to govern to communicate the content of a directive before formally enacting it,[13] with the possibility that the directive will be given *retroactive* effect. The need for quick action may result in directives burdened with unanticipated *ambiguities*, some of which may emerge in debates surrounding enforcement. And this same need for quick action in response to rapidly changing circumstances may disrupt any sense of *stability* in the state of the law, such that the community's members may have little confidence that yesterday's set of directives remains the same today.[14]

Such departures from the Rule of Law may be expected when it comes to the exercise of extraordinary powers. The law-making procedure established for the normal situation privileges deliberation so as to guard against error and misjudgment, including errors with respect to Rule of Law requirements. Having set such procedure aside in favour of extraordinary powers, rapid decision-making is liable to depart from the Rule of Law. The exigencies of the situation may excuse many such departures, where failures in promulgation, clarity, coherence, non-retroactivity, and stability all have their source in the need to respond to circumstances.

Yet, even when excused by the exigencies of the circumstances, departures from the Rule of Law cannot be total or far-reaching, for, if they are, the government's directives will fail to achieve what all

13. See Daly, this volume, Chapter B-6, for how the Government of Ontario's emergency alert notice in April 2020 predated the corresponding regulation.
14. A compendium of the many orders issued by federal, provincial, territorial, municipal, and First Nations' authorities helps to illustrate the possible risks for the Rule of Law: see Craig Forcese, "Repository of Canadian COVID-19 Emergency Orders" (updated on 25 May 2020), online (blog): *Intrepid* <www.intrepidpodcast.com/blog/2020/3/19/repository-of-canadian-covid-19-emergency-orders>.

sound directives seek to achieve: the direction of human conduct by those willing to do their part. The requirements of the Rule of Law are not exclusive to law in the normal situation, but are required by all reasonable attempts to guide human conduct by rules. Good members of a community are willing to do their part in patterns of collaboration, but such willingness requires directives that are apt to be followed. Departures from the Rule of Law, no matter their justification, may frustrate the capacity of the community's members to assist in efforts to respond to the emergency situation. Indeed, given the need to settle a pattern of coordination to address the COVID-19 pandemic, departures from the Rule of Law may frustrate the community's ability to achieve coordinated action and so frustrate the community's pursuit of its various health, economic, and other ends.

Conclusion: Between Normal and Exceptional

Even though forecasts for the COVID-19 pandemic range from the medium to long term, there is every reason to resist concluding that extraordinary powers are a "new normal."[15] The emergency situation contemplated by a well-formed legal system is often contrasted with the normal situation in terms analogous to night and day. Yet, like dusk and dawn, there are situations that are neither quite normal nor exceptional. Despite this reality, the law vesting extraordinary powers may not anticipate such in-between situations.

In situations that are between normal and exceptional, extraordinary powers may need to be maintained, but those with the responsibility to rule should seek to re-establish the normal legal order where and to the extent possible. The need for rapid decision-making may wane with time, thereby allowing the more considered and deliberate law-making process of the legislature to resume. In turn, even if the normal situation has not yet resumed such that those with extraordinary powers have not yet exhausted their commission, some aspects of their commission may now be spent so that the normal legal order may resume its place in part. Much here falls, as with so much in government, to the sound exercise of authority by those with the duty to govern, a duty that recalls that all authority is for the benefit of those for whom the ruler has a responsibility to govern well.

15. For an argument along similar lines, but developed for a different purpose, see Giorgio Agamben, *State of Exception* (Chicago: University of Chicago Press, 2005).

CHAPTER B-4

Does Debunking Work? Correcting COVID-19 Misinformation on Social Media*

Timothy Caulfield**

Abstract

A defining characteristic of this pandemic has been the spread of misinformation. The World Health Organization (WHO) famously called the crisis not just a pandemic, but also an "infodemic." Why and how misinformation spreads and has an impact on behaviours and beliefs is a complex and multidimensional phenomenon. There is an emerging rich academic literature on misinformation, particularly in the context of social media. In this chapter, I focus on two questions: Is debunking an effective strategy? If so, what kind of counter-messaging is most effective? While the data remain complex and, at times, contradictory, there is little doubt that efforts to correct misinformation are worthwhile. In fact, fighting the spread of misinformation should be viewed as an important health and science policy priority.

* I would like to thank Gordon Pennycook, Kate Starbird, Briony Swire-Thompson, Robyn Hyde-Lay, Sandro Marcon, Darren Wagner, and the rest of our CIHR COVID-19 rapid response team. I am also grateful for the funding support from the Canadian Institutes of Health Research, Alberta Innovates, the Ministry of Economic Development, Trade and Tourism, the Government of Alberta, and the Government of Canada for their generous support of the following projects: *Coronavirus Outbreak: Mapping and Countering Misinformation* and *Critical Thinking in the Digital Age: Countering Coronavirus Misinformation*.

** Canada Research Chair in Health Law and Policy, Professor, Faculty of Law and School of Public Health, Research Director, Health Law Institute, University of Alberta.

Résumé

La démystification fonctionne-t-elle ? Rectifier la désinformation sur les médias sociaux au sujet de la COVID-19

Cette pandémie est marquée par la propagation de la désinformation. L'Organisation mondiale de la santé a qualifié cette crise non seulement de pandémie, mais aussi d'« infodémie ». Pourquoi et comment la désinformation se propage-t-elle et a-t-elle une incidence sur les comportements et les croyances ? Il s'agit d'un phénomène complexe et multidimensionnel. On assiste à l'émergence d'une riche littérature universitaire sur le sujet, en particulier dans le contexte des médias sociaux. Dans ce chapitre, je me concentre sur deux questions : la démystification est-elle une stratégie utile ? Si oui, quel type de contre-message est le plus efficace ? Si les données restent complexes et parfois contradictoires, il apparaît néanmoins que les efforts visant à corriger la désinformation en valent la peine. En fait, la lutte contre la diffusion de fausses informations devrait être considérée comme une priorité des politiques sanitaires et scientifiques.

A defining characteristic of the COVID-19 pandemic has been the spread of misinformation.[1] The WHO famously called the crisis not just a pandemic, but also an "infodemic."[2] Misinformation includes the suggestions that the coronavirus is both caused by 5G wireless technology and is a bioweapon. Cow urine and bleach have been put forward as cures. And enumerable wellness gurus have pushed immune-boosting supplements and diets—all science-free nonsense, of course. It has been suggested that this noise has already, *inter alia*, caused physical harm[3] and financial loss,[4] impacted health and science

1. Areeb Mian & Shujhat Khan, "Coronavirus: The Spread of Misinformation" [2020] BMC Medicine, online: *BMC Medicine* <https://bmcmedicine.biomedcentral.com/articles/10.1186/s12916-020-01556-3>.
2. World Health Organization, "Infodemic Management" (15 April 2020), online: *World Health Organization* <https://www.who.int/teams/risk-communication/infodemic-management>.
3. Alistair Smout & Paul Sandle, "Misinformation Ruins Lives, UK Fact-Checker Says", *National Post* (30 April 2020), online: <https://nationalpost.com/pmn/entertainment-pmn/misinformation-ruins-lives-uk-fact-checker-says>.
4. Greg Iacurci, "Americans Have Lost $13.4 Million to Fraud Linked to Covid-19", *CNBC* (15 April 2020), online: <https://www.cnbc.com/2020/04/15/americans-have-lost-13point4-million-to-fraud-linked-to-covid-19.html>.

policy,[5] added confusion and distraction to an already chaotic information environment,[6] heightened stigma and prejudice,[7] and made it more difficult to implement needed health policy initiatives.[8]

Much of this misinformation is spreading on social media,[9] which has included the use of bots and strategic disinformation campaigns.[10]

It is worth noting that social media has also played a constructive role. It has, for instance, been used as a tool for communicating preventative strategies and mapping the spread of the virus.[11] And

5. Michael Liu et al, "Internet Searches for Unproven COVID-19 Therapies in the United States" Research Letter (29 April 2020) JAMA Intern Medicine at E1 DOI: <10.1001/jamainternmed.2020.1764>: "Demand for chloroquine and hydroxychloroquine increased substantially following endorsements by high-profile figures and remained high even after a death attributable to chloroquine-containing products was reported".
6. See generally Amy Mitchell, J Baxter Oliphant & Elisa Shearer, "About Seven-in-Ten U.S. Adults Say They Need to Take Breaks From COVID-19 News" (29 April 2020) at 4, online: *Pew Research Center* <https://www.journalism.org/2020/04/29/about-seven-in-ten-u-s-adults-say-they-need-to-take-breaks-from-covid-19-news/> (it was found that 86% believe that misinformation is causing either a great deal (49%) or some (37%) confusion about basic facts). See also Michael Sean Pepper & Stephanie Burton, "Sheer Volume of Misinformation Risks Diverting Focus from Fighting Coronavirus", *The Conversation* (29 April 2020), online: <https://theconversation.com/sheer-volume-of-misinformation-risks-diverting-focus-from-fighting-coronavirus-137408>.
7. Harrison Mantas, "COVID-19 Infodemic Exacerbates Existing Religious and Racial Prejudices" (1 May 2020), online: *Poynter* <https://www.poynter.org/reporting-editing/2020/covid-19-infodemic-exacerbates-existing-religious-and-racial-prejudices/> ("COVID-19 has inflamed fears of outsiders across the globe").
8. See Leonardo Bursztyn et al, "Misinformation During a Pandemic" (2020) Becker Friedman Institute [working paper] at abstract: "While our findings cannot yet speak to long-term effects, they indicate that provision of misinformation in the early stages of a pandemic can have important consequences for how a disease ultimately affects the population." See also Mian & Khan, "Public Confusion Leaves Citizens Unprepared for Combatting a Public Health Crisis", *supra* note 1 at 2.
9. See Soroush Vosoughi, Deb Roy & Sinan Aral, "The Spread of True and False News Online" (2018) 359:6380 Science 1141 at 1141, DOI: <10.1126/science.aap9559>, where the authors analyzed millions of social media shares and came to the grim conclusion that "falsehood diffused significantly farther, faster, deeper, and more broadly than the truth in all categories of information."
10. Ryan Ko, "Social Media Is Full of Bots Spreading COVID-19 Anxiety. Don't Fall for It" (2 April 2020), online: *Science Alert* <https://www.sciencealert.com/bots-are-causing-anxiety-by-spreading-coronavirus-misinformation>: "These fake accounts are common on Twitter, Facebook, and Instagram. They have one goal: to spread fear and fake news."
11. Katherine Ellison, "Social Media Posts and Online Searches Hold Vital Clues about Pandemic Spread", *Scientific American* (30 March 2020), online: <https://

it has served as a primary source of news for many in the general public.[12] Indeed, more and more people are turning to social media to keep up-to-date on developments surrounding the pandemic.[13] It has been reported that Twitter had about "12 million more daily users in the first three months of 2020 than in the last three of 2019."[14]

Still, in the context of the "infodemic," social media platforms have been the focus of much of the concern and policy activity.[15] There is some suggestion that the spread of overt misinformation—that is, misinformation provided by known "fake news" sources—on some platforms, such as Facebook, has decreased since the implementation of platform countermeasures, including removing fake accounts and tweaking their algorithm to reduce the reach of debunked articles.[16] But on other platforms, including Twitter, the situation has

www.scientificamerican.com/article/social-media-posts-and-online-searches-hold-vital-clues-about-pandemic-spread/>.

12. See e.g. Alaa Abd-Alrazaq et al, "Top Concerns of Tweeters During the COVID-19 Pandemic: Infoveillance Study" (2020) 22:4 J Medicine Internet Research e19016, DOI: <10.2196/19016>, where the authors analyzed 2.8 million tweets on the pandemic and found tweets on issues such as the source, cause, economic consequences, and treatments and cures, concluding: "Social media provides an opportunity to directly communicate health information to the public."

13. Jeffrey Gottfried & Elisa Shearer, "News Use Across Social Media Platforms 2016" (16 May 2016), online: *Pew Research Center* <https://www.journalism.org/2016/05/ 26/news-use-across-social-media-platforms-2016/>.

14. Jon-Patrick Allem, "Social Media Fuels Wave of Coronavirus Misinformation as Users Focus on Popularity, Not Accuracy", *The Conversation* (6 April 2020), online: <https://theconversation.com/social-media-fuels-wave-of-coronavirus-misinformation-as-users-focus-on-popularity-not-accuracy-135179>. See also Vengattil Munsif & Dave Paresh, "Twitter Ad Sales Hit by Coronavirus but Active Users Soar" (23 March 2020), online: *Reuters* <https://www.reuters.com/article/us-health-coronavirus-twitter/twitter-ad-sales-hit-by-coronavirus-but-active-users-soar-idUSKBN21A3HY>.

15. Ramez Kouzy et al, "Coronavirus Goes Viral: Quantifying the COVID-19 Misinformation Epidemic on Twitter" (2020) 12:3 Cureus e7255, DOI: <10.7759/cureus.7255>.

16. Hunt Allcott, Matthew Gentzkow & Chuan Yu, "Trends in the Diffusion of Misinformation on Social Media" (2019) 6:2 Research & Politics 1 at abstract: "Our results suggest that the relative magnitude of the misinformation problem on Facebook has declined since its peak." See also Paul Resnick, Aviv Ovadya & Garlin Gilchrist, "Iffy Quotient: A Platform Health Metric for Misinformation" (18 October 2018) at 1, online: *School of Information Center for Social Media Responsibility, University of Michigan* <https://csmr.umich.edu/wp-content/uploads/2018/10/UMSI-CSMR-Iffy-Quotient-Whitepaper-810084.pdf>: "there has been gradual improvement in Facebook's Iffy Quotient since mid-2017, with a substantial cumulative impact. [...] In 2016 the Iffy sites' share of attention was about twice as high on Facebook as Twitter; now it is 50% higher on Twitter."

worsened.[17] Much of the misinformation about the coronavirus remains unchecked and continues to circulate, especially on Twitter.[18]

Why and how misinformation spreads and has an impact on behaviours and beliefs is a complex and multidimensional phenomenon.[19] There is an emerging rich academic literature on misinformation, particularly in the context of social media.[20] Here, I make no attempt to provide a comprehensive overview of that work. Rather, I focus on two relatively narrow questions: Is debunking an effective strategy; If so, what kind of counter-messaging is most effective? The goal of this article is to bring together relevant empirical research and expert commentary to serve as a resource and guide in the battle against misinformation (hence the heavy referencing) and to stand as a defence of these efforts.[21]

---

17. Allcott, Gentzkow & Yu, *supra* note 16.
18. J Scott Brennen et al, "Types, Sources, and Claims of COVID-19 Misinformation" (7 April 2020) at 1, online: *Reuters Institute for the Study of Journalism, University of Oxford* <https://reutersinstitute.politics.ox.ac.uk/types-sources-and-claims-covid-19-misinformation>: "On Twitter, 59% of posts rated as false in our sample by fact-checkers remain up." See also Craig Timberg, "On Twitter, Almost 60 Percent of False Claims about Coronavirus Remain Online—Without a Warning Label", *Washington Post* (7 April 2020), online: <https://www.washingtonpost.com/technology/2020/04/07/twitter-almost-60-percent-false-claims-about-coronavirus-remain-online-without-warning-label/>.
19. Dietram A Scheufele & Nicole M Krause, "Science Audiences, Misinformation, and Fake News" (2019) 116:16 PNAS 7662 at 7662, DOI: <10.1073/pnas.1805871115>: "[W]e show how being misinformed is a function of a person's ability and motivation to spot falsehoods, but also of other group-level and societal factors that increase the chances of citizens to be exposed to correct(ive) information."
20. See generally Yuxi Wang et al, "Systematic Literature Review on the Spread of Health-related Misinformation on Social Media" (2019) 240:112552 Social Science & Medicine 1 at 1, DOI: <10.1016/j.socscimed.2019.112552>: "Overall, we observe an increasing trend in published articles on health-related misinformation and the role of social media in its propagation." See also Denise-Marie Ordway, "Fake News and the Spread of Misinformation: A Research Roundup" (1 September 2017), online: *Journalist's Resource* <https://journalistsresource.org/studies/society/internet/fake-news-conspiracy-theories-journalism-research/>.
21. The word "debunking" is less than ideal, as some may feel it fails to capture the need to listen to and engage the public. It can also be associated with a more aggressive, or mocking, approach (a strategy I criticize below). However, in total, with those critiques noted, I still feel it is a good catch-all word that, as defined by Amy Sippitt, can be used to refer to "factual messages which seek to rebut inaccurate factual claims." See Amy Sippitt, "The Backfire Effect: Does It Exist? And Does It Matter for Factcheckers?" (March 2019) at 7, online: *Full Fact* <https://fullfact.org/blog/2019/mar/does-backfire-effect-exist/>.

Is It Worth It?

Let's start with two of most frequently raised arguments *against* vigorously countering the spread of misinformation. One is that correcting misinformation online is simply ineffective. Dumping more science on people has little impact, it is often said, because attempting to correct a misperception can cause individuals to become *more* entrenched in their beliefs. This phenomenon—usually called the "backfire effect"—has received a lot of attention and is often noted whenever there is a call for more individuals to get actively involved in the countering of misinformation. Debunking doesn't work, it is argued.[22]

But how strong is the backfire phenomenon? There are several well-known studies associated with the birth of this concern. Probably the most influential is a study published in 2010 where the researchers explored the impact of corrected news articles that contained a misleading claim by a politician. It was found that "corrections frequently fail to reduce misperceptions among the targeted ideological group" and there were "several instances of a 'backfire effect' in which corrections actually increase misperceptions among the group in question."[23] As a result of this and several other studies, there now seems to be a widely accepted belief that the backfire effect is a dominant phenomenon that makes debunking a near futile exercise.[24]

22. See, for example, Christian Bokhove, "Beware: Debunking Research Myths Can Backfire on You" (19 July 2019), online: *Tes* <https://www.tes.com/magazine/article/beware-debunking-research-myths-can-backfire-you>.
23. Brendan Nyhan & Jason Reifler, "When Corrections Fail: The Persistence of Political Misperceptions" (2010) 32 Political Behaviour 303, DOI: <10.1007/s11109-010-9112-2>.
24. See, for example, Julie Beck, "This Article Won't Change Your Mind", *The Atlantic* (11 December 2019), online: <https://www.theatlantic.com/science/archive/2017/03/this-article-wont-change-your-mind/519093/>; "The Backfire Effect: Why Facts Don't Win Arguments" (15 October 2013), online: *Big Think* <https://bigthink.com/think-tank/the-backfire-effect-why-facts-dont-win-arguments>. See also Erin Brodwin, "Facebook's Covid-19 Misinformation Campaign Is Based on Research. The Authors Worry Facebook Missed the Message" (1 May 2020), online: *StatNews* <https://www.statnews.com/2020/05/01/facebooks-covid-19-misinformation-campaign-is-based-on-research-the-authors-worry-facebook-missed-the-message/>, where it is noted that Facebook's coronavirus misinformation strategy is "designed to avoid what's known as the backfire effect." Why the "backfire effect" gained so much traction is an interesting question on its own, one which is beyond the scope of this piece. But I think that the fact it feels intuitively correct is a big part of its appeal. It is hard to change opinions.

In reality, the backfire effect seems to be a relatively rare occurrence.[25] Indeed, Brendan Nyhan, the lead author of the 2010 study, has noted that their results often have "been overstated and oversold,"[26] in part because their conclusions may be quite context specific.[27] A 2019 comprehensive analysis of the available research concluded that the existing body of evidence—much of it published after the 2010 study—found no backfire effect and that "most recent studies now suggest that generally debunks can make beliefs in specific claims more accurate."[28] For example, a study published in 2019 found that "evidence of factual backfire is far more tenuous than prior research suggests. By and large, citizens heed factual information, even when such information challenges their ideological commitments."[29] Another study from 2019 found that "debunking" works—if done using appropriate strategies (more on that below)—and "no evidence" that "rebutting science denialism in public discussions backfires, not even in vulnerable groups (for example, U.S. conservatives)."[30] To be fair, motivated reasoning (constructing rationales to fit a pre-existing position) and other cognitive biases (for example, confirmation bias) have been shown to influence what information we see online and elsewhere.[31] Still, for many areas of science, at least some research has found that differences in scientific belief are driven mostly by levels of

---

25. Indeed, some have gone so far as to call its existence a myth. See, for example, Laura Hazard Owen, "The 'Backfire Effect' Is Mostly a Myth" (22 March 2019), online: *NiemanLab* <https://www.niemanlab.org/2019/03/the-backfire-effect-is-mostly-a-myth-a-broad-look-at-the-research-suggests/>.
26. See 8 January 2018 tweet by lead author Brendan Nyhan, where he states: "[T]he research findings, including accounts of my own backfire effect paper with @jasonreifler, have often been overstated and oversold" (3 January 2020 at 8:21), online: *Twitter* <https://twitter.com/brendannyhan/status/948544775799607296?lang=en>.
27. For example, see Sippitt, *supra* note 21 at 10, who notes that the experiment "purposefully covered a highly controversial topic in American politics [WMD in Iraq] where people would have prior beliefs" and as such "it's arguably unsurprising that individuals were unpersuaded by a single news item."
28. See *ibid* at 5.
29. Thomas Wood & Ethan Porter, "The Elusive Backfire Effect: Mass Attitudes' Steadfast Factual Adherence" (2019) 41 Political Behaviour 135.
30. Philipp Schmid & Cornelia Betsch, "Effective Strategies for Rebutting Science Denialism in Public Discussions" (2019) 3 Nature Human Behaviour 931 at abstract.
31. For example, see Dan Kahan, "The Politically Motivated Reasoning Paradigm, Part 1: What Politically Motivated Reasoning Is and How to Measure It" in RA Scott and SM Kosslyn, eds, *Emerging Trends in the Social & Behavioral Sciences* (Wiley Library Online, 2016), DOI: <10.1002/9781118900772.etrds0417>.

scientific knowledge and not motivated reasoning.[32] So while a backfire effect may occur in some circumstances—this is an area where more research would be helpful—it certainly isn't such a robust and measurable phenomenon that it should stop us from mounting efforts to counter misinformation on social media.

The second and perhaps more challenging critique of correcting and debunking is that it may inadvertently help to spread misinformation.[33] Specifically, there might an "illusory truth" effect.[34] Studies have consistently found that merely exposing people to an idea increases the believability of that idea.[35] In many ways this is how "fake news" works.[36] A study by Gordon Pennycook et al, for

32. Jonathon McPhetres & Gordon Pennycook, "Science Beliefs, Political Ideology, And Cognitive Sophistication" (2020) at abstract, online: *OSF Preprints* <https://osf.io/ad9v7/>: "We also found little evidence of motivated reasoning; reasoning ability was instead broadly associated with pro-science beliefs. Finally, one's level of basic science knowledge was the most consistent predictor of people's beliefs about science. Results suggest educators and policymakers should focus on increasing basic science literacy and critical thinking rather than the ideologies that purportedly divide people."
33. This is also often called the backfire effect, though it is a different phenomenon than that described by Nyhan & Reifler in "When Corrections Fail," who coined the phrase. As such, I usually treat them as distinct and refer to this as the "spreading" concern.
34. Melissa Healy, "Misinformation About the Coronavirus Abounds, but Correcting It Can Backfire", *Los Angeles Times* (8 February 2020), online: <https://www.latimes.com/science/story/2020-02-08/coronavirus-outbreak-false-information-psychology>: "Sometimes the effort to correct misinformation involves repeating the lie. That repetition seems to establish it in our memories more firmly than the truth."
35. See Jonas De keersmaecker, David Dunning & Gordon Pennycook, "Investigating the Robustness of the Illusory Truth Effect Across Individual Differences in Cognitive Ability, Need for Cognitive Closure, and Cognitive Style" (2020) 46:2 Personality and Social Psychology Bulletin 204. Indeed, this effect can still have an impact even if the information runs counter to an existing knowledge base. See, for example, Lisa K Fazio et al, "Knowledge Does Not Protect Against Illusory Truth" (2015) 144 J Experimental Psychology 993 at 993: "Contrary to prior suppositions, illusory truth effects occurred even when participants knew better."
36. See, for example, Danielle C Polage, "Making Up History: False Memories of Fake News Stories" (2012) 8:2 Europe's J Psychology 245; Christopher Paul & Miriam Matthews, "The Russian 'Firehose of Falsehood' Propaganda Model: Why It Might Work and Options to Counter It" (2016), online: *RAND* <https://www.rand.org/pubs/perspectives/PE198.html>. I have argued that this is also one reason that celebrities can have such a large impact on the spread of misinformation. See, for example, Timothy Caulfield, "Celebrities like Gwyneth Paltrow Made the 2010s the Decade of Health and Wellness Misinformation", *NBC News* (27 December 2019), online: <https://www.nbcnews.com/think/opinion/

example, found that even a single exposure to misinformation could increase subsequent perceptions of accuracy.[37]

So, does this mean that debunking misinformation and conspiracy theories on social media—which often, of necessity, will include a restatement of the problematic belief—has the potential to do more harm than good? While the speculation about the problem of spreading is rooted in evidence about the possible impact of exposure to misinformation, there does not appear to be much direct empirical evidence that debunking actually has this problematic impact. Indeed, a recent study (still in preprint at time of this writing) explored this exact concern by analyzing whether a debunking of a new piece of misinformation—a not widely known and novel myth or conspiracy theory—led to an increase in beliefs about the claim. They found that corrections that "repeated novel misinformation claims did not lead to stronger misconceptions compared to a control group never exposed to the false claims or corrections."[38] As a result of this finding—which fits with other works on this point[39]—the authors conclude, "it is safe to repeat misinformation when correcting it, even when the audience might be unfamiliar with the misinformation."[40]

The timing of a correction may also be relevant here. Claire Wardle, executive director of an institute dedicated to fighting misinformation, suggests that if you debunk a bit of misinformation too early, you may give it unintended oxygen and allow it to spread further.[41] But once the public awareness of a particular myth, conspiracy

---

celebrities-gwyneth-paltrow-made-2010s-decade-health-wellness-misinformation-ncna1107501>. See also Mathew Ingram, "Amplifying the Coronavirus Protests", *Columbia Journalism Review* (22 April 2020), online: <https://www.cjr.org/the_media_today/amplifying-coronavirus-protests.php>, where it is noted that less-than-ideal reporting of lockdown protests may have given them more legitimacy than the objective numbers might have suggested was appropriate.

37. Gordon Pennycook, Tyrone D Cannon & David G Rand, "Prior Exposure Increases Perceived Accuracy of Fake News" (2018) 147:12 J Experimental Psychology: General 1865, DOI: <10.1037/xge0000465>.
38. Ullrich KH Ecker, Stephan Lewandowsky & Matthew Chadwick, "Can Corrections Spread Misinformation to New Audiences? Testing for the Elusive Familiarity Backfire Effect" (2020) [working paper], DOI: <10.31219/osf.io/et4p3>.
39. Ullrich KH Ecker et al, "The Effectiveness of Short-Format Refutational Fact-Checks" (2020) 111:1 British J Psychology 36 at 36: "[W]e found no evidence for a familiarity-driven backfire effect."
40. *Ibid.*
41. Claire Wardle, "What Role Should Newsrooms Play in Debunking COVID-19 Misinformation?", *Nieman Reports* (8 April 2020), online: <https://niemanreports.org/articles/what-role-should-newsrooms-play-in-debunking-covid-19-mis-

theory, or item of misinformation hits a tipping point—that is, the item is starting to be shared more widely—it is important to vigorously counter. If we wait too long to attempt a correction, it may become increasingly difficult to stop the momentum of the misinformation.[42] As we have seen with issues like the myths surrounding vaccination, once a conspiracy theory gets a strong foothold in the public conscious, it can be difficult to dislodge.

A better interpretation of the existing literature is that while we need to be cognizant of the spreading concern, the evidence is far from definitive and what evidence is available suggests it doesn't often happen. There are, of course, many other challenges associated with efforts to correct misinformation, such as the possibility for a range of additional unintended consequences (for example, general warning tags skewing how people perceive legitimate news).[43] But despite the need for more research, there is nothing in the existing research to suggest debunking is a futile exercise. On the contrary, as we will see, there is a growing body of evidence that tells us correcting

information/>. See also Whitney Phillips, "The Oxygen of Amplification: Better Practices for Reporting on Extremists, Antagonists, and Manipulators Online" (2012), online: *Data & Society* <https://datasociety.net/library/oxygen-of-amplification/>; Susan Benkelmam, "Getting it Right: Strategies for Truth-Telling in a Time of Misinformation and Polarization" (11 December 2019), online: *American Press Institute* <https://www.americanpressinstitute.org/publications/reports/strategy-studies/truth-telling-in-a-time-of-misinformation-and-polarization/>: "Journalists must ask themselves whether a falsehood has become so significant that it needs to be knocked down."

42. There is some recent evidence to support this view. See e.g. Wasim Ahmed et al, "COVID-19 and the 5G Conspiracy Theory: Social Network Analysis of Twitter Data" (2020) 22:5 J Medicine Internet Research e19458 at abstract: The authors found that "there was a lack of an authority figure who was actively combating such [5g] misinformation" on social media. What is needed, they conclude, is the "combination of quick and targeted interventions oriented to delegitimize the sources of fake information."

43. John M Carey et al, "The Effects of Corrective Information about Disease Epidemics and Outbreaks: Evidence from Zika and Yellow Fever in Brazil" (2020) 6:5 Science Advances 1 at 9, DOI: <10.1126/sciadv.aaw7449>: "[A] general warning about the presence of fake news has been found to decrease belief in the accuracy of both false and legitimate news headlines." For a study that found the opposite effect, see Gordon Pennycook et al, "The Implied Truth Effect: Attaching Warnings to a Subset of Fake News Headlines Increases Perceived Accuracy of Headlines Without Warnings" (2020) Management Science [forthcoming], DOI: <10.2139/ssrn.3035384>. While placing "fake news" warnings on social media content can have a positive impact, this study found that "the presence of warnings caused untagged headlines to be seen as more accurate than in the control" (at abstract).

misinformation should be viewed as a vitally important science and health policy activity.

What Kind of Counter-Messaging Works?

As with the research on the challenges associated with correcting misinformation, the data surrounding effective debunking strategies is messy and context-dependent. More research on how best to deal with misinformation is clearly needed,[44] but there is little doubt that countering misinformation can have a positive impact.[45] Indeed, silence in the face of misinformation seems likely to be the worst strategy. A 2019 study, for example, found that not responding to misinformation "has a negative effect on attitudes towards behaviours favoured by science."[46] But what kind of social media counter is likely to have the biggest positive result? Below is a list of some of the general themes that have emerged in the research regarding the tone and style of debunking messaging that is relevant to all social media platforms. Here, I focus on the actual content of a social media debunk. Obviously, not every approach will work for every corrective

---

44. See Gordon Pennycook & David Rand, "The Right Way to Fight Fake News", *New York Times* (24 March 2020), online: <https://www.nytimes.com/2020/03/24/opinion/fake-news-social-media.html>: "The obvious conclusion to draw from all this evidence is that social media platforms should rigorously test their ideas for combating fake news and not just rely on common sense or intuition about what will work."
45. For the benefits of debunking in the context of a pandemic, see Toni GLA van der Meer & Yan Jin, "Seeking Formula for Misinformation Treatment in Public Health Crises: The Effects of Corrective Information Type and Source" (2020) 35:5 Health Communications 560 at 560: "Results show that, if corrective information is present rather than absent, incorrect beliefs based on misinformation are debunked and the exposure to factual elaboration, compared to simple rebuttal, stimulates intentions to take protective actions." See generally Nathan Walter & Sheila T Murphy, "How to Unring the Bell: A Meta-Analytic Approach to Correction of Misinformation" (2018) 85:3 Communications Monographs 423 at 436. A meta-analysis of existing data concludes that: "corrective attempts can reduce misinformation across diverse domains, audiences, and designs"; Man-pui Sally Chan et al, "Debunking: A Meta-Analysis of the Psychological Efficacy of Messages Countering Misinformation" (2017) 28:11 Psychological Science 1531; Brendan Nyhan et al, "Taking Fact-Checks Literally But Not Seriously? The Effects of Journalistic Fact-Checking on Factual Beliefs and Candidate Favorability" (2019) Political Behaviour [forthcoming], DOI: <10.1007/s11109-019-09528-x>; Victoria L Rubin, "Deception Detection and Rumor Debunking for Social Media" in L Sloan & A Quan-Haase, eds, *The SAGE Handbook of Social Media Research Methods* (London: SAGE, 2017).
46. Schmid & Betsch, *supra* note 30 at abstract.

message—a tweet is, after all, just 280 characters. But these evidence-informed general principles can help to maximize the impact of efforts to correct online misinformation.

First, use facts. Despite all the concern regarding the impotence of facts to change minds, most studies have found that providing corrective information can be effective,[47] especially if the alterative explanation—the science-informed facts—fills in the gap in understanding caused by the debunk and (when appropriate and possible) provides a causal explanation.[48] This approach can also nudge people to think more critically generally, which may help to shield them against related forms of misinformation.[49]

Second, provide clear, straightforward, and shareable content.[50] Studies have shown that the use of scientific jargon will cause people to disengage, even if explanatory language is also provided in the text.[51]

---

47. Leticia Bode & Emily K Vraga, "In Related News, That Was Wrong: The Correction of Misinformation Through Related Stories Functionality in Social Media" (2015) 65:4 J Communication 619 at 630: "Our experimental evidence suggests that attitude change related to GMOs can be achieved with regard to misperceptions by virtue of exposure to corrective information within social media." See also Emily Falk & Molly Crockett, "You Can Help Slow the Virus if You Talk about it Accurately Online", *Washington Post* (28 April 2020), online: <https://www.washingtonpost.com/outlook/2020/04/28/you-can-help-slow-virus-if-you-talk-about-it-accurately-online/>; *ibid.*
48. See Walter & Murphy, *supra* note 45 at 436: "[C]orrective messages that integrate retractions with alternative explanations (i.e., coherence) emerge as an effective strategy to debunk falsehoods." See also Briony Swire & Ullrich Ecker, "Misinformation and its Correction: Cognitive Mechanisms and Recommendations for Mass Communication" in Brian G. Southwell, Emily A Thorson & Laura Sheble, eds, *Misinformation and Mass Audiences* (Austin: University of Texas Press, 2018): The alternative explanation effectively plugs the model gap left by the retraction. See also Brendan Nyhan & Jason Reifler, "Displacing Misinformation about Events: An Experimental Test of Causal Corrections" (2015) 2:1 J Experimental Political Science 81.
49. See Ecker et al, *supra* note 39 at 49: "We can thus conclude that embedding a rebuttal in a fact-oriented context has beneficial implications beyond specific belief reduction, fostering a more sceptical and evidence-based approach to the issue at hand."
50. Samantha Yammine, "Going Viral: How to Boost the Spread of Coronavirus Science on Social Media", *Nature* (5 May 2020), online: <https://www.nature.com/articles/d41586-020-01356-y>.
51. See e.g. Hillary C Shulman et al, "The Effects of Jargon on Processing Fluency, Self- Perceptions, and Scientific Engagement" (2020) J Language and Social Psychology 1 at 13: "Jargon can then serve as exclusionary language that disengages meaningful relationships between public and expert communities from forming."

Third, use trustworthy and independent sources. Evidence perceived to be removed from an agenda (and the profit motive) is more likely to be trusted and persuasive.[52] While it can be a challenge to find sources that are trusted by all—there has been a significant erosion in trust in many public institutions[53]—public health authorities and independent scientists still retain a relatively high level of trustworthiness, particularly during times of crisis.[54]

Fourth, if applicable and available, emphasize the scientific consensus.[55] Ideally, this tactic should be accompanied by a recognition that science evolves and, as such, the consensus can change.

---

52. Susan T Fiske & Cydney Dupree, "Gaining Trust as Well as Respect in Communicating to Motivated Audiences about Science Topics" (2014) 111:4 PNAS 13593.

53. Timothy Caulfield, "Now More Than Ever, We Must Fight Misinformation. Trust in Science Is Essential", *The Globe and Mail* (20 March 2020), online: <https://www.theglobeandmail.com/opinion/article-now-more-than-ever-we-must-fight-misinformation-trust-in-science-is>. Not surprisingly, studies have found that debunking has a more modest effect if people view the original source of misinformation favourably. But even in this situation, debunking efforts can help. See Jeong-woo Jang, Eun-Ju Lee & Soo Yun Shin, "What Debunking of Misinformation Does and Doesn't" (2019) 22:6 Cyberpsychology, Behavior, & Social Networking 423 at 426: "Overall, the results showed that when the falsehood of information was exposed, participants became less favorable toward the immediate source who shared the misinformation, but their initial source attitude also moderated their reactions by inducing different attribution processes." For another commentary on the impact of low trust, see Mike Caulfield, "Cynicism, Not Gullibility, Will Kill Our Humanity" (27 November 2018), online: *Hapgood* <https://hapgood.us/2018/11/27/cynicism-not-gullibility-will-kill-our-humanity/>.

54. See Pew Research Centre, "Public Holds Broadly Favorable Views of Many Federal Agencies, Including CDC and HHS" (9 April 2020), online: *Pew Research Centre* <https://www.people-press.org/2020/04/09/public-holds-broadly-favorable-views-of-many-federal-agencies-including-cdc-and-hhs/>: "Currently, 79% of U.S. adults express a favorable opinion of the CDC…"; Hannah Fingerhut, "AP-NORC Poll: High Use, Mild Trust of News Media on COVID-19", *Associated Press* (30 April 2020), online: <https://apnews.com/4e2a20bd01bd2352009c3281b657375d>: "Americans are especially likely to trust information about the coronavirus that comes from the CDC or from personal health care providers," See van der Meer & Jin, *supra* note 45 at 560, where it is summarized that during times of crisis "government agency and news media sources are found to be more successful in improving belief accuracy compared to social peers."

55. See Sander L van der Linden, Chris E Clarke & Edward W Maibach, "Highlighting Consensus among Medical Scientists Increases Public Support for Vaccines: Evidence from a Randomized Experiment" (2015) 15:1207 BMC Public Health; Jeremy D Sloane & Jason R Wiles, "Communicating the Consensus on Climate Change to College Biology Majors: The Importance of Preaching to the Choir" (2020) 10:2 Ecology and Evolution 594; Sander L van der Linden et al, "The Scientific Consensus on Climate Change as a Gateway Belief: Experimental Evidence" 10:2 PLoS ONE e0118489, DOI: <10.1371/journal.pone.0118489>; and Sander L van der Linden, "Why Doctors Should Convey the Medical Consensus

Fifth, be nice and be authentic. Research has found that an aggressive language style is perceived to be both less credible and less trustworthy.[56] Don't shame, ridicule, or marginalize members of the public who are looking for answers (though I have less patience for those pushing bunk for profit, brand enhancement, and ideological spin).[57] In addition, messaging that comes from someone who is seen to be a unique and authentic individual—that is, not just a talking head associated with an institution—can also enhance trust, credibility, and the persuasiveness of the message.[58]

Sixth, consider using a narrative. Humans are wired to respond to stories.[59] Indeed, there is some evidence that an engaging anecdote can overwhelm our ability to think scientifically.[60] This is one reason that testimonials are such an effective strategy for marketing unproven therapies.[61] But a narrative can also be used to convey science—and information about critical thinking and the scientific process[62]—in a way that is compelling and memorable.[63]

---

on Vaccine Safety" (2016) 21:3 Evidence Based Medicine 119, DOI: <10.1136/ebmed-2016-110435>.

56. See Lars König & Regina Jucks, "Hot Topics in Science Communication: Aggressive Language Decreases Trustworthiness and Credibility in Scientific Debates" (2019) 28:4 Public Understanding of Science 401. See also Fisk & Dupree, *supra* note 52.

57. Anand Ram, "How to (Tactfully) Discourage Spread of False Pandemic Information", *CBC News* (19 April 2020), online: <https://www.cbc.ca/news/canada/covid-19-misinformation-rumour-1.5532302>, where misinformation expert Claire Wardle notes the value of being empathetic and using words that "put yourself in the same perspective."

58. See Lise Saffran et al, "Constructing and Influencing Perceived Authenticity in Science Communication" (2020) 15:1 PLoS ONE e0226711; Sara Reardon, "Adding a Personal Backstory Could Boost Your Scientific Credibility with the Public", *Nature Career News* (2020), DOI: <10.1038/d41586-020-00857-0>.

59. Michael F Dahlstrom, "Using Narratives and Storytelling to Communicate Science with Nonexpert Audiences" (2014) 111:4 PNAS 13614.

60. Fernando Rodriguez et al, "Examining the Influence of Anecdotal Stories and the Interplay of Individual Differences on Reasoning" (2016) 22:3 Thinking & Reasoning 274 at 274: "[A]necdotal stories decreased the ability to reason scientifically even when controlling for education level and thinking dispositions."

61. Bethany Hawke et al, "How to Peddle Hope: An Analysis of YouTube Patient Testimonials of Unproven Stem Cell Treatments" (2019) 12:6 Stem Cell Reports 1186.

62. See Michael F Dahlstrom & Dietram A Scheufele, "(Escaping) the Paradox of Scientific Storytelling" (2018) 16:10 PLoS Biology e2006720: "[N]arratives might have most of their power not in conveying facts or building excitement but in rebuilding the foundation of understanding scientific reasoning."

63. For an overview of the evidence on point, see Timothy Caulfield et al, "Health Misinformation and the Power of Narrative Messaging in the Public Sphere"

Seventh, emphasize the gaps in logic and the flawed strategies used by those pushing misinformation. Several studies have found that using rational arguments, such as highlighting the rhetorical tools used to spread misinformation (for example, relying on conspiracy theories, misrepresenting risks, using false "experts"), can be an effective debunking strategy.[64]

Eighth, make the facts the hook, not the misinformation. While the evidence about whether debunking can inadvertently spread misinformation is mixed, it makes sense to frame debunking in a manner that makes the correct information—not the misinformation, myth, or conspiracy theory—the memorable part of the messaging.[65] Make sure the misinformation is clearly flagged as wrong so the debunk is the key takeaway.

Finally, the audience should be the general public, not the hard-core believer. This should be the case even if the debunk is triggered by information circulated by a hard-core believer or someone who is pushing misinformation for personal gain.[66] It is difficult to change the mind of someone who is heavily invested in a particular myth or conspiracy theory. As noted by the WHO, the probability of changing a vocal science denier is extremely low.[67] For this reason,

(2019) 2:2 Can J Bioethics 52.

64. See Schmid & Betsch, *supra* note 30; Stephan Lewandowsky & John Cook, *The Conspiracy Theory Handbook* (Fairfax: George Mason University, 2020); Gábor Orosz et al, "Changing Conspiracy Beliefs through Rationality and Ridiculing" (2016) 7:1525 Frontiers in Psychology 8: "[U]ncovering arguments regarding the logical inconsistencies of CT beliefs can be an effective way to discredit them."

65. Some have called this the "truth sandwich" strategy. See Benkelmam, *supra* note 41 at sum: "There are a number of strategies for reporting on falsehoods without amplifying them. One is the 'truth sandwich,' which involves stating a true fact, then the falsehood, then the true fact again." While this approach makes sense, once again there isn't that much direct empirical evidence on point. And there is some research that suggests order may not be that significant. See Evan R Anderson, William S Horton & David N Rapp, "Hungry for the Truth: Evaluating the Utility of 'Truth Sandwiches'" (July 2019), online: *ResearchGate* <www.researchgate.net/publication/334491502_Hungry_for_the_Truth_Evaluating_the_Utility_of_Truth_Sandwiches_as_Refutations>, where it was found that "the truth sandwich structure did not significantly affect the likelihood of readers' endorsing false claims relative to a more typical refutation structure."

66. I will often use a pop culture moment—the spread of misinformation by a celebrity, for example—as an opportunity to create sharable content about science and the problems associated with the spread of health misinformation.

67. World Health Organization, "Best Practices Guidance: How to Respond to Vocal Vaccine Deniers in Public" (Copenhagen: Regional Office for Europe of the World Health Organization, 2016): "Rule 1: The general public is your target audience, not the vocal vaccine denier."

the correct information should be framed as if the general public is the audience.

Empowering Users

Fighting the spread of misinformation will, of course, require more than just carefully crafted debunks on social media. We need to come at this issue from every angle.[68] We need, for instance, social media platforms to adopt evidence-informed strategies that will both remove the most harmful content and heighten user vigilance. Studies have found, for example, that the use of warning tags—such as those "rated false"—on social media posts can be an effective strategy to inform the public about potential problems with accuracy with specific content.[69] And we need a more robust policy response against individuals who are pushing unproven products and ideas on social media platforms in a manner that infringes existing laws and regulations.[70]

Perhaps the most important strategy will be to empower people with the tools necessary to be more critical consumers of information. This should incorporate teaching both critical thinking skills and media literacy,[71] including inoculating (or "pre-bunking") people

68. See e.g. Kate Starbird, "Disinformation's Spread: Bots, Trolls and All of Us" (2019) 571 Nature World View 449, DOI: <10.1038/d41586-019-02235-x>: "But effective disinformation campaigns involve diverse participants; they might even include a majority of 'unwitting agents' who are unaware of their role."

69. Katherine Clayton et al, "Real Solutions for Fake News? Measuring the Effectiveness of General Warnings and Fact-Check Tags in Reducing Belief in False Stories on Social Media" (2019) Political Behaviour at abstract, " … indicate that false headlines are perceived as less accurate when people receive a general warning." While warning tags seem to have a role to play, they need to be deployed sensibly. Research has found, for example, that general warnings telling readers to beware of misinformation can have an unintended spillover of effect of decreasing "belief in the accuracy of true headlines…" Pennycook et al, *supra* note 43 highlights that using warning tags can lead to an inappropriate implication that posts without warnings are *more* accurate. See also Melanie Freeze et al, "Fake Claims of Fake News: Political Misinformation, Warnings, and the Tainted Truth Effect" (2020) Political Behaviour, DOI: 10.1007/s11109-020-09597-3>.

70. For an example of regulatory action, see Health Canada, *Health Products that Make False or Misleading Claims to Prevent, Treat or Cure COVID-19 May Put Your Health at Risk,* (Advisory RA-72659) (Ottawa: Health Canada, 27 March 2020); Federal Trade Commission, Press Release, "FTC Sends 45 More Letters Warning Marketers to Stop Making Unsupported Claims That Their Products and Therapies Can Effectively Prevent or Treat COVID-19" (7 May 2020).

71. See e.g. Michelle A Amazeen & Erik P Bucy, "Conferring Resistance to Digital Disinformation: The Inoculating Influence of Procedural News Knowledge"

against misinformation[72] and simply reminding them to think about accuracy before sharing.[73] A growing body of literature has found that, in general, people want to be accurate and want to share only factual material.[74] Most users do not fall for or share misinformation due to a malevolent agenda or, even, a partisan bias.[75] If we can nudge people to think about accuracy before they share social media content, we may be able to have a significant impact on the spread of misinformation.[76] A 2020 study that specifically looked at misinformation in the context of the coronavirus found exactly this effect, concluding

(2019) 63:3 J Broadcasting & Electronic Media 415 at 429: "[A]dditional educational campaigns to inform citizens about mainstream news media operations could yield significant benefits." See also Viren Swami et al, "Analytic Thinking Reduces Belief in Conspiracy Theories" (2014) 133:3 Cognition 572.

72. See e.g. Jon Roozenbeek & Sander van der Linden, "The New Science of Prebunking: How to Inoculate against the Spread of Misinformation" (7 October 2019), online (blog): *BMC On Society* <http://blogs.biomedcentral.com/on-society/2019/10/07/the-new-science-of-prebunking-how-to-inoculate-against-the-spread-of-misinformation/>; Jon Roozenbeek & Sander van der Linden, "Fake News Game Confers Psychological Resistance against Online Misinformation" (2019) 5:65 Palgrave Communications at abstract, DOI: 10.1057/s41599-019-0279-9>: "We provide initial evidence that people's ability to spot and resist misinformation improves after gameplay [which is teaching about misinformation], irrespective of education, age, political ideology, and cognitive style."

73. Bence Bago, David G Rand & Gordon Pennycook, "Fake News, Fast and Slow: Deliberation Reduces Belief in False (But Not True) News Headlines" J Experimental Psychology: General, Advance online publication, online: *NCBI* <https://www.ncbi.nlm.nih.gov/pubmed/31916834> at abstract: "Our data suggest that, in the context of fake news, deliberation facilitates accurate belief formation and not partisan bias."

74. Emma Young, "Most People Who Share 'Fake News' Do Care About the Accuracy of News Items—They're Just Distracted" (16 January 2020), online: *Research Digest (The British Psychological Society)* <https://digest.bps.org.uk/2020/01/16/most-people-who-share-fake-news-do-care-about-the-accuracy-of-news-items-theyre-just-distracted/>.

75. Gordon Pennycook & David G Rand, "Lazy, Not Biased: Susceptibility to Partisan Fake News is Better Explained by Lack of Reasoning Than By Motivated Reasoning" (2019) 188 Cognition 39 at abstract: "Our findings therefore suggest that susceptibility to fake news is driven more by lazy thinking than it is by partisan bias per se—a finding that opens potential avenues for fighting fake news."

76. See e.g. Lisa Fazio, "Pausing to Consider Why a Headline is True or False Can Help Reduce the Sharing of False News" (10 February 2020), online: *Misinformation Review* <https://misinforeview.hks.harvard.edu/article/pausing-reduce-false-news/>: "This research suggests that forcing people to pause and think can reduce shares of false information"; Gordon Pennycook et al, "Understanding and Reducing the Spread of Misinformation Online" (25 November 2019) at abstract [working paper], online: <https://psyarxiv.com/3n9u8/>: "we find that subtly inducing people to think about the concept of accuracy increases the quality of the news they share."

that "nudging people to think about accuracy is a simple way to improve choices about what to share on social media."[77]

Conclusion

There is a growing body of research on both the phenomenon of online misinformation and the best way counter it. While the data remain complex and, at times, contradictory, there is little doubt that efforts to correct misinformation are worthwhile. In fact, fighting the spread of misinformation should be viewed as a critical health and science policy priority.

77. Gordon Pennycook, "Fighting COVID-19 Misinformation on Social Media: Experimental Evidence for a Scalable Accuracy Nudge Intervention" (2020) [working paper], online: <https://psyarxiv.com/uhbk9/>.

CHAPTER B-5

The Media Paradox and the COVID-19 Pandemic

Jeffrey Simpson*

Abstract

The COVID-19 pandemic struck the media financially, depressing advertising revenues and imperiling already shaky balance sheets. At the very moment when demand for news rose, as it usually does in crises, the media had fewer financial and personnel resources to meet that demand. Similarly, the media generally has few reporters and editors educated and experienced in science, as opposed to politics, economics, and culture. Nonetheless, the media mobilized the resources it had and did a creditable job covering the facts of the crisis as provided by public health officials and political leaders, who took their cue from those officials. Perhaps belatedly, the media did focus on problems revealed by the crisis, notably in the long-term care and nursing home sectors.

Résumé
Le paradoxe médiatique et la pandémie de COVID-19

La pandémie de COVID-19 a secoué les médias sur le plan financier, entraînant une baisse des recettes publicitaires et mettant en péril des bilans déjà fragiles. Au moment même où la demande d'informations

* Author of seven books, including one on the Canadian health care system, which won the Donner Prize for the best book on Canadian public policy.

augmentait, comme c'est généralement le cas lors d'une crise, les médias avaient moins de ressources financières et humaines pour y répondre. De même, ils disposaient généralement de peu de journalistes et de rédacteurs en chef formés et expérimentés dans le domaine scientifique, contrairement à la politique, à l'économie et à la culture. Malgré tout, les médias ont mobilisé les ressources auxquelles ils avaient accès et ont fait un travail honorable en couvrant les faits de la crise qui leur étaient présentés par les responsables de la santé publique et les dirigeants politiques, eux-mêmes guidés par ces responsables. Les médias se sont intéressés, bien que tardivement, aux problèmes révélés par la crise, notamment dans les résidences de soins de longue durée et les maisons de retraite.

The COVID-19 crisis has highlighted a paradox for today's media. Seldom was the thirst for information greater than during this crisis; never was the news media's financial wherewithal thinner for providing information about it.

Crises heighten worries about the unknown. Think of 9/11. Who does not remember the news of those attacks? The shock produced fear. Were terrorists going to strike elsewhere? Were they part of a larger assault for which we were not prepared? Who were these people, and what did they want?

Canada closed its airspace to commercial flights for four days after the planes crashed into buildings in New York and Washington, DC, in contrast to the prolonged shutdown during the coronavirus crisis. After swift and adroit diplomatic efforts by the Chrétien government, notably senior minister John Manley, Canada presented ideas to a stunned U.S. government about how and why to keep open the Canada–U.S. border. By contrast, the Canada–U.S. border remained closed for months, except for "essential travel," which included commerce. Normal travel by people was forbidden. The aftermath of the 9/11 attacks inflicted very modest economic damage on Canada but no public health woes. The coronavirus has produced both a public health crisis and an economic meltdown.

News about terrorism continued for years after 9/11. But at home, terrorism news was eventually relegated to the back pages, except when separate terrorist incidents occurred on Parliament Hill and in Quebec. Just as long waiting lines for airport security continue to remind us of terrorism and those 9/11 attacks, too willl certain long-term institutional and attitudinal changes be woven into our lives after COVID-19. Just which ones, when and how, remains unclear.

COVID-19 is different from 9/11. Instead of one unexpected blow, as with 9/11, the virus crept up on the country: vague, early reports about a virus in faraway China; comments and concerns from the World Health Organization (WHO); dismissive remarks from a loud, foolish voice in the White House; and few early alarm bells in Ottawa or provincial capitals. Outbreaks then occurred in places Canadians knew better: Italy, Spain, and elsewhere in Europe, until finally, slowly at first, then with growing and deadly rapidity, the coronavirus took hold here. Canada became part of a worldwide pandemic.

The Canadian media took its cue from international reports about the coronavirus overseas from foreign sources, because Canadian reporting about and from the world has almost completely disappeared. Twenty years ago, Canadian correspondents were sprinkled around the world. A gaggle of them, some very perspicacious, were posted in China. Only *The Globe and Mail* today maintains a bureau in China. The *Globe*'s Beijing correspondent Nathan VanderKlippe was alive to the COVID-19 story in Wuhan early.

If events that might directly affect Canadians happen elsewhere, except in Washington, chances are Canadians will not hear about them from their own foreign correspondents, because only *The Globe and Mail* and the state-subsidized Canadian Broadcasting Corporation/Radio-Canada deploy them.

The shrivelling of foreign coverage by and for Canadians is part of a wider story of the decline of the traditional media, as opposed to the digital media. COVID-19 exacerbated this decline with consequences that are already apparent and will intensify whenever the crisis ends.

Newspapers, radio, and television have been losing revenues in recent years as the digital age unfolds. Younger people turn elsewhere; advertisers look elsewhere to reach consumers; digital giants such as Google suck up advertising. Digital advertising revenues are increasing, but traditional advertising is declining faster. A thorough, detailed report about the media from the Public Policy Forum in 2017 stated: "Journalism's economic model has collapsed, profoundly and structurally." For example, newspaper classified ads attracted $819 million in revenues in 2009 but only $119 million in 2015.[1] The downdraught hit other forms of print advertising—careers, retail, entertainment, company announcements. It also struck radio and television, with the result that companies reduced their reporting and behind-the-scenes personnel. The number of reporters and technical staff required to cover the news, let alone to analyze it, declined.

Along came COVID-19. Its effects on the media were immediate. Postmedia Network closed 15 community newspapers in Ontario and Manitoba, furloughed some staff, and imposed salary reductions for employees earning more than $60,000. Print and digital advertising had experienced "very significant" declines, the company said.[2] Torstar eliminated 85 positions and cut its operating budget. The readership of The Toronto Star.com and other Torstar websites increased, but not enough to offset "substantial" declines in advertising, the company explained.[3] Saltwire Media, Atlantic Canada's largest newspaper chain, laid off 40% of its staff and shut down all its weekly newspapers.[4] The desire to consume news during the crisis was not matched by an increase in revenues. Indeed, *The Globe and Mail* made news about the crisis free as a public service, rather than charging digital subscribers for it. Governments, it is true, helped by buying large amounts of advertising instructing citizens about the disease and what should be done to prevent its spread. But this income, although undoubtedly useful, could not staunch the flow of red ink.

The COVID-19 story challenged the media beyond coping with fewer staff and reduced revenues. Few journalists have any scientific or medical training. Most are generalists. Some might have

1. "The Shattered Mirror: News, Democracy and Trust in the Digital Age" (January 2017), online (pdf): *Public Policy Forum* <shatteredmirror.ca/wp-content/uploads/theShatteredMirror.pdf>.
2. Aleksandra Sagan, "Postmedia to Lay Off 80 Employees, Permanently Close 15 Newspapers as COVID-19 Hits Revenue", *The Globe and Mail* (28 April 2020), online: <www.theglobeandmail.com/business/article-postmedia-to-lay-off-80-employees-permanently-close-15-newspapers-as>.
3. "Torstar Eliminates 85 Positions as Coronavirus Cuts into Ad Revenue", *Financial Post* (7 April 2020), online: <business.financialpost.com/telecom/media/torstar-eliminates-85-positions-as-coronavirus-cuts-into-ad-revenue>.
4. Anjuli Patil, "Atlantic Canada's Largest Newspaper Chain Temporarily Lays Off 40% of Staff", *CBC News* (24 March 2020), online: <www.cbc.ca/news/canada/nova-scotia/saltwire-network-announces-temporary-layoffs-covid-19-1.5508396>.

experience, academic or actual, in understanding politics or economics, the courts, or the broad outline of the health care system, or culture or sports or whatever—but not medicine per se, and certainly not pandemics. Who can blame them? Do elected officials have this knowledge? Pandemics do not happen often. Outbreaks in recent times have sometimes been rather localized—SARS in Toronto, Ebola in Africa—and based on different viruses than the coronavirus. SARS caused 774 deaths worldwide in 2003 and only 43 in Canada.[5] The WHO declared that pandemic over six months after it began.[6] Once it became obvious that COVID-19 was a virus many times more serious than SARS, the media was thrust perforce into reporting and explaining something new, ubiquitous, challenging, and foreign.

The media is at an immediate disadvantage when faced with such stories, since only a handful of reporters are knowledgeable about public health and diseases. Any journalist can gab about politics, even if they do not really know much about what is going on, but such gabbing is essentially harmless background noise. Reporting on a pandemic where lives are at stake and the economy shudders is a different matter.

Lacking expertise in reporting on pandemics (with a few notable exceptions), the media performed, as best it could and sometimes admirably, the essential duty of reporting the "facts" as they could be known. The media reported daily what public health officials and political actors said, and why they said it. Since public figures throughout the crisis spoke with forthrightness and dignity, sticking to facts however unpalatable, the media did not feel, as in other instances, that partisan or tactical considerations lay behind public utterances. The media, by and large, trusted these non-partisan public figures because the media itself had no access to conflicting information and did not ascribe ulterior motives to those in positions of authority.

In general, trust in public figures is especially pronounced when it comes to medical and provincial officers of health, most of whom are women. These officers spoke frankly but with empathy and won almost universal respect. Political leaders are enjoying a jump in popularity. Prime Minister Justin Trudeau's and most of the provincial

---

5. "Summary of Probable SARS Cases with Onset of Illness from 1 November 2002 to 31 July 2003" (last visited 27 May 2020), online: *World Health Organization* <www.who.int/csr/sars/country/table2004_04_21/en>.
6. "SARS Outbreak Contained Worldwide" (5 July 2003), online: *World Health Organization* <www.who.int/mediacentre/news/releases/2003/pr56/en/>.

premiers' polling numbers have improved since the beginning of the crisis.[7] International polling is showing increases in support for incumbents in many countries, except in the United States and Brazil.[8]

In Canada, health care is a responsibility divided between the federal and provincial governments. Even municipalities have medical officers of health. In contrast to the U.S., it was striking to see how the two senior levels of government cooperated and avoided useless political point-scoring. The federation worked well. Journalists who are accustomed to covering federal–provincial conflicts had few serious tensions to report. There were grumblings about access to equipment and some confusion about which government was responsible for what but compared with the frequent federal–provincial blame game, these were modest indeed. The oft-used slogan "We are all in this together" underscored the lack of appetite for partisan debate. The media that inherently defines news as conflict therefore could not display its preference for partisan skirmishing.

Elements of the media did contribute through editorial skepticism to the federal government changing course on several proposed policies. Commentators complained the first iteration of the government's wage subsidy was too low. It was subsequently raised. The government, criticized in Parliament and by the media, abandoned the notion that it could authorize all spending without parliamentary approval. Media voices raised questions about the efficacy of certain government remedial programs, but on the issue of public health media largely supported the policies of the medical officers of health and the politicians who followed their advice. Was the media too supine about public health decisions and proclamations? In a few cases, perhaps; overall, no.

7. "Federal Politics: Justin Trudeau's Handling of COVID-19 Crisis Lifts His Approval to Highest Level Since 2017" (22 April 2020), online: *Angus Reid Institute* <angusreid.org/federal-issues-april-2020>; Philippe J Fournier, "388Canada: Canadians Are Overwhelmingly Satisfied with Their Governments' COVID-19 Responses", *Maclean's* (13 April 2020), online: <www.macleans.ca/news/canada/338canada-canadians-are-overwhelmingly-satisfied-with-their-governments-covid-19-responses>; Robert Benzie, "Political Leaders Have Seen Approval Ratings Surge During the COVID-19 Pandemic, Poll Finds", *Toronto Star* (6 May 2020), online: <www.thestar.com/politics/provincial/2020/05/06/political-leaders-have-seen-approval-ratings-surge-during-the-covid-19-pandemic-poll-finds.html>.
8. "Covid-19 Has Given Most World Leaders a Temporary Rise in Popularity", *The Economist* (9 May 2020), online: <www.economist.com/graphic-detail/2020/05/09/covid-19-has-given-most-world-leaders-a-temporary-rise-in-popularity>.

It might be argued that the media missed anticipating one of the important, tragic elements of the COVID-19 pandemic: the outbreaks of the disease that struck with often fatal consequences in nursing and long-term care facilities. Perhaps a more alert media would have understood early on that such facilities, with so many frail patients and staff in close proximity, would become "hot spots" for the disease. But that kind of prescience would have taken sustained commitment to cover health care in all of its dimensions, something the media does not do well, dwindling resources and ephemeral attention spans, among other reasons. The media often plays catch-up; that is, when something suddenly pops up on the public radar screen, as with the pandemic's appearance in nursing homes and long-term care institutions, the media reported the outbreaks, the reaction of loved ones, and the reaction of governments. And when cries went up to take private institutions into public ownership, the media reported the cries, but then ignored a discussion of what such a move would entail—billions of dollars expropriating private property and the bottom-line costs of running the institutions. This debate, now launched by the New Democratic Party and the Canadian Labour Congress, will likely go on for some time, with evidence from some shoddy for-profit institutions being raised as justification for more public ownership.

Skepticism is part of the media's obligation to hold public authorities to account. It does this, among other methods, by asking if better ways exist to achieve objectives or questioning whether the objectives themselves are valid. In the case of COVID-19, the objectives seemed almost universally agreed upon: the maximization of the public health of the population and the eventual re-opening of the economy. The means to achieve those objectives will continue to be debated, as they should be, in the media. And various options will be given full coverage, including the ones that might, in the opinion of frequently quoted experts, increase chances of a second wave of the virus developing in the fall.

The primary objective of keeping people safe raised various questions that the media asked but did not pursue; notably whether those in authority had missed or minimized signals coming from overseas about the seriousness of COVID-19. Similarly, in the aftermath of SARS, had Canada prepared itself adequately for another pandemic? The answer is evidently no. But the media, by and large, did not belabour this lack of preparation, because SARS was by many orders of magnitude less menacing than COVID-19 and the viruses were different. Preparations for something akin to SARS would have been inadequate for COVID-19. Moreover, electoral cycles are four years. Pandemic preparations for the unknown take much longer.

Here is a failing not only of the media but of the body politic: forgetfulness as events rush forward. In theory, the media should be the public's reminder of matters come-and-gone but nonetheless serious, as in pandemic preparations. After SARS, former University of Toronto President and medical doctor David Naylor reported on lessons learned and proposals for better preparation.[9] It was reported on, then largely forgotten. The occasional writer would pen a commentary reminding us of the perils of pandemics. A 2015 report on pandemic preparedness by a group of civil servants did not produce sustained action.[10] The question therefore is why the media did not follow up and pester elected officials, to which the perhaps unsatisfactory answer is a combination of the previously mentioned shrinking of resources and, of greater importance, the rush of events otherwise known as the "news." The urgent too often trumps the important in the media business, now operating on a 24-hour news cycle for audiences with fleeting attention spans. Preparing for something that might happen, somewhere, sometime, with unknown consequences does not at all fit into the paradigm of what constitutes "news." Of importance, yes; of "news" value, no—until a pandemic happens, at which point the lack of preparation becomes "news."

The media did fall into the trap of putting too much faith in long-term predictions that any experienced journalist should be inured to treat with great skepticism, be it in economics, politics, or anything else involving the human condition. For instance, who can really predict with accuracy three years from voting day which party will form a government? Where will the stock market be in two or three years? What will economic growth be three years hence? Will war break out somewhere? Or, as a former bank economist predicted in a book *The End of Oil*, when will the price of oil hit $200 a barrel? Answer: it did not and will not. Oil is still with us in such abundance that the price has plummeted, even to entering negative numbers at one point.

9. *Learning from SARS: Renewal of Public Health in Canada—Report of the National Advisory Committee on SARS and Public* (Ottawa: Health Canada, 2003).
10. "Canadian Pandemic Influenza Preparedness: Planning Guidance for the Health Sector" (last modified 9 September 2019), online: *Public Health Agency of Canada* <www.canada.ca/en/public-health/services/flu-influenza/canadian-pandemic-influenza-preparedness-planning-guidance-health-sector.html>.

Not being knowledgeable in things scientific, the media reported gloomy, even apocalyptic, projections without asking skeptical questions. The media may thereby have contributed to public misunderstanding of the seriousness of the outbreak. That COVID-19 was literally deadly serious all right, with a dispiriting ability to be transmitted easily; that it would reach the infection and death levels projected in worst-case scenarios would have presumed failure in policy by governments and lack of fidelity to proposed measures by citizens. Neither occurred.

Early studies of COVID-19's infection rates and possible death totals, including an influential one from the Imperial College COVID-19 Response Team in Britain, produced alarmist projections, including its "best-case" scenario, wherein even if Britain took all possible restraining measures the National Health System (NHS) would be "overwhelmed." (The study projected that by the second week of April, the NHS would need 30 times the available number of beds. Instead, the NHS has had plenty of empty beds.) Short of these measures, the Imperial College study suggested that perhaps 500,000 Britons and 2.2 million Americans would die.[11] The same sort of early, ugly scenarios appeared in Canadian reports. Anticipated "surges" caused hospitals to move patients to other facilities and clear operating rooms that, as things turned out, were not needed for COVID-19 patients. The patients who suffered from idle beds were those for whom operations for other medical problems had been delayed—delays of the sort that plague the Canadian health care system according to various international, comparative studies. The British Columbia government acknowledged, for example, that *before* the COVID-19 crisis 90,000 patients had been awaiting surgery.[12]

Given the rush of events, the uncertainty of the virus's trajectory, the cascading effects on the economy (that is, on the lives of millions of people), the dwindling of reportorial resources, and the international dimensions of the crisis, the media performed as well as could

11. Neil Ferguson et al, "Impact of Non-Pharmaceutical Interventions (NPIs) to Reduce COVID19 Mortality and Healthcare Demand" (16 March 2020), online (pdf): *Imperial College COVID-19 Response Team* <www.imperial.ac.uk/media/imperial-college/medicine/sph/ide/gida-fellowships/Imperial-College-COVID19-NPI-modelling-16-03-2020.pdf>.

12. Kelly Grant & Justine Hunter, "Provinces Face Big Backlogs as They Resume Elective Operations", *The Globe and Mail* (7 May 2020), online: <www.theglobeandmail.com/canada/article-provinces-face-big-backlogs-as-they-resume-elective-surgeries>.

be expected, maybe even better. That the public had a high degree of knowledge of how to behave and supported government measures and entreaties to influence behaviour suggests citizens did pay attention to the media and were not misled by the nature and seriousness of the virus.

CHAPTER B-6

Governmental Power and COVID-19: The Limits of Judicial Review*

Paul Daly**

Abstract

This paper argues that anyone hoping for a high level of judicial engagement with the forms of power being used to combat the cultural, economic, medical, social, and other impacts from the current pandemic is likely to be disappointed. First, I explain the different forms of power being used in Canada to respond to the pandemic: *imperium* (general norms with the force of law), *dominium* (government contracting and distribution of resources), and *suasion* (information provided to the citizenry). Second, I explain why judges are unlikely to enforce public law principles, such as reasonableness, procedural fairness, and compliance with constitutional norms, on the uses of these different forms of power. As to imperium, any judicial engagement is likely to be at the margins; as to dominium and suasion, there is a long tradition of courts refusing to judicially review contractual decisions and non-binding guidance. Those concerned about the difficulty of holding Canadian governments to account in these trying times would be better advised to look to improving the channels of political accountability than trying to navigate those of legal accountability.

* Thanks to Kseniya Kudischeva for research assistance, to Marie-France Fortin, Jennifer A. Quaid, and Mel Cappe for discussion, and to the editors and anonymous reviewers for comments.

** University Research Chair in Administrative Law & Governance, University of Ottawa.

Résumé
Pouvoirs publics et COVID-19 : les limites du contrôle judiciaire

Ce texte affirme que quiconque aspire à un niveau élevé d'engagement judiciaire de la part des divers pouvoirs responsables de contrer les répercussions culturelles, économiques, médicales, sociales et autres de la pandémie actuelle risque fort d'être déçu. Tout d'abord, je présente les différentes formes de pouvoir employées au Canada pour répondre à la pandémie : *imperium* (normes générales ayant force de loi), *dominium* (passation des marchés publics et distribution des ressources) et *persuasion* (informations fournies aux citoyens). Puis, j'explique pourquoi il est peu probable que les juges appliquent les principes de droit public, comme le caractère raisonnable, l'équité procédurale et le respect des normes constitutionnelles, à l'utilisation de ces différentes formes de pouvoir. En ce qui concerne l'imperium, tout engagement judiciaire est susceptible de se trouver à la marge ; quant au dominium et à la persuasion, il existe une longue tradition de refus par les tribunaux de revoir les décisions contractuelles et les orientations non contraignantes. Ceux qui s'inquiètent de la difficulté à tenir les gouvernements canadiens responsables en ces temps difficiles seraient mieux avisés de chercher à améliorer les canaux de la responsabilité politique plutôt que d'essayer de naviguer sur ceux de la responsabilité juridique.

In Westminster-style systems, such as Canada, there are two primary forms of accountability, political and legal.[1] Legal accountability emphasizes the role of courts in imposing constraints of law and due process on the freedom of action of those in the political branches of government. Political accountability relies on individual interests and the public good being safeguarded by robust debate within the political process, supported by an active media, civil society organizations, and engaged private citizens.[2]

Current conditions are hardly ideal for political accountability. If legislatures are sitting at all, they are doing so in reduced numbers

1. See e.g. Paul Daly, "*Miller*: Legal and Political Fault Lines" (2017) Public L (Brexit Special Issue) 73 at 86-90; Yee-Fui Ng, "Political Constitutionalism: Individual Responsibility and Collective Restraint" (2020) Federal L Rev [forthcoming in 2020].
2. See further Vanessa MacDonnell, this volume, Chapter B-1.

or remotely, with parliamentarians having to adjust to Zoom and other electronic meeting platforms. And, of course, governments have insisted that pandemic conditions require rapid responses, reducing the time available for parliamentary scrutiny. Moreover, media, civil society organizations, and citizens face an information deficit, as our understanding of COVID-19 remains a work-in-progress and official statistics about tests, infections, hospitalizations, deaths, and recoveries are difficult to decipher.[3] The resultant shortfall in terms of political accountability might be thought to create a heightened need for legal accountability, in the form of rigorous judicial oversight of governmental responses to the COVID-19 crisis. This could take the form of robust controls holding governments—and private actors aiding governments—to public law principles: the high standards of substantive reasonableness, procedural fairness, and human rights protections developed by the courts in recent decades.[4] With acceptable levels of political accountability hard to achieve, perhaps courts could help to ensure that emergency powers, state largesse, and official guidance are being used appropriately and are achieving governmental objectives. However, those who hope for a high level of judicial engagement with the forms of power being used to combat the cultural, economic, medical, social, and other impacts from the current pandemic are likely to be disappointed.

In this first section of this chapter, I explain the different forms of power being used in Canada, at the federal and provincial levels, to respond to the pandemic. In the second section, I explain why judicial control of these forms of power is likely to be limited. Judicial control of public administration is carried out through judicial review, which allows the courts to impose public law principles on governmental decision makers. These public law principles include reasonableness, procedural fairness, and compliance with the Constitution of Canada, including the *Charter of Rights and Freedoms*. Where governmental decision-makers fail to comply with public law principles, their decisions can be invalidated by the courts. But as I will explain, there is little prospect of muscular judicial engagement with governmental responses to the pandemic.[5] This is not because the courts are inaccessible—though

3. See Colleen M Flood & Bryan Thomas, this volume, Chapter A-6.
4. Jennifer A Quaid suggests, for instance, in her contribution to this section that legal controls should be adapted to the exigencies of the current situation, improving accountability. See Quaid, this volume, Chapter B-8.
5. See also Marie-France Fortin, this volume, Chapter B-7.

this is often a problem[6]—but because of the forms of power being used by governments to respond to the current crisis. Accordingly, with legal accountability likely to be limited, there is a pressing need for robust political scrutiny of Canadian governments.

Forms of Power

Governments can use different forms of power to achieve their objectives. Terence Daintith makes an analytically useful distinction between *imperium*, *dominium*, and *suasion*. *Imperium* denotes "the government's use of the command of law in aid of its policy objectives" taking the familiar form of statute and delegated legislation; *dominium* concerns "the employment of the wealth of government," used to enter into contracts and otherwise spend money; and *suasion* relates to the use of information to enlighten and persuade the citizenry.[7] Canada's federal and provincial governments have used the force of law (*imperium*), the force of money (*dominium*), and the force of information (*suasion*) to respond to the COVID-19 pandemic.

At the federal level, Parliament has adopted economic emergency legislation to respond to the crisis. Bill C-13 provides significant fiscal authority to the federal government to respond to the economic fallout from the pandemic.[8] Provincial legislation has also been passed at speed.[9] Moreover, the provinces have invoked emergency powers under public health legislation.[10] Some of these powers are

6. MacDonnell, *supra* note 2.
7. "The Techniques of Government" in Jeffrey Jowell & Dawn Oliver, eds, *The Changing Constitution* (Oxford: Clarendon Press, 1995) at 212-13, as summarized in Jo Shaw, Jo Hunt & Chloe Wallace, *Economic and Social Law of the European Union* (Basingstoke, UK: Palgrave Macmillan, 2007).
8. See *COVID-19 Emergency Response Act*, SC 2020, c 5.
9. The Alberta Legislature modified existing public health emergency legislation through the *Public Health (Emergency Powers) Amendment Act*, SA 2020 c 5 to give Ministers the ability to amend other parts of the statute book and to make orders with retroactive effect; see especially Shaun Fluker, "COVID-19 and Retroactive Law-Making in the *Public Health (Emergency Powers) Amendment Act* (Alberta)" (6 April 2020), online (blog): *ABlawg* <www.ablawg.ca/2020/04/06/COVID-19-and-retroactive-law-making-in-the-public-health-emergency-powers-amendment-act-alberta/>. Perhaps this was motivated by a concern that emergency orders already made might not have had a sufficiently firm legal basis; see Shaun Fluker, "COVID-19 and the *Public Health Act* (Alberta)" (31 March 2020), online (blog): *ABlawg* <ablawg.ca/2020/03/31/COVID-19-and-the-public-health-act-alberta/>.
10. In Ontario, the government has invoked the *Emergency Management and Civil Protection Act*, RSO 1990, c E.9, which has given it the power to close all businesses

quite sweeping. For example, Quebec's emergency decree purports to modify judicial orders relating to child custody arrangements;[11] at the federal level, although most of Bill C-13's important provisions are subject to sunset clauses and will expire before the end of the year, the Minister of Finance has been given the power to create and capitalize a Crown corporation (which is exempted from the usual statutory rules on Crown corporations) for whatever pandemic-related purpose he deems fit.[12]

Both the federal government and provincial governments have entered into contractual arrangements to secure necessary medical supplies, existing stockpiles proving insufficient to meet current needs.[13] On occasion, private bodies have been co-opted into the emergency response. Airlines flying into and within Canada, for instance, are obliged to check passengers for symptoms of COVID-19.[14] There is little doubt that *dominium* will continue to play a prominent role as the COVID-19 crisis drags on, with governments entering into further contracts for supplies, antiviral drugs, and vaccines.

Lastly, the technique of *suasion* has been very much in evidence. Since before the pandemic swept Canada, public health officials have regularly been providing advice and guidance on matters such as travel and personal safety.[15] Daily newspapers in Ontario invariably feature government advertisements urging residents to stay home to "flatten the curve" of viral spread and to protect vital public services.

save those that are essential and limit gatherings of groups of people; see *Closure of Places of Non-Essential Businesses*, O Reg 119/20.

11. See e.g. *Ordering of measures to protect the health of the population during the COVID-19 pandemic situation*, OIC 2020-006 (2020) GOQ II, 778A (*Public Health Act*).
12. See Paul Daly, "Emergency Economic Powers in Canada: Bill C-13's Crown Corporation" (1 April 2020), online (blog): *Administrative Law Matters* <www.administrativelawmatters.com/blog/2020/04/01/emergency-economic-powers/>.
13. See e.g. Elizabeth Thompson, "How the Federal Government Can Fast-track Medical Supplies in a Crisis", *CBC News* (18 March 2020), online: <www.cbc.ca/news/politics/covid-emergency-procurement-supplies-1.5500984>; Bartley Kives, "Manitoba Plans to Purchase $35M Worth of Masks, Sanitizers and Other Gear to Protect Against COVID-19", *CBC News* (10 March 2020), online: <www.cbc.ca/news/canada/manitoba/manitoba-covid-equipment-1.5492577>.
14. See "Coronavirus Disease (COVID-19): Travel Restrictions, Exemptions and Advice" (last modified 22 May 2020), online: *Government of Canada* <www.canada.ca/en/public-health/services/diseases/2019-novel-coronavirus-infection/latest-travel-health-advice.html#domestic>.
15. See e.g. Rachael D'Amore, "Stopping All Canada-China Flights Won't Stop Spread of Coronavirus—Here's Why", *Global News* (last updated 14 February 2020), online: <www.globalnews.ca/news/6546569/china-coronavirus-flights-canada/>.

In early April, smartphones blared out an emergency alert[16] (sent once in English, once in French) warning Ontarians to stay home unless "absolutely necessary." Slightly more formally, governments at the federal and provincial level have resorted to soft law, in the form of non-binding guidance. Innovation, Science and Economic Development Canada has published new guidelines[17] on the "enhanced scrutiny" of foreign investment in Canada. Specifically, close attention will be paid to investment in "Canadian businesses that are related to public health or involved in the supply of critical goods and services to Canadians or to the Government," a policy that will continue, "until the economy recovers from the effects of the COVID-19 pandemic." Ontario has published pages upon pages of guidance on COVID-19, including documents explaining what is expected of care homes and pharmacies, guidance which is of great import to those affected.[18]

How are *imperium, dominium,* and *suasion* to be controlled? Given their prominent role in the crisis so far—which they are likely to maintain going forward—this is an urgent question. As I explain in the next section, however, it is unlikely that judges will impose substantial controls on the exercise of these forms of power. A renewed emphasis on ensuring robust political accountability is much more likely to bear fruit.

Controlling Government Power

Imperium

Parliamentary sovereignty forms part of the constitutional bedrock of Westminster-style systems. As Canada is a federation with an entrenched *Charter* of fundamental rights, parliamentary sovereignty

16. Lauren O'Neil, "Ontario Emergency Alert Telling Everyone to Stay Home Sparks Anger and Frustration" (4 April 2020), online (blog): *blogTO* <www.blogto.com/city/2020/04/ontario-emergency-alert/>.
17. "Policy Statement on Foreign Investment Review and COVID-19" (18 April 2020), online: *Innovation, Science and Economic Development Canada* <www.ic.gc.ca/eic/site/ica-lic.nsf/eng/lk81224.html>.
18. See for example, "COVID-19 Guidance for the Health Sector" (last modified 5 May 2020), online: *Ontario Ministry of Health and Long-term Care* <www.health.gov.on.ca/en/pro/programs/publichealth/coronavirus/2019_guidance.aspx>; "COVID-19 Guidance: Community Pharmacies" (15 March 2020) at 1, online (pdf): *Ontario Ministry of Health and Long-term Care* <www.health.gov.on.ca/en/pro/programs/publichealth/coronavirus/docs/2019_pharmacies_guidance.pdf>; "COVID-19 Guidance: Long-Term Care Homes" (15 April 2020) at 1, online (pdf): *Ontario Ministry of Health* <www.health.gov.on.ca/en/pro/programs/publichealth/coronavirus/docs/2019_long_term_care_guidance.pdf>.

subsists in modified form. Nonetheless, subject to the limits imposed by the *Charter*, Parliament and the provincial legislatures have plenary authority "within their respective spheres of jurisdiction."[19]

The scope for legal challenges to emergency legislation is, accordingly, limited. Reasonableness and procedural fairness do not come into it.[20] Even broad delegations of authority to ministers are constitutionally valid,[21] as long as a legislature does not abdicate its powers[22] or breach a distinct constitutional provision.[23] Such delegations may be "constitutionally suspect" when they vest plenary powers in ministers, but Canadian courts have no authority to invalidate legislative delegations of power.[24] Powerful arguments have been mounted for a more forceful judicial role in policing delegations of authority,[25] but these are likely to fall on deaf ears in the context of an ongoing pandemic—indeed, the most prominent Canadian statements in relation to a legislature's ability to delegate power to ministers in the most sweeping terms have been made in times of crisis.[26]

Courts can certainly police the boundaries of delegated power; however, ensuring that authority is exercised reasonably and procedurally fairly is an uncontroversial part of the judicial function. Judges might even narrow broad delegations of authority to bring these delegations into line with fundamental constitutional principles; for example, Quebec's emergency legislation might be held not to authorize interference with extant judicial orders.[27] *Charter* concerns might

19. *Reference re PanCanadian Securities Regulation*, 2018 SCC 48 at para 56.
20. See especially *Reference Re Canada Assistance Plan (BC)*, [1991] 2 SCR 525, [1991] 6 WWR 1.
21. See *Chemicals Reference*, [1943] SCR 1, [1943] 1 DLR 248 [*Chemicals Reference*].
22. See *Re Grey*, (1918) 57 SCR 150 at 158, [1918] 3 WWR 111 [*Re Grey*].
23. For example, the taxation provisions of the *Constitution Act, 1867*: see Paul Daly, "Emergency Taxation Legislation: The Constitutional Framework" (24 March 2020), online (blog): *Administrative Law Matters* <www.administrativelawmatters.com/blog/2020/03/24/emergency-taxation-legislation-the-constitutional-framework>.
24. *Ontario Public School Boards' Association v Ontario (Attorney General)* (1997), 151 DLR (4th) 346 at para 51, 45 CRR (2d) 341.
25. See James Johnson, "The Case for a Canadian Nondelegation Doctrine" (2019) 53:3 UBC L Rev 817.
26. *Re Grey*, *supra* note 22; *Chemicals Reference*, *supra* note 21. Moreover, it is not at all clear that the solution to the accountability problems caused by broad delegations of authority, which reduce the ability of legislatures to hold ministers to account, is to increase the powers of the judiciary.
27. See Martine Valois, "Droit et urgence ne font pas bien ménage", *La Presse* (14 April 2020), online: <www.lapresse.ca/debats/opinions/202004/13/01-5269169-droit-et-urgence-ne-font-pas-bon-menage.php>.

cause limits to be read into legislative responses to the emergency and judges may take a dim view at trial of the validity of tickets issued by officious municipal officers. Important as such judicial activity would be, it would occur at the margins, as judges are singularly unlikely in the current context to invalidate legislation that empowers ministers and other officials to take emergency action to combat a public health crisis.

Dominium

Government power to enter into contracts and distribute largesse is subject to few limits. The ordinary rules of contract, property, tort law and so on apply, but the principles of public law—reasonableness and procedural fairness—backed up by remedies that invalidate government action are unlikely to extend to the exercise of *dominium* in response to COVID-19.

Governments can rely on broad statutory and inherent powers in responding to the economic fallout from the pandemic. Section 60.3(1) of Bill C-13 empowers the Minister of Finance to establish and capitalize a Crown corporation where, in his opinion "It is necessary to promote the stability or maintain the efficiency of the financial system in Canada." Any such corporation is exempt from the usual rules relating to the management and oversight of Crown corporations.[28] Rather, under subsections 4-8, the Minister may issue directives to the corporation which, in turn, its directors must follow, make regulations concerning the corporation's operations, and set out terms and conditions relating to transactions in which the corporation can engage. This legislative grant of almost unconstrained power is not especially anomalous. The Crown—that is, the federal and provincial governments—"enjoys a general capacity to contract in accordance with the rule of ordinary law."[29] Once monies have been lawfully appropriated, governments can put them to use in the pursuit of their policy objectives.[30] Given that "the Crown has the capacities and powers of a

28. These are contained in the *Financial Administration Act*, RSC 1985, c F-11, Part X but excluded by s 60.3(3) of Bill C-13, *An Act respecting certain measures in response to COVID-19*, 1st Sess, 42nd Parl, 2020 (assented to 25 March 2020), SC 2020, c 5.
29. *Attorney General of Quebec v Labrecque*, [1980] SCR 1057 at 1082, 125 DLR (3d) 545.
30. See e.g. *Pharmaceutical Manufacturers Assn of Canada v British Columbia (Attorney General)* (1997), 149 DLR (4th) 613, [1998] 1 WWR 702; *Canadian Doctors for Refugee Care v Canada (Attorney General)*, 2014 FC 651.

natural person,"[31] it has the inherent authority to enter into contracts, take out newspaper advertisements, and publish guidelines as to how its powers will be exercised.

It would be difficult to successfully seek a judicial review of any decision made by the Crown corporation envisaged by Bill C-13 or any contract entered into by the federal or provincial governments in the pursuit of medical supplies or vaccines. Judicial review, which permits the invalidation of governmental decisions, "is reserved for state action."[32] Courts typically weigh several factors in the balance in determining whether a particular decision is subject to judicial review,[33] but, in general, decisions to enter into contracts are singularly unlikely to qualify as state action.[34] Absent a violation of a statutory provision, allegations of "fraud, bribery, corruption or other kinds of grave misconduct,"[35] or some other special marker of public importance, courts will not be able to justify subjecting exercises of *dominium* to judicial review.

There is a recent strand of Commonwealth case law that suggests the principles of public law can be injected into contractual arrangements. Where contractual discretionary powers exist, they must be exercised in accordance with public law principles.[36] This strand has not yet been woven into the tapestry of Canadian law.[37] Even if Canadian courts were to do so, it is not clear that contracts for the supply of vital medical equipment, antiviral drugs, or vaccines would contain any discretionary powers into which courts could inject principles of public law. And, of course, such principles could only be invoked by an unhappy party to a contract with the federal or provincial governments, who would be seeking to advance its commercial interests, not the public interest.

31. *Pharmaceutical Manufacturers Assn of Canada v British Columbia (Attorney General)* (1997), 149 DLR (4th) 613 at para 27, [1998] 1 WWR 702.
32. *Highwood Congregation of Jehovah's Witnesses (Judicial Committee) v Wall*, 2018 SCC 26 at para 12.
33. See *Air Canada v Toronto Port Authority and Porter Airlines Inc*, 2011 FCA 347 at para 60 [*Air Canada*].
34. See e.g. *ibid* at para 52 (contract for janitorial services); *Ferme ViBer inc v Financière agricole du Québec*, 2016 SCC 34 at para 46 (government stabilization program); *People for the Ethical Treatment of Animals, Inc v City of Toronto*, 2020 ONSC 2356 at paras 38-49 (contract for advertising on bus shelters).
35. *Irving Shipbuilding Inc v Canada (Attorney General)*, 2009 FCA 116 at para 62.
36. See *Braganza v BP Shipping Ltd*, [2015] UKSC 17, [2015] 1 WLR 1661.
37. See Paul Daly, "The Limits of Public Law: *JW v Canada (Attorney General)*, 2019 SCC 20" (2019) 32:3 Can J of Admin L & Prac 231.

Suasion

Judicial review remedies are available in respect of decisions that have an impact on "the rights, interests, property, privileges, or liberties of any person."[38] This list is not to be parsed like a taxing statute but rather is to be given a large and liberal interpretation such that any modification to an individual's legal position can be scrutinized for conformity with public law principles of reasonableness and fairness.

It is not boundless, however. For example, government pronouncements do not, in any sense, modify the legal position of any individuals. Consider Ontario's use of the emergency alert system in April 2020, blaring a message out across the province's smartphones. The emergency alert suggested that residents of Ontario should not leave their homes at all-in fact, circulating freely was and is still not prohibited[39] as long as large gatherings are avoided; indeed, non-essential businesses were not ordered to close until the day after the alert was sent out.[40] Nonetheless, although the terms of the alert might be debated as a matter of political propriety, it would be difficult if not impossible to persuade a court to judicially review an alert that did not impose any obligations or otherwise modify anyone's legal position.

As for government guidance, it has long been difficult to seek a judicial review of soft law instruments. A clue lies in the term: although such instruments are designed to guide (hence "law"), they do not bind (hence "soft"). Accordingly, they are subject to judicial review only in a relatively limited set of circumstances, such as where they conflict with legislation or delegated legislation,[41] prevent a decision maker from exercising a discretionary power,[42] or violate *Charter* rights (but only in situations where the soft law instrument has binding force).[43]

---

38. *Martineau v Matsqui Institution Disciplinary Board (No 2)*, [1980] 1 SCR 602 at 623, Dickson J, dissenting.
39. See Government of Ontario, News Release, "Ontario Prohibits Gatherings of More Than Five People with Strict Exceptions" 28 March 2020), online: Ontario Newsroom <news.ontario.ca/opo/en/2020/03/ontario-prohibits-gatherings-of-five-people-or-more-with-strict-exceptions.html?utm_source=ondemand&utm_medium=email&utm_campaign=p>.
40. See O Reg 119/20.
41. See for example *Ishaq v Canada (Minister of Citizenship and Immigration)*, 2015 FC 156.
42. See *Maple Lodge Farms v Government of Canada*, [1982] 2 SCR 2, 137 DLR (3d) 558.
43. See *Greater Vancouver Transportation Authority v Canadian Federation of Students—British Columbia Component*, 2009 SCC 31.

The recent decision in *Sprague v. Her Majesty the Queen in right of Ontario*[44] is highly instructive. This was an application for judicial review brought in the Divisional Court on behalf of an inpatient at the York General Hospital. The applicant was the inpatient's son. The inpatient, who suffered from an acquired brain injury, had been moved to the hospital from a long-term care facility for reasons unrelated to COVID-19. At the hospital, the inpatient was assigned to a ward of patients particularly vulnerable to COVID-19. After the inpatient's hospitalization, the Chief Medical Officer of Health for Ontario issued a memorandum to hospitals strongly recommending that only essential visitors be permitted. On foot of the memorandum, the hospital instituted a "no visitors" policy, which prevented the inpatient's son from visiting his father. The Divisional Court rejected the applicant's attempts to judicially review the memorandum and policy. As for the policy, it was not a public act subject to judicial review but rather a private act relating to the hospital's management of access to its premises.[45] As for the memorandum, it was not issued pursuant to a statutory power, had no legal force, coerced no one, and did not require anyone to do or refrain from doing anything; it was a mere recommendation over which the courts have no supervisory jurisdiction. For much the same reasons, the memorandum was not subject to review for compliance with the *Charter*.[46]

A different factual and legal matrix might lead to a different result in terms of the susceptibility of government guidance to judicial review, but there is no doubt that the circumstances in which pandemic-related soft law instruments will be reviewed for compliance with public law principles (including the *Charter*) are limited.

Conclusion

In the first section of this chapter, I outlined the different forms that governmental power can take—*imperium*, *dominium*, and *suasion*—and identified how each has been used in response to the pandemic. In the second section, I turned my attention to judicial oversight of these different forms of governmental power, concluding that any such oversight will probably be strictly limited. Accordingly, any shortcomings

44. 2020 ONSC 2335 [*Sprague*].
45. It was also not issued in the exercise of a statutory power of decision as per the *Judicial Review Procedure Act*, RSO 1990, c J.1.
46. *Sprague*, *supra* note 44 at para 60.

in the political accountability during the current crisis are unlikely to be remedied by increased legal accountability. Those concerned about the difficulty of holding Canadian governments to account in these trying times would be better advised to look to improving the channels of political accountability than trying to navigate those of legal accountability. If these channels are improved, public law principles such as reasonableness, fairness, and proportionality may well flow through them to nourish debate and discussion,[47] but the necessary dredging is unlikely to be done by the judiciary.

47. See for example Paul Daly, "The Covid-19 Pandemic and Proportionality: A Framework" (31 March 2020), online (blog): *Administrative Law Matters* <www.administrativelawmatters.com/blog/2020/03/31/the-covid-19-pandemic-and-proportionality-a-framework/>.

CHAPTER B-7

Liability of the Crown in Times of Pandemic

Marie-France Fortin*

Abstract

While both federal and provincial governments are accountable before the courts for violations of individuals' rights and freedoms constitutionally protected in the *Canadian Charter of Rights and Freedoms*, their civil liability in tort for damages is a different matter. This chapter addresses the issue of the suitability of these actions in light of the immunity from suit that the federal and provincial governments ("the Crown") enjoy. In the first section of this chapter, the state of the law and recent developments in relation to the Crown's liability in Canada are discussed. The meaning and consequences of the Supreme Court of Canada's most recent decisions in relation to the Crown's liability in the context of the COVID-19 pandemic—including for the acts of its departments, servants, agents, corporations, and independent contractors—are discussed in the second section.

Résumé
Responsabilité de la Couronne en période de pandémie

Si les gouvernements fédéral et provinciaux doivent répondre devant les tribunaux de toute violation des droits et libertés des individus protégés par la *Charte canadienne des droits et libertés*, leur responsabilité

* Assistant Professor, Faculty of Law, University of Ottawa.

civile en matière de dommages-intérêts est différente. Le présent chapitre traite de la pertinence de ces actions à la lumière de l'immunité judiciaire dont jouissent les gouvernements fédéral et provinciaux (« la Couronne »). La première section de ce chapitre aborde l'état du droit et les derniers développements en matière de responsabilité de la Couronne au Canada. Puis, la signification et les conséquences des plus récentes décisions de la Cour suprême du Canada concernant la responsabilité de l'État dans le contexte de la pandémie de COVID-19, y compris pour les agissements de ses ministères, fonctionnaires, agents, sociétés et entrepreneurs indépendants, sont examinées dans la deuxième section.

The COVID-19 pandemic has already led to legal proceedings being initiated against long-term care homes. It is reasonable to assume that lawsuits against public and governmental institutions will follow, led for example by aggrieved families or essential workers. Doctors, nurses, and long-term care home workers who were infected with COVID-19 because of a lack of personal protective equipment (PPE), patients who were infected due to the back and forth from long-term care homes to hospitals, and individuals who caught COVID-19 in the community due to lack of testing or lack of precautionary measures are some of the examples of possible lawsuits against public and governmental entities. This chapter addresses the likely success of these actions in light of the immunity from lawsuits that the federal and provincial governments ("the Crown") enjoy. While the federal and provincial governments are accountable before the courts for violations of the *Canadian Charter of Rights and Freedoms*, the Crown's liability in tort for damages because it was negligent is a different matter. As I will demonstrate in this chapter, establishing the contours of the "Crown" in the context of its civil liability for a tort is important for understanding the likelihood of success of lawsuits brought against it, as well as the applicability of Crown immunity from suit.

In the first section, I discuss the state of the law and recent developments in relation to the Crown's liability in Canada. In the second section, I discuss the meaning and consequences of the Supreme Court of Canada's most recent decisions for the Crown's liability in the context of the COVID-19 pandemic. My conclusion is that prospective plaintiffs are likely to face significant hurdles in initiating proceedings against the Crown, even in the context of a global pandemic.

Crown Immunity from Suit and Public Law Immunity

The Crown's Immunity from Suit: The Common Law

The principle that the Crown understood as the government—Ministers and Crown officers in their official capacity and government departments—cannot be sued as common law became an important feature of legal thinking at the turn of the 20th century.[1]

In 1947, the United Kingdom Parliament enacted the *Crown Proceedings Act, 1947*,[2] abolishing in part the Crown's immunity from suit. The Parliament of Canada followed suit shortly thereafter and enacted the *Uniform Model Act of 1950*—now the *Crown Liability and Proceedings Act* (CLPA).[3] Provinces throughout Canada have also enacted statutes limiting provincial Crowns' immunity from suit. Ontario's *Crown Liability and Proceedings Act, 2019*[4] represents the latest reform in that regard. By contrast, in Quebec, the Crown[5] is subject, like any ordinary individual, to the general provisions of the *Civil Code of Quebec* relating to liability.[6]

While such statutes are thought to have marked the end of the Crown's immunity from suit,[7] important caveats remain. First, various public and governmental entities benefit from statutory immunities, which are granted to them by the legislature, often on the condition that they act in good faith. For instance, under the *Public Health Act* in Quebec, "The Government, the Minister or another person may not be

1. The belief that the Crown's immunity from suit is historically entrenched is inaccurate; see Marie-France Fortin, *A Historical Constitutional Approach to the King Can Do No Wrong: Revisiting Crown Liability* (PhD, University of Cambridge, 2020) [unpublished].
2. (UK), 1947, 10 & 11 Geo VI, c 44 [*CAP*].
3. *Crown Liability and Proceedings Act*, RSC 1985, c C-50 [*CLPA*]. In *The King v Cliche*, [1935] SCR 561, [1936] 1 DLR 195, the Supreme Court of Canada found that art 1011 *CCP*—introduced as s 886a by the *Petition of Right Act*, SQ 1883, c 27—created a right of action against the Crown.
4. SO 2019, c 7, sch 17 [*Ontario CLPA*].
5. More widely referred to as the State in that province, a difference in semantic acknowledged in the CLPA, s. 1 "État."
6. CQLR c CCQ-1991, arts 1376, 1457.
7. Similar statutes have been adopted, albeit at different times, throughout the Commonwealth: Peter W Hogg, Patrick Monahan & Wade K Wright, *Liability of the Crown*, 4th ed (Toronto: Carswell, 2011) at 8-11.

prosecuted by reason of an act performed in good faith in or in relation to the exercise of [the] powers [provided for in the Act]."[8]

Second, the Crown—federal or provincial—continue to benefit from important procedural advantages and immunities, which range from the exclusion of certain types of evidence to immunity against the enforcement of judgments, thus making it impossible to take action to force the Crown to execute the judgment.[9] "Public" common law immunities—notably the Crown's immunity from suit for policy decisions it has made—remain and can be invoked by the government, including in Quebec.[10]

Third, statutes partly abolishing the Crown's immunity from suit can be repealed or their scope modified by Parliament. This has led courts to interpret statutory provisions subjecting the Crown to various proceedings narrowly, on the basis that upon repeal the Crown would regain its full common law immunity, the Crown's blanket immunity being perceived as the default position.[11]

Fourth, the CLPA created vicarious liability only for the fault of Crown servants. Indeed, under section 3, the Crown is liable for the fault of its servant.[12] However, the Crown is not liable if the tort committed by the servant is not included in the definition of the act.[13] In addition, if the act or omission of the servant herself cannot give rise to a cause of action for liability because the servant benefits from immunity, then the Crown cannot be sued for the servant's tortious

8. CQLR c S-2.2, s 123.
9. *Canada (Attorney General) v Thouin*, 2017 SCC 46 at para 23. See Hogg, Monahan & Wright, *supra* note 7. On the immunity from execution of judgments, see Daniel Mockle & HR Eddy, *Immunity from Execution* (Ottawa: Law Reform Commission of Canada, 1987). The Ontario CLPA maintains many of the Crown's immunities, see e.g. *Ontario CLPA, supra* note 4, ss 3, 5, 10.
10. *Prud'homme v Prud'homme*, 2002 SCC 85.
11. See *Thouin, supra* note 9 at para 23. See also, in the Australian context, *Commonwealth v Mewett* (1997), 191 CLR 471 at 502, Dawson J, concurring; *Georgiadis v Australian and Overseas Telecommunications Corporation* (1994), 179 CLR 297 at 305-06; Mason CJ, Deane and Gaudron JJ [*Georgiadis*]; *Georgiadis, supra* note 11 at 325-26, McHugh J, dissenting.
12. *CLPA, supra* note 3, s 3: The Crown is liable for the damages for which, if it were a person, it would be liable: (a) in the Province of Quebec, in respect of: (i) the damage caused by the fault of a servant of the Crown, or (ii) the damage resulting from the act of a thing in the custody of or owned by the Crown or by the fault of the Crown as custodian or owner; and (b) in any other province, in respect of (i) a tort committed by a servant of the Crown, or (ii) a breach of duty attaching to the ownership, occupation, possession or control of property.
13. See *Morgan v Ministry of Justice*, [2010] EWHC 2248 (QB).

behaviour either.[14] The Ontario CLPA states clearly under section 8(2): "For greater certainty, nothing in clause (1) (a) subjects the Crown to liability for a tort that is not attributable to the acts or omissions of an officer, employee or agent of the Crown." In short, if the servant cannot be sued, the chain is broken and the Crown is free from liability.

Servants of the Crown are not immune from suit and can be sued before ordinary courts according to ordinary law.[15] But individual civil servants are not likely to have the deep pockets necessary to make large payouts after successful lawsuits. Moreover, under the CLPA, the Crown is not liable for its own fault. Therefore, where harm is caused by institutional failures that cannot be attributed to identifiable individuals over long periods of time the Crown is not liable—as was the case in *Hinse*, where a claim for damages based on the Federal Minister of Justice's refusal to exercise Crown's power of mercy failed.[16] Following *Hinse*, it would not be possible, for example, to sue the "Minister" or the "Government" generally for a series of decisions taken over the years in relation to, for instance, the funding of research on novel coronaviruses.

Public Law Immunity: Immunity for Policy Decisions

The belief in current legal thinking that the Crown is immune at common law also subverts the CLPA and its provincial equivalents in a different way. While these statutes clearly establish recourse in tort against the Crown, courts have nevertheless developed a substantial body of law distinguishing governmental policy decisions (which are shielded from judicial scrutiny) from operational aspects. Moreover, the scope of "policy" decisions continues to grow, to the detriment of "operational" measures.

In *R v Imperial Tobacco Canada Ltd. (Imperial)*, the Court defined "core policy" decisions shielded from suit as, "decisions as to a course or principle of action that are based on public policy considerations, such as economic, social and political factors, provided they are neither irrational nor taken in bad faith."[17] This description is potentially very broad. As has been noted before, "Policy and operational acts

14. *CLPA*, *supra* note 3, s 10.
15. Albert Venn Dicey, *The Oxford Edition of Dicey*, ed by JWF Allison (Oxford: Oxford University Press, 2013) at 100.
16. *Hinse v Canada (Attorney General)*, 2015 SCC 35 [*Hinse*].
17. 2011 SCC 42 at para 90 [*Imperial*].

are closely linked and the decision to do an operational act may easily involve and flow from a policy decision."[18] In *Imperial*, for instance, the Court found that the federal government's decisions to promote low-tar cigarettes and develop new strains of tobacco based on public considerations such as economic, social, and political factors were core policy decisions. As such, these decisions and the acts taken in furtherance of them constituted "core policy" and were immune.[19]

By leaving the contours of its new category of "core policies" undefined, the Supreme Court in *Imperial* created a thoroughly vague zone of action in which the Crown cannot be sued.[20] This is likely to encroach substantially on the operational realm that was previously open to scrutiny, and could possibly lead to unlimited immunity for the Crown where it would previously have been held liable.[21] It will be difficult for prospective plaintiffs to demonstrate that the Crown's actions in the context of COVID-19—for example, decisions on the level of testing or stockpiling of PPE; decisions to ease lock-down measures; or decisions to close or re-open schools—were not decisions as to a course of action that were based on public policy considerations. As a result of the uncertainty surrounding what used to be the policy/operational distinction, courses of action taken in accordance with policy decisions are also susceptible of falling under the umbrella of immunity covering policy decisions. The immunity can be overcome if it can be proven that the government's policy decisions were irrational or taken in bad faith, but that is a threshold that is difficult to meet. It is possible that the courts will find that the lack of care and the treatment endured by patients in long-term care homes did not flow from policy decisions taken in the context of the pandemic, and therefore fall at the other end of the spectrum, into what used to be the operational realm. However, the care and treatment provided at long-term care homes were to be inspected by the government, and the manner in which those inspections were carried out is likely to be

18. *Barrett v Enfield London Borough Council*, [2001] 2 AC 550 at 571, Lord Slynn of Hadley LJ.
19. This finding was found to also apply in the context of Quebec law: *Canada (Procureur général) c Imperial Tobacco Ltd*, 2012 QCCA 2034.
20. Bruce Feldthusen, "Simplifying Canadian Negligence Action Against Public Authorities—Or Maybe Not" (2012) 20 Tort L Rev 176; Bruce Feldthusen, "Public Authority Immunity from Negligence Liability: Uncertain, Unnecessary, and Unjustified" (2013) 92:2 Can Bar Rev 211.
21. For an example of an operational aspect, see *Laurentide Motels Ltd v Beauport (City)*, [1989] 1 SCR 705, 23 QAC 1.

characterized as a policy decision resulting from assessing and allocating resources.[22] Lastly, whether a provincial Crown can be sued for the actions taken by long-term care homes will depend on statutory provisions on Crown liability and the degree of control exercised by the Crown over them, as discussed further below.

Added to the public law immunity flowing from policy decisions is the fact that common law courts rarely find that there was a duty of care between the authority and the plaintiff.[23] This is also likely to be true in the context of the current pandemic,[24] where multifaceted factors—relating to health care, the allocation of resources, and other social and economic aspects—are taken into account. As the existence of a duty of care is necessary to find that anyone is liable, the absence of such a duty of care means that tortious liability cannot be established and that a plaintiff's claim must fail.

Defining the Contours of the Crown and Its Liability in the Context of COVID-19

What are the implications of the current state of the law on Crown immunity in the context of the COVID-19 pandemic?

The difficulty in suing the federal government as the Crown directly for the decisions it took in relation to stockpiling medical supplies, funding research into novel coronaviruses, testing, or other areas of policy is likely to be two-fold. First, as per the *Hinse* decision, the Crown cannot be sued directly; it cannot, therefore, be sued for institutional inertia. Individual or specific wrongdoing will have to be identified. Second, core policy decisions attract immunity. Decisions that were taken by considering the allocation of finite resources and evaluating the risk that there would be a new virus—in short, these are conflicting policy considerations—may also fall in the "core policy" category following the Court's ruling in *Imperial*. The Court cautioned in *Imperial* that it did not purport to provide a litmus test, and that "[d]ifficult cases may be expected to arise from time to time where it

22. Even where the government had a duty to inspect long-term care homes, failing to meet a statutory duty does not entail liability when the duty is owed to the population at large: *Cooper v Hobart*, 2001 SCC 79; *Edwards v Law Society of Upper Canada*, 2001 SCC 80; *Fullowka v Pinkerton's of Canada Ltd.*, 2010 SCC 5; *Alberta v Elder Advocates of Alberta Society*, 2011 SCC 24.
23. Feldthusen, "Public Authority Immunity", *supra* note 20 at 213.
24. Lara Khoury, "Crises sanitaires et responsabilité étatique envers la collectivité" (2016) 46:2 RDUS 261.

is not easy to decide whether the degree of 'policy' involved suffices for protection from negligence liability."[25] However, the Court added that "most government decisions that represent a course or principle of action based on a balancing of economic, social and political considerations will be readily identifiable."[26] Unless governments' decisions in Canada were taken in bad faith or can be proven to be irrational,[27] it appears unlikely that they will attract liability.

Courts conduct a control test to determine if a Crown corporation is part of the Crown and therefore can benefit or not from the various immunities the Crown can claim.[28] The status of each individual Crown corporation, Crown agent, or other public entities will depend on its enabling statute and the relevant legislative framework and regulatory scheme. In the case of lawsuits against long-term care homes themselves, the issue of whether they can rely on public law immunities—because they are part of the "Crown"—will depend on that test. Whether claimants will be able to sue provincial or local governments for actions that were taken or not taken at long-term care homes, for example, will also depend on that care home's status and the degree of control exercised by the government over it.

In Ontario, the *Crown Liability and Proceedings Act* maintains the Crown's immunity for torts committed by Crown agencies, Crown corporations, municipalities, hospitals, universities, colleges, boards of education, community health facilities, long-term care homes, along with independent contractors providing services to the Crown for any purpose.[29]

Crown agencies and other Crown corporations, as well as all other entities funded by the Ontario government listed above, must therefore be sued individually. Under the Ontario CLPA, the Government of Ontario cannot be sued for the tort they committed, or for their regulatory or policy decisions taken in good faith—or their failure to make such a decision. Under the Ontario CLPA, a policy

25. *Imperial*, *supra* note 17 at para 90.
26. *Ibid*.
27. *Ibid*.
28. Hogg, Monahan & Wright, *supra* note 7 at 465.
29. *Ontario CLPA*, *supra* note 4, ss 1, 9(1)(a)–(b). Crown corporations are defined broadly as "a corporation having 50 per cent or more of its issued and outstanding shares vested in the Crown or having the appointment of a majority of its board of directors made or approved by the Lieutenant Governor in Council or by one or more members of the Executive Council" and "a wholly-owned subsidiary" of such a corporation.

decision includes not only the manner in which a program, project, or other initiatives are carried out, but also changes to their scope and their termination. The Ontario CLPA provides more specifically that where programs, projects, or other initiatives are carried out on behalf of the Ontario government by "another person or entity"—including a Crown agency, Crown corporation, public body funded by the Ontario government, or an independent contractor—the government itself cannot be sued.[30]

By contrast, in Quebec, all public corporations—government departments, local authorities, and Crown corporations—are subject to the *Civil Code* and can be sued by individuals,[31] subject to the various procedural and statutory advantages and immunities they can claim. Public entities that are not directly or sufficiently overseen by ministers and that otherwise fail the control test, as well as local authorities such as municipalities, which are creatures of statute and are therefore not part of the "Crown," can be sued individually. Generally, the government will not be held accountable for their actions or omissions. This is likely to also be true of independent contractors if their contractual relationship with the government is such that the degree of governmental oversight does not reach the threshold of the control test.

Conclusion

The immunities benefiting the Crown when it is sued in tort is not negligible. Although it is possible to sue individual civil servants, suing the Crown is not straightforward. Since the Crown is immune from suit at common law, the only possible recourse against it are those provided for by statute. Statutes creating such recourse against the Crown have been interpreted narrowly. The difficulty in suing the Crown is compounded by the courts' jurisprudence on the policy/operational distinction, which has lately moved to cover a broader range of governmental actions.

The difficulty in suing the Crown raises the issue of the non-applicability of the rule of law to the Crown from the standpoint of legal theory. In the context of the COVID-19 pandemic, it also raises the issue of accountability. As claims in tort against the Crown involve

30. *Ontario CLPA*, *supra* note 4, s 11(5)(c).
31. *Civil Code of Quebec*, *supra* note 6, art 1376. For a recent example, see *Kosoian v Société de transport de Montréal*, 2019 SCC 59.

significant hurdles and are unlikely to succeed if they are tied to policy decisions that were made in the lead-up to the pandemic and its aftermath, the courts in civil liability cases are unlikely to serve as an effective accountability mechanism.

CHAPTER B-8

Balancing Risk and Reward in the Time of COVID-19: Bridging the Gap Between Public Interest and the "Best Interests of the Corporation"

Jennifer A. Quaid*

Abstract

The scale of the COVID-19 pandemic has shown that business organizations have a key role to play in supporting public health efforts to contain the virus. Corporate managers have been called upon to make proactive decisions about risk reduction that are the right thing to do but which may be costly and difficult to implement. However corporate law does not dictate what should be done, so long as it is in the "best interests of the corporation." In this chapter, I discuss how the pandemic situation exposes the limits of this permissive approach. Uncontrolled outbreaks of the virus in certain sectors of the economy deemed essential suggest that where corporate decisions have a significant and unavoidable impact on the wider public interest, such as the protection of human life and health, current manager accountability mechanisms are inadequate. I suggest that bridging this accountability gap may be possible if we are prepared to recognize more explicitly that sometimes what is best for the corporation can properly extend to protecting the public interest.

* Vice-Dean Research and Communications in the Faculty of Law (Civil Law Section) at the University of Ottawa, where she teaches criminal law, competition law, and corporate law.

Résumé
Entre risques et récompenses à l'ère de la COVID-19 : combler l'écart entre l'intérêt public et l'intérêt de l'entreprise

L'ampleur de la pandémie de COVID-19 a montré que les organisations commerciales ont un rôle clé à jouer pour soutenir les efforts en matière de santé publique visant à contenir le virus. Les dirigeants d'entreprise ont été appelés à prendre des décisions proactives relatives à la réduction des risques. S'il s'agit assurément de la bonne chose à faire, cela peut s'avérer coûteux et difficile à mettre en œuvre. Cependant, le droit des sociétés ne dicte pas ce qu'il convient de faire, pourvu que ce soit au mieux des intérêts de l'entreprise. Dans ce chapitre, j'examine comment la situation de pandémie expose les limites de cette approche permissive. La propagation incontrôlée du virus dans certains secteurs de l'économie jugés essentiels laisse à penser que lorsque les décisions des entreprises ont un impact considérable et inéluctable sur l'intérêt public en général, comme la protection de la vie et de la santé humaines, les mécanismes actuels de responsabilisation des dirigeants sont inadéquats. Je soutiens qu'il est possible de combler cet écart si nous sommes prêts à reconnaître plus explicitement que ce qui est mieux pour l'entreprise peut parfois englober la protection de l'intérêt public.

There has long been a deep discomfort at the notion of telling business what to do. The mantra is: Keep government out of business, let business make the decisions that are right for them, and apply mandatory rules only where essential. What serves the best interests of the corporation is context-specific, and so regulation should allow for a range of approaches and solutions. Managers who make the "wrong" choices are subject to market discipline—through loss of customers, investors, and talented employees. If they make enough mistakes, they could end up out of a job. More serious negligence that violates specific legal obligations could expose them to action by corporate stakeholders or liability under regulatory or criminal statutes. The COVID-19 pandemic is forcing an urgent reckoning with the notion that businesses are free to take risks so long as they are held accountable when things go wrong. What if the mistakes have wide-ranging and possibly catastrophic effects that cannot be reversed or remedied by damages? What if the costs of poor risk management decisions are not necessarily borne—at least not completely—by the corporation and its stakeholders?

This mismatch between risk and reward points to the practical inadequacy of a reliance on conventional accountability mechanisms that apply *ex post* when these are a poor substitute for *ex ante* prevention. In this chapter, I draw on two contrasting stories of pandemic response by corporations to make the argument that the time is ripe for a bold response to this accountability gap—thus reframing the duty of corporate managers to act in the "best interests of the corporation" to reflect the critical role that corporations play in protecting broader interests like public health.

Setting the Stage: When Doing the Right Thing Is Imperative

The emergence of a highly infectious virus to which no one is immune has thrust Canada, and the world, into an unprecedented situation. Government responses must be coordinated to contain the spread of infection until an effective vaccine is developed, but decisions are being made in the face of significant uncertainty about the virus and the efficacy of containment strategies. Moreover, the successful implementation of these public health measures depends entirely on the willingness of individuals and organizations to abide by significant restrictions and to take proactive measures to promote safe behaviours. In liberal democracies like Canada's, encouraging voluntary compliance is vital;[1] reliance on extensive recourse to coercion is both impractical and lacks legitimacy.

Just like individuals, business organizations are being called upon to do the "right" thing. There is an unexpressed expectation that risk assessment decisions should extend beyond the usual frame of reference used by those who exercise corporate management duties. And just like individuals, how businesses are expected to "do their part" varies based on what they do. Some businesses have been asked to continue their operations because they are too important to close or provide essential goods and services. Others have been forced to suspend operations because they are not deemed essential and cannot

1. For a fascinating study of the critical role that social motivations play in supporting voluntary cooperation, especially where this cooperation may be at odds with an individual's personal interest, see Tom R Tyler, *Why People Cooperate: The Role of Social Motivations* (Princeton: Princeton University Press, 2011).

be operated safely. Still others have been expected to transform—very quickly—most or all of their operations to a virtual/distance setting for an indeterminate period. Each of these situations has forced corporate managers to make decisions with important consequences, not just for their traditional stakeholders, but for the public at large.

In being asked to put the collective public welfare at the centre of their decision-making, corporate managers are being pushed into uncharted and uncomfortable territory. Some are handling it better than others. The following two contrasting stories of pandemic response highlight how corporate risk assessment decisions can have significant impacts beyond the conventional confines of the corporation.

A Tale of Two Companies

Dollarama

Dollarama is a family-run Canadian public company traded on the Toronto Stock Exchange.[2] It operates "dollar" retail stores that specialize in selling low-priced goods across Canada and in Latin America.[3] A profitable company, at the end of its fiscal year ending February 2, 2020, it reported $3.8 billion in revenues and net earnings of $564 million.[4]

Dollarama reacted quickly to the COVID-19 pandemic. Its first press release issued on March 20, 2020, affirmed its decision to keep stores open while adopting several preventive measures such as extra

2. Dollarama, "Annual Information Form—Fiscal Year Ended February 2, 2020" (29 April 2020) at 3, online (pdf): *Dollarama* <www.dollarama.com/en-CA/corp/wp-content/uploads/2020/05/2020-Annual-Information-Form-vFINAL.pdf>. Dollarama was founded in 1992 and incorporated in 2004 under the *Canada Business Corporations Act*, RSC 1985, c C-44 [*CBCA*].
3. Dollarama. "About Us: Proudly Serving Customers from Coast to Coast" (last visited 27 May 2020), online: *Dollarama* <www.dollarama.com/en-CA/corp/about-us>.
4. Dollarama, "Dollarama Reports Fourth Quarter and Fiscal Year 2020 Results", News Release (1 April 2020) at 1, online (pdf): *Dollarama* <www.dollarama.com/en-CA/corp/wp-content/uploads/2019/06/Press-Release-FINAL.pdf>. At the time it released its annual report, Dollarama made the decision not to issue the customary guidance that public companies offer as to expected earnings for the coming year, underscoring that it was impossible to predict the impact of the COVID-19 pandemic on its business: Susan K Robertson, "Dollarama Suspends Guidance for Expected Performance Amid COVID-19 Pandemic", *The Globe and Mail* (1 April 2020), online: <www.theglobeandmail.com/business/article-dollarama-suspends-guidance-for-expected-performance-amid-covid-1/>.

cleaning and special hours for seniors.[5] Once designated an essential business in Ontario and Quebec on March 24, 2020, Dollarama published an update explaining the extensive measures being taken to protect the safety of employees and customers, and committing to keep prices at pre-pandemic levels.[6] Since then, Dollarama's website includes a special pop-up update from CEO Neil Rossy about the company's COVID-19 measures and news.[7] In a special interview published on April 30, 2020, Rossy explained that Dollarama's designation as an essential business was top of mind in making decisions about managing the company. The company was spending what was needed on preventive measures for staff and customers, wage increases,[8] additional hiring and allowing employee time off for those unable or unwilling to work, without regard for the bottom line, because it was the right thing to do.[9] Rossy also continued to place orders in the usual quantities to support his suppliers, even if it was unclear what the retail demand would be going forward. Despite a few bumps, he was satisfied with how the company had adjusted to the crisis (fewer than 10 employees had become infected with COVID-19).[10]

Cargill

Cargill is a U.S.-based, private, family-run multinational corporation founded in 1865.[11] It operates in a wide range of industries related to

5. Dollarama, "Dollarama Reaffirms Commitment to Serving Canadians" (20 March 2020), online: *Dollarama* <www.dollarama.com/en-CA/corp/news-release?id=122656>.
6. Dollarama, News Release, "Dollarama Recognized as Essential Business" (24 March 2020), online: *Dollarama* <www.dollarama.com/en-CA/corp/news-release?id=122657>.
7. Neil Rossy, "Message to Customers: COVID-19 Update" (1 May 2020), online: *Dollarama* <www.dollarama.com/en-CA/>.
8. Aleksandra Sagan, "Dollarama, Walmart Canada Boost Employee Pay Amid Coronavirus Outbreak", *The Globe and Mail* (24 March 2020), online: <www.theglobeandmail.com/business/article-dollarama-says-stores-recognised-as-essential-service-in-ontario-and/>.
9. Nicolas Van Praet, "Dollarama's CEO on Protecting Staff, Navigating Supply Chains and Sacrificing Profits in a Pandemic", *The Globe and Mail* (30 April 2020), online: <www.theglobeandmail.com/business/article-dollarama-ceo-admits-mistakes-during-pandemic-but-sees-companys-long/>.
10. *Ibid*.
11. Cargill, "Cargill Timeline" (2019) at 1, online (pdf): *Cargill* <www.cargill.com/doc/1432078093613/pdf-cargill-timeline.pdf>.

food, food production, and food processing.[12] It reported revenues of $113.5 billion and a profit of $2.82 billion in the year ending May 31, 2019.[13] Cargill Canada employs about 8,000 people in the food and agriculture industries, including meat processing in Alberta, Ontario, and Quebec.[14] Its High River beef processing plant, which employs 2000,[15] accounts for about 35% of the beef processing capacity in Canada.[16]

Given their prominence in the Canadian food production system, Cargill's Canadian operations were also deemed essential.[17] Unlike Dollarama, the company provided scant information about preventive measures at its plants until an April 29, 2020, press release[18] on the U.S. parent website. The post was clearly responding to negative publicity following revelations that several hundred workers at the High River plant were infected with COVID-19 and one had died.[19] An investigation by *The Globe and Mail* reported that protective measures were not fully implemented until mid-April despite the first cases of infection being reported in March; curiously, an inspection by Alberta regulators, conducted by video call on April 15, concluded that the site was safe.[20] While accounts differ, employees reported

12. Cargill, "About Cargill" (last visited 27 May 2020), online: *Cargill* <www.cargill.com/about>.
13. As a private company, Cargill's financial information is not subject to the reporting requirements of securities law and regulations, but it does publish a form of annual report on its website. See Cargill, "Cargill Annual Report—Year Ended May 31, 2019)" (30 July 2019) at 2, online (pdf): *Cargill* <www.cargill.com/doc 1432144962450/2019-annual-report.pdf>.
14. Cargill, "Products and Services" (last visited 27 May 2020), online: *Cargill* <www.cargill.ca/en/products-and-services>.
15. Cargill, "Meat Processing" (last visited 27 May 2020), online: *Cargill* <www.cargill.ca/en/meat-processing>.
16. Bill Graveland, "Cargill is Shuttering its High River Meat-Packing Plant After it Was Linked to More than 350 Cases of Coronavirus", *Financial Post* (20 April 2020), online: <business.financialpost.com/commodities/agriculture/newsalert-high-river-alta-meat-packing-plant-temporarily-stopping-production>.
17. Cargill, "Cargill Statement on Reopening High River Alberta Protein Facility" (29 April 2020), online: *Cargill* <www.cargill.com/story/cargill-statement-reopening-high-river-alberta-protein-facility>.
18. *Ibid*. A full company statement on its COVID-19 response was published on April 30, 2020, see Cargill, "Cargill's Response to the COVID-19 Global Pandemic" (30 April 2020), online: *Cargill* <www.cargill.com/story/cargills-response-to-the-covid-19-global-pandemic>.
19. Graveland, *supra* note 16.
20. Katherine B Brown, Carrie Tait & Tavia Grant, "How Cargill Became the Site of Canada's Largest Single Outbreak of COVID-19", *The Globe and*

being fearful of being fired if they refused to work because they felt unsafe.[21] High River rapidly became a COVID-19 hot spot.[22] The High River plant was shut down on April 20 for two weeks but by then the infection rate among employees had surpassed 50% and two more deaths were connected to the plant.[23] The plant reopened on May 4, but lingering safety concerns remain and Alberta Health and Safety is investigating.[24] Outbreaks among Cargill employees have also been reported at its plants in Chambly[25] and Guelph.[26]

It is too early to say if Cargill's handling of the COVID-19 risk will lead to some form of accountability. Since its shares are not publicly traded, Cargill is shielded from stock market discipline and is not subject to the obligation to disclose material information, such as corrective measures and investments in safety, to investors. Though it operates in a highly regulated industry and could face regulatory or criminal liability, investigations take time and are not guaranteed to lead to charges. And, while Cargill may seem like an extreme case linked to an industry with pre-existing safety problems and a vulnerable workforce of foreign workers,[27] there are examples of companies

Mail (2 May 2020), online: <www.theglobeandmail.com/business/article-how-cargill-became-the-site-of-canadas-largest-single-outbreak-of/>.

21. *Ibid*.
22. James Keller & Christine Dobby, "Hundreds of Alberta Infections Linked to Meat-Processing Plant", *The Globe and Mail* (19 April 2020), online: <www.theglobeandmail.com/canada/alberta/article-covid-19-outbreak-in-high-river-linked-to-infections-at-nearby/>.
23. Carrie Tait, "Cargill Employee Dies of COVID-19 after Month-Long Hospitalization", *The Globe and Mail* (12 May 2020), online: <www.theglobeandmail.com/canada/alberta/article-cargill-employee-dies-of-covid-19-after-month-long-hospitalization/>.
24. Joel Dryden, "Safety Investigation of COVID-19 in Cargill slaughterhouse Didn't Include Worker Representation, OHS Finds", *CBC News* (9 May 2020), online: <www.cbc.ca/news/canada/calgary/cargill-michael-hughes-ohs-occupational-health-and-safety-1.5562931>.
25. Morgan Lowrie, "Cargill Meat-Packing Plant Closes in Montreal after 64 Workers Test Positive for COVID-19", *Financial Post* (11 May 2020), online: <business.financialpost.com/commodities/agriculture/another-cargill-plant-closes-after-covid-19-outbreak>.
26. Kenneth Armstrong, "Now Three Confirmed Cases of COVID-19 at Cargill Plant in Guelph, Says Union", *Guelph Today* (13 May 2020), online: <www.guelphtoday.com/coronavirus-covid-19-local-news/now-three-confirmed-cases-of-covid-19-at-cargill-plant-in-guelph-says-union-2349157>.
27. Ian Mosby & Sarah Rotz, "As Meat Plants Shut Down, COVID-19 Reveals the Extreme Concentration of Our Food Supply", *The Globe and Mail* (29 April 2020), online: <www.theglobeandmail.com/opinion/article-as-meat-plants-shut-down-covid-19-reveals-the-extreme-concentration/>; Brown, Tait & Grant, *supra*

in other industries whose slow reaction to the pandemic and poor risk management has led to important outbreaks and community spread.[28]

Two companies with official permission to remain operating while much of the economy was put on hold to contain the virus, both with workforces who were at an increased risk of infection as well as being potential vectors of transmission. Two very different outcomes for their workers and the public. Could the essential difference lie in the fact that in making decisions about risk, Dollarama applied a broader view of its interests, one that extended to the public interest in protecting public health?

In the context of a public health crisis where prevention is critical to reducing negative outcomes, promoting a proactive response to risk, such as that adopted by Dollarama, is vastly superior to relying on a reactive *ex post* corrective accountability dependent on scarce regulatory resources. Could the key to bridging this gap between hard enforcement and voluntary cooperation be as simple as framing the best interests of the corporation to reflect Dollarama's approach? Is the time ripe to recognize explicitly that private interests can and should cede to the public interest where the corporation plays a key role in protecting the common good?

Corporations and the Public Interest

Corporations are vehicles of commerce that make it easier to bring people and resources together in the pursuit of common objectives, chief among them generating a profit. While hardly revolutionary itself, there has always been debate about whether the pursuit of profit is the defining and perhaps singular feature of a corporation, or whether it is or should be bounded by outer limits. The answers to these questions inform how the standard applicable to management decisions is framed and identify to whom managers are answerable.

For many years, it was an article of faith that private wealth maximization would translate into increased total welfare. In this respect,

note 20; Joel Dryden & Sarah Rieger, "Inside the Slaughterhouse", *CBC News* (6 May 2020), online: <newsinteractives.cbc.ca/longform/cargill-covid19-outbreak>. For a discussion of the working conditions in meat-processing plants in Canada, see Sarah Berger Richardson, this volume, Chapter E-5.

28. Emma McIntosh, "'Alberta Didn't Contain It': COVID-19 Outbreak at Oilsands Camp Has Spread Across the Country", *National Observer* (13 May 2020), online: <www.nationalobserver.com/2020/05/13/news/alberta-didnt-contain-it-covid-19-outbreak-oilsands-camp-has-spread-across-country>.

these questions should be answered by "yes" and "no." Manager accountability to shareholders was sufficient to promote good decisions about risk.[29] This is still the guiding rationale behind the permissive structure of corporate law in Canada—to create a framework to ensure corporate officers and directors ("corporate managers"[30]) evaluate the best interests of the corporation rationally, based on the factors they consider relevant. Against that backdrop, where the decision-making *process* seems reasonable in the circumstances, courts tend to be highly deferential to management regarding the *soundness* of business decisions, absent strong indications to the contrary.[31]

This approach is tailored to the context in which business decisions are scrutinized—where there is a conflict between "corporate" stakeholders (managers and shareholders or between majority and minority shareholders), though they may also arise where corporate decisions affect other stakeholders with an "interest" in the corporation.[32] This latter situation was at the heart of the *BCE* case, in which the Supreme Court of Canada recognized that sometimes corporate decisions will trigger unavoidable negative effects for some stakeholders. In *BCE*, the Court recognized the need for a more flexible concept of best interests of the corporation, one in which managers could consider factors and interests beyond those of the limited categories of stakeholders expressly dealt with in corporate law (directors and officers, majority shareholders, minority shareholders), including those of employees, suppliers, creditors, consumers, governments, and the environment.[33]

In framing "best interests" primarily as the corporation's long-term interests as a going concern and as a responsible corporate citizen, the Court implicitly integrated some elements of theories of the

---

29. Henry Hansmann & Reiner Kraakman, "The End of History for Corporate Law" (2000) 89:2 Geo LJ 439 at 439-68.
30. For ease of exposition, I use the term "manager" to refer collectively to directors and officers of the corporation. Directors are invested with the power to manage the corporation, but they can delegate most of their powers to officers. Those who exercise these powers are subject to two special duties: the duty of loyalty (or the fiduciary duty to manage in the best interests of the corporation) and the duty of care to act in a prudent and diligence manner. See e.g. *CBCA*, *supra* note 2, ss 122(1)(a)–(b); Art 322 CCQ; *Business Corporations Act*, CQLR c S-31.1, s 119.
31. *BCE Inc v 1976 Debentureholders*, 2008 SCC 69 at para 40 [*BCE*]; *Unique Broadband Systems Inc, Re*, 2014 ONCA 538 at para 72.
32. *BCE*, *supra* note 31 at paras 41-46, 81-82.
33. *Ibid* at para 42.

corporation as a public institution.[34] But while the Court's approach does not *mandate* shareholder value maximization, it does not clearly banish it either.[35] Not surprisingly then, *BCE* did not usher in a new era of corporate decision-making aligned to principles of corporate social responsibility. Expanding the list of stakeholders whose interests could be considered when assessing the best interests of the corporation on its own does not address the limited way in which corporate duties were applied. Despite appearance to the contrary, duties of corporate directors did not extend outside the scope of traditional corporate law.[36] As such, only those stakeholders with specific private economic interests in the corporation had an enforceable remedy. As Carol Liao has observed, this means that it is only where the state deems consideration of other factors to be *imperative,* and mandates accountability through *express regulation,* that there will be an independent basis on which to intervene outside this narrow range. This leaves an important gap because it enables corporations to externalize costs that do not directly affect shareholder wealth, such as environmental or consumer harms, where these are insufficiently enforced by regulation.[37]

Even before the pandemic, there was an increasingly loud chorus of voices, many of whom were proponents of sustainable governance,[38] who challenged the view that corporations are entitled to ignore this kind of collateral effect of their decisions.[39] Since a stable market economy depends on state support of the underlying rights

---

34. A prominent proponent of this view advocates for treating corporate law as a branch of public law: Kent Greenfield, *The Failure of Corporate Law* (Chicago: University of Chicago Press, 2007).

35. In a key decision on corporate remedies, the Ontario Court of Appeal cited *BCE* in support of the view that most of the time, the best interests of the corporation are those of shareholders, taken collectively. *Rea v Wildeboer,* 2015 ONCA 373.

36. For one of the most quoted defences of the shareholder primacy model, see Hansmann & Kraakman, *supra* note 29.

37. Carol Liao, "Power and the Gender Imbalance in Corporate Law" in Beate Sjåfjell & Irene Lynch Fannon, eds, *Creating Corporate Sustainability: Gender as an Agent for Change* (Cambridge, UK: Cambridge University Press, 2018) 282 at 289-90.

38. See e.g. Beate Sjåfjell & Irene Lynch Fannon, *Creating Corporate Sustainability: Gender as Agents for Change* (Cambridge, UK: Cambridge University Press, 2018); Lynn Stout, *The Shareholder Value Myth: How Putting Shareholders First Harms Investors, Corporations, and the Public* (San Francisco: Berrett-Koehler, 2012); Margaret Blair & Lynn Stout, "A Team Production Theory of Corporate Law" (1999) 85:2 Va L Rev 247 at 248-328; Kelly Testy, "Linking Progressive Corporate Law and Progressive Social Movements" (2002) 76:5/6 Tul L Rev 1227 at 1227-52.

39. Liao, *supra* note 37 at 290.

of property and contract without which commerce cannot exist,[40] it is fair to expect that the privilege of incorporation and its associated rights is granted so long as the pursuit of private commerce promotes the broader public interest.

The pandemic has raised this point squarely. Just as with matters of climate change and sustainable governance, absent of hard rules to mandate that decisions integrate specific considerations, relying on corporate law duties that provide the option, but not the obligation, to do the right thing seems hopelessly optimistic. As the Cargill example shows, even when it could be argued it would be rational from a long-term perspective for the corporation to take preventive measures and address externalities like risk factors linked to the socio-economic circumstances of its vulnerable workforce (carpooling, living arrangements) and the risk of community spread, short-term thinking is all too common; the temptation to take a chance and underspend on prevention is high. And this temptation only increases when the benefits of these preventive measures do not accrue to the corporation. The result is an accountability gap in those areas where there is no regulation specifically mandating that interests external to the corporation be considered. And the reality is that even where there is regulation, enforcement capacity tends to be limited and highly dependent on self-regulation.

A Way Forward?

Though not prepared with this in mind, a recent amendment to the *Canada Business Corporations Act*[41] that expressly recognizes and expands on the more inclusive view of stakeholder interests relevant to corporate decision-making set down in *BCE*[42] could be leveraged

40. Scholars like Cass Sunstein have argued that private rights of contract and property do not exist without state support through enforceable remedies and legal recognition of rights. Cass R Sunstein, "State Action Is Always Present" (2002) 3 Chicago J Intl L 465. Sunstein's position suggests that in discussions of horizontal distribution of rights, nothing is exempt from scrutiny *a priori*, though other factors, such as cost, may make it impractical, even for an activist state, to assure meaningful protection of certain social and economic rights, like the right to housing.

41. *CBCA*, *supra* note 2, s 122(1.1).

42. Charles-Étienne Borduas & Petra Vrtkova, "Stakeholders' Primacy: Paradigm Shift Confirmed" (September 2019), online: *Norton Rose* <www.nortonrosefulbright.com/en-ca/knowledge/publications/a979357b/stakeholders-primacy-paradigm-shift-confirmed>.

to support a broader duty of corporate managers. This amendment is part of a suite of changes (not all of which are in force) aimed at promoting corporate governance aligned with broader societal values, such as diversity and sustainability, that is gaining traction in other jurisdictions as well.[43]

While it has yet to be interpreted, the way the new paragraph 122 (1.1) *CBCA* is drafted lays the foundation for an expanded corporate duty that extends beyond private interests. Rather than simply codifying the list of interests set out by the Court in *BCE*, new par (1.1) is parsed into three distinct clauses. The first makes specific reference to stakeholder groups attached to a specific constituency: shareholders, employees, retirees and pensioners, creditors, consumers, and governments.[44] The final clause refers to the long-term interests of the corporation.[45] The second clause refers to the environment alone. Why segregate this clause from the first? A plausible interpretation is that the interests of the environment are different from the interests outlined in the first clause. They relate to a social good, the benefits of which are not exclusive to and indeed transcend the specific interests of stakeholder groups, but the protection of which demands contributions from all. Indeed, there is an increasing consensus that the promotion of a healthy environment is a collective good that is aligned with the best interests of the corporation, even if the corporation does not reap the entirety of the benefits of its protective actions. Given this, it is a small step to say that clause 122 (1.1)(b) is a broader legislative recognition for the need to incorporate concern for public, intangible goods into the decision-making of commercial entities that are supported by the state on the expectation their actions promote the public welfare. The paragraph in the *CBCA* should be amended to extend beyond the environment and expressly recognize the duty of corporate managers to consider other public interests, such as public health.

43. "Business Roundtable Redefines the Purpose of a Corporation to Promote 'An Economy That Serves All Americans'" (19 August 2019), online: *Business Roundtable* <www.businessroundtable.org/business-roundtable-redefines-the-purpose-of-a-corporation-to-promote-an-economy-that-serves-all-americans>.

44. It is noteworthy that this list adds two categories not included in the original *BCE* list: retirees and pensioners.

45. Some have questioned the wisdom of focusing only on the long-term interests of corporations. Borduas & Vrtkova, *supra* note 42.

Conclusion

The COVID-19 pandemic has laid bare, in a way that a slow-moving crisis like climate change could not, the cost of tolerating the externalization of risks that are within the control of corporations to prevent, but which fall outside current corporate law accountability mechanisms. It is no longer enough to implore corporate managers to do the right thing when it suits them. The time has come for private economic interests to be subject to the obligation to be proactive about managing risk where some, or even most, of the impacts will be felt outside the corporation.

This is not just about the pandemic. This is about the future of responsible corporate citizenship. While calls for greater recognition of the impact that corporations have beyond their immediate private economic interests have been brewing for some time, I am cautiously optimistic that the convergence of the *CBCA* amendment and the pandemic may finally create the impetus for a new vision of the role and purpose of the corporation to take root—one that sees the promotion of the public interest as fundamentally aligned with the successful pursuit of the corporation's own interests.

SECTION C

CIVIL LIBERTIES VS. IDEAS OF PUBLIC HEALTH

CHAPTER C-1

Civil Liberties vs. Public Health

Colleen M. Flood,* Bryan Thomas,** and Dr. Kumanan Wilson***

Abstract

The COVID-19 pandemic highlights the challenges governments face in balancing civil liberties against the exigencies of public health, amid the chaos of a public health emergency. A key question concerns the evidentiary standards for justifying interferences with civil liberties. Superficially, civil liberties law and public health appear to invoke opposite evidentiary standards: under the principle of proportionality, civil libertarians demand strong evidence of the necessity of interference with civil liberties, while public health officials, invoking the precautionary principle, urge that intrusive measures be taken—limits on social gatherings, for example—even without conclusive evidence of their necessity. In this chapter, we argue that the two principles are not so oppositional in practice. In testing for proportionality, courts recognize the need to defer to governments on complex policy matters, especially where the interests of vulnerable populations are at stake. For their part, public health experts have incorporated ideas of

* University Research Chair and Director of the Centre for Health Law, Policy & Ethics, University of Ottawa.

** Senior Research Associate and Adjunct Professor, Centre for Health Law, Policy & Ethics, University of Ottawa.

*** Physician Scientist, The Ottawa Hospital, Professor of Medicine, University of Ottawa, and member of the University of Ottawa Centre for Health Law, Policy and Ethics.

proportionality in their evolving understanding of the precautionary principle. We emphasize the importance of agility in the COVID-19 response, pointing to strategies that might simultaneously satisfy the proportionality and precautionary principles.

Résumé
Libertés civiles et santé publique

La pandémie de COVID-19 témoigne des défis que doivent surmonter les gouvernements, appelés à chercher un certain équilibre entre les libertés civiles et les exigences de santé publique, au cœur du chaos qui règne en situation d'urgence. Les normes de preuve pour justifier les atteintes aux libertés civiles constituent une question clé. En apparence, le droit des libertés civiles et la santé publique semblent invoquer des normes de preuve opposées : en vertu du principe de proportionnalité, les défenseurs des libertés civiles exigent des preuves solides de la nécessité de porter atteinte aux libertés civiles, tandis que les responsables de la santé publique, citant le principe de précaution, exhortent à prendre des mesures intrusives – par exemple, limiter les rassemblements sociaux – même sans preuve définitive de leur utilité. Dans ce chapitre, nous soutenons que ces deux principes ne sont pas si opposés en pratique. Mettant à l'essai le critère de proportionnalité, les tribunaux reconnaissent le besoin de s'en remettre aux gouvernements sur des questions politiques complexes, en particulier lorsque les intérêts des populations vulnérables sont en jeu. Pour leur part, les experts de la santé publique ont intégré la notion de proportionnalité dans leur compréhension évolutive du principe de précaution. Nous soulignons l'importance de faire preuve d'agilité lorsqu'il s'agit d'intervenir en temps de pandémie, en présentant des stratégies qui pourraient satisfaire simultanément aux principes de proportionnalité et de précaution.

Government responses to public health emergencies often involve apparent trade-offs between individual civil liberties and public health goals.[1] These apparent trade-offs are reflected in federal,

1. Lawrence O Gostin & Lindsay F Wiley, *Public Health Law: Power, Duty, Restraint*, 3rd ed (Berkeley: University of California Press, 2016) at chapter 2.

provincial, and municipal responses to COVID-19. As discussed in the first part of this volume dealing with federalism, Canadian provinces and municipalities have imposed various restrictions: limiting public gatherings; locking down prisons and mental health facilities; stopping visitors to long-term care homes; closing all but essential businesses; restricting recreational amenities; and imposing mandatory quarantine orders against specific individuals.[2] The federal government, employing the *Quarantine Act*, has limited entry into the country and now imposes a two-week quarantine on citizens returning from abroad. Many of these measures are enforced by significant fines (for example, up to $100,000 for a first offence and $500,000 for a second offence in Alberta)[3] and even imprisonment (Ontario's limitation on social gatherings is punishable by a fine of up to $100,000 and up to a year's imprisonment).[4]

On their face, many of these measures seem to interfere with *Charter* rights to freedom of assembly, freedom of mobility, and freedom of religion for would-be churchgoers. Further, as the pandemic has unfolded, it has become clearer that significant testing and contact tracing using cell phone GPS records may be an important tool to battle COVID-19, yet absent consent, this conflicts with privacy rights.[5] Similarly, as hope for the end of the pandemic centres on developing a vaccine or treatment, the future prospect of mandatory vaccination regimes (even if limited to essential workers and at-risk populations) may raise questions of conscience and religious freedom.[6] There has also been some discussion of introducing legal penalties for individuals spreading harmful misinformation about the disease and treatment—a move that would no doubt engage the *Charter* right to freedom of expression.[7] In this chapter, we contrast and evaluate

2. Rob Ferguson, "Use Law to Impose COVID-19 Quarantines, Ontario's Chief Medical Officer Tells Local Health Officials", *Toronto Star* (1 April 2020), online: <www.thestar.com/politics/provincial/2020/04/01/ontarios-chief-medical-officer-dr-david-williams-strongly-urging-law-restricting-movements-of-covid-19-patients.html>; *Health Protection and Promotion Act*, RSO 1990, c H.7, s 22.
3. *Public Health Act*, RSA 2000, c P-37, s 73(3); Bill 10, *Public Health (Emergency Powers) Amendment Act*, 2nd Sess, 30th Leg, Alberta, 2020, s 9(b)(ii)—(iii) (assented to 2 April 2020).
4. *Emergency Management and Civil Protection Act*, RSO 1990, c E.9, s 7.0.11(1)(a).
5. See Teresa Scassa, Jason Millar & Kelly Bronson, this volume, Chapter C-2.
6. Richard Moon, *Freedom of Conscience and Religion* (Toronto: Irwin Law, 2014).
7. Elizabeth Thompson, "Federal Government Open to New Law to Fight Pandemic Misinformation", *CBC News* (15 April 2020), online: <www.cbc.ca/news/politics/covid-misinformation-disinformation-law-1.5532325>.

two overarching principles in evaluating these apparent trade-offs: the principle of proportionality, central to Canadian *Charter* jurisprudence; and the precautionary principle, used in public health.

As traditionally conceived, the discourses of civil rights and public health rest on opposite assumptions about the burden of proof. In the discourse of civil and political rights—of the sort guaranteed under the Canadian *Charter of Rights and Freedoms*[8]—the onus rests primarily on government to show a "pressing and substantial" objective for interfering with protected rights and freedoms; moreover, governments are obliged to use rational, minimally intrusive, and proportionate means of achieving that objective. By contrast, public health discourse centres on the precautionary principle which holds that action should be taken—even actions that impact civil rights—to mitigate potentially catastrophic risks, even in the absence of complete evidence of the benefits of the intervention or of the nature of the risk. Dr. Anthony Fauci, Director of the U.S. National Institute of Allergy and Infectious Diseases, captures the precautionary principle with his now-famous maxim, "If it looks like you're overreacting, you're probably doing the right thing."[9]

In non-emergency policy-making scenarios, where governments have time to gather social science evidence before enacting and enforcing laws, it is often possible to reconcile this conflict between civil liberties and public health. In a fast-moving pandemic, governments are forced to make urgent policy maneuvers that impact civil liberties in a vortex of uncertainty, without the luxury of prolonged deliberation; often, actions are taken on the basis of executive orders, pursuant to emergency legislation, even without legislative debate.[10] In such situations, decision makers may be forced to lean more heavily on first principles—whether employing restrictive measures that may ultimately prove unnecessary, overreaching in deference to the precautionary principle, or hesitating to act in deference to civil liberties.

---

8. *Canadian Charter of Rights and Freedoms*, Part I of the Constitution Act, 1982, being Schedule B to the *Canada Act 1982* (UK), 1982, c 11.
9. Interview of Dr. Anthony Fauci (15 March 2020) on *Face the Nation*, CBS News, Chicago, online (video): *CBS News* <www.cbsnews.com/news/transcript-dr-anthony-fauci-discusses-coronavirus-on-face-the-nation-march-15-2020/>.
10. For a discussion of the near-complete absence of deliberation to date, see Vanessa MacDonnell, this volume, Chapter B-1. See also Craig Forcese, "Repository of Canadian COVID-19 Emergency Orders" (last visited 13 May 2020), online (blog): *Intrepid* <www.intrepidpodcast.com/blog/2020/3/19/repository-of-canadian-covid-19-emergency-orders>.

As we will explain, the ideological contrast between civil liberties and public health is not as stark as it first appears. In the domain of civil liberties and *Charter* rights, courts acknowledge the need for governments to act under conditions of uncertainty.[11] Meanwhile, in the domain of public health, the precautionary principle has, in practice, evolved to incorporate elements of proportionality testing. For example, the European Commission's recent guidance on the precautionary principle[12] incorporates various sub-principles that echo the commitments of *Charter* law, including the principles of proportionality, non-discrimination, and consistency with measures taken in areas where scientific data are available.

Precautionary Principle (and its Evolution) Explained

As traditionally understood, the precautionary principle is the idea that measures should be taken to protect against a risk even if there is uncertainty over the benefit of the measures or the level of risk; the burden of proof rests on those who argue against the measures.[13] Applied to the issue at hand, it stands for the proposition that one does not require *complete evidence* of the efficacy of, for example, near-universal, mandatory physical distancing or closure of provincial borders before implementing such measures. Indeed, as the risk to the population increases, the evidentiary threshold for taking precautions lowers. The principle reflects a recognition of the limitations of scientific models to accurately describe complex issues pertaining to environmental harm or health risks, and the need for policy-makers to act notwithstanding those limitations.

While emerging out of the European environmental movement, the principle has increasingly been applied to public health matters. In Canada, the primary impetus for its use in public health in Canada was the Krever Inquiry.[14] In criticizing Canada's decision not to intro-

11. The Supreme Court has not been altogether consistent in the degree of deference shown to governments legislating under conditions of uncertainty. For an excellent, if slightly dated, discussion, see Sujit Choudhry, "So What is the Real Legacy of *Oakes*? Two Decades of Proportionality Analysis under the Canadian *Charter's* Section 1" (2006) 34:1 SCLR 501.
12. "EU's Communication on Precautionary Principle" (2000), online: *The Global Development Research Center* <www.gdrc.org/u-gov/precaution-4.html>.
13. D Kriebel et al, "The Precautionary Principle in Environmental Science" (2001) 109:9 Environmental Health Perspectives 871.
14. H Krever, *Commission of Inquiry on the Blood System in Canada: Final Report*, vol 1 (Ottawa: Government of Canada Publications, 1997).

duce surrogate testing of blood donations for hepatitis C, Justice Krever stated: "The safety of the blood supply is an aspect of public health, and, therefore, the blood supply system must be governed by the public health philosophy, which rejects the view that complete knowledge of a public health hazard is a prerequisite for action."[15]

However, the application of precautions to public health has been problematic, as the reflexive application of precautions to prevent one health risk can cause another health risk. For example, banning the use of lower-dose DDT for malaria prevention in Africa because of bioaccumulation concerns related to high-dose agricultural use in North America has led to malaria outbreaks. This dilemma has been all too evident with COVID-19: precautionary measures such as physical distancing are criticized for their accompanying risks, both to the economy and to public health, particularly to the most vulnerable, and to the risk of deepening social inequalities. Critics argue that the rational path forward is to attend, as best we can, to the risks on all sides rather than take refuge in a principle that reflexively favours precautionary measures. Some argue that we should move from precaution to risk—risk analyses in these scenarios.[16]

Given these challenges, the EU has provided more modern guidance, clarifying that the application of the precautionary principle should be:

- *proportional* to the chosen level of protection;
- *non-discriminatory;*
- *consistent* with similar measures already taken;
- *based on an examination of the potential benefits and costs* of action or lack of action (including, where appropriate and feasible, an economic cost/benefit analysis);
- *subject to review,* in the light of new scientific data; and
- *capable of assigning responsibility for producing the scientific evidence* necessary for a more comprehensive risk assessment.

In assessing any emerging threat, one must be cognizant that these are scientifically and socially dynamic situations with emerging evidence continually altering the level of uncertainty. This has been true of the COVID-19 pandemic. At the outset, with little known

15. *Ibid* at 1049.
16. Indur Goklany, "From Precautionary Principle to Risk—Risk Analysis" (2002) 20:11 Nature Biotechnology 1075.

about the pathogen, decision-making was guided by models out of Imperial College London, which suggested the U.K. could experience 500,000 deaths and the U.S. 2.2 million. Thus, the COVID-19 pandemic met the criteria of a potentially catastrophic risk, justifying the introduction of significant precautionary measures, such as travel restrictions and widespread lockdowns, with evidence of their benefit unclear and each with clear associated harms. As the availability of scientific evidence changed, and uncertainty lessened, these measures could be recalibrated. As such, countries are now attempting to introduce less restrictive measures to balance health protection concerns with the need to mitigate economic and other associated harms. In doing so, it will also be important to balance health protection with a healthy respect for civil liberties. It is in this evolution that Canadian governments may fall short, both from the perspective of a modern take on the precautionary principle and as part of a proportional response under s 1 of the *Charter*. In other words, Canadian policymakers need to be sufficiently reflective and responsive to changing public health evidence and adopt public health measures that curb a pandemic while respecting *Charter* rights.

Sometimes governments may not respond to the extant evidence and sufficiently loosen the restrictions they have put in place that are intrusive of civil liberties. There are factors *apart from epidemiological efficacy* that may play a role in government decision-making over COVID-19 responses. Public health officials may hesitate to shift direction for fear of undermining public trust in their expertise (as has arguably resulted from shifting opinions on border closures), or for fear of opening the floodgates to interventions that are costly and difficult to claw back once promised (for example, a shift from targeted to universal testing). Thus, one of the challenges of precautionary decision-making is to lift or modify restrictions as evidence emerges against the necessity of keeping them—a clear example being the maintenance of blood donation bans on men having sex with men long after screening tests for HIV emerged.[17]

On the other hand, a move to reopen may be driven by pure economic imperatives rather than public health evidence that a less intrusive stance is viable. In that case, civil liberties may be "respected" but at the risk of other human rights (such as the right to life and right to

17. Kumanan Wilson et al, "Three Decades of MSM Donor Deferral: What Have We Learnt?" (2014) 18 Intl J of Infectious Diseases 1.

health), although these latter rights, while recognized in many countries, are not recognized as free-standing rights under the Canadian *Charter*.[18]

Charter Proportionality Explained

Charter law, and civil liberties generally, have a different centre of gravity than public health law—their primary commitment is to secure protected rights and freedoms of individuals against incursions by the state. There is a popular misconception that rights are *trumps* against government action—that once a rights infringement has been identified, the offending government action must cease, though the heavens may fall. With some possible exceptions,[19] this is not how rights operate in Canada. Indeed, the possibility of limitations on individual rights is made explicit in section 1 of the *Charter*,[20] which clarifies that the enumerated rights and freedoms are subject to "such reasonable limits prescribed by law as can be demonstrably justified in a free and democratic society." What *Charter* rights provide, then, is not some fixed and all-purpose licence to do x, y, and z. What the *Charter* guarantees, first and foremost, is a requirement of demonstrable *justification* of government interference with enumerated rights (and the remediation of unjustifiable government actions).

The culture of justification mandated by the *Charter* manifests itself at various levels. The requirement that government actions infringing rights be "prescribed by law" is a safeguard against arbitrariness,[21] ensures that rules are communicated to the public, and offers initial assurance that some legislative debate has taken place. Of course, with the use of emergency powers invoked by all provinces, the executive may issue orders profoundly impinging upon civil liberties without the sunlight of parliament scrutiny.

In response to these incursions, in theory individuals have recourse to the courts, to press the case that some government action

18. For further discussion see Martha Jackman, this volume, Chapter D-3.
19. As an example, some have argued that the right to be free from torture is absolute, though this is debatable and arguably belied by the Supreme Court of Canada's jurisprudence.
20. There are also similar limitations within s 7 itself: any deprivation of "life, liberty, or security" must not occur except in accordance with the "principles of fundamental justice." This has been interpreted to include, among other things, that the law cannot be "arbitrary" or "over-broad."
21. *R v Therens*, [1985] 1 SCR 613, 18 DLR (4th) 655.

infringes their *Charter* rights. In *Charter* jurisprudence, the question of whether a rights infringement has occurred is separated from whether that infringement is justifiable. The infringement question is asked first, and the burden is on the claimant to show that an infringement has occurred. At this stage, the guiding principle is that rights should be given a "large and liberal interpretation at this stage.[22] The rationale for this, partly, is that the onus on *Charter* claimants should be eased to compensate for government's vastly superior legal resources. Under this large and liberal approach, it suffices in freedom of expression cases, for example, for the claimant to establish that some content-bearing expressive activity—no matter how trivial or ignoble—has been interfered with by government. Thus, for example, cigarette advertising has been found to fall within the right to free expression.[23]

If a claimant succeeds at that task, the government then bears the onus, under s 1, of showing that the infringement is demonstrably justified in a free and democratic society. *R v Oakes*[24] is perhaps the most important of all *Charter* decisions, providing the framework for the application of section 1. The *Oakes* test specifies that the infringement of a *Charter* right will be justified provided:

1. the government's objective in infringing the right is pressing and substantial;
2. the infringement is rationally connected with (1);
3. the right is minimally impaired; and
4. the value of the objective, and the actual costs and benefits associated with pursuing it, are proportionate to the costs of the infringement.

---

22. *Hunter et al v Southam Inc*, [1984] 2 SCR 145, 11 DLR (4th) 641. The scope given at the infringement stage varies by *Charter* guarantee. For example, the s 2(a) protection of freedom of religion has been read broadly to protect against any non-trivial state interference with activities the claimant sincerely believes are connected to their faith; *Syndicat Northcrest v Amselem*, 2004 SCC 47. By contrast, the courts have circumscribed the s 7 protection of "life, liberty and security of the person" to activities of a deeply personal nature (for example, the decision to have an abortion) as opposed to less-integral lifestyle choices (for example, recreational marijuana use); see, respectively, *R v Morgentaler*, [1988] 1 SCR 30, 44 DLR (4th) 385 and *R v Malmo-Levine*, 2003 SCC 74; *R v Caine*, 2003 SCC 74.
23. *RJR-MacDonald Inc v Canada (Attorney General)*, [1994] 1 SCR 311, 111 DLR (4th) 385.
24. [1986] 1 SCR 103, 26 DLR (4th) 200.

Ideally, when governments develop legislation, they invest considerable time in anticipating potential effects on *Charter* rights, ensuring there is some evidence available to answer a court challenge. This is a luxury that may be unavailable as governments confront an unprecedented pandemic.

Often, when governments fail at the *Oakes* test, it is at the *minimal impairment* stage: courts will point to some *less intrusive* policy alternative as evidence that government has overstepped its powers. Rare is the case where merely contemplating policy alternatives in the abstract will suggest less-impairing alternatives—particularly when it comes to complex, polycentric questions such as choices involving public health measures or the design features of complex health systems. Thus, the courts will at times look at measures taken in other jurisdictions—whether other provinces or other countries—to assess whether the government action is truly minimally impairing.[25]

It would be a mistake to suppose that the courts apply *uniform* evidentiary standards to all s 1 analysis. In some (but by no means all) cases, the courts impose a heavier burden of proof on government, at the s 1 stage, such as in criminal law matters—an area where the court feels most confident in its institutional competence, and where the state is the "singular antagonist" of the claimant's rights. By contrast, the courts can be more deferential to government in *Charter* cases that involve complex, polycentric trade-offs between multiple individuals[26]—particularly *vulnerable* individuals (for example, low-skilled workers,[27] children[28]). This reflects, first, a recognition that courts lack institutional competence over polycentric questions, and, second, that laws protecting vulnerable people should be shown special deference lest the *Charter* "simply become an instrument of better situated individuals to roll back legislation which has as its object the improvement of the condition of less advantaged persons."[29] The

25. *Chaoulli v Quebec (Attorney General)*, 2005 SCC 35 [*Chaoulli*].
26. Christopher P Manfredi & Antonia Maioni, "Judicializing Health Policy: Unexpected Lessons and an Inconvenient Truth" in James B Kelly & Christopher P Manfredi, eds, *Contested Constitutionalism: Reflections on the Canadian Charter of Rights and Freedoms* (Vancouver: University of British Columbia Press, 2010) at 129; Kent Roach, "The Challenges of Crafting Remedies for Violations of Socio-economic Rights" in Malcolm Langford, ed, *Social Rights Jurisprudence: Emerging Trends in International and Comparative Law* (Cambridge, UK: Cambridge University Press, 2008) at 46.
27. *R v Edwards Books and Art Ltd*, [1986] 2 SCR 713, 35 DLR (4th) 1 [*Edwards Books*].
28. *Irwin Toy Ltd v Quebec (Attorney General)*, [1989] 1 SCR 927, 58 DLR (4th) 577.
29. *Edwards Books*, supra note 27.

Supreme Court of Canada has also indicated that government should be granted wider latitude to justify measures enacted in response to national emergencies.[30]

These considerations suggest that courts are likely to be deferential to government actions taken in response to COVID-19.[31] Such measures, designed to flatten the curve and achieve statistical improvements in survival rates, are quintessentially complex and polycentric. Likewise, the primary intended beneficiaries are paradigmatically vulnerable populations—the elderly and immunocompromised.

Proportionality and Precaution Compared

There are points of both convergence and divergence between the orientation of civil rights laws and public health law. As noted, *Charter* rights do not operate as *trumps,* but instead entitle people to a reasoned justification for government actions that interfere with their enumerated rights. This overarching commitment to reasoned justification is echoed in the precautionary principle, as elaborated by the European Commission, in its sub-principle that restrictive measures should be subject to review in light of further scientific evidence. Whether in the domain of law or science, it is naïve to assume that arguments, evidence, and conclusions are ever *final,* and it is therefore appropriate that both domains have this commitment to *ongoing* justification, as new evidence emerges regarding the efficacy or necessity of specific responses. We have seen that courts are cognizant of the need to govern under conditions of uncertainty and will defer to governments that make good-faith efforts at striking a reasonable balance between individual rights and collective societal interests. Governments can expect—and deserve—that deference when they scrupulously consider and reconsider the necessity of incursions into civil liberties, ensuring in real time that they are carefully tailored.

Likewise, the *Oakes* test's *minimal impairment* stage has clear parallels in the precautionary principle's sub-test of "consistency

30. *R v Heywood,* [1994] 3 SCR 761 at 802-03, 120 DLR (4th) 348; *Reference Re BC Motor Vehicle Act,* [1985] 2 SCR 486 at 518, 24 DLR (4th) 536.
31. Section 7 rights are rarely saved under s1. In part, this is because a similar analysis to s 1 is conducted within s 7 itself, namely an examination of whether the deprivation of a "right" is in accordance with the "principles of fundamental justice." For example, the latter requires that the law or policy not be "over-broad," which is similar to one part of the s 1 analysis that examines whether the law or policy is "minimally impairing."

with measures already successfully taken in other jurisdictions." As explained, in carrying out the minimal impairment analysis, the courts will often look at what has been tried in other jurisdictions; this is tantamount to testing for consistency with measures successfully undertaken elsewhere. There are, of course, limitations to this method of analysis: it may be the case, particularly with a rapidly spreading infectious disease that all countries are grasping in the dark or attempting multiple policy responses simultaneously, making it difficult to identify which measures are having an impact. One expects (and hopes) the courts will be especially deferential in these initial scenarios and ratchet up scrutiny of government actions as evidence emerges. Another important limitation is that measures employed elsewhere may be less feasible in the Canadian context, due to our federal system, the design features of our health and long-term care system, and so on.

An example of the "play" in minimal impairment testing can perhaps be found in current employment standards for health care workers (HCWs).[32] Seasonal influenza poses a threat to HCWs as well as, more notably, the health of vulnerable patients for whom they care. As influenza can be transmitted in the asymptomatic stage, precluding HCWs with symptoms from working will not in and of itself be fully successful in preventing hospital-acquired infections (nosocomial transmission). As such, several jurisdictions have attempted to bring in policies that require influenza vaccination of HCWs to wear a mask at work—despite the lack of complete certainty that this reduces patient morbidity and mortality. This approach is arguably consistent with both the *Oakes* minimal impairment test as well as the precautionary principle. Complete evidence of benefit is not necessary to introduce a measure that can protect against an important risk. Reasonable minds can disagree, of course, and it bears noting that some labour tribunals have overturned hospital vaccine or mask policies, deeming them an unreasonable exercise of management rights and finding no evidence of benefit from a policy of mandatory masking.[33]

As explained, the final stage of the *Oakes* test inquires whether the costs and benefits of the government action are, on the whole, proportionate to the infringement of individual rights. Some legal theorists

32. R Rodal, NM Ries & K Wilson, "Influenza Vaccination for Health Care Workers: Towards a Workable and Effective Standard" (2009) 17 Health LJ 297.
33. Sault Area Hospital and Ontario Hospital Association v Ontario Nurses' Association, [2015] OLAA No 339; 124 CLAS 244.

have construed this as "a very conventional 'utilitarian' standard."[34] This branch of the *Oakes* test ensures the court is not *merely* engaged in an instrumentalist assessment of whether the government's actions are appropriately tailored to its aims, but also asks the deeper question of *what those ends are worth*, and whether the game is worth the candle when it comes to rights infringements. A similar utilitarian logic infuses the precautionary principle through the commitment to examining costs and benefits. One can imagine responses to an infectious disease outbreak that, despite being well targeted and effective epidemiologically, would strike many as unacceptable—for example, vaccination or quarantine orders that target individuals on the basis of their religious beliefs.[35] Needless to say, the evidentiary challenges associated with demonstrating minimal impairment are at play at this stage as well; indeed, there is the added challenge of measuring the costs to rights holders, necessary to show that the impugned government action is net beneficial.

In some areas, however, *Charter* logic deviates from the guidance offered under the precautionary principle. Shifting from a civil liberties frame to an equality frame (more fully explored in the next section, Equity, of this volume), we note the European Commission's guidance defines its non-discrimination principle as requiring that "comparable situations should not be treated differently, and that different situations should not be treated in the same way, unless there are objective grounds for doing so." Canadian courts have explicitly rejected this conception of equality in s 15 *Charter* jurisprudence as overly formalistic: "[T]he concept of equality does not necessarily mean identical treatment and that the formal 'like treatment' model of discrimination may in fact produce inequality."[36] COVID-19 responses that seem on their face non-discriminatory per the European Commission's definition—such as heavy fines or imprisonment for violators of shelter-at-home orders—may offend the *Charter* conception of equality, unless accommodations are made for vulnerable groups such as the homeless.[37]

34. David Beatty, "The End of Law: At Least as We Have Known It" in Richard Devlin, ed, *Canadian Perspectives on Legal Theory* (Toronto: Emond Montgomery, 1991) at 393.
35. Lawrence O Gostin & SG Hodge Jr, "Potential Discrimination in NYC's Measles Public Health Emergency Order", *The Hill* (11 April 2019), online: <thehill.com/opinion/healthcare/438301-potential-discrimination-in-nycs-measles-public-health-emergency-order>.
36. *R v Kapp*, 2008 SCC 41 at para 15.
37. See Terry Skolnik, this volume, Chapter C-4.

Applying the Proportionality and Precautionary Principles to COVID-19 Responses

A number of measures to prevent a bush fire spread of COVID-19 interfere with personal freedoms, and take a heavy toll on people who find lockdown conditions intolerable because of their particular circumstances. While s 7 of the *Charter* protects life, liberty and security of the person, it is generally understood that *economic* rights are not protected—except perhaps in the limiting case where government interferences with market freedoms jeopardize health, or life, or security.[38] Many Canadians have felt severe economic distress from lockdown measures, but it seems unlikely that a s 7 challenge would pass the infringement stage, especially given the countervailing relief measures in place (for example, expanded Employment Insurance benefits, employment subsidization packages for some businesses, mortgage deferral programs, eviction moratoria).

It is, nevertheless, worthwhile reflecting on the proportionality of these measures.[39] These measures were likely justified at the outset of the pandemic—given its scientific uncertainty and its potentially catastrophic nature. As the scientific uncertainty reduces and we have a better understanding of the nature, severity, and extent of the threat, there may be opportunities to strike a better balance between public health measures and rights and freedoms. Currently, a calibrated reopening of society based on detected cases and health care capacity is the approach in most jurisdictions; nevertheless, unless there is a change in the nature of the pathogen to be less harmful, these approaches are problematic, as a high percentage of the population remains susceptible (95%). Furthermore, front line workers are particularly at risk as society is reopened, given the inability to effectively physically distance in their work environments and the likelihood of exposure to a high viral load in a confined setting.

A paradox of the current situation is that the imposition of economic hardship and restrictions on personal freedom may be prolonged out of concern that alternative responses raise legal/ethical concerns of their own. Two technological solutions—immunity passports and digital contact tracing—could address these challenges but, so far, have been delayed due to legal/ethical concerns and scientific

38. *Chaoulli*, *supra* note 25.

39. Proportionality testing under s 7 is less straightforward than other *Charter* provisions. See *supra* note 31.

uncertainty over their benefits. For example, immunity passports, which identify those who have antibodies in their blood that may confer immunity, could permit further protection for front line workers in meat-packing plants or long-term care homes, where either social distancing isn't possible or transmission affects the vulnerable.[40] Differing views of this technology have prevented its adoption, and thus we are potentially at risk of repeating the error that Justice Krever identified—waiting for clear evidence before acting.[41] We may wish that we had acted earlier, but what is unclear is how to weigh the potential benefits of lifting restrictions with essential rights and values such as privacy and equity.

Conclusion

As we write, the COVID-19 pandemic is still unfolding. One of the major challenges is to settle on durable framing of the issues—in full knowledge that the facts are changing every day, and will have evolved considerably before this book is published. As we have pointed out, both proportionality analysis and the precautionary principle may offer shifting conclusions as new evidence and responses emerge. While this may disappoint rights-absolutists, it is surely a good thing, as it signals that these methods of analysis are in dialogue with our evolving understanding of the facts on the ground.

From a civil rights perspective, the legal permissibility of COVID-19 responses may turn partly on *when* legal challenges emerge. In the early stages of a global pandemic, as governments scramble to develop a response, it seems unlikely that courts would overturn restrictions on social gatherings or non-essential work. One expects deference from courts in these situations, given their limited institutional competence in public health and the potential risks to vulnerable populations. Even if courts were to find a *Charter* infringement, one expects they might opt for a *remedy* that offers government some latitude. Canadian courts have been at the forefront in using

40. JS Weitz et al, "Modeling Shield Immunity to Reduce COVID-19 Epidemic Spread" (2020), online: *Nature Medicine* DOI: <doi.org/10.1038/s41591-020-0895-3>.
41. For opposing viewpoints on digital passports, see Kumanan Wilson, Sophie Moreau & Sabine Tsuruda, "The Big Debate: Should Those With Immunity Get a COVID-19 Digital Passport?", *Toronto Star* (12 May 2020), online: <www.thestar.com/opinion/contributors/thebigdebate/2020/05/12/the-big-debate-should-those-with-immunity-get-a-covid-19-digital-passport.html>.

"suspended declarations of invalidity"—a remedy where a government action is deemed invalid, but is allowed to remain operative for month or even years as the government develops alternative plans. Assuming that some legal challenge to COVID-19 responses had traction in the courts, it is possible that the pandemic may have run its course and that the infringing measures are lifted voluntarily before any court order vindicating civil rights comes into effect.

On the other hand, as time passes and evidence gathers on effective responses, courts may become more demanding. Take, for example, excluding family members from seeing their dying relatives—a heartbreaking scenario where a loved one is left to die alone, potentially engaging the *Charter*'s s 7 right to liberty and security of the person. As we reset to a new normal where we mitigate risks as best as possible, courts may demand of governments that their precautionary measures evolve with changing evidence to better protect such fundamental rights.

We believe that there is an opportunity to reconcile these conflicts, as there are many parallels between the *Oakes* test and the EU guidance on the precautionary principle. Ultimately, an agile policy is needed, one that recognizes the changing level of scientific uncertainty and the changing balance between civil liberties and precautionary measures. In fact, the importance of civil liberties can encourage the timely revisiting of precautionary measures—something that has been a challenge in its application to public health. Conversely, the inclusion of the public health perspective can be a corrective against extremist interpretations of rights and freedoms—scenarios where individuals "die with their rights on." As such, ultimately a dynamic policy approach would be consistent with both the *Charter* and the appropriate application of precaution, and the two would work together to both protect the public's health and ensure protection of an individual's rights and freedoms.

CHAPTER C-2

Privacy, Ethics, and Contact-Tracing Apps

Teresa Scassa,* Jason Millar,** and Kelly Bronson***

Abstract

Data and analytics are being enlisted to play a role in understanding and preventing the spread of COVID-19. This chapter focuses on digital "apps," which are being deployed by governments around the world to supplement the manual contact-tracing efforts typically performed by public health officials. Contact-tracing apps have been developed rapidly, with little time for user testing, and their adoption raises important privacy and ethical concerns. In this chapter, we outline some of these potential concerns. We begin by tracing the history of contact tracing as a pre-digital, or manual, method and then detail the current contact-tracing efforts, distinguishing among different types of apps and data use approaches. We then draw from our complementary expertise in law, ethics, and sociology to outline potential risks of contact-tracing apps along these dimensions. Risks include

* Canada Research Chair in Information Law and Policy and Professor, Faculty of Law (Common Law Section), University of Ottawa.

** Canada Research Chair in The Ethical Engineering of Robotics and Artificial Intelligence and Assistant Professor in the School of Electrical Engineering and Computer Science, University of Ottawa.

*** Canada Research Chair in Science and Society and Assistant Professor in the School of Sociological and Anthropological Studies, University of Ottawa. We gratefully acknowledge the support of the Scotiabank AI & Society Initiative and the SSHRC Canada Research Chairs program.

misuse of personal data for surveillance and insufficient uptake leading to inaccurate information for individuals, which could lead to increased infection. Risks also include differential access and thus the reproduction of vulnerability among marginalized communities. Overall, the chapter identifies issues relevant to the responsible development and use of big data and AI for COVID-19 mitigation efforts.

Résumé
Vie privée, éthique et applications de recherche de contacts

Les données et les analyses sont mises à contribution pour comprendre et prévenir la propagation de la COVID-19. Ce chapitre porte sur les applications numériques déployées par les gouvernements du monde entier pour appuyer les efforts de recherche manuelle des contacts généralement consentis par les responsables de la santé publique. Les applications de recherche de contacts ont été développées rapidement, sans que les utilisateurs aient le temps de les tester, et leur adoption soulève d'importantes questions en matière d'éthique et de respect de la vie privée. Dans ce chapitre, nous présentons certaines de ces préoccupations. Nous commençons par retracer l'historique de la recherche de contacts en tant que méthode prénumérique, ou manuelle, puis nous détaillons les efforts actuels en la matière, en distinguant différents types d'applications et d'approches quant à l'utilisation des données. Nous nous appuyons ensuite sur nos compétences complémentaires en droit, en éthique et en sociologie pour exposer les risques potentiels des applications de recherche de contacts en fonction de ces dimensions. Parmi ces risques, nommons l'utilisation inappropriée des données personnelles à des fins de surveillance et leur application insuffisante, qui pourrait conduire à des informations inexactes sur les personnes et, par conséquent, à une augmentation des infections. Les risques incluent également l'inégalité d'accès, susceptible de reproduire la vulnérabilité parmi les communautés marginalisées. Dans l'ensemble, ce chapitre recense les questions relatives au développement et à l'utilisation responsables de mégadonnées et de l'IA pour atténuer les effets de la COVID-19.

Many people today carry smartphones—powerful devices capable of, among other things, recording and communicating both their geographic location and their physical proximity to other devices. It is perhaps not surprising, then, that data about our movements and contacts collected by these devices are being enlisted to play a role in the battle against COVID-19. Governments around the world have shown interest in the potential for cellphone applications, or "apps," to assist in contact tracing normally performed by public health officials and to better enable the gradual lifting of physical distancing restrictions.

Developers have produced these apps rapidly, with little time for user testing. Adopting them raises important privacy and ethical concerns.[1] This chapter identifies and examines a number of these. We begin by tracing the history of contact tracing as a manual method and then detail the current digital contact-tracing efforts, which include different types of apps and data use approaches. The core of the paper draws from our complementary expertise in privacy law, ethics, and sociology to outline some potential limitations of these contact-tracing apps along these dimensions. We end with an argument that data privacy, technology ethics, and social justice must guide the development and use of contact-tracing apps.

Contact Tracing as a Public Health Measure

Contact tracing is a well-established public health practice for slowing the spread of an infectious disease within a community.[2] Typically, a person who tests positive for a given disease is questioned by public health officials to determine those with whom that person had contact during the period in which they would have been contagious. Officials then contact those at-risk individuals, at which point they may direct them to seek immediate medical treatment if they are symptomatic or instruct them to get tested. If the infected person travelled on a bus

1. Although privacy has an ethical dimension, we treat it separately because privacy rights are legally protected under the *Canadian Charter of Rights and Freedoms* and in provincial and federal privacy legislation. In our view it is important to distinguish between issues of legal compliance and broader questions about how to do the right thing in concert with the law and wider social values. See e.g. Emanuel Moss, "Too Big a Word, What Does it Mean to do 'Ethics' in the Technology Industry?" (29 April 2020), online: *Points, Data & Society* <points.datasociety.net/too-big-a-word-13e66e62a5bf>.
2. "Contact Tracing: Part of a Multipronged Approach to Fight the COVID-19 Pandemic" (29 April 2020), online: *Centers for Disease Control and Prevention* <www.cdc.gov/coronavirus/2019-ncov/php/principles-contact-tracing.html>.

during the contagious period, there may even be a public announcement directing people on the same bus trip to get tested for the disease. Where an outbreak is small, and a disease is not particularly contagious, contact tracing can be highly effective in containing its spread.

Manual contact tracing has proven extremely challenging in the COVID-19 crisis. The disease is highly contagious and spreads rapidly. Many people with COVID-19 are contagious despite being asymptomatic, and even those who develop symptoms may be contagious days before symptoms appear. In many jurisdictions, including Canada, there has been insufficient testing, test results may be substantially delayed, and an already strained medical system limits the human resources required for widespread manual contact tracing. The question has become whether data-driven technologies might supplement, or even replace, manual contact tracing.

Contact-Tracing Apps

Early and rather blunt uses of technology to assist in contact tracing relied on cellphone global positioning system (GPS) data to track individuals. In mid-March 2020, for example, Israel announced that it would use cellphone geolocation data to monitor those who tested positive for COVID-19, and would use text messaging to notify those who might have come in contact with them.[3] This emergency measure raised constitutional concerns, faced stiff opposition, and was eventually suspended in late April.[4]

A major trend in contact-tracing apps has been to rely on Bluetooth technology. Bluetooth offers better privacy features for users, focusing on the assessment of proximity between devices rather than a GPS-determined location.

Two overarching issues emerged as interest in contact-tracing apps increased. One pits privacy against the need or desire of government and the public to have data collected via these apps for public health purposes. Because of the different privacy/necessity balances struck by different governments, a second broad issue has been

3. Natasha Lomas, "Israel Passes Emergency Law to Use Mobile Data for COVID-19 Contact Tracing" (18 March 2020), online: *TechCrunch* <techcrunch.com/2020/03/18/israel-passes-emergency-law-to-use-mobile-data-for-covid-19-contact-tracing/>.
4. "Coronavirus: Israel Halts Police Phone Tracking Over Privacy Concerns", *BBC News* (23 April 2020), online: <www.bbc.com/news/technology-52395886>.

interoperability.[5] Apps are adopted by specific national or regional governments. As restrictions lift and people begin once again to cross borders, interoperability of different apps across jurisdictions becomes important.[6]

Centralized vs Decentralized Data Storage

Apple and Google have sought to address both privacy and interoperability by collaborating on an exposure notification system that could be used as a foundation for Bluetooth-enabled contact-tracing apps.[7] With input from privacy scholars and advocates,[8] this system was designed for decentralized data storage. A decentralized data storage approach keeps information about contacts stored locally on a user's phone, rather than automatically uploading it to a central database.[9] A person who tests positive for COVID-19 can enable public health authorities to notify significant contacts without actually identifying them.

Some governments were unwilling to adopt a fully decentralized contact-tracing app, preferring a centralized model in which data about users and/or contacts is stored on a central server accessible to public authorities. Centralized data solutions have the benefit of allowing governments (or app developers) to access de-identified data about proximity and infection that might be useful in modelling and analytics to better understand the disease and its spread. Some governments have sought a compromise solution that allows for decentralized storage of contact data only up until the point of a user's

5. Leila Abboud, Joe Miller & Javier Espinoza, "How Europe Splintered over Contact Tracing Apps", *Financial Times* (10 May 2020), online: <www.ft.com/content/7416269b-0477-4a29-815d-7e4ee8100c10>.
6. Teresa Scassa, "One App per Province? How Canada's Federalism Complicates Digital Contact Tracing", *Heinrich Böll Stiftung* (13 May 2020), online: <us.boell.org/en/2020/05/13/one-app-province-how-canadas-federalism-complicates-digital-contact-tracing>.
7. Apple/Google, "Privacy-Preserving Contact Tracing" (last visited 11 May 2020), online: <www.apple.com/covid19/contacttracing/>; Andy Greenberg, "Google and Apple Reveal How Covid-19 Alert Apps Might Look", *Wired* (4 May 2020), online: <www.wired.com/story/apple-google-covid-19-contact-tracing-interface/>.
8. DP-3T, "Decentralized Privacy-Preserving Proximity Tracing—Documents", *GitHub* (last visited 11 May 2020), online: <github.com/DP-3T/documents>.
9. Carmela Troncoso et al, "Decentralized Privacy-Preserving Proximity Tracing—White Paper" (12 April 2020), online (pdf): <github.com/DP-3T/documents/blob/master/DP3T%20White%20Paper.pdf>.

positive COVID-19 test.[10] At that point, contact data would be shared with public health authorities, who would notify those judged to have been in sufficient proximity to the infected person.

The ability of governments to find new purposes for shared data—including purposes in which individuals might be made identifiable—was one reason why many privacy advocates pushed for a decentralized model. The decentralized model gained traction in the EU, although France has remained a notable standout. Germany reluctantly adopted a decentralized model, but added a feature to allow users to voluntarily contribute data for research purposes.[11] The U.K. has opted for a centralized model.[12] Both Australia[13] and the Canadian province of Alberta[14] have chosen models that are initially decentralized but that give users diagnosed with COVID-19 the option to upload their contact data to a centralized system to enable contact tracing.

The centralization or decentralization of data storage can impact the extent to which an app is integrated with public health efforts, as well as the extent to which de-identified data regarding the movements of the population can be used in modelling and other data analytics.

AI-enabled Contact Tracing

Another type of contact-tracing app would use artificial intelligence (AI) to supplement disease testing. In countries like Canada, where there have been substantial challenges with testing—including lack of testing equipment and slow lab results—even symptomatic

---

10. Leo Kelion, "Apple and Google Accelerate Coronavirus Contact Tracing Apps Plan", *BBC News* (24 April 2020), online: <www.bbc.com/news/technology-52415593>.
11. Douglas Busvine & Andreas Rinke, "Germany Flips to Apple-Google Approach on Smartphone Contact Tracing", *Reuters* (26 April 2020), online: <www.reuters.com/article/us-health-coronavirus-europe-tech/germany-flips-to-apple-google-approach-on-smartphone-contact-tracing-idUSKCN22807J>.
12. Kieran McCarthy, "UK Finds Itself Almost Alone with Centralized Virus Contact-Tracing App that Probably Won't Work Well, Asks for Your Location, May Be Illegal", *The Register* (5 May 2020), online: <www.theregister.co.uk/2020/05/05/uk_coronavirus_app/>.
13. "COVIDSafe App" (last modified 27 May 2020), online: *Australian Government Department of Health* <www.health.gov.au/resources/apps-and-tools/covidsafe-app>.
14. "ABTraceTogether" (last visited 11 May 2020), online: *Government of Alberta* <www.alberta.ca/ab-trace-together.aspx>.

individuals have not been tested due to lack of capacity.[15] The app being developed for the U.K. will use user-reported symptoms to determine likelihood of infection.[16] An AI-enabled assessment can then trigger contact notification functions. To continue to develop and enhance the AI, and to use the data collected for other AI analytics related to understanding or modelling the disease, user-contributed data could be treated differently, with users being asked to consent to the inclusion of their de-identified self-reporting data in a central database. An app under development in Canada would also use AI and machine learning to supplement low rates of testing in order to develop targeted risk profiles for individuals.[17] With all AI-enabled apps, the additional data collected would have research applications that go beyond contact tracing.

Uptake and Use

Contact-tracing apps are not a magic bullet. In fact, many depend upon considerable uptake and use by the public before they can have meaningful impact. An Oxford University study of the U.K. app determined that 56% uptake was required.[18] The Australian government assessed the necessary uptake rate for their app at 40%.[19] The more privacy-protective Bluetooth-only apps require greater rates of uptake since these apps record only proximity with other app users. Apps that use GPS or a combination of GPS and Bluetooth can provide data useful

15. Tonda MacCharles, "Canada Must Triple its COVID-19 Testing Before Loosening Restrictions, Experts Say", *Toronto Star* (23 April 2020), online: <www.thestar.com/politics/federal/2020/04/22/canada-must-triple-its-covid-19-testing-before-loosening-restrictions-experts-say.html>.
16. Hasan Chowdhury, Matthew Field & Margi Murphy, "NHS Contact Tracing App: How Does it Work and When Can You Download It?", *The Telegraph* (10 May 2020), online: <www.telegraph.co.uk/technology/2020/05/10/nhs-contact-tracing-app-download/>.
17. Martin Patriquin, "Montreal Computer Scientists Expect to Launch Contact-Tracing App in Less than a Week", *The Logic* (9 April 2020), online: <thelogic.co/news/montreal-computer-scientists-expect-to-launch-contact-tracing-app-in-less-than-a-week/>.
18. Robert Hinch et al, "Effective Configurations of a Digital Contact Tracing App: A report to NHSX" (16 April 2020), online (pdf): *University of Oxford* <cdn.theconversation.com/static_files/files/1009/Report_-_Effective_App_Configurations.pdf?1587531217>.
19. Asha Barbaschow, "Morrison Says Using COVID-19 Tracing App a Matter of 'National Service'" (17 April 2020), online: *ZDNet* <www.zdnet.com/article/morrison-says-using-covid-19-tracing-app-a-matter-of-national-service/>.

for manual contact tracing even with lower uptake. Where a separate function of a contact-tracing app is to collect self-reported symptom data for AI, a much smaller percentage of users may still make the data collected useful for research purposes, even if that small percentage renders the contact-tracing functions ineffective.

Most governments that have adopted contact-tracing apps have made them voluntary, in spite of the need for significant uptake to be effective. Requiring all citizens to download and use an app that collects information about their movements or proximity to other individuals raises serious civil liberties concerns. It is also not practicable or equitable in a context in which not every member of the population has a cellphone. While data from Statistics Canada suggest that a high number of Canadians have smartphones, the number of smartphones is significantly lower for seniors, with only 60.4% of those over the age of 65 reporting having a smartphone.[20] Beyond this, the limitations of relying on cellphone-collected data to guide policy have been revealed in early experiments that used such data to guide local policing and other municipal services, for example.[21]

Privacy

It is evident that the architecture of contact-tracing apps has been influenced by privacy concerns. Initial use of GPS data raised the potential for surveillance. Bluetooth-based solutions aim to solve the surveillance problem by not capturing or sharing location data. Instead, when two phones using the Bluetooth-enabled app are in proximity, the devices exchange digital "tokens" that are stored only on users' phones. These tokens record data about the device encountered, as well as the degree of proximity and the duration of the encounter. A concern with Bluetooth models is that even de-identified contact data could be used to create a "social graph" mapping an

20. "Smartphone Use and Smartphone Habits by Gender and Age Group" (last modified 27 May 2020), online: *Statistics Canada* <doi.org/10.25318/2210011501-eng>.
21. See for example Kate Crawford, "The Hidden Biases in Big Data" (1 April 2013), online: *Harvard Business Review* <hbr.org/2013/04/the-hidden-biases-in-big-data>; Stephen Goldsmith & Susan Crawford, "The Responsive City: Engaging Communities through Data-smart Governance" (2014) 39:3 J Urban Affairs 458; Alred Tat-Kei Ho et al, "Big Data and Local Performance Management: The Experience of Kansas City, Missouri" In Yu-Che Chen & Michael Ahn, eds, *Routledge Handbook on Information Technology in Government* (Routledge, 2017) 95.

individual's contacts, which could enable surveillance by the state or a bad actor.[22]

The more rigorous the privacy protection, the less that data are available to public health authorities. Some governments want contact-tracing apps to also provide data that might be useful for modelling and understanding the spread of COVID-19. Thus, not all jurisdictions will opt for the least privacy-intrusive apps.

A privacy impact assessment (PIA) carried out on the Australian COVIDSafe app[23] raised several important issues relevant to all contact-tracing apps. These included a need for data minimization in the collection of registrant data, as well as in the sharing with authorities of data about the duration and proximity of encounters after a positive test. The PIA recommended that if technically feasible, only those contacts of sufficient proximity and duration to create risk of infection should be reported. The PIA also recommended that the government provide assurances that the data collected would be deleted after the end of the emergency period. It also recommended obtaining free and informed consent not just at the time of registration for the app, but also at the point when authorizing public health officials to collect digital handshake data (for example, the exchanged Bluetooth tokens) after a positive test. The PIA raised concerns about obtaining appropriate consent from users under the age of 16. Finally, it recommended clear communications about any future changes to the app beyond its original purpose to protect against "function creep."

AI-enabled contact-tracing apps will raise additional privacy concerns, particularly since one of their goals is to collect symptom data from users for analytics purposes. Potentially, researchers could use these data (in de-identified format) in other AI applications. However, good privacy practice, requiring multiple consents (for sharing of information on registration; for sharing contact details

22. Danny Palmer, "Security Experts Warn: Don't Let Contact-Tracing App Lead to Surveillance" (7 May 2020), online: *ZDNet* <www.zdnet.com/article/security-experts-warn-dont-let-contact-tracing-app-lead-to-surveillance/>.

23. "The COVIDSafe Application: A Privacy Impact Assessment" (24 April 2020), online (pdf): *Australian Government Department of Health* <www.health.gov.au/sites/default/files/documents/2020/04/covidsafe-application-privacy-impact-assessment-covidsafe-application-privacy-impact-assessment.pdf>. For a critique of Australia's app, see Graham Greenleaf & Katharine Kemp, "Australia's 'COVIDSafe App': An Experiment in Surveillance, Trust and Law" (30 April 2020), online (pdf): *University of New South Wales Law Research Series* <ssrn.com/abstract=3589317>.

after testing positive or receiving a high-risk rating; and for sharing symptom data for further AI purposes) may lead to user confusion. The use of symptom data in combination with other data in unspecified analytics may also create a re-identification risk.

Socio-ethics

Contact-tracing apps also raise social and ethical concerns. One concern is that these technologies are being rolled out on whole populations in a time of crisis and vulnerability. Technologies always present societal risks, but developers have an ethical obligation to anticipate these when possible; arguably, their responsibility is greater in a time when vulnerable populations are being asked to use untested and unproven technology. Bluetooth apps may err in assessing the significance of proximity, for example if a physical wall/barrier exists between two phones.[24] AI-enabled apps may miscalculate infection risk. Such errors could have important adverse consequences for users of the apps and, subsequently, for population health. Security experts have warned of trolling that could disrupt the functioning of such apps, including entering false symptom data and carrying the phone around areas where there are many people, such as grocery stores.[25] Bluetooth also raises significant security concerns which may leave users vulnerable to other types of hacking and attack.[26]

As noted earlier, Bluetooth-enabled contact-tracing apps require a significant uptake within the population to make a difference. If uptake is insufficient, those who do adopt the app will be relying on an inaccurate tool to provide them with information about their risk of infection. Over-reliance by users is also possible given what we know of "automation bias," or people's tendency to place unwarranted faith

24. Rob Kitchin, "Using Digital Technologies to Tackle the Spread of the Coronavirus: Panacea or Folly" (21 April 2020), online (pdf): *Maynooth University* <progcity.maynoothuniversity.ie/wp-content/uploads/2020/04/Digital-tech-spread-of-coronavirus-Rob-Kitchin-PC-WP44.pdf>.

25. Andrew Crocker, Kurt Opsahl & Bennett Cyphers, "The Challenge of Proximity Apps for COVID-19 Contact Tracing" (10 April 2020), online: *Electronic Frontier Foundation* <www.eff.org/deeplinks/2020/04/challenge-proximity-apps-covid-19-contact-tracing>; Ross Anderson, "Contact Tracing in the Real World" (12 April 2020), online: *Light Blue Touchpaper Cambridge University* <www.lightbluetouchpaper.org/2020/04/12/contact-tracing-in-the-real-world/>.

26. Anderson, *supra* note 25.

in automated systems.[27] A similar problematic impact could then be users relaxing their risk management approach, even shirking public health messaging, because of this false sense of security.[28]

For contact-tracing apps with an AI dimension, even if uptake is well under 60%, the app may be useful for analytics purposes or to support AI research and development because of the personal data collected. Even if the app allows, through consent agreements, for transparency regarding the uses of personal data (for contact tracing or analytics), questions linger about whether this is equitable and fair, again in this context of widespread anxiety and vulnerability.

There are a host of justice-related questions raised by all types of contact-tracing apps. Employers may refuse to allow employees to return to work, or businesses may deny access to individuals who cannot demonstrate that they are using the app. The dual use of contact-tracing apps as so-called "COVID passports" would undermine the voluntary and consent-based approach underpinning these apps' ethical uptake.[29] This problem was flagged in the Australian PIA, and it was recommended that the risk be dealt with as part of a specific legislative framework for the app.[30] It is also possible that not all people will have access to contact-tracing apps given an existing "digital divide" where not all individuals have cellphones, and some cellphones may not be capable of running the app.[31] There may also be issues of accessibility in the use of the interface. Accessibility could include access for the visually impaired, as well as access for those without the necessary language skills to use the apps.[32] Language barriers may make text-heavy notifications (such as privacy policies, consents, or information about the limitations of the app) inaccessible to some users. There is a wealth of research showing that most people

27. Linda J Skitka, Kathleen Mosier & Mark D Burdick, "Accountability and Automation Bias" (2000) 52:4 Intl J of Human-Computer Studies 701 at 701-17.
28. Jason Millar, "Five Ways a COVID-19 Contact-Tracing App Could Make Things Worse" (15 April 2020), online: *Policy Opinions* <policyoptions.irpp.org/magazines/april-2020/five-ways-a-covid-19-contact-tracing-app-could-make-things-worse/>.
29. "Social, legal, and ethical issues of Test-trace-isolate-quarantine strategies" (9 May 2020), online: *Swiss National COVID-19 Science Task Force* <ncs-tf.ch/de/policy-briefs>.
30. See *Australian Department of Health, supra* note 13.
31. See Kelion, *supra* note 10.
32. See e.g. Tess Sheldon and Ravi Malhotra, "Not All In This Together: Disability Rights and COVID-19", in Flood et al, eds, *Law, Policy and Ethics of COVID-19* (Ottawa: University of Ottawa Press) [forthcoming in July 2020].

have difficulty interpreting consent or user agreements. Last, with AI-enabled contact-tracing apps, language or literacy barriers may impact symptom collection. Not only may some users not be able to fully understand the questionnaires, the interpretation of one's symptoms is necessarily subjective and can be influenced by anxiety, a tendency toward hypochondria or its opposite, or a perceived need to not be identified as symptomatic in order to be able to return to work, for example.

Conclusion

In sum, the issues raised by contact-tracing apps include privacy and security risks, but also broader issues of ethics and social justice. These issues must be carefully considered by developers and adopting governments. Privacy impact assessments and algorithmic impact assessments are one way to identify and address issues. Transparency as to the results of these assessments can build public trust. A failure to carefully consider and address the legal, ethical, and social implications of contact-tracing apps could lead to legitimacy failures for public health and technology firms, and stall our collective desire to mitigate fallout from COVID-19.

CHAPTER C-3

Should Immunity Licences be an Ingredient in our Policy Response to COVID-19?

Daniel Weinstock* and Vardit Ravitsky**

Abstract

According to their advocates, immunity licences in the post-confinement phase of the COVID-19 pandemic should be granted to those who have been exposed to the virus and as a result have (presumably) developed immunity. This would allow them to go back to work, engage in leisure activities, and travel. Those who are in favour of such licences argue that the ability of some to return to work would be of benefit to all. Opponents of the proposal point to their lack of scientific basis, to the perverse incentives that their introduction might generate, and to the risk that they might exacerbate existing inequalities. But should we consider them as wrong *per se*, that is, independent of the negative consequences that they might produce in present circumstances, consequences that might be neutralized by scientific advances and by an appropriate regulatory apparatus? They would still be morally deficient because they violate the principle of "least infringement" relative to the value of equality. Reorganizing the spaces in which we work and play, and create is one way in which the task of emerging from confinement safely could be accomplished in a more egalitarian manner.

* Katharine A. Pearson Chair in Civil Society and Public Policy, Faculty of Law and Faculty of Arts, McGill University.

** Full Professor, Bioethics Program, Department of Social and Preventive Medicine, School of Public Health, Université de Montréal.

Résumé
Les licences d'immunité devraient-elles faire partie de notre réponse politique à la COVID-19?

Selon leurs partisans, des licences d'immunité devraient être accordées, en phase postconfinement de la pandémie de COVID-19, aux personnes qui ont été exposées au virus et qui, de ce fait, ont (probablement) développé une immunité. Cela leur permettrait de retourner au travail, de s'adonner à des activités de loisirs et de voyager. Ceux qui sont en faveur de ces licences font valoir que le retour au travail d'une partie de la population serait bénéfique pour tous. Les opposants à la proposition soulignent quant à eux son absence de fondement scientifique, les incitations perverses que l'instauration de ces licences pourrait engendrer et le risque qu'elles exacerbent les inégalités existantes. Mais devrions-nous les considérer comme mauvaises en soi, indépendamment des conséquences négatives qu'elles pourraient produire dans les circonstances actuelles, conséquences qui pourraient être neutralisées par les progrès scientifiques et par un mécanisme de régulation approprié ? Elles demeureraient malgré tout moralement déficientes parce qu'elles violent le principe de « moindre atteinte » par rapport à la valeur de l'égalité. Réorganiser les espaces dans lesquels nous travaillons et profitons des activités de loisirs est un moyen de mettre un terme à notre confinement en toute sécurité et de manière plus égalitaire.

The public health response to the COVID-19 pandemic initially required restrictive measures to "flatten the curve." While posing grave limitations to personal freedoms, these measures were ethically and politically justified given the urgency of the goal to be achieved. However, as we gradually emerge from this restrictive phase and are yet nowhere near the end of the pandemic, we must navigate a more complex policy terrain in which we gradually open up society, but do so in an environment of managed risk.

To open society in ways that do not take us back to a phase of massive, uncontrolled community transmission and high death rates, governments will choose among several policy tools, ranging from low-tech interventions such as selective confinement to high-tech tools such as advanced contact tracing based on big data and machine learning. These tools should be assessed based on their capacity to help us safely navigate this new risk environment, as well as with respect to their compatibility with core moral values of our liberal democratic society, such as freedom, equality, and transparency of the political process.[1] Since many of the dilemmas facing us involve a tension between safety, on the one hand, and freedom (for example, forcing confinement) or equality (for example accepting the differential impact of these restrictions on people's lives) on the other, a key principle of public health ethics during this challenging period will be the *least infringement* principle, which says that "a proposed policy ... should seek to minimize the infringement of general moral considerations."[2] We interpret this principle as applying to both freedom and equality as fundamental values. Policies will be justified if they represent the least offensive ways, relative to these core values, to attain the policy goal of limiting virus spread.

Immunity Licences

One of the tools currently at the centre of discussions is immunity passports, more appropriately referred to as "immunity licences."[3] These would be conferred on individuals who are found to have immunity to the disease based on a serological test, and would grant their holders the right to return to normal life while continuing to restrict those who do not possess immunity. The advantages are clear. Immunity licences would allow a portion of the population to safely work, travel, and engage in social and cultural activities of various kinds. A significant proportion of the population of most countries going back to work without risk would benefit all of us, since we have all suffered from the economic downturn wrought by the COVID-19 pandemic.

Given what seems to be a strong *prima facie* case, why then have immunity licences ignited such controversy? In this chapter, we

1. For the importance of democratic norms in the context of pandemics, see Vanessa MacDonnell, this volume, Chapter B-1.
2. James Childress et al, "Public Health Ethics: Mapping the Terrain" (2002) 30:2 JL Med & Ethics 170 at 170-78.
3. Persad and Emanuel persuasively argue that "licence" is a better term than "passport," as the latter term implies an all-or-nothing access to a territory, whereas licences are granted in specific contexts, for specific purposes. Govind Persad & Ezekiel Emanuel, "The Ethics of COVID-19 Immunity-Based Licenses ('Immunity Passports')" (6 May 2020), online: *JAMA Network* <jamanetwork.com/journals/jama/fullarticle/2765836>.

aim to contribute conceptual clarity to this debate by distinguishing between empirical and normative arguments that are being employed in opposition to this tool. We conclude by focusing on some normative objections that, we will argue, need to be taken quite seriously before we decide whether or not to adopt immunity licences as part of our overall mix of policy responses to COVID-19.

Empirical Objections

The first set of empirical objections concerns the reliability of the serological tests currently available. Such tests would require a high level of accuracy for their widespread use to be morally justifiable. If they generate too many false positives, they will only serve to give false assurance to people actually at risk of infection. Currently, we also lack an evidence base that the presence of antibodies confers immunity, and whether the immunity it might confer is long-lasting. Such empirical uncertainty is at the basis of the World Health Organization's current opposition to the use of such licences.[4]

The second set of empirical objections relates to possible perverse incentives that the use of immunity licences might generate. If they were to become a condition of employment, travel, or access to highly prized leisure or cultural activities, one could imagine a black market of counterfeit licences emerging, or even people becoming so desperate to acquire one that they voluntarily seek to infect themselves, with all of the attendant risks this would give rise to at the individual and collective levels. Moreover, if immunity licences were to acquire widespread currency, they could become a tool in the arsenal of states to police and impose surveillance on their citizenry, in a manner that would, moreover, most likely target already marginalized or racialized communities disproportionately.[5]

The third and final set of empirical objections relates to the regulatory challenges of ensuring fair access. Minimal fairness would require that citizens have equitable access to serological tests and to

---

4. "'Immunity Passports' in the Context of COVID-19" (24 April 2020), online: *World Health Organization* <www.who.int/news-room/commentaries/detail/immunity-passports-in-the-context-of-covid-19>.
5. Françoise Baylis & Natalie Kofler, "Why Canadians Should Fight Tooth and Nail Against Proof-of-Immunity Cards", *CBC News Opinion* (7 May 2020), online: <www.cbc.ca/news/opinion/opinion-pandemic-coronavirus-immunity-passport-1.5551528>.

the process of issuing such licences, regardless of their geographic location or socio-economic status. Otherwise, the distribution of immunity licences would be based not only on the presence of immunity, but also on antecedent patterns of advantage.[6] But, the objection goes, these fair background conditions are unlikely to be met, especially given the paucity of such tests and the structural injustices already in place.

These objections are weighty. Taken together, they may be sufficient to seal the case against immunity licences under present circumstances, and possibly for the foreseeable future. But note that they constitute a powerful *contingent* case against immunity licences. They do not amount to an argument that there is anything wrong with them *as such*, but only that for empirical reasons they are either scientifically premature or would engender more negative than positive consequences. These arguments tell us it would be immoral to implement them as part of our policy response because we cannot effectively and ethically regulate their use *at this time*—not that their use would be wrong if we *could* effectively regulate them.

Categorical Arguments

Let's consider the possible normative arguments that there is something *categorically* wrong with immunity licences, which would defeat the *prima facie* case for their adoption. What might such arguments look like? Let us assume that if there is something wrong with them as such, it is because they offend values that are foundational to a liberal-democratic order, such as liberty and equality.

On the face of it, immunity licences would seem to involve a restriction of liberty, because though the liberty of licence holders would be greatly increased, the liberty of all others would be restricted. However, in the present context, the (temporary) restriction of liberty is justified on public health grounds. While a broader perspective would require the justification of both immunity licences *and* confinement, we are asking a narrower question here: can licences be justified *given* the assumed justification of temporary confinement

6. Françoise Baylis & Natalie Kofler, "Covid-19 Immunity Testing: A Passport to Inequity" (29 April 2020), online: *Center for Genetics and Society* <www.who.int/news-room/commentaries/detail/immunity-passports-in-the-context-of-covid-19>.

measures?[7] From this more limited point of view (though not from the other), licences represent a gain in the space of liberty.

Clearly, however, the adoption of immunity licences would create two categories of citizens with respect to the practices to which they would allow access. Holders of such licences would possess a range of opportunities that would be restricted for others, potentially across a wide range of domains. Would this inequality be ethically unjustified? Would it be an inequity? There are powerful arguments to the effect that it would not be.

First, the objection to the effect that if *everyone* cannot be released from confinement, then *no one* should, is subject to the "levelling down" objection.[8] In other words, immunity licences would make some people better off, without making anyone worse off. They are therefore Pareto-superior to the *status quo* of continued confinement. To object to such a Pareto improvement is, according to this objection, to fetishize equality as a formal rather than a substantive value and to forget that the moral point of egalitarianism is, after all, to make people better off than they would otherwise be.[9]

Second, the inequality that would be created by the deployment of immunity licences does not seem to be grounded in any kind of invidious comparisons among persons or categories of persons. There are objective grounds for everyone to prefer that immunity licence-holders go back to work. The possession of relevant antibodies is not the same as reference to gender, race, religion, sexual orientation, and the like in objectionably discriminatory social policies. As noted by Persad and Emanuel, they are similar to the age limitations on driver's licences: a way of protecting individuals and society as a whole from persons who do not possess relevant characteristics. In the context of a pandemic, not putting others at risk of infection counts as a relevant characteristic.

The (Qualified) Normative Case Against Immunity Licences

This pair of arguments would seem to dispose of the claim that immunity licences ought to be rejected due to their inegalitarian implications.

7. For the broader perspective, see for example Lawrence O. Gostin, Eric A Friedman & Sarah A Wetter, "How to Navigate a Public Health Emergency Legally and Ethically" (26 March 2020), online: *Hastings Center Report* DOI: <doi.org/10.1002/hast.1090>.
8. Persad & Emanuel, *supra* note 3.
9. Harry Frankfurt, "Equality as a Moral Ideal", (1987) 98:1 Ethics 21.

In our view, this is a too hasty conclusion. The claim we want to explore in the final section of this chapter is that the defence of immunity licences against the equality argument holds only if no other policy tools can achieve these goals while being less costly with respect to the value of equality. Going back to our interpretation of the principle of "least infringement," immunity licences would be ethically acceptable only if they did in fact pose the least threat to equality, compared with other policy tools that have the ability to achieve similar safety objectives.

Are immunity licences "least infringing" with respect to the value of equality? The primacy afforded the value of equality—both in the general ethics of a liberal democracy and in its constitutional order—means that before we opt for a measure that is offensive to that value, we should look for measures that do not offend against it, or that do so in a more minimal way. There should be a presumption in favour of equality-promoting or at the very least inequality-minimizing measures. Clearly, the goal of policy measures in the post-confinement, pre-vaccine, or pre-herd immunity phase of the pandemic is to control the spread of the virus, and the level of restriction that is required to achieve this goal may vary as new evidence comes in.[10] As we emerge from confinement, we should choose the most egalitarian policies available, taking into account that confinement is, in and of itself, an inegalitarian policy that trades on a resource that is massively unequally distributed—namely, the quality of the spaces in which people confine. Emerging from this situation should not exacerbate inequity if alternatives exist.

Are there ways to achieve safety goals that are less offensive to the value of equality? We think there are. Governments can reduce the potential spread of the virus, not by limiting individuals but rather through a community approach that redesigns the context of our interactions to make them (safely) equally accessible to all. Such an approach would for example favour the efficient use of space and time through creative and thoughtful redesign. For example, the expansion of shared spaces and the time they are available, physical distancing, and the wearing of face coverings within these spaces are among the tools that we can use to emerge from confinement together—united in a shared predicament and a shared fate—rather than conferring privileges on those who can prove immunity.[11]

---

10. Colleen M Flood & Bryan Thomas, this volume, Chapter A-6.
11. Daniel Weinstock, "A Harm Reduction Approach to Physical Distancing", in Meredith Schwartz, ed, *The Ethics of Pandemics* (Peterborough: Broadview Press, 2020) [forthcoming in August 2020].

There are intimations of this approach around the world even in this early phase of deconfinement. For example, municipal authorities in Vilnius, Lithuania, have allowed bars and restaurants to spill out into urban spaces like parks and squares so residents can dine while distancing, in an outdoor context less likely to facilitate the spread of the virus.[12] The mayor of Montréal recently announced an ambitious plan to deliver 1,200 kilometres of roads to pedestrians and cyclists to make it easier for them to physically distance. We believe that making both our indoor and our outdoor spaces as compatible as possible with the imperative of limiting virus spread should be a policy avenue of choice for egalitarians. Such avenues target community-based rather than individual-based solutions and thus represent a lesser infringement on the value of equality than do immunity licences in a post-confinement society.

Naturally, certain settings do not lend themselves to such inequality-mitigating measures. Obvious examples are health care settings, where providers must come into close contact with possibly infected patients, and hairdressing salons. A selective use of immunity licences for those who work in such sectors would be ethically appropriate, because in this case the presumption in favour of equality would be defeated by the unavailability of equality-preserving measures.

Conclusion

Even if science were to advance to a point where immunity licences might be viewed as reliable indicators of immunity, and even if we were able to put a regulatory framework in place that would avoid morally problematic results, there would still be reasons to oppose them in most settings. Specifically, they violate the "least infringement" principle relative to the value of equality.

It is perilous to attempt to "translate" the kind of ethical analysis we have conducted here into Canadian constitutional terms. It is unclear whether legislation imposing the use of immunity licences would pass *Charter* scrutiny. If the Supreme Court of Canada is convinced that distinguishing on the basis of immunity status is analogous to other permissible exclusionary criteria, such as age limits on driver's licences, and not to invidious discrimination, such as that

12. Stacey Lastoe, "Lithuanian City Flirts with Becoming One Large Outdoor Café", *CNN* (28 April 2020), online: <www.cnn.com/travel/article/outdoor-dining-vilnius-lithuania-pandemic/index.html>.

based on race, religion, or sexual orientation, then it might be difficult to establish that immunity licences constitute an infringement of Canadians' constitutionally guaranteed rights. Ethical and legal analysis would then point in different directions.

It would still be possible to propose that discriminating between immune and non-immune persons is analogous to the constitutionally prohibited grounds of disability, which would constitute an infringement of section 15.[13] In this case, the question would become that of determining whether the infringement could be saved by the various tests that make up the *Oakes Test*, in particular the proportionality test that it includes. Our analysis suggests that it could not, since, in effect, we have shown that in the pursuit of public health goals, the policy goes further in the limitation of equality than is necessary.

13. *Canadian Charter of Rights and Freedoms*, s 15(1), Part 1 of the *Constitution Act, 1982*, being Schedule B to the *Canada Act 1982* (UK), 1982, c 11.

CHAPTER C-4

The Punitive Impact of Physical Distancing Laws on Homeless People*

Terry Skolnik**

Abstract

One of the hallmarks of COVID-19 is that it disproportionately impacts vulnerable individuals and groups. The State's punitive legal responses to the pandemic are no different. This chapter shows why coercive physical distancing laws disparately impact homeless people. It argues that harsh financial penalties for violating these laws can constitute cruel and unusual punishments that contravene s. 12 of the *Canadian Charter of Rights and Freedoms*. It challenges prevailing s. 12 *Charter* jurisprudence and demonstrates why expensive fines amount to cruel and unusual punishments even when judges have discretion to modify their severity. After situating the regulation of homelessness within its historical context, it concludes by setting out why homeless people are uniquely vulnerable to over-policing. Ultimately, this chapter elucidates why a public health approach to both COVID-19 and homelessness are necessary and why neither can be punished out of existence.

* I thank Anna Maria Konewka, Michelle Biddulph, Nayla El Zir, Mary Roberts, Vanessa MacDonnell, and the anonymous reviewers for comments on prior drafts. All mistakes are my own.

** Assistant Professor, University of Ottawa, Faculty of Law, Civil Law Section.

Résumé
L'impact punitif des mesures de distanciation physique sur les sans-abri

L'une des caractéristiques de la COVID-19 est qu'elle a un impact disproportionné sur les individus et les groupes vulnérables. Les interventions juridiques punitives de l'État en réaction à la pandémie ne sont pas différentes. Ce chapitre illustre les raisons pour lesquelles les mesures de distanciation physique coercitives ont des effets différents sur les sans-abri. Il avance que des sanctions pécuniaires sévères en cas de violation de ces règles peuvent représenter des peines cruelles et inusitées qui contreviennent à l'article 12 de la *Charte canadienne des droits et libertés*. Ce chapitre remet en cause la jurisprudence relative à l'article 12 de la *Charte* et démontre pourquoi des amendes coûteuses constituent des peines cruelles et inusitées, même lorsque les juges ont le pouvoir discrétionnaire d'en modifier la sévérité. Après avoir replacé la réglementation applicable aux sans-abri dans son contexte historique, il conclut en exposant les raisons pour lesquelles les personnes sans domicile sont particulièrement vulnérables en cas de surveillance policière accrue. Enfin, ce chapitre explique pourquoi il est nécessaire d'adopter une approche de santé publique pour la COVID-19 et l'itinérance avec des sanctions.

Homeless people face unique personal, systemic, and legal disadvantages. They have higher mortality rates compared to the general population.[1] Many homeless people also endure important physical and mental health challenges, which the pandemic has exacerbated significantly.[2] In addition to these difficulties, the condition of homelessness is also highly stigmatized.[3]

Many legal responses to homelessness have only worsened the lives of homeless people. For centuries, the law regulated the condition of homelessness through vagrancy statutes that punished

1. James Frankish, Stephen Hwang & Darryl Quantz, "Homelessness and Health in Canada" (2005) 96:2 Can J Public Health 523 at 524-26.
2. *Ibid;* Jack Tsai & Michal Wilson, "COVID-19: A Potential Public Health Problem for Homeless Populations" (2020) 5:4 Lancet Public Health at e186.
3. Jo Phelan et al, "The Stigma of Homelessness: The Impact of the Label 'Homeless' on Attitudes Toward Poor Persons" (1997) 60:4 Soc Psychology Quarterly 323 at 324-26, 332.

acts such as sleeping on public property, wandering without giving an adequate account of one's conduct, and not having a visible means of employment. Within the past several decades, the rise of quality-of-life offences—ordinances that regulate low-level incivilities to promote residents' quality-of-life—has led to an explosion in the number of fines that are issued to homeless people in many Canadian cities.[4]

There have been few positive legal developments for homeless people in the courts. Some judges have struck down municipal by-laws that prohibited homeless people from erecting temporary shelters on public property when there were insufficient shelter spaces available to them.[5] Courts have ruled that certain mandatory financial penalties constitute cruel and unusual punishments in violation of s 12 of the *Canadian Charter of Rights and Freedoms*.[6] Yet outside of these contexts, the state continues to have significant power to regulate homeless people's most rudimentary acts and further entrench them in homelessness.[7]

The *Charter* has failed to bring about changes that would require the state to alleviate homelessness and address its root causes.[8] Courts have rejected poverty and homelessness as analogous grounds of discrimination, such that groups experiencing these conditions lack constitutionally protected status under s 15 of the *Charter*.[9] Courts have also concluded that there is no constitutional right to housing encompassed within s 7.[10] Since judges interpret the scope of homeless people's rights restrictively and recognize that the state's power to regulate homelessness is broad, homeless people continue to be subject to unique legal and social vulnerabilities.

In this chapter, I show why punitive legal responses to the COVID-19 pandemic will exacerbate these vulnerabilities. I argue that

---

4. See for example Céline Bellot & Marie-Ève Sylvestre, "La judiciarisation de l'itinérance à Montréal : les dérives sécuritaires de la gestion pénale de la pauvreté" (2017) 47 RGD 11 at 19-22.
5. *Victoria (City) v Adams*, 2009 BCCA 563; *Abbotsford (City) v Shantz*, 2015 BCSC 1909 [*Shantz*].
6. *R v Boudreault*, 2018 SCC 58 [*Boudreault*].
7. Terry Skolnik, "Rethinking Homeless People's Punishments" (2019) 22:1 New Crim L Rev 73 at 81-84.
8. Marie-Ève Sylvestre, "The Redistributive Potential of Section 7 of the *Canadian Charter*: Incorporating Socio-economic Context in Criminal Law and in the Adjudication of Rights" (2012) 42:3 Ottawa L Rev 389 at 401-08.
9. *Tanudjaja v Canada (Attorney General)*, 2013 ONSC 5410 at paras 122-37 [*Tanudjaja*]; *Shantz*, *supra* note 5 at para 231.
10. *Tanudjaja*, *supra* note 9.

laws governing physical distancing will disproportionately impact homeless people and shows why these laws raise serious constitutional concerns. Building on existing case law, I demonstrate why financial penalties for breaching physical distancing laws can constitute a cruel and unusual punishment for indigent and homeless persons. I then situate the regulation of homelessness within its historical context, explaining how laws that govern homeless people emerged following the Black Plague—a pandemic that occurred in the 1300s. After discussing how the notion of public health continues to play a role in justifying laws that regulate homeless people, I conclude by setting out why people experiencing homelessness are particularly vulnerable to coercion from laws that are enforced to prevent the transmission of COVID-19.

Punitive Responses to COVID-19: An Overview

The COVID-19 pandemic has led to unprecedented governmental responses that aim to curb its spread. State-sanctioned coercion and punishment are playing a fundamental role in ensuring that individuals obey physical distancing guidelines to prevent COVID-19 infections, complications, and deaths.

Alexander McClelland and Alex Luscombe explain that in response to COVID-19, governments and the police enforce three types of punitive laws: the *Criminal Code*, provincial health laws, and municipal ordinances.[11] First, with respect to the *Criminal Code*, defendants charged with COVID-19-related crimes are often accused of assault for coughing on others, especially police officers.[12] Second, many individuals are issued harsh fines for violating public health legislation that mandates physical distancing—financial penalties that can cost upwards of roughly $1,500 in Quebec and a minimum fine of $750 in Ontario. Third, some municipalities, such as Brampton, Ontario, have adopted their own municipal by-laws that result in a minimum fine of $500 and a maximum fine of $100,000: twice the maximum fine that

11. Alex Luscombe & Alexander McClelland, "Enforcement Report April 14 2020-May 1 2020" (2020) at 1-6, online (pdf): *Policing the Pandemic* <static1.squarespace.com/static/5e8396f40824381145ff603a/t/5eae43d69d70876a67c26421/1588478934909/Police_the_Pandemic_Report_1May2020.pdf>.

12. *Ibid* at 4-5. See also Alex Luscombe & Alexander McClelland, "Searchable Database" (2020), online: *Policing the Pandemic* <policingthepandemic.github.io/table/>.

is imposed for careless driving causing bodily harm or death under Ontario's *Highway Traffic Act.*[13]

Homeless people have received harsh fines for violating public health acts or municipal by-laws. *The Hamilton Spectator* reported that the city's police force issued $750 fines to a group of 10 homeless people who were allegedly passing around a bottle of alcohol.[14] In the City of Montréal, a group of homeless youth were ticketed $1,546 each for failing to obey physical distancing measures.[15]

Prior to the pandemic, empirical research showed that the vast majority of municipal and transportation by-law offences in Montréal were issued to homeless people, even though they made up less than 1% of the city's population.[16] Most could not afford to pay their fines, which in many cases tallied thousands of dollars and hung over their heads for years. These financial penalties entrench people in homelessness in several ways. They must pay money that would otherwise go toward their rent or basic necessities, such as food, clothing, and medication. Criminal justice debt adversely impacts one's credit rating, which decreases one's prospect of securing housing, obtaining utilities, and receiving bank loans.[17] As Canada approaches an inevitable recession and an increase in unemployment, these financial penalties will impact homeless people more than ever.

These fines raise serious legal concerns. In *R v Boudreault,* the Supreme Court of Canada decided that mandatory victim surcharges constitute a cruel and unusual punishment because they result in *de facto* indeterminate sentences for indigent persons.[18] The amount of the surcharge was $100 for summary conviction offences and $200

13. City of Brampton, by-law MO 1-2020, *Physical Distancing By-law MO* (2020), s 12(2); *Highway Traffic Act*, RSO 1990, c H.8, ss 130(3)–(4).
14. Teviah Moro, "COVID-19: 'Physical Distancing' Fines of $750 Issued to Homeless People by Hamilton Police", *Hamilton Spectator* (6 April 2020), online: <www.thespec.com/news/hamilton-region/2020/04/06/covid-19-hamilton-police-urged-to-not-ticket-homeless-during-pandemic.html>.
15. Ugo Giguère, "Des contraventions données aux jeunes sans-abris", *La Presse* (11 April 2020), online: <https://www.lapresse.ca/covid-19/2020-04-11/des-contraventions-donnees-aux-jeunes-sans-abris>.
16. Commission des droits de la personne et des droits de la jeunesse, *The Judiciarization of the Homeless in Montréal: A Case of Social Profiling. Executive Summary of the Opinion of the Commission,* cat 2.120-8.61.2 (Montréal: CDPDJ, 6 November 2009) at 2.
17. Catherine T Chesnay, Celine Bellot & Marie-Eve Sylvestre, "Taming Disorderly People One Ticket at a Time: The Penalization of Homelessness in Ontario and British Columbia" (2013) 55:2 Can J Corr 161 at 178-79.
18. *Boudreault, supra* note 6 at para 76.

for indictable offences. The Supreme Court of Canada observed that many homeless defendants cannot afford to pay these fines, which can result in additional fees, unsurmountable civil debts, and imprisonment for default.[19]

Many of these same considerations apply to fines that are issued to homeless people for violating physical distancing guidelines. First, the quantum of COVID-19-related fines (roughly $1,500 in Quebec) is substantially higher than the mandatory victim surcharge (between $100 and $200), which exemplifies the grossly disproportionate nature of these fines for homeless people. Second, individual and systemic barriers make it more difficult for homeless people to successfully challenge these financial penalties even where judges retain discretion to modify them.[20] As the Supreme Court of Canada observed in *Boudreault,* many homeless people have mental health problems, addiction issues, and other circumstances that make it more difficult to attend court and navigate their way through the justice system.[21] This is further complicated by the fact that most courts are currently closed and will have to clear months of backlogs attributable to the pandemic, which will further limit access to justice. Third, the realities of homelessness complicate evidentiary issues. For instance, in Ontario, accused persons can be convicted of provincial offences without a hearing. If an individual wishes to challenge such convictions, they must swear an affidavit that explains that they did not receive a delivery notice or describes why they could not attend a prior court date.[22] This additional burden complicates the process for self-represented litigants and may hinder a successful defence.[23]

One might argue that harsh financial penalties do not constitute cruel and unusual punishments, because judges retain some discretion to modify the quantum of fines in certain circumstances. The Supreme Court of Canada suggested in *R v Lloyd* and in *R v Boudreault* that the presence of discretion might prevent an otherwise mandatory punishment from being found to be cruel and unusual.[24] Yet financial

19. *Ibid* at paras 69-73.
20. Terry Skolnik, "Beyond *Boudreault*: Challenging Choice, Culpability, and Punishment" (2019) 50 Crim R (7th) 283 at 289-91.
21. *Boudreault, supra* note 6 at para 70.
22. *Provincial Offences Act,* RSO 1990, c P.33, s 11(1).
23. Deborah Doherty, "Promoting Access to Family Justice by Educating the Self-Representing Litigant" (2012) 63 UNBLJ 85 at 86.
24. *R v* Lloyd, 2016 SCC 13 at para 36; *Boudreault, supra* note 6 at para 97.

penalties can still be cruel and unusual even where judges have discretion to modify them.

If judicial discretion were sufficient to ensure that financial penalties respect s 12 of the *Charter*, it would lead to the absurd consequence that a $100,000 fine imposed on a homeless person is not a cruel and unusual punishment, even where personal and systemic circumstances prevent them from accessing the justice system to challenge the fine. Homeless people experience serious stress and anxiety from these fines, and there is no guarantee that judges will exercise their discretion in homeless people's favour. Furthermore, as the Supreme Court of Canada noted in *Boudreault*, homeless people are subject to threats of imprisonment for their criminal justice debts.[25] Unpaid fines also carry significant collateral consequences, such as a destroyed credit rating, which entrenches them in poverty.

For these reasons, notwithstanding judicial discretion, harsh financial penalties may constitute cruel and unusual punishments for society's most economically disadvantaged members of society who lack access to justice. Homeless people already face significant stigma, social exclusion, and marginalization—realities that the pandemic has worsened considerably.

Situating Punitive Responses to COVID in Their Historical Context

The historical context surrounding the criminalization of homelessness shows why homeless people risk being over-policed and disproportionately punished during the pandemic. Historically, homeless people were regulated by vagrancy laws that originated in England after the Black Plague.[26] The pandemic arrived as feudalism was breaking down and workers were gaining greater economic autonomy.[27] The Black Plague killed a significant portion of the country's working population. The resulting labour shortages allowed workers

25. *Boudreault*, *supra* note 6 at paras 69-73.
26. For a historical overview of vagrancy statutes and their connection to quality-of-life laws, see Marie-Eve Sylvestre & Céline Bellot, "Challenging Discriminatory and Punitive Responses to Homelessness in Canada" in Martha Jackman & Bruce Porter, eds, *Advancing Social Rights in Canada* (Toronto: Irwin Law, 2014) at 162-67.
27. Bertha Haven Putnam, *The Enforcement of the Statutes Labourers During the First Decade after the Black Death, 1349-1359* (New York: Columbia University, 1908) at 1-5.

to demand higher than normal wages.[28] King Edward III responded by passing the *Statute of Labourers 1351*, a largely economic measure that fixed wages and limited the ability of people to travel and seek higher pay.[29]

During the centuries that followed, laws that criminalized vagrancy were enforced against homeless people, the indigent, and other marginalized groups as a means of social control. The hallmarks of vagrancy statutes were that they were vague, accorded sweeping police discretion, and were disproportionately enforced against vulnerable individuals and groups.[30] Although vagrancy laws emerged following a public health crisis, public health justifications for regulating homeless people persisted after the Black Plague resolved. Even centuries later, many construed homelessness as a form of social malady and drew connections between homelessness, disease, and filth—depictions that underpinned law enforcement policies and were employed to justify homeless people's exclusion from public spaces.[31]

If vagrancy statutes seem like some irrelevant relic of the past, they are not. One of the most important U.S. constitutional decisions that governs procedural due process arose from a successful constitutional challenge to a vagrancy statute—a decision that served to subsequently invalidate loitering laws that were enforced against minority communities.[32] In England and Wales, the *Vagrancy Act* still prohibits sleeping on public property and panhandling.[33] Canada's *Criminal Code* prohibited the crime of vagrancy until 2019. Once vagrancy laws were struck down as unconstitutional in the U.S. as being void for vagueness and in Canada for overbreadth, cities responded by drafting more narrowly tailored and precise quality-of-life laws, which the police still enforce.[34] Today, quality-of-life offences continue to

28. *Ibid.*
29. *Ibid.*
30. Deborah Livingston, "Police Discretion and the Quality of Life in Public Places: Courts, Communities, and the New Policing" (1997) 97:3 Colum L Rev 551 at 584-85.
31. See for example Sir George Nicolls, Thomas Mackay & HG Wilink, *A History of the English Poor Law in Connection with the State of the Country and the Condition of the People* (London: King & Son, 1904) at 22, 248, 377; Ronald Amster, "Patterns of Exclusion: Sanitizing Space, Criminalizing Homelessness" (2003) 30:1 Social Justice 195 at 198.
32. *Papachristou v Jacksonville*, 405 US 156 (1972). See also: *Chicago v Morales*, (1999) 527 US 41 at 53-54; *Kolender* v Lawson, (1983) 461 US 352 at 357-58.
33. *The Vagrancy Act* 1824 (UK), 5 Geo IV, c 83, ss 3-4.
34. Rita Goluboff, "Dispatch from the Supreme Court Archives: Vagrancy, Abortion,

prohibit homeless people's most rudimentary human acts: sheltering themselves, sleeping in public parks or in subway stations, and public urination.

Before COVID-19 became a new reality, cities were already selectively enforcing these ordinances against homeless people. The pandemic has significantly altered the climate in which the state deploys criminal laws and regulatory offences. Emergency contexts characteristically result in two consequences: individuals experience greater fear and the state restricts civil liberties.[35] These consequences are aggravated when the scope of a crisis is unclear and crucial information is unavailable.[36] As discussed below, this partly explains why homeless people's rights may increasingly shrink as fears about their role in perpetuating COVID-19 grow. Indeed, law enforcement practises show that the police perceive that some homeless people constitute a public health risk that can be coerced and punished out of the public sphere. In this sense, vagrancy laws' historical underpinnings and justifications are at work here too. Although the state continues to direct everyone to stay at home, it continues to impose harsh fines that will prevent homeless people from securing access to housing.

Problems and Pitfalls of Enforcing Physical Distancing Guidelines

There are many reasons why punitive responses to COVID-19 impact homeless people in unique ways. First, since homeless people lack real private property rights, they are vulnerable to various forms of police coercion to which individuals with access to housing are not. Homeless people must spend a significant portion of their time in public spaces—the very places where quality-of-life offences and COVID-19-related laws apply and where police officers spend their time patrolling. Because homeless people lack real private property rights, they do not have legal protections against state power that a home affords. The police can easily surveil, coerce, and punish homeless people for violating physical distancing laws that characteristically apply on public property because homeless people generally

and What the Links between Them Reveal About the History of Fundamental Rights" (2010) 62:5 Stan L Rev 1361 at 1374.

35. See for example Eric Posner & Adrian Vermeule, "Accommodating Emergencies" (2003) 56:3 Stan L Rev 605.

36. Colleen M Flood, Bryan Thomas & Kumanan Wilson, this volume, Chapter C-1.

have no refuge from these laws. This makes it extremely difficult—if not impossible—for homeless people to comply with certain laws that govern public property.[37]

The second reason why COVID-19-related laws disproportionately affect homeless people is rooted in the fact that police officers enjoy particularly broad discretion when enforcing these laws. Before the pandemic, homeless people were issued significant fines for conduct such as sleeping on a picnic table and sitting on the edge of a water fountain. These financial penalties were imposed for the ambiguous offence of "us[ing] street furniture for a purpose other than the one for which it is intended" (whatever that means).[38] COVID-19 laws generate similar concerns about the scope of police officers' discretion. In response to the pandemic, the Government of Quebec issued an Order in Council that prohibits "outdoor assemblies," even though the decree does not define that term, leaving individual officers to determine its meaning.[39] Police have also encouraged individuals to denounce others who disobey physical distancing guidelines.[40] This creates an added risk of discriminatory enforcement, especially given how subconscious biases and prejudice can influence both individuals' decisions to denounce others and officers' discretion to enforce fines. Furthermore, it adds to the harassment that many homeless people already experience.[41]

Finally, the cumulative effect of quality-of-life offences and COVID-19-related laws place many homeless people in the untenable position of having to sleep in a shelter and expose themselves to the virus, or risk receiving a fine for occupying public space. It is important to note that even prior to the pandemic, many homeless shelters had unsanitary conditions. There are many documented cases of tuberculosis and other communicable disease outbreaks in shelters

37. Terry Skolnik, "Homelessness and the Impossibility to Obey the Law" (2016) 43:3 Fordham Urb LJ 741 at 750-76.
38. *Ibid* at 771; City of Montréal, by-law 99-102, *By-Law Concerning Cleanliness and Protection of Public Property and Street Furniture* (17 May 1999), s 20; Sylvestre & Bellot, *supra* note 26 at 173.
39. OIC 222-2020, (2020) GOQ II, 771A (*concerning renewal of the public health emergency under section 119 of* Public Health Act *and certain measures to protect the health of the population*).
40. Luscombe & McClelland, *supra* note 11 at 4.
41. See for example Bill O'Grady, Stephen Gaetz & Kristy Buccieri, "Can I See Your ID? The Policing of Youth Homelessness in Toronto" (2011) at 11, online (pdf): *Homelessness Hub* <www.homelesshub.ca/sites/default/files/attachments/CanISeeYourID_nov9.pdf>.

because they are confined spaces with poor air circulation.[42] The sanitation risks in homeless shelters have only increased since the pandemic and have materialized in many cases. There have been major COVID-19 outbreaks in homeless shelters in Toronto—the only available alternative to sleeping in public for many individuals without access to housing.[43] Homeless people therefore face the particularly unpalatable choice of endangering their well-being in shelters or risking financial penalties for violating COVID-19-related laws.

Conclusion

Hegel once suggested that history teaches us that we learn nothing from history.[44] Canada's legal responses to homelessness during COVID-19 are part of a larger historical story about how coercion and punishment cannot resolve society's most persistent social problems. Canadian cities are increasingly confronted with the choice between employing a predominantly public health response to homelessness during the pandemic or resorting to the criminal law and public welfare offences. The pandemic is making homeless people's lives immeasurably more difficult and is exposing them to additional health risks. All levels of government thus should choose to avoid coercive legal responses to homelessness that entrench individuals in that condition. More than ever, the state should use the law as a tool to lift individuals out of extreme poverty and homelessness, improve access to affordable housing, and affirm homeless people's dignity. Ultimately, the state's legal responses to homelessness both during and after COVID-19 should be rooted in an enduring truism. Similar to how we cannot police our way out of a pandemic, we cannot punish our way out of homelessness.[45] History shows this to be true.

---

42. See for example Kamran Khan et al, "Active Tuberculosis among Homeless Persons, Toronto, Ontario, Canada, 1998-2007" (2011) 17:3 Emerging Infectious Diseases 357.
43. The Canadian Press, "COVID-19 Spreads in Homeless Shelter, WHO Seeks Funds", *National Post* (25 April 2020), online: <nationalpost.com/pmn/news-pmn/canada-news-pmn/covid-19-spreads-in-homeless-shelter-who-seeks-funds-in-the-news-for-april-25>.
44. Georg Wilhelm Friedrich Hegel, *The Philosophy of History* (New York: Colonial Press, 1900) at 6.
45. Alexander McClelland "We Cannot Police Our Way Out of a Pandemic", *NOW* (30 March 2020), online: <nowtoronto.com/news/coronavirus-we-cant-police-our-way-out-of-pandemic/>.

CHAPTER C-5

The Right of Citizens Abroad to Return During a Pandemic*

Yves Le Bouthillier** and Delphine Nakache***

Abstract

To prevent the spread of COVID-19 Canada has, like most other states, temporarily limited access to its territory. It has, as requested by international law, allowed the return of its own citizens. However, in contrast to other countries, Canada has opted for a more restrictive approach by requesting air carriers to deny boarding to any passengers abroad, citizen or not, with symptoms suggestive of COVID-19. In this article, we assess the legality of Canada's approach regarding the return of citizens, both under international human rights law and Canadian constitutional law.

Résumé

Le droit de retour des citoyens durant une pandémie

Pour empêcher la propagation de la COVID-19, le Canada, comme la plupart des autres pays, a temporairement limité l'accès à son territoire. Il a toutefois, comme le prescrit le droit international, autorisé

* The second part of this article draws on: Yves Le Bouthillier & Delphine Nakache, "Is it Constitutional to Screen Canadians Trying to Board Flights Home?", *Policy Options* (7 April 2020), online: <policyoptions.irpp.org/magazines/april-2020/is-it-constitutional-to-screen-canadians-trying-to-board-flights-home>.

** Full Professor, Faculty of Law, University of Ottawa.

*** Associate Professor, Faculty of Law, University of Ottawa.

le retour de ses propres citoyens. Cependant, contrairement à d'autres pays, le Canada a opté pour une approche plus restrictive en demandant aux transporteurs aériens de refuser l'embarquement de tout passager à l'étranger, citoyen canadien ou non, présentant des symptômes apparentés à la COVID-19. Dans cet article, nous analysons la légalité de l'approche du Canada concernant le retour de ses citoyens au pays, tant au regard du droit international des droits de la personne qu'en vertu du droit constitutionnel canadien.

To prevent the spread of COVID-19, states around the world have temporarily limited access to their territory. While some, such as Morocco,[1] decided to ban entry to everyone—including their own citizens who are stranded abroad—most allowed their own citizens to return, often through repatriation efforts. In doing so, these states acted in a manner consistent with a citizen's right in international law to return to their country, as explained in the first part of this chapter. Once on national soil, citizens were assessed to determine if they would need to self-isolate or be directed to a quarantine facility. However, in contrast to other countries such as Australia and New Zealand, Canada opted for control both on foreign soil and on arrival. It requested that air carriers deny boarding to any passengers abroad, citizen or not, with symptoms suggestive of COVID-19. In choosing this more restrictive approach, Canada was an outlier. Whether this approach was consistent with both Canada's international obligations and the constitutionally protected right for citizens to return to Canada is the focus of the second part of this chapter.

The "Right to Return" in International Law

In international law, "freedom of movement" is a generic term covering movements of individuals within a state as well as from one state

1. On March 13, 2020, Morocco suspended all international passenger flights to and from its territory and announced its intention to not repatriate the estimated 18,000 Moroccans stranded abroad. It committed, instead, to providing, through its consular officers, basic assistance for accommodation, food, and medicines. See Samir Bennis, "Morocco Should Move to Repatriate Moroccans Stranded Overseas", *Morocco World News* (19 April 2020), online: <www.moroccoworldnews.com/2020/04/300036/morocco-should-move-to-repatriate-moroccans-stranded-overseas>.

to another. While the former embraces the right of persons to move freely and to choose a place of residence within the territory of a state (the internal aspect of freedom of movement), the latter covers the right to leave any country (including one's own), either temporarily or permanently, and to enter or return to one's own country (the external aspect of freedom of movement). The rights to leave and return are closely connected "in that the existence of one allows for the effective exercise of the other,"[2] but they respond to different needs.[3] The person leaving a country may be doing so out of a desire to travel, emigrate, or seek refuge; whereas the person seeking to return to their country is usually motivated by a desire to return "home," to the "place where he or she belongs, to his or her roots."[4]

The right to enter or return to one's own country is embodied in numerous international and regional human rights instruments, including Article 12(4) of the International Covenant on Civil and Political Rights (ICCPR) ("no one shall be arbitrarily deprived of the right to enter his own country").[5] With the exception of Article 12(4) of the ICCPR, all other instruments envisage no particular restriction to its application. Moreover, while Article 12(3) of the ICCPR contemplates permissible limitations to a citizen's right to move or leave their state (when such limitations are "necessary to protect national security, public order, public health or morals or the rights and freedoms of others"), no such limitations apply to the right to return in Article 12(4). The only limitation to the right to return found in Article 12(4) is in relation to the term "arbitrarily." In 1999, the UN Human Rights Committee (UNHRC), a body of experts that monitors the implementation of the Covenant, interpreted this term very restrictively, stating "there are few, if any, circumstances in which deprivation of the right to enter one's own country could be reasonable."[6] Therefore, in

2. Sander Agterhuis, "The Right to Return and its Practical Application" (2005) 58:1 RHDI 165 at 168.
3. It is also worth highlighting that the "right to return" was originally considered as a means for strengthening the "right to leave," rather than as an independent right in and of itself. See *Report of the Third Committee*, UNGAOR, 3rd Sess, UN Doc A/777 (1948).
4. Agterhuis, *supra* note 2 at 168.
5. For more on these instruments, see François Crépeau & Delphine Nakache, "The Right to Leave and Return" in Rhona K M Smith & Christien van den Anker, eds, *Essentials of Human Rights* (London: Hodder Arnold, 2005), 222-24.
6. International Covenant on Civil and Political Rights, *General Comment 27, Freedom of movement (Art 12)*, UNHRCOR, 1999, 67th Sess, UN Doc CCPR/C/21/Rev 1/Add 9 (1999), at para 19.

international law, it appears that it would be only in exceptional circumstances, none of which have been identified by the committee, that the right to return could possibly be legally limited in ordinary times.[7]

One legally possible justification for states to obstruct the exercise of the right to return is through the derogation clause found at Article 4(1) of the ICCPR. This article permits states parties to derogate temporarily from some of their ICCPR obligations in times of public emergency. It reads as follows:

> In time of public emergency which threatens the life of the nation and the existence of which is officially proclaimed, the States Parties to the present Covenant may take measures derogating from their obligations under the present Covenant to the extent strictly required by the exigencies of the situation, provided that such measures are not inconsistent with their other obligations under international law and do not involve discrimination solely on the ground of race, colour, sex, language, religion or social origin.[8]

As Sarah Joseph notes, this provision is not a "blank cheque."[9] Derogations measures are only permitted in extreme circumstances and must be proportionate and consistent with other international human rights obligations. Furthermore, there are rights (listed in Article 4(2)) from which a state may never derogate.[10] Finally, the state

7. The Travaux Préparatoires to the ICCPR reveal that the only limitation on this right, expressed with the word "arbitrarily," was intended to apply exclusively to cases of lawful exile as punishment for a crime, whether accompanied by a revocation of citizenship or not. However, in its concluding observations on the Dominican Republic, the UNHRC stated in 1993 that "punishment by exile is not compatible with the Covenant." See Sara Joseph & Melissa Castan, *The International Covenant on Civil and Political Rights*, 3rd ed (Oxford: Oxford University Press, 2013). See also: Marc J Bossuyt, *Guide to the 'Travaux Préparatoires' of the International Covenant on Civil and Political Rights* (Dordrecht: Martinus Nijhoff Publishers, 1987), at 260-63; Manfred Nowak, *UN Covenant on Civil and Political Rights: CCPR Commentary* (Kehl & Rhein, Germany: NP Engel, 1993) at 219.
8. *International Covenant on Civil and Political Rights*, GA Res 2200A (XXI), 21 UNGAOR, Supp No 16, UN Doc A/6316 (1966) at 52.
9. Sarah Joseph, "A Timeline of COVID 19 and Human Rights: Derogations in Time of Public Emergency", *Griffith News* (5 May 2020), online: <news.griffith.edu.au/2020/05/05/a-timeline-of-covid-19-and-human-rights-derogations-in-time-of-public-emergency>.
10. These are the right to life, the prohibition of torture and other cruel, inhuman, or degrading treatment or punishment, the prohibition of slavery and servitude,

has important procedural obligations with regard to derogations. First, it must "officially proclaim" the state of emergency (Article 4(1)), using its own domestic mechanisms for doing so. Second, it must immediately notify the UN of any derogation (Article 4(3)).

Recently, the UNHRC and the UN Office of the High Commissioner for Human Rights clarified the specific requirements that states must meet when derogating from human rights with respect to COVID-19.[11] Recognizing that the pandemic may satisfy the description of a "public emergency," they highlighted that derogation measures must be "strictly required by the exigencies of the public health situation" and "limited…in respect of their duration, geographical coverage and…scope."[12] As well, states' derogation legislation and measures must be the "least intrusive option among those to achieve the stated public health goals" and provide "safeguards" that guarantee the return to normal laws "as soon as the emergency situation is over."[13] Finally, the UNHRC noted that a derogation is not necessary when states parties "can attain their public health objectives" by limiting a right "in conformity with the provisions for such restrictions set out in the Covenant."[14] In other words, when limitations on human rights are permissible, states should not resort to derogation to protect their public health.

Limitations on international human rights are permissible in "ordinary times," provided they are proportionate measures prescribed by law to protect public health and abide by the principles of equality and non-discrimination. As noted earlier, however, these limitations cannot justify a restriction to the right to return. The only permissible limitation to the right to return for reasons of "public health" is through the derogation clause, an "extraordinary measure" by which the right to return can be temporarily suspended or restricted in response to a "full-fledged national emergency—not a

---

the prohibition of imprisonment for inability to fulfill a contractual obligation, the prohibition against the retrospective operation of criminal laws, and the right to recognition before the law.

11. Human Rights Committee, *Statement on Derogations from the Covenant in Connection with the COVID-19 Pandemic*, UNHRCOR, 2020, UN Doc CCPR/C/128/2 [UNHRCOR]; "Emergency Measures and COVID-19: Guidance" (2020), online (pdf): *UN Office of the High Commissioner for Human Rights* <www.ohchr.org/Documents/Events/EmergencyMeasures_COVID19.pdf>.
12. UNHRCOR, *ibid*, at para 2(b).
13. UN Office of the High Commissioner for Human Rights, *supra* note 11 at 2.
14. UNHRCOR, *supra* note 11, at para 2(c).

mere public health emergency."[15] As of today, only a few states parties to the ICCPR have complied with the strict procedural requirements in relation to measures adopted to combat COVID 19.[16] Therefore, all other non-compliant states that have resorted to emergency measures—including Canada as discussed below—can be seen as having already "derogated from their [procedural] obligations under the ICCPR."[17] Beyond the fact that procedural requirements are not followed, the above discussion reveals, more importantly, that it is not legally possible under international law for states to obstruct the exercise of citizens' right to return unless it is truly justified in an emergency situation.

Limits to the "Right to Return" in Canada During the COVID-19 pandemic

Starting in February 2020, Canada adopted a number of orders under its *Quarantine Act*[18] empowering its Chief Public Health Officer to compel any returning passenger to self-isolate at home or, for those exhibiting signs of COVID-19, in a designated quarantine facility.[19] On March 18, 2020, Canada took a more restrictive step, prohibiting, through an interim order adopted under the Aeronautics Act,[20] air

15. Adina Ponta, "Human Rights Law in the Time of the Coronavirus" (20 April 2020), online: *ASIL Insights* <www.asil.org/insights/volume/24/issue/5/human-rights-law-time-coronavirus>.
16. These states are Armenia, Chile, Colombia, Ecuador, El Salvador, Estonia, Georgia, Guatemala, Kyrgyzstan, Latvia, Palestine, Peru, and Romania. See "OCHR & Human Rights Committee Address Derogations During Covid-19" (29 April 2020), online: *International Justice Resource Center* <ijrcenter.org/2020/04/29/ohchr-human-rights-committee-address-derogations-during-covid-19>.
17. Joseph, *supra* note 9.
18. *Quarantine Act*, SC 2005, c 20.
19. PC numbers 2020-0059 (3 February 2020); 2020-0070 (17 February 2020); 2020-0071 (19 February 2020); 2020-0157 (18 March 2020); 2020-061 (20 March 2020); 2020-0162 (22 March 2020); 2020-0175 (24 March 2020); 2020-0184 (26 March 2020); 2020-0185 (26 March 2020); 2020-0260 (14 April 2020); 2020-0263 (20 April 2020). See Government of Canada, "Orders in Council Division" (30 April 2017), online: *Orders in Council online database* <orders-in-council.canada.ca/results.php?pageNum=4&lang=en>.
20. "Interim Order to Prevent Certain Persons from Boarding Flights to Canada due to COVID-19" (18 March 2020), online: *Transport Canada* <www.tc.gc.ca/eng/mediaroom/interim-order-prevent-certain-persons-boarding-flights-canada-covid-19.html>. This order was updated a number of times after March 18. The latest version is dated May 26, 2020. See "Interim Order to Prevent Certain Persons from Boarding Flights to Canada due to COVID-19, No. 9", online:

carriers from allowing foreign nationals from boarding an aircraft bound for Canada. Citizens and permanent residents were excluded to entry. Exemptions were also provided for their immediate family members and a number of other categories, including persons with refugee status in Canada. On March 24, more stringent quarantine measures were adopted. Persons who had no other options than public transport (bus, train) to get to their residence to self-isolate would be directed instead to quarantine facilities, as were those who could not self-isolate without being in contact with vulnerable persons (for instance, a returning passenger who shares a residence with an elderly person) or without having access to basic necessities (such as food).[21]

Canada's first series of measures were similar to those taken by other states, such as Australia and New Zealand, whose immigration regimes are often compared to Canada's regime given that all three are countries of immigration and have comparable legal traditions. In Australia, borders were closed to international travellers on March 19, 2020, with the exception of citizens and permanent residents from Australia as well members of their families. By reciprocal arrangement with New Zealand, it also allowed for the entry of citizens from New Zealand habitually residing in Australia. There were other exceptions that could be considered by the Australian Border Force, for instance, for compassionate reasons or for COVID-19-related medical services.[22] All travellers arriving in Australia had to isolate for 14 days at a designated facility at their point of entry.[23] The same day, New Zealand adopted similar measures with slight differences in terms of exceptions to the bar to entry.[24] Since April 9, all returning passengers are required to isolate for 14 days in managed facilities. Those identified

Transport Canada <www.tc.gc.ca/eng/mediaroom/interim-order-prevent-certain-persons-boarding-flights-canada-covid-19-no-9.html>. See also: *Aeronautics Act*, RSC, 1985, c A-2.

21. PC number 2020-0175 (24 March 2020). See Government of Canada, *supra* at note 19.
22. "Coming to Australia | Covid-19 and the Border" (last visited 24 April 2020), online: *Australian Government Department of Home Affairs* <covid19.homeaffairs.gov.au/coming-australia>.
23. "COVID-19 Information" (last visited 12 May 2020), online: *US Embassy & Consulates in Australia* <au.usembassy.gov/covid-19-information>.
24. "Border Closures and Exceptions" (last visited 13 May 2020), online: *Immigration New Zealand*<www.immigration.govt.nz/about-us/covid-19/border-closures-and-exceptions>.

as being at high-risk of COVID-19 are placed in special quarantine facilities.[25] Many other countries did the same.

However, Canada went one step further. Starting on March 19, 2020, the government requested air carriers to prevent all travellers abroad, including Canadian citizens, from boarding if they showed symptoms suggestive of COVID-19.[26] Air carriers had to conduct health checks, relying on questions from a World Health Organization (WHO) document that offers guidance for the management of ill travellers at points of entry.[27] However, here, the government was requiring air carriers to ask those questions *before* the plane departed from a foreign country. This order was subsequently updated a number of times. Later versions do not refer to the WHO document.[28]

Persons prohibited from boarding could not get on an aircraft for at least 14 days unless they had a medical note certifying that their symptoms were not related to COVID-19. Yet, the risk was real that 14 days later they could no longer leave a country either because there were no longer flights available or because that country had closed its borders.

Section 6(1) of the Canadian Charter of Rights and Freedoms[29] provides that "[e]very citizen of Canada has the right to enter, remain in, and leave Canada," a right some citizens could no longer exercise since the government's March 19, 2020, order to air carriers. The government could, however, justify this violation if, as provided for in s 1 of the *Charter*, these limits can "be demonstrably justified in a free and democratic society." To do so, the government has the burden to establish 1) that the measure is taken to address a pressing and substantial objective; 2) that the measure is rationally connected to the objective; 3) that the measure impairs as little as possible the right in question; and 4) that the measure's overall

25. Government of New Zealand, "COVID-19: Key Updates" (last visited 13 May 2020), online: *Immigration New Zealand* <www.immigration.govt.nz/about-us/covid-19/coronavirus-update-inz-response>.
26. PC number 2020-0175 (24 March 2020). See Government of Canada, *supra* note 19.
27. "Management of Ill Travellers at Points of Entry—International Airports, Seaports and Ground Crossings—in the Context of COVID -19 Outbreak" (19 March 2020), online: *World Health Organization* <www.who.int/publications-detail/management-of-ill-travellers-at-points-of-entry-international-airports-seaports-and-ground-crossings-in-the-context-of-covid--19-outbreak>.
28. Government of Canada, *supra*, note 19.
29. Part I of the *Constitution Act*, 1982, being Schedule B to the *Canada Act 1982* (UK), 1982, c 11.

effects on the right protected is not disproportionate to the government's objective.[30]

There is little doubt that the Government of Canada could meet the first two hurdles. The objective to protect the health of the Canadian population was pressing and urgent, and the measure to ban travellers exhibiting signs or symptoms of COVID-19 was rationally linked to this objective. However, it is questionable whether the government could meet the other two conditions. This measure did not impair the right in question as little as possible, as it was both over- and under-inclusive. It targeted Canadian citizens exhibiting symptoms that could be indicative of COVID-19 but that could also be associated with many other conditions, such as other infectious pulmonary diseases, non-infectious pulmonary diseases, a common cold, or flu. The Government of Canada was asking for an assessment to be made by airlines representatives who are not medically trained. As such, they could deny boarding to Canadian citizens who were not COVID-19 positive and accept on board citizens who could have been COVID-19 positive but were asymptomatic. This measure also had the perverse effect of leading some travellers to hide their condition out of fear of being refused boarding, as has been reported by the media.[31] Finally, critics claim that the transfer of migration management to private carriers increases risks of arbitrariness and discriminatory practices (racial profiling).[32]

Contrary to other situations where the measure chosen was the only means by which the government could meet its pressing and substantial objectives,[33] in this case there were a range of options that would have allowed for the repatriation of all Canadian citizens. For example, on regular flights, airlines could have isolated the few citizens exhibiting symptoms. Apart from having to wear masks,[34] these

30. *R v Oakes* [1986] 1 SCR 103, 26 DLR (4th) 200.
31. Dave Seglins, Lisa Mayor & Linda Guerriero "How Sick Canadian Travellers Are Masking COVID-19 Symptoms to Get Through Airport Screening", *CBC News* (25 March 2020), online: <www.cbc.ca/news/investigates/how-sick-canadian-travellers-are-masking-covid-19-symptoms-to-get-through-airport-screening-1.5508276>.
32. Anna Tims, "Barred from Flying from a British Airport—Over a Visa He Didn't Need", *The Guardian* (22 October 2018), online: <www.theguardian.com/money/2018/oct/22/airlines-bar-passengers-visa-rules-no-recourse>.
33. *Alberta v Hutterian Brethren of Wilson Colony*, 2009 SCC 37 at para 62.
34. The obligation to wear a face mask during a flight was only imposed on April 19, 2020, a month after the initial interim order. See Transport Canada, *supra* note 20.

passengers could have been distanced by one or two rows from other passengers, as suggested by some studies.[35] As well, special flights could have been arranged to repatriate these citizens. It is interesting to note that as early as February 17, 2020, in the second quarantine order adopted by the government to prevent the spread of COVID-19, the government provided for measures to bring travellers back on flights "organized by the Government of Canada or a foreign government for the purpose of transporting persons from the foreign country who have or may have been exposed to that disease."[36] The government subsequently did organize flights to repatriate Canadians, but not, to our knowledge, specifically for those exposed to the COVID-19 virus. These alternatives could have been costly and have taken some time to implement, but that, in and of itself, should not have been sufficient reason to justify infringing Canadian citizens' fundamental rights. Admittedly, increased deference should be given to governments' choices when, in the midst of a pandemic, it is urgent to act.[37] In such moments, the range of what should be considered as reasonable limits on *Charter*'s rights might be widened, because of uncertainty as to the effectiveness of various measures taken to protect public health. However, this still does not shift the onus of establishing the reasonableness of the measure.[38] Neither does it justify more intrusive measures that are no less certain to achieve the desired goal than other available measures, while increasing uncertainty for those affected by those measures. Moreover, uncertainty or not, deference or not, it is particularly important to carefully scrutinize limitations on rights in emergency situations.

As for whether the effects on the constitutionally protected rights were disproportionate to the government's objective, this measure was preventing vulnerable Canadian citizens from getting back to their country. Apart from the fact that these citizens needed care if they were indeed COVID-19 positive, many of them could have suffered from other conditions requiring continued access to medical

35. Michael Laris, "Scientists Know Ways to Help Stop Viruses from Spreading on Airplanes. They're Too Late for This Pandemic", *The Washington Post* (29 April 2020), online: <www.washingtonpost.com/local/trafficandcommuting/scientists-think-they-know-ways-to-combat-viruses-on-airplanes-theyre-too-late-for-this-pandemic/2020/04/20/83279318-76ab-11ea-87da-77a8136c1a6d_story.html>.
36. PC number 2020-0070 (17 February 2020); See Government of Canada, *supra* note 19.
37. See Colleen M Flood, Bryan Thomas & Kumanan Wilson, this volume, Chapter C-1.
38. For more on this topic, see *Carter v Canada (AG)*, 2015 SCC 5 at para 102.

care and medications. That access was not a given for anyone suddenly forced to remain in another country, especially if this other country was facing or soon would face a crisis in its health sector. How can a measure that directly affects the most vulnerable, and that risks excluding from boarding some citizens who are not COVID-19 positive while allowing others who are, be proportionate?

In writing this, we do not wish to diminish the effort that the Government of Canada has deployed to bring back citizens, permanent residents, and others stranded abroad. It is estimated that, as of April 23, 2020, the government had coordinated the repatriation of approximately 20,000 persons on 160 flights from 76 countries.[39] One assumes that a great percentage of those were Canadian citizens. However, some were also refused boarding. How many were left behind on the basis that they had symptoms suggestive of COVID-19 is unknown at this point. Likewise, we do not know how many of those proved later to be indeed COVID-19 positive, nor do we know how many passengers were allowed to board and, within 14 days of arrival, tested positive for COVID-19.

Given its obligations both in international and domestic law, Canada must ensure at all times that it does not create disproportionate hurdles on the ability of its citizens to exercise their right to return home. As the current Prime Minister has repeated on numerous occasions in the past: "A Canadian is a Canadian is a Canadian."[40]

---

39. Brian Hermon & Scott McTaggart, "The Canadian Consular Service and Response to COVID-19" (24 April 2020), online (blog): *Library of Parliament, Hillnotes* <hillnotes.ca/2020/04/24/the-canadian-consular-service-and-response-to-covid-19/>.
40. Faiha Naqvi-Mohamed, "'A Canadian Is a Canadian Is a Canadian", *Huffington Post* (last modified 20 October 2016), online: <www.huffingtonpost.ca/fariha-naqvimohamed/a-canadian-is-a-canadian-is-a-canadian_b_8337718.html>.

SECTION D

EQUITY AND COVID-19

CHAPTER D-1

How Should We Allocate Health and Social Resources During a Pandemic?

Sridhar Venkatapuram*

Abstract

In this chapter, I argue that the particular use and applications of two scientific ideas profoundly affected national pandemic responses, including the allocation of resources, with significant harmful implications for social and health equity. First, the familiar "contain and control" approach to infectious diseases was applied maximally by countries (through national lockdowns) and was without precedent. Second, the epidemic forecasting models and modelling that were so influential early on were mono-dimensional; they modelled scenarios of how human bodies will likely spread infections, and of the biological impacts (infected, recovered, or dead) over time. These models erased acute and endemic vulnerabilities, and were not capable of identifying the impacts of policies to reduce virus transmissions on other health and well-being issues, or on other important social domains (for example, the economy).

* Associate Professor, King's College London, UK.

Résumé
Comment répartir les ressources en santé et services sociaux pendant une pandémie ?

Dans ce chapitre, je soutiens que l'utilisation et les applications particulières de deux idées scientifiques ont profondément influencé les stratégies nationales de lutte contre la pandémie, y compris la répartition des ressources, entraînant des conséquences néfastes majeures pour l'équité sociale et l'équité en matière de santé. Tout d'abord, l'approche familière consistant à « contenir et contrôler » les maladies infectieuses a été appliquée rigoureusement par de nombreux pays (par le confinement des populations) et était sans précédent. Ensuite, les modèles de prévision et la modélisation des épidémies qui ont eu tant d'influence au départ étaient unidimensionnels ; ils présentaient des scénarios sur la manière dont le corps humain est susceptible de propager l'infection et sur les impacts biologiques (infecté, rétabli ou décédé) au fil du temps. Ces modèles ont ignoré les vulnérabilités sévères et endémiques, et n'ont pas permis de cerner les effets des politiques visant à réduire la transmission du virus sur d'autres questions de santé et de bien-être, ou sur d'autres domaines sociaux importants (par exemple, l'économie).

A pandemic such as this was expected. In fact, many of the world's richest countries had been preparing for years by commissioning pandemic preparedness plans (PPPs), creating new agencies, and even conducting major simulations. A significant part of the national pandemic responses involves "surge capacity" entailing the rapid allocation of health and other social resources, including financial, intellectual, scientific, labour, military, and infrastructure. The world over, trillions of dollars have been marshalled to address issues ranging from increasing health care capacity, procuring testing kits and protective wear, building additional hospitals, providing food rations, helping businesses stay solvent, supporting and investing in scientific research and the development of vaccines, and so forth. How a country allocates resources, or does not, during a pandemic affects how the pandemic evolves within the country, sometimes in other countries, and in the world. Yet, alongside increasing surge capacity to control the pandemic—in terms of the spread of infections as well as managing consequent illnesses and deaths—how a society allocates resources also reflects and impacts the parallel social concern of equity.

The following discussion argues that the particular use and applications of two scientific ideas profoundly affected national pandemic responses, including the allocation of resources, with significant harmful implications for social and health equity. First, the familiar "contain and control" approach to infectious diseases was applied maximally by countries (through national lockdowns) and was without precedent. Second, the epidemic forecasting models and modelling that were so influential early on were mono-dimensional; they modelled scenarios of how human bodies will likely spread infections and of the biological impacts infected, recovered, or dead) over time. They used assumptions about equal susceptibility and probability of death, which then motivated the society-wide lockdowns. The assumptions obfuscated inequalities in the vulnerabilities of social groups to exposures, infections, and death. Plus, used in isolation, with a focus on only one dimension, these models could not identify the impacts of policies to reduce virus transmissions on other health and well-being issues or on other important social domains (for example, the economy). In light of this argument, a partial answer to the question "how should we allocate resources during a pandemic" is that we should allocate resources with greater attention paid to social equity, particularly through more close scrutiny of the proposed use and application of infectious disease science and control methods.

For many readers, the social concern around equity during this pandemic might initially and most easily be recognizable regarding the distribution of limited health care in the face of overwhelming need. Equity as a concept is often used in relation to the distribution of valuable things. Indeed, the ethical or fair allocation of limited ICU beds, ventilators, and protective equipment rose to prominence in the media and scientific journals early on in the pandemic as the infections spread to high-income countries, particularly in the United States.[1] Concerns are also being expressed around equity related to the future distribution of treatments or vaccines, both domestically and globally, which are currently being researched and developed.[2]

1. Ezekiel J Emanuel et al, "Fair Allocation of Scarce Medical Resources in the Time of Covid-19" (2020) 382:21 N Engl J Med 2049.
2. David Pilling & Andrew Jack, "'People's Vaccine' for Coronavirus Must be Free, Leaders Urge", *Financial Times* (13 May 2020), online: <www.ft.com/content/af929941-7c02-415a-a692-bf8443ede58a>.

The fair social distribution of valuable health care resources is a coherent concern, and speaks to the question of how nations should allocate resources during a pandemic. But concerns about equity or fairness have also been raised regarding the high proportion of deaths among older people and racial and ethnic minorities, the impacts of lockdowns and gender inequalities, and the economic impacts due to loss of incomes and jobs. Beyond the allocation of health care resources, the equity concerns raised by this pandemic go to the very foundations of how the 260-plus countries and territories in the world are organized and function.

Health Equity and Social Determinants of Health

During normal times, the health and well-being of both individuals and a national population, as well as health inequalities across individuals and social groups, are created overwhelmingly by social determinants. Across all high-, middle-, and low-income countries, social determinants of health are what have been described as "the conditions in which people are born, grow, live, work and age."[3] These conditions include such things as early infant care and stimulation, safe and secure employment, housing conditions, discrimination, self-respect, personal relationships, community cohesion, and income inequality, among others. Access to health care for prevention and care is important, but it is only one of the many social determinants of health, illness, impairments, and premature death. Furthermore, these determinants operate at levels ranging from the micro, such as interpersonal interactions affecting neuropsycho-biological pathways, to the meso and macro, such as community cultures, national political regimes, and global processes affecting trade—and, as this pandemic shows, global organizations, governance structures, and norms.

Social determinants of health, unlike the proximate determinants of individual biology, personal behaviours, and exposure to harmful agents (for example, pathogens) are most often the long chain of causes setting up these proximate determinants. A third key aspect of social determinants of health is that health, with life expectancy

3. WHO Commission on Social Determinants of Health & World Health Organization, "Closing the Gap in a Generation: Health Equity Through Action on the Social Determinants of Health: Final Report of the Commission on Social Determinants of Health" (2008), online (pdf): *World Health Organization* <www.who.int/social_determinants/final_report/csdh_finalreport_2008.pdf>.

as a good proxy, is distributed along a social gradient in every society; every socio-economic group is healthier and lives longer than the group below.[4]

In sum, the way we organize our societies, how we treat and relate to each other, the social choices we make in policies, and the persistent neglect of issues and groups all contribute to creating and distributing health and health inequalities along a social gradient within and across societies. The broad social bases of health and health inequalities make health and its determinants a central concern for social equity and justice.[5] In the same vein, the broad social bases of the determinants of health and health inequalities that operate across countries puts them squarely at the centre of the scope of deliberations on global equity and justice.

Social Bases of Infectious Diseases

Given such an understanding of the social bases of health as well as of individual and social group health inequalities, it should be easy to recognize the social bases of infectious disease outbreaks and potential epidemics and pandemics. While the origin of the virus SARS-CoV-2 is still yet to be confirmed, we already know that the conditions that enabled its formation were socially determined. It was not a natural disaster or an act of God, but because of how human-animal interactions were addressed or neglected, through policy choices and social practices. The spread of the virus from person to person is a social phenomenon, and conditions that enable or restrict those social interactions are socially determined. The spread of the virus across countries, initially carried by persons along busy international flight paths to major global cities, is socially determined. And, to press the point to its conclusion, how infections take root and spread in other countries as well as how they are or are not being controlled are determined by social choices or, indeed, neglect.[6]

4. Michael Marmot, *The Health Gap: The Challenge of an Unequal World* (New York; London: Bloomsbury Press, 2015).
5. Sridhar Venkatapuram, *Health Justice: An Argument from the Capabilities Approach* (Cambridge, U.K. & Malden, MA: Polity, 2011).
6. Isaac Chotiner, "The Interwoven Threads of Inequality and Health", *The New Yorker* (14 April 2020), online: <www.newyorker.com/news/q-and-a/the-coronavirus-and-the-interwoven-threads-of-inequality-and-health>; Michael Marmot, "Society and the Slow Burn of Inequality" (2 May 2020) 395:10234 The Lancet 1413.

Just as in normal times, equity concerns related to the pandemic are not only related to access to health care when people are sick with COVID-19 or to claims of new discoveries such as vaccines. We care about equity or fairness in multiple dimensions of health, including the causes, levels, distribution patterns, health consequences, non-health consequences, health care experiences, differences in outcomes, and even how the dead are treated. The difference is that during epidemics and pandemics, the aim of containing infections seemingly dominates any other considerations of equity in health or other social domains. In normal times, this would be like pursuing policies to maximize health outcomes above all other considerations. Such a position is unacceptable because maximizing health outcomes is not the only equity goal within health care, nor is it the only equity concern across all social domains. Ethics and equity concerns are not novel to infectious disease control; we do not cull human beings like we might a herd of farm animals when infections start to spread. However, equity has not been a foremost concern or as prominent as it needs to be.

Vulnerability and Equity

In most countries, even when the infections may be starting to get under control, the national responses to control the COVID-19 pandemic have been negatively affecting the health and well-being of individuals and groups, and making health inequalities worse.[7] This is true even in countries where the pandemic looks as if it is being managed well. Importantly, the harmful impacts of both the infections and national responses are not being distributed evenly or randomly. Instead, the negative impacts are most visible among the most socially disadvantaged, and they are likely to track and make the extant socio-economic gradient in health worse in all countries.[8] And while standard measurement tools are able to capture health outcomes and other social and economic facts, the uneven increase in vulnerability to diverse harms is less measurable—but it is visible. Vulnerability to harms of individuals and groups is a coherent concept; it is akin

7. Yuwa Hedrick-Wong, "The Great Lockdown Is Saving Lives While Increasing Poverty and Hunger Globally", *Forbes* (28 April 2020), online: <www.forbes.com/sites/yuwahedrickwong/2020/04/28/the-great-lockdown-is-saving-lives-while-increasing-poverty-and-hunger-globally/>.
8. Marmot, *supra* note 6.

to the vulnerability of countries to an attack or pandemic threat. However, while national vulnerability has been measured, studied, and addressed, individual and community vulnerability to health risks and threats has not been a focus of comparable efforts.

While all human beings have been made newly vulnerable to the harms of COVID-19, the extent of this new vulnerability varies enormously across individuals and social groups according to their existing vulnerabilities. Vulnerability to COVID-19 disease and to other diverse harms has disproportionately increased for certain individuals and social groups, within and across countries, numbering in the billions. The national responses, while aiming to reduce the new vulnerability to COVID-19, have contributed to even more vulnerabilities—the most direct evidence of this is reflected in the more than 300,000 premature deaths from COVID-19 as of June 2020, and especially in the distinct socio-demographic distribution patterns of those deaths.[9] By far, more older people have died than any other social group, and in many countries where socio-demographic data are being collected and reported, more socially disadvantaged racial and ethnic minorities are dying. There are millions more who are suffering non-COVID harms invisibly, particularly in low- and middle-income countries, beyond the reach of cameras, journalists, government agencies, and researchers.[10]

These layers of vulnerabilities, including existing vulnerabilities, the new vulnerability to COVID-19, and further new vulnerabilities created by the varying national pandemic responses, are all socially created, through certain kinds of policies, or are due to wilful or benign neglect. One form of neglect is to ignore or erase diversity when considering the vulnerabilities of citizens and human beings, all while implementing policies that carry significant burdens.[11] But among the range of social choices, two applications of scientific ideas

9. "COVID-19 Dashboard" (21 May 2020), online: *Centre for Systems Science and Engineering at Johns Hopkins University* <www.arcgis.com/apps/opsdashboard/index.html#/bda7594740fd40299423467b48e9ecf6>.

10. Maria Abi-Habib, "Millions Had Risen Out of Poverty. Coronavirus Is Pulling Them Back", *The New York Times* (30 April 2020), online: <www.nytimes.com/2020/04/30/world/asia/coronavirus-poverty-unemployment.html>; Maria Abi-Habib & Sameer Yasir, "India's Coronavirus Lockdown Leaves Vast Numbers Stranded and Hungry", *The New York Times* (29 March 2020), online: <www.nytimes.com/2020/03/29/world/asia/coronavirus-india-migrants.html> [*Abi-Habib & Yasir*].

11. Chotiner, *supra* note 6.

stand out as causing significant and unequal increase in vulnerabilities to harms, even while aiming to control infections. The unprecedented scale of the "contain and control" approach to its maximum scope, with the aim of reducing vulnerability to COVID-19 among as many people as possible, has also created enormous harms and greater vulnerability to harms. Second, epidemiological models and modelling, particularly those initially produced at Imperial College, UK, only makes use of "natural facts" regarding human bodies and pathogens.[12] This is standard to infectious disease epidemiology. However, without being able to recognize the role of social factors in increasing vulnerability to exposures, or to death, the models have in fact given rise to incomplete analyses and policy recommendations. Indeed, one of the main concerns raised by the models was that a sudden rise in serious disease cases would collapse the health care system, which is crucial to the response. Decreasing pressure on the health care system thus became a focus, which in turn increased vulnerabilities of dying outside of hospitals for many. Furthermore, the modelling only considered the impacts of policy interventions on disease dynamics, and not the impacts on other socially important dimensions (for example, non-COVID-19 health care, the economy, unemployment, gender roles). Consequently, the policies implemented, such as national lockdowns, were focused largely on slowing transmissions and "protecting" the health care system. But the policies seemed to have been blind or willfully tolerant of the potential unequal burdens they would produce and distribute, as well as the potential social distribution patterns of deaths.

Consequently, while few countries have been able to actively control the pandemic, significant burdens have been placed on national populations while also disproportionately affecting the most socially disadvantaged within and across countries. The other chapters in this section discuss what the implications have been for older people and the rise in virulent and structural ageism; for people with inadequate housing; for prisoners who have little ability to control their environment; for the rise of racism against those who are thought to be carriers; for groups who are already constrained in their health abilities, such as Indigenous Peoples, people with disabilities, and those with

---

12. N Ferguson et al, "Report 9: Impact of Non-Pharmaceutical Interventions (NPIs) to Reduce COVID19 Mortality and Healthcare Demand" (2020), online (pdf): Imperial College COVID-19 Response Team <spiral.imperial.ac.uk:8443/bitstream/10044/1/77482/14/2020-03-16-COVID19-Report-9.pdf>.

mental health impairments. The devastating impact reflected in these chapters is only a partial story. And the argument here is not meant to lead to the conclusion that governments should not vigorously act to control pandemics or deploy scientific resources. Rather, much of the incredible deprivations can be traced back to the lack of sufficient concern for equity by national leaders, and to the use and expansive influence of a particular set of scientific ideas and tools. The science could have been better.

The remaining discussion in this chapter focuses on the large-scale application of the contain-and-control approach to infectious diseases, followed by an examination of the use of epidemiological models and the impact on equity. The fourth section concludes the chapter.

Contain-and-Control Approach to the Max

The first and foremost national capacity identified by any PPP is epidemiology, which is the study of the causes, frequency, and distribution of disease and disability. Epidemiology is the informational engine that drives all biomedical sciences and health care as well as public and global health. From infectious disease epidemiology, we get the standard "contain-and-control" approach to outbreaks. This approach involves identifying the pathogen, source, or vector of infections and all carriers; isolating carriers so they do not transmit the infections further; and treating them, if possible. Because the contain-and-control approach is seen to be so effective, it is the standard approach. Pathogens, vectors, and routes of transmissions have an impact on the biological parts and processes, and the treatments that address infection and biological parts and processes are accepted as sufficient information. Other biological facts such as age and sex are also recorded, as they can be important facts when it comes to documenting transmission, discovering which biological parts and processes are affected, and determining the natural progression of disease, behaviours, and so forth.

The contain-and-control approach was applied to the outbreak in Wuhan, China, but it did not contain the spread of infection. Likely, the approach was implemented too late, after too many infections had spread. The decision to quarantine an entire city of over 11 million people was decided based on the likelihood that the spread of infection was beyond a few people, families, or a neighbourhood. And there is enough evidence to conclude that individuals reporting early on during a potential outbreak were harassed or censored.[13] This undermined the possibility of an earlier effective containment of a smaller area. But Wuhan is also a major transport hub in China, as well as a major international trade centre with frequent inbound and outbound international flights. For this reason, it is possible that infections had been spreading widely even before some doctors began seeing pneumonia-like symptoms in patients. Nevertheless, the scale of the quarantine that China implemented around Wuhan and then around 10 other cities set a significant global precedent. Importantly, the scale was also new to infectious disease science; nothing of that scale and force had been attempted since the advent of epidemiological science.

The scale of the Chinese quarantines is mind-boggling and also raises questions about justification, effectiveness, plausibility, and equity. Since the 14th century, when the quarantine measure is often cited as being first practised, it has been recognized that isolating individuals or groups for the sake of infectious disease control implies additional burdens on those individuals being isolated. And the long-standing justification for the burdens of those in quarantine has been that it is necessary to protect the health and lives of the larger segment of the uninfected population. In Wuhan, there was a quarantine placed around 11 million people for the sake of protecting the rest of the 1 billion or so Chinese population. International observers viewed the excess burdens of those in quarantine as justified for the sake of protecting the rest of the global population. The quarantine drew admiration for the government's ability to implement this measure, as well as criticism that the measure reflected authoritarian power; it can only move boldly and forcefully when it does act. The lack of transparency and international trust in Chinese data also makes it unclear as to whether the quarantine was needed, was effective, or will be needed again.

For the residents of Wuhan, quarantine meant no travel and a lockdown that reduced social interactions to a bare minimum. Authorities also implemented massive testing and tracing programs, including the mandatory use of a mobile phone app.[14] And while ris-

13. Tom Mitchell, "China's Martyred Coronavirus Doctor Poses Problems for Beijing", *Financial Times* (7 February 2020), online: <www.ft.com/content/413353ae-4995-11ea-aee2-9ddbdc86190d>.

14. Paul Mozur, Raymond Zhong & Aaron Krolik, "In Coronavirus Fight, China Gives Citizens a Color Code, With Red Flags", *The New York Times* (1 March

ing cases were being reported in various countries such as Iran and Spain, the Italian government decided to adopt China's contain-and-control approach on a large scale by implementing quarantines around various regions. On March 9, Italy then implemented a nationwide lockdown.[15] Perhaps the rising number of deaths, and uncertainty of transmission rates and case fatality rates, moved the Italians to err on the side of precaution. Plus, infectious epidemiological models and modelling at this time began to gain traction in public and policy discussions.[16] Perhaps, guided by China and Italy precedents, as well as by these modelling exercises, by the end of March, the majority of countries worldwide had implemented some form of border closure and national lockdowns.[17]

So far in human history, the contain-and-control approach has primarily been used in relation to individuals or small geographical areas. Nationwide lockdowns—unknown until now—are first and foremost meant to reduce social interactions. Citizens and people were told to work from home, public gatherings were not allowed, and universities and schools were asked to move classes online. It was clear that health care workers had to move in the opposite direction. As many as possible were asked to work in hospitals and new field hospitals being built. Beyond health care workers, countries also began to identify certain groups of workers as essential and required to work during the lockdowns. These included those in education and child care, transportation, justice and safety, public utilities, food and essential goods, and so forth. However, it became clear that health care workers were also becoming sick and dying at higher rates from hospital exposures. And many of these other essential workers faced frequent social interactions in their jobs. In addition to bearing a higher burden of risk of infection and death, many of these essential jobs are low paying and often done by people lower down on

---

2020), online: <www.nytimes.com/2020/03/01/business/china-coronavirus-surveillance.html>.

15. William Feuer, "Italy Expands its Quarantine to the Entire Country as Coronavirus Cases and Deaths Surge", *CNBC* (9 March 2020), online: <www.cnbc.com/2020/03/09/italy-extends-its-quarantine-to-the-entire-country-pm-asks-residents-to-stay-at-home.html>.
16. David Adam, "Special Report: The Simulations Driving the World's Response to COVID-19" (2020) 580:7803 Nature 316.
17. University of Oxford, Blavatnik School of Government, "Coronavirus Government Response Tracker" (2020), online: *University of Oxford* <www.bsg.ox.ac.uk/research/research-projects/coronavirus-government-response-tracker>.

the socio-economic ladder. In many countries, these people are also among racial and ethnic minority groups, women, migrants, and other socially disadvantaged groups.[18]

A second dimension to the mega-lockdowns, particularly in some high-income countries, was that the expectation that hospitals would be overwhelmed with COVID-19 patients led to the transfer of non-COVID-19 patients, such as older people to nursing homes—a decision that has resulted in an alarming spread of infections and deaths.[19] Paramedics responding to health emergency calls raised the threshold for people being admitted to hospitals.[20] Moreover, as news spread of hospitals focusing their efforts on the COVID-19 response, of health care workers dying of COVID-19, and the uncertainty expressed by individuals wondering whether they would get adequate care, the end result was people deciding not to go to a hospital despite needing care. Nursing homes in the U.S., the U.K., France, Spain, and Canada saw infections spread among patients, but were unable to provide sufficient care, nor did they seem to be able to easily transfer nursing home residents needing care to hospitals. While much attention focused on hospitals' daily death toll due to COVID-19, the number of people dying at home and in nursing homes increased dramatically. By May, "excess mortality" due to non-COVID-19 causes was also increasing dramatically.[21] More people were dying from other causes well beyond normal as there were people dying from COVID-19.

A third dimension of the lockdowns is the increase in various harms to health and well-being, particularly for those with variety of social disadvantages and vulnerabilities. For example, in India, the Prime Minister gave a few hours' notice before implementing a national lockdown.[22] As a result, millions of people, especially migrants who live on a daily cash wage, were left without any ability to pay for food, housing, and other living costs. Without any social

18. The Lancet Editors, "The Plight of Essential Workers During the COVID-19 Pandemic" (23 May 2020) 395:10237 The Lancet 1587.
19. Kelly Grant & Tu Thanh Ha, "How Shoring up Hospitals for COVID-19 Contributed to Canada's Long-Term Care Crisis", *The Globe and Mail* (20 May 2020), online: <www.theglobeandmail.com/canada/article-how-shoring-up-hospitals-for-covid-19-contributed-to-canadas-long/>.
20. Sarah Bloch-Budzier, "Fears Some COVID Patients 'Not Taken to Hospital,'" *BBC News* (23 April 2020), online: <www.bbc.com/news/health-52317781>.
21. "Tracking COVID-19 Excess Deaths Across Countries", *The Economist* (16 April 2020), online: <www.economist.com/graphic-detail/2020/04/16/tracking-covid-19-excess-deaths-across-countries>.
22. Abi-Habib & Yasir, *supra* note 10.

safety net, millions took to the roads, often walking hundreds of kilometres to go home to their ancestral towns and villages. Public transportation had been shut down. Similar impacts on the poor were seen in some African countries. Moreover, in many low- and middle-income countries, police harassment and brutality increased as they sought to enforce lockdowns. Reports of violence against women and children also increased around the world.[23]

In low-income countries, adequate housing, access to clean water and toilets, household savings, and other COVID-19 prevention necessities are simply unavailable to millions of people. Moreover, unlike in high-income countries, COVID-19 is not the only epidemic to impact many low- and middle-income countries. There are ongoing epidemics of tuberculosis, malaria, Lassa fever, Ebola, and others. All of those programs were brought to a halt because of lockdowns. In fact, as in high-income countries, hospitals situated in low- and middle-income countries have been converted into COVID-19 hospitals. The excess mortality in these countries is likely to be enormous, and many of the gains in infectious disease control are likely to be lost.

The enormous devastation that has been caused, particularly in low- and middle-income countries, because of the application of the contain-and-control approach at a national scale have raised fundamental questions about the one-size-fits-all approach implicit in scientific guidance. From here on in, it is likely that universal scientific guidance will not be applied without scrutiny when responding to the next waves or when dealing with other health issues. When applied to a small group of people or even to a region, additional burdens resulting from the contain-and-control approach seem justifiable; it benefits the greater good. But the appropriateness and effectiveness of the geometric scaling up to the national level have yet to be evaluated. This approach has created enormous harms to certain communities, as well as the population as a whole. In high-income countries, particularly the United States, the enormous harm to economic activity has resulted great scepticism of scientific expertise, and even, its clear rejection by political leadership.

23. "Human Rights Dimensions of COVID-19 Response" (19 March 2020), online: *Human Rights Watch* <www.hrw.org/news/2020/03/19/human-rights-dimensions-covid-19-response>.

Biological Models at the Individual Level

Aside from the precedent set by China, another impetus for the plausibility or necessity of national lockdowns was the application of infectious disease epidemiological models and modelling. A few models gained prominence, including those used at Imperial College, the London School of Hygiene & Tropical Medicine, and Oxford in the United Kingdom, and at Harvard University in the United States.[24] In mid-March the modellers at Imperial projected 500,000 deaths in the U.K. and 2.2 million deaths in the U.S. if no action were taken. Furthermore, and most importantly, the modellers were able to share their projections directly with the U.K. Prime Minister's Office as well as U.S. Presidential advisors.

The influence of the projections was enormous, and resulted in lockdown policies in the U.K. They also may have propelled the U.S. President to take the pandemic more seriously. The models used to simulate new diseases are informed by characteristics of previous epidemics, but are unique to each research group. Even when different research groups try to produce forecasts of the same epidemic, their modelling can vary in numerous ways, including the assumptions for regarding transmission rates, incubation periods, case fatality rates, and so forth. Some groups may add more complexity such as geographical space, density, age, and so forth. Different projections reflect all the underlying differences in assumptions and informational bases. But what seems to be true, at least of the Imperial Model, are the types of assumptions made and narrow informational bases used. For example, in the initial Imperial Model, all individuals are equally susceptible to risk to infection, equally infectious when they do become infected, and completely immune when they recover.

Two aspects of such assumptions in the models are worth remarking on, as they have direct bearing on the unequal burdens and vulnerabilities people are facing. First, vulnerability to infections is clearly not equal among all human beings, or even within a country. Such differences in vulnerability can be created from existing health conditions, frailty from being older, as well as from social conditions such as lack of clean water or the inability to afford soap. The evening-out of inequality of vulnerability to infection, in turn, also produces an analysis that erases the unequal abilities, thus indicating a benefit from the intervention to reduce transmission. This evening-out obfuscates the

24. Adam, *supra* note 16.

possibility of the intervention actually creating more vulnerabilities. It is the same with assuming that all individuals develop immunity once infected. The modellers might easily reply that the assumptions are meant to produce approximations rather than exact projections, or that they could introduce variations of vulnerability to become infected. The issue here is that they did not in February 2020. While it may be possible to assume equal vulnerability in a small group of people to assist with a small outbreak, modelling an entire national population of millions should have made the issue of inequality in vulnerability to exposures, infection, and deaths both obvious and required.

The second aspect to note is that as this particular model assumed generic biological bodies, it was not able to present any analysis on social distribution patterns. The analysis was only able to present aggregate numbers of infected and immune, infected and dead, and susceptible before the pandemic dies out. Once again, rather than just increase the population size to the country level, if the model was also able to project vulnerability for death by social group or social class variables, it may have been able to project the scale of deaths of vulnerable populations. Moreover, if that were to have been done, it seems plausible to imagine that the national response, at least in the U.K., may have marshalled additional resources early enough to prevent deaths among vulnerable groups. Instead, only after deaths began to occur, and it was obvious that the people dying were older and from racial and ethnic minority groups, that socio-demographic data started to be collected and analyzed.

Mathematical modelling of infectious diseases have suddenly become influential scientific evidence in the U.K., U.S., and many other countries. While important, even the modellers agree that they have severe limitations; forecasts have to be presented, and received, with caution. To be more reflective of the context, and hopefully more accurate, some research groups incorporate more information into their models, including more diversity of individuals. But even those models are limited in their ability to incorporate inequalities in vulnerabilities to infections created by a range of natural and social causes. Without doing so, these infectious disease models will continue to erase vulnerabilities and, in turn, recommend policies that are generic. Furthermore, they will be unable to recognize the potential additional burdens that interventions such as physical distancing might distribute to those already vulnerable as well as across many social domains.

Conclusion

As stated in the introduction, a partial answer to the question of how a nation should allocate its resources during a pandemic is that it should seek to deploy a pandemic response that aims to effectively control the epidemic, but with attention to equity. Such attention entails giving greater scrutiny to the scientific ideas at play. The implementation of national lockdowns reflects the use of the contain-and-control approach to infectious diseases to its maximum and unprecedented extent.

While the deployment of quarantine measures at such a large scale was designed to protect the health care systems and save as many lives as possible, it also distributed burdens across the population, and disproportionately to those who are already vulnerable. Every country may have its particular vulnerable groups, and some groups may cut across all countries, but it is clear that the background vulnerabilities prior to the pandemic, the new vulnerability created by COVID-19, and the further vulnerabilities created by national pandemic responses have resulted in hundreds of thousands of deaths and greater deprivations for millions. We are now entering a difficult period, one that is expected to last one to two years. Thus, low- and middle-income countries are likely to experience the impact of this approach for a longer duration, perhaps even decades.

The discussion also aimed to show that basic infectious disease modelling so influential early in this pandemic actually erased inequalities in vulnerabilities. Such erasure of inequalities in vulnerabilities then produces recommendations for policies such as lockdowns, which do not recognize acute vulnerability, or the further burdens and vulnerabilities from the interventions. Nor does such modelling provide any indication of the social distributions of immunity and deaths. One potentially practicable and impactful use of resources would be to combine infectious disease modelling and social epidemiology to produce better forecasts that incorporate differences in vulnerability and show social distribution patterns of impacts of infections as well as social responses. This is not a novel assertion. Such a call to improve infectious disease modelling and epidemiology by incorporating social determinants of unequal vulnerability was raised in the mid 1990s in response to HIV/AIDS modelling. But it went unheeded. This shows again how the devastation from this COVID-19 pandemic has a long chain of causes rooted in social choices and neglect, going back decades.

CHAPITRE D-2

COVID-19 et âgisme : crise annoncée dans les centres de soins de longue durée et réponse improvisée ?

Martine Lagacé*, Linda Garcia** et Louise Bélanger-Hardy***

Résumé

Au Canada, la crise de la COVID-19 a frappé très lourdement les résidents des centres de soins de longue durée (CSLD) au pays. Un très grand nombre de personnes âgées y sont décédées, souvent dans des conditions lamentables. Comment en sommes-nous arrivés là ? N'était-il pas possible de prévenir le désastre ? Le présent chapitre se penche sur ces questions et suggère que l'une des causes de cette triste situation est l'âgisme, soit les stéréotypes associés aux personnes âgées et la discrimination qui s'ensuit. Après avoir défini l'âgisme, ses manifestations et ses retombées, le texte analyse certains des enjeux et problématiques bien connus des centres de soins de longue durée : l'âge avancé des résidents, leur comorbidité, la précarité du milieu de travail pour le personnel soignant et l'absence d'équipement de protection approprié. Somme toute, la crise sanitaire causée par la COVID-19 a permis d'exposer une réalité troublante, soit que les adultes âgés les plus vulnérables vivent dans des milieux où les préposés sont débordés, mal rémunérés et où leurs compétences spécialisées ne sont ni reconnues, ni valorisées. Bien

* Professeure titulaire au Département de communication et membre de l'Institut de recherche LIFE à l'Université d'Ottawa.

** Professeure titulaire à l'École interdisciplinaire des sciences de la santé et directrice de l'Institut de recherche LIFE à l'Université d'Ottawa.

*** Professeure titulaire à la Faculté de droit, Section de common law, membre de l'Institut de recherche LIFE à l'Université d'Ottawa.

qu'il semble clair que l'absence d'un financement adéquat soit l'une des causes du problème, le portrait des conditions de travail, des enjeux et des problématiques auxquels sont confrontés les CSLD depuis de nombreuses années suggèrent que les attitudes sociétales envers le vieillissement, particulièrement envers les personnes les plus âgées et les plus vulnérables, sont peut-être la véritable pierre angulaire du problème.

Abstract
COVID-19 and ageism: a predictable crisis in long-term care centres and an impromptu response?

In Canada, the COVID-19 crisis has hit residents of long-term care centres hard. A very high number of seniors have passed away in these facilities, often in deplorable conditions. How did we end up here? Was this disaster not preventable? This chapter addresses these issues and suggests that one of the causes of this predicament is ageism, which is the stereotyping of individuals based on their age and the discrimination that ensues. After defining ageism and exploring its effects and consequences, the text delves into certain well-known challenges and problems of long-term care facilities: the advanced age of residents, their comorbidity, the precarious work environments health-care personnel face, and the lack of proper personal protective equipment. Overall, the COVID-19 health crisis has helped expose a troubling reality: the most vulnerable seniors live in environments where personal support workers are overworked and underpaid, and where their specialized skills are neither recognized nor valued. While it may seem obvious that a lack of adequate funding is one of the causes of the problem, a look at long-term care facilities' working conditions, challenges, and concerns over the years suggests that societal attitudes on aging, particularly regarding our oldest and most vulnerable citizens, are possibly the true root of the problem.

Au jour du 2 mai 2020, au plus fort de la crise sanitaire au Canada, l'Ontario comptait un total de 17 553 cas de COVID-19, dont 2 488 (14 %) dans les centres de soins de longue durée (CSLD)[1]. Des

1. Les centres de soins de longue durée réfèrent aux établissements où résident des personnes nécessitant des soins continus et un soutien personnel pour la réalisation des activités quotidiennes.

1 216 personnes décédées des suites du virus, 590 (49 %) étaient des résidents de ces mêmes centres[2]. La province voisine, le Québec, affichait un scénario d'autant plus inquiétant : les données du 26 avril 2020 révélaient que parmi les 1 859 personnes décédées, 1 469 (79 %) d'entre elles résidaient en CSLD[3]. De fait, il n'a fallu que quelques semaines suivant le début de la pandémie à la mi-mars 2020 pour que la situation dans les CSLD se dégrade rapidement ; à un point tel que les dirigeants ont dû faire appel à des citoyens volontaires ainsi qu'à du personnel soignant de l'armée canadienne pour prêter main-forte aux équipes soignantes. L'abondante couverture médiatique a d'ailleurs levé le voile sur une situation quasi inimaginable, montrant la détresse des résidents en CSLD, contraints à un confinement des plus stricts, voire à un isolement physique et social quasi absolu et un personnel soignant à bout de souffle, bien souvent mal équipé.

Comment en est-on arrivé là ? La rapide dégradation de la situation aurait-elle pu être évitée, en partie du moins ? La question est importante, car d'une part, dès les premiers cas de la COVID-19 en Chine, il est devenu manifeste que le nombre de décès était plus élevé chez les adultes plus âgés[4]. D'autre part, les données européennes, notamment celles provenant de l'Italie, montraient clairement que les résidents de CSLD étaient parmi les plus nombreuses victimes de la maladie. Pourquoi alors les efforts de contention du virus n'ont-ils pas été dirigés, dès le début de la pandémie au Canada vers ces centres ? Pourquoi l'expérience des pays confrontés à la crise sanitaire, avant son déploiement sur le continent nord-américain, n'a-t-elle pas mené les autorités sanitaires canadiennes à concentrer leurs efforts vers le cas des personnes âgées résidant en CSLD ?

Dans ce chapitre, nous suggérons que l'une des explications possibles de ce phénomène découle de la problématique de l'âgisme à l'égard des personnes âgées, particulièrement les plus vulnérables, en l'occurrence celles habitant dans les CSLD. Dans les sections qui suivent, nous définissons d'abord l'âgisme, ses manifestations et ses retombées. Ensuite, nous présentons un état des lieux des CSLD, en

2. Public Health Ontario, « Epidemiologic Summary—COVID-19 in Ontario: January 15, 2020 to May 2, 2020 » (4 mai 2020), en ligne (pdf) : *Public Health Ontario* <files.ontario.ca/moh-covid-19-report-en-2020-05-03.pdf>.

3. Gabrielle Duchaine, « COVID-19 : 69 nouveaux décès au Québec », *La Presse* (26 avril 2020), en ligne : <www.lapresse.ca/covid-19/202004/26/01-5270972-covid-19-69-nouveaux-deces-au-quebec.php>.

4. Robert Verity et al, « Estimates of the Severity of Coronavirus Disease 2019: A Model-Based Analysis » (2020) 20:6 The Lancet Infectious Diseases 669.

amont de la pandémie. Enfin, nous soutenons que cet état des lieux résulte, en partie du moins, d'attitudes et de pratiques âgistes, et proposons des pistes de réflexion pour contrer ces dernières.

Vieillissement : le regard âgiste des sociétés occidentales

En Occident, le processus du vieillissement comme celui de la vieillesse repose sur une construction plutôt négative, associant l'avancement en âge à la perte et au déclin[5]. Le corollaire d'une telle construction est d'ailleurs celui d'un culte de la jeunesse, d'un vouloir rester jeune et de ne pas être catégorisée comme « personne âgée ». Et c'est là le paradoxe des sociétés occidentales : si le temps de vie physique s'est allongé, le temps de vie sociale s'en trouve réduit par cette construction négative du vieillissement. Robert N. Butler a conceptualisé ce profond malaise des jeunes et des adultes face à la vieillesse en référant à l'âgisme[6]. Ce concept sous-tend notamment une composante cognitive et comportementale, soit a) les stéréotypes négatifs associés aux personnes âgées (fragilité, inutilité, impuissance, dépendance) et b) la discrimination, l'exclusion, voire l'abandon des personnes âgées. Ces stéréotypes et cette discrimination âgistes se manifestent de manière consciente/volontaire ou inconsciente/involontaire ainsi qu'au niveau individuel ou systémique[7]. C'est, par exemple, la personne âgée qui est infantilisée ou brimée dans sa capacité de dire et d'agir, ou plus encore, ignorée quant à ses besoins et droits, sur le plan physique, psychologique et social. L'âgisme est une forme de violence, mais aussi de négligence exercées par les individus et la société sur les personnes âgées[8].

Les travaux des deux dernières décennies ont permis de documenter les manifestations comme les retombées de l'âgisme dans plusieurs sphères de la société. Le milieu du travail en témoigne par des

5. Nick M Wisdom et al, « The Relationship of Anxiety and Beliefs Toward Aging in Ageism » (2014) J of Scientific Psychology 10; Jacqueline Trincaz et Bernadette Puijalon, « Vieillir en terre hostile » dans Sylvie Carbonnelle, dir, *Penser les vieillesses. Regards sociologiques et anthropologiques sur l'avancée en âge*, Paris, Éditions Seli Arslan, 2010, 21 à la p 21.
6. Robert N Butler, « Age-ism: Another Form of Bigotry » (1969) 9:4 The Gerontologist 243.
7. Valérian Boudjemad et Kamel Gana, « L'âgisme : adaptation française d'une mesure et test d'un modèle structural des effets de l'empathie, l'orientation à la dominance sociale et le dogmatisme sur l'âgisme » (2009) 28:4 Can J on Aging / La Rev can du vieillissement 371.
8. Daphne Nasmiash, « Powerlessness and Neglect of Older Adults » (2002) 14:1 J of Elder Abuse and Neglect 21.

conditions d'embauche et de rétention difficiles pour les personnes âgées de 50 ans et plus[9]. Le domaine des soins de santé n'échappe pas non plus à l'âgisme. Des travaux empiriques suggèrent en effet l'omniprésence de stéréotypes et de pratiques âgistes, au niveau individuel comme systémique. Par exemple, les études sur la communication interpersonnelle dans un contexte de soins suggèrent que le personnel soignant adopte parfois (volontairement ou involontairement) un mode de communication infantilisant[10] et cela, particulièrement dans un contexte de soins de longue durée[11]. Cette communication âgiste résulterait en partie du regard stéréotypé posé sur les personnes âgées : fragilité, dépendance, impuissance. En outre, l'infantilisation aurait un effet délétère sur la santé psychologique des personnes âgées, entraînant une baisse de leur estime de soi et de leurs interactions sociales ainsi qu'une augmentation de symptômes dépressifs[12]. Au niveau systémique, des chercheurs soutiennent que l'âgisme et les représentations négatives du vieillissement s'inscriraient comme facteurs de risque majeur quant aux différents types d'abus et de négligence – physique, psychologique, social et financier – envers les personnes âgées[13]. Il est intéressant de noter que certains travaux récents sur l'âgisme suggèrent que les personnes les plus âgées et nécessitant des soins de longue durée seraient désormais les plus ciblées en termes de stéréotypes et de pratiques âgistes[14]. Pour paraphraser les propos de Higgs et al, ces grands aînés fragilisés représenteraient une sorte de

9. Kelly Harris et al, « Ageism and the Older Worker: A Scoping Review » (2017) 58:2 The Gerontologist e1.
10. La communication infantilisante se traduit par un parler plus lent, une intonation exagérée, une répétition de mots et une structure grammaticale simplifiée.
11. Jaye L Atkinson et Robin G Sloan, « Exploring the Impact of Age, Race, and Stereotypes on Perceptions of Language Performance and Patronizing Speech » (2016) 36:3 J of Language and Social Psychology 287 ; Martine Lagacé et al, « À mots couverts : le regard des aînés et des soignants sur la communication quotidienne et ses manifestations d'âgisme implicite » (2011) 20 Can J on Aging/La R Can du vieillissement 185.
12. Shaughan A Keaton et Howard Giles, « Subjective Health: The Role of Communication, Language, Aging, Stereotypes, and Culture » (2016) 4:2 Intl J of Society, Culture and Language 1.
13. Lucio Bizzinin et Charles-Henri Rapin, « L'âgisme. Une forme de discrimination qui porte préjudice aux personnes âgées et prépare le terrain de la négligence et de la violence » (2007) 123 Gérontologie et Société 263.
14. Martine Lagacé et Najat Firzly, « Who's "Really" Old?: Addressing Shifting Targets of Ageism Through Intragroup and Intergroup Perceptions of Aging » (2017) 7:3 Intl J of Aging and Society 35 ; Paul Higgs et Chris Gilleard, *Rethinking Old Age. Theorising The Fourth Age*, Londres (R-U), Macmillan Publishers, 2015 à la p 172.

« distorsion dans le miroir » des plus jeunes par rapport à leur propre vieillissement et à leur peur de l'impuissance et de l'inutilité[15]. La voie semble alors pavée pour celles et ceux résidant en CSLD, dépeints comme des individus avec peu de pouvoir de se dire et d'agir.

L'âgisme est donc une réalité sociale indéniable qui s'immisce dans plusieurs facettes de la société, particulièrement celle des soins de santé, et particulièrement à l'égard des plus âgés et des plus vulnérables. La COVID-19, en frappant de plein fouet les CSLD, a-t-elle surligné des problèmes auxquels sont confrontés depuis longtemps les résidents de ces centres et les personnes y travaillant ? Plus précisément, a-t-elle magnifié des attitudes âgistes, suscitant un questionnement essentiel sur les valeurs qui sous-tendent les choix politiques et sociaux face aux aînés depuis les dernières décennies ?

COVID-19 et centres de soins de longue durée : une loupe braquée sur l'âgisme ?

Les conséquences tragiques de la pandémie COVID-19 ont exposé les multiples défis tout autant que les failles du système des CSLD au Canada. Bien que les difficultés fussent connues des autorités, elles semblent avoir été ignorées. En effet, des facteurs tels l'âge avancé des résidents, leur comorbidité et la précarité de la main-d'œuvre qui les appuient sont documentés depuis longtemps dans les rapports officiels sur la santé et le bien-être des personnes habitant ces centres[16].

L'âge a été l'un des premiers facteurs liés à l'apparition de maladies graves et à un nombre élevé de décès pendant la pandémie. Pourtant, nous savons depuis des années que les résidents des CSLD comptent un nombre important de personnes très âgées. L'*Ontario Long-Term Care Association* (OLTA), l'association la plus importante en son genre au pays, confirme dans l'un de ses récents rapports[17] que 82 % des résidents (établissements publics et privés combinés) ont plus de 75 ans et que 55 % d'entre eux sont âgés de plus de 85 ans. Ces statistiques, représentatives de la situation canadienne dans son ensemble, démontrent que contrairement à la situation d'il y a 30 ou

15. *Higgs et Gilleard, supra* note 14.
16. Hugh Armstrong, Tamara J Daly et Jacqueline A Choinière, « Policies and Practices: The Case of RAI-MDS in Canadian Long-Term Care Homes » (2016) 50:2 J of Can Studies 348.
17. « This is Long-Term Care 2019 » (2019), en ligne (pdf) : *Ontario Long-Term Care Association* <www.oltca.com/OLTCA/Documents/Reports/TILTC2019web.pdf>.

40 ans, les CSLD doivent composer avec une population de plus en plus âgée, ayant des besoins complexes et nécessitant des soins de plus en plus spécialisés[18].

En fait, au-delà de l'âge, la présence et la nature de deux ou plusieurs problèmes de santé chroniques, c'est-à-dire la comorbidité, a pour effet d'accroître la vulnérabilité des personnes résidant en CSLD. Il semble d'ailleurs que ces comorbidités, en particulier celles affectant le système cardiovasculaire, augmentent le risque de développer une forme grave d'infection chez les personnes atteintes de la COVID-19[19]. Or, rappelons qu'en Chine et en Italie notamment, ce sont aussi les plus âgés, affrontant plusieurs problèmes de santé chroniques et vivant en CSLD, qui ont été les plus touchés par le virus. Pourquoi, au Canada, ne pas avoir anticipé une crise dans ces milieux et, surtout, mis en oeuvre un plan pour la maîtriser ? Voilà la question qui nous préoccupe.

Une autre réalité bien connue avant la pandémie est celle des conditions de travail des préposés aux soins des bénéficiaires. Au Canada, les préposés aux soins ne font pas partie d'une profession autonome autoréglementée. Leur salaire est peu élevé et leur situation précaire les amène à travailler dans plusieurs centres de soins[20]. L'un des problèmes les plus publicisés de la pandémie de la COVID-19 a été celui de la rétention des préposés aux soins qui ont, dans certains cas, quitté leur lieu de travail pour cause d'épuisement ou parce que les mesures de prévention de la contamination n'étaient pas adéquates. Pourtant, la situation actuelle ne doit surprendre personne, car les problèmes ne datent pas d'hier[21]. L'absence de plusieurs employés oblige ceux qui restent en place à continuer de travailler dans des

18. Voir aussi les statistiques dans Armstrong, Armstrong et Bourgeault, ce volume, chapitre E-1.

19. Wei-jie Guan et al, « Comorbidity and its impact on 1590 patients with Covid-19 in China: A Nationwide Analysis » (2020) 55:5 European Respiratory J e1; Steven Gjerstad et Andrea Molle, « Comorbidity Factors (such as heart disease and diabetes) Influence COVID-19 Mortality More Than Age » (21 mars 2020), en ligne : *Start Insight* <www.startinsight.eu/en/comorbidity-factors-covid19/>.

20. Gordon Cooke et al, « Zero Hours and Near Zero Hours Work in Canada » dans Michelle O'Sullivan et al, dir, *Zero Hours and On-call Work in Anglo-Saxon Countries*, Singapore, Springer, 2019, 137.

21. Janet E Squires et al, « Job Satisfaction Among Care Aides in Residential Long-Term Care: A Systematic Review of Contributing Factors, Both Individual and Organizational » (2015) Nursing Research and Practice e1 ; Mary Halter et al, « The Determinants and Consequences of Adult Nursing Staff Turnover: A Systematic Review of Systematic Reviews » (2017) 17:824 BMC Health Services Research e1 ; Zenobia CY Chan et al, « A Systematic Literature Review of Nurse Shortage and the Intention to Leave » (2013) 21 J of Nursing Management 605.

conditions non seulement très difficiles, mais plus propices à la contamination des résidents. En effet, les préposés qui prodiguent des soins sur plusieurs étages d'un CSLD ou qui comblent des postes dans plusieurs centres contribuent à faciliter la transmission des maladies. Dès le début de la pandémie au Canada, les autorités sanitaires savaient que le virus de la COVID-19 était très contagieux et qu'il pouvait se transmettre via une personne asymptomatique. Ces autorités savaient aussi qu'il y avait une pénurie de personnel infirmier et de préposés aux soins dans les CSLD[22]. Pourquoi, étant donné ces faits, n'était-il pas possible de prévoir les conséquences de l'absence d'une intervention ciblée visant à promouvoir la santé des plus vulnérables ?

Enfin, il s'est avéré très clair, au moment où la pandémie a été déclarée à la mi-mars 2020, que les mesures de protection y compris les masques et les autres équipements de protection individuelle n'étaient pas disponibles en nombres suffisants. Il faut décrier l'absence de planification et de mesures préventives dans les CSLD alors que les autorités savaient que ces lieux étaient très vulnérables à la propagation du virus et que la maladie risquait d'y faire des ravages auprès des résidents.

Au final, la crise sanitaire causée par la COVID-19 a permis d'exposer une réalité troublante : les adultes âgés les plus vulnérables vivent dans des milieux où les préposés sont débordés, mal rémunérés et où leurs compétences spécialisées ne sont ni reconnues, ni valorisées.

Les facteurs menant à une telle situation sont complexes. D'emblée, il semble clair que l'absence d'un financement adéquat est l'une des causes du problème. Toutefois, le portrait des enjeux et des problématiques – en particulier les conditions de travail – auxquels les CSLD sont confrontés depuis de nombreuses années suggère que les attitudes sociétales envers le vieillissement, particulièrement envers les personnes les plus âgées et les plus vulnérables, sont peut-être la véritable pierre angulaire du problème. C'est l'hypothèse que nous soutenons : malgré une évolution démographique prévisible marquée par le vieillissement de la population et l'augmentation du nombre de personnes âgées en perte d'autonomie, s'en sont suivis des choix politiques et sociaux à l'égard des aînés les plus vulnérables qui pourraient résulter, en partie à tout le moins, d'une culture âgiste.

---

22. Ontario Health Coalition et Unifor, « Caring in Crisis: Ontario's Long-Term Care PSW Shortage » (2019), en ligne (pdf) : *Unifor* <www.unifor.org/sites/default/files/documents/document/final_psw_report.pdf>.

Quelle société vieillissante post-COVID ?

La pandémie actuelle prendra éventuellement fin. Déjà, deux mois après le début de la crise au Canada, des mesures de déconfinement progressif étaient envisagées. Que se passera-t-il dans les CSLD une fois le pire passé ? Des mesures seront peut-être proposées pour améliorer le taux de rétention des travailleurs ou pour restructurer la façon dont les soins sont fournis. Les gouvernements ouvriront peut-être leurs bourses pour injecter des fonds permettant de parer au manque de personnel ou pour améliorer l'état physique de certains lieux, répondant ainsi à celles et ceux qui réclament depuis longtemps de tels changements. Certes, ces améliorations d'ordre structurel, organisationnel et administratif seraient bienvenues, mais nous suggérons qu'elles resteront insuffisantes si elles ne sont pas portées par une profonde réflexion, sociale comme politique, sur les valeurs qui nous animent face au vieillissement et aux personnes âgées. Cette réflexion exige en premier lieu de reconnaître la prévalence de l'âgisme et d'admettre que ce phénomène a pu orienter et oriente toujours nos choix de société. Demandons-nous ceci : la situation de grande vulnérabilité dans laquelle sont plongés les CSLD depuis plusieurs années résulte-t-elle, en partie, des choix de société âgistes, témoignant d'indifférence, voire de négligence ? Nous répondons par l'affirmative.

Réfléchir à notre système de valeurs face au vieillissement et remettre en question l'âgisme sont des tâches colossales, mais elles sont réalisables. Nous proposons en particulier une mesure en amont. Comme l'âgisme est affaire de représentations qui s'acquièrent tôt dans la vie, il est essentiel d'intégrer dans le parcours éducationnel des plus jeunes une sensibilisation quant aux préjugés et à la discrimination âgistes. En outre, en milieu de travail, et particulièrement en contexte de soins de longue durée, cette sensibilisation à l'âgisme est une condition *sine qua non* à la fois pour le personnel soignant, les dirigeants et les résidents[23]. Il est plausible de penser que la sensibilisation à l'âgisme via la formation serait le point de départ d'un changement au système de valeurs.

Par ailleurs, pour concrétiser ce changement de valeurs, il faut franchir un pas de plus et mettre en place des dispositifs politiques et

23. Ashley Lytle et Sheri R Levy, « Reducing Ageism: Education About Aging and Extended Contact With Older Adults » (2019) 59:3 Gerontologist 580 ; Brian J Gleberzon, « Combating Ageism Through Student Education » (2002) 9:2 Topics in Clinical Chiropractic 41.

légaux qui pourront servir de tremplin pour le déploiement d'initiatives visant à contrer l'âgisme. Tel est l'objectif derrière, par exemple, une convention internationale protégeant les droits des personnes âgées[24], un instrument qui pourrait leur donner une voix, des choix et *de facto* la possibilité d'exiger des acteurs sociaux le respect de leur personne et de leur santé.

---

24. HelpAge International, « A New Convention on the Rights of Older People: A Concrete Proposal » (2015), en ligne (pdf) : *United Nations* <social.un.org/ageing-working-group/documents/sixth/HelpAgeInternational.pdf>.

CHAPTER D-3

Fault Lines: COVID-19, the *Charter*, and Long-term Care*

Martha Jackman**

Abstract

COVID-19 has underscored the crucial role of the single-payer health care system in ensuring access to care based on need, consistent with the *Canadian Charter of Rights and Freedoms* (the *Charter*) and international human rights guarantees. But significant fault lines were exposed when health authorities across the country concentrated their pandemic readiness efforts on maximizing hospitals' capacity to deal with the anticipated surge of COVID-19 patients, without considering the potentially disastrous consequences for an already struggling long-term care system. COVID-19 laid bare the reality that barriers to care continue to exist as a function of who patients are and where they are being treated. Focussing on COVID-19 hospital transfer decisions and their impact on the life, liberty, and security of the person and the equality rights of long-term care residents, this chapter argues that governments and health care decision makers in Canada must recognize that access to a comprehensive range of care is a fundamental right, and that human rights–based accountability is urgently needed in the battle against COVID-19, and beyond.

* This paper is dedicated to Robert Bycraft, Anna Babey, and the many other grandparents, parents, and friends whose lives have been cut short by the COVID-19 pandemic./Ce chapitre est dédié à Robert Bycraft et Anna Babey, ainsi qu'aux nombreux autres grands-parents, parents, amis et amies qui ont perdu la vie en raison de la pandémie de COVID-19.

** Professor of Constitutional Law in the Faculty of Law, University of Ottawa.

Résumé
Les failles : la COVID-19, la *Charte* et les soins de longue durée

La COVID-19 a souligné le rôle crucial du système de soins de santé à payeur unique pour assurer l'accès aux soins en fonction des besoins, conformément à la *Charte canadienne des droits et libertés* et aux garanties internationales relatives aux droits de la personne. Mais d'importantes failles ont été mises au jour lorsque les autorités sanitaires de tout le pays ont concentré leurs efforts sur l'optimisation de la capacité des hôpitaux en prévision de l'augmentation du nombre de patients et de patientes atteints de la COVID-19, sans tenir compte des conséquences potentiellement désastreuses sur un système de soins de longue durée déjà en difficulté. La pandémie a révélé qu'il existe toujours des obstacles aux soins en fonction de l'identité des patients et des patientes et de l'endroit où ils et elles sont traités. Ce chapitre porte sur les décisions en matière de transfert hospitalier dans le contexte de la COVID-19, ainsi que sur leurs répercussions sur la vie, la liberté et la sécurité des personnes et sur les droits à l'égalité des résidents et résidentes des centres de soins de longue durée. Il soutient que les gouvernements et les décideurs en matière de soins de santé au Canada doivent reconnaître que l'accès à une gamme complète de soins est un droit fondamental et qu'il est urgent de miser sur une responsabilisation fondée sur les droits de la personne dans la lutte contre la COVID-19, et au cours des années qui viennent.

COVID-19 has underscored the crucial role of Canada's single-payer system[1] in ensuring that everyone has access to care based on need, in keeping with the *Canada Health Act*,[2] the *Canadian Charter of Rights and Freedoms* (the *Charter*),[3] and international human rights guarantees.[4] But significant fault lines in our system were also exposed when health authorities across the country concentrated their pandemic

1. Ian Austen, "Two Medical Systems, Two Pandemic Responses", *New York Times* (1 May 2020), online: <www.nytimes.com/2020/05/01/world/canada/america-canada-coronavirus-comparison.html>.
2. *Canada Health Act*, RSC 1985, c C-6.
3. *Canadian Charter of Rights and Freedoms*, Part I of the *Constitution Act, 1982*, being Schedule B to the *Canada Act 1982* (UK), 1982, c 11 [*Charter*].
4. See generally Martha Jackman, "*Charter* Review of Health Care Access" in Joanna Erdman, Vanessa Gruben & Erin Nelson, eds, *Canadian Health Law and Policy*, 5th ed (Toronto: LexisNexis Canada, 2017) 71.

readiness efforts on maximizing the capacity of hospitals to treat those who fell critically ill.[5] In pursuit of that objective, non-emergency surgeries (including for cancer, cardiac, and other serious illnesses) were cancelled, and diagnostic testing, clinical trials, palliative care, medically assisted death, and other hospital services were suspended.[6] The resulting costs to life and health are only now being calculated.[7]

Beyond hospitals, the pandemic also deepened pre-existing access problems within the broader health care system. As other chapters in this book document, long-standing inequalities in health services for Indigenous people on reserves and in rural and remote areas were amplified,[8] as were barriers to prison health,[9]

5. Kelly Grant & Thu Thanh Ha, "How Shoring up Hospitals for COVID-19 Contributed to Canada's Long-term Care Crisis", *Globe and Mail* (20 May 2020), online: <www.theglobeandmail.com/canada/article-how-shoring-up-hospitals-for-covid-19-contributed-to-canadas-long/>; Karen Howlett, "With an Early Focus on Seniors' Residences, Kingston Has So Far Avoided the Brunt of COVID-19", *Globe and Mail* (28 April 2020), online: <www.theglobeandmail.com/canada/article-with-an-early-focus-on-seniors-residences-kingston-has-so-far/>.
6. Avis Favaro, Elizabeth St Phillips & Ben Cousins, "Canadian Hospitals Take Drastic Measures Amid COVID-19 Crisis", *CTV News* (16 March 2020), online: <www.ctvnews.ca/health/coronavirus/canadian-hospitals-take-drastic-measures-amid-covid-19-crisis-1.4855849>; Financial Accountability Office of Ontario, *Ontario Health Sector: A Preliminary Review of the Impact of the COVID-19 Outbreak on Hospital Capacity* (Toronto: Queen's Printer for Ontario, 2020) at 9; Charlie Pinkerton, "Ontario Inches Closer to Allowing More Doctor Support at Long-term Care Homes", *iPolitics* (6 May 2020), online: <ipolitics.ca/2020/05/06/ontario-inches-closer-to-allowing-more-doctor-support-at-long-term-care-homes/>; Tom Blackwell, "In Scramble over COVID, the Patients We Forgot", *Ottawa Citizen* (9 May 2020) NP1, 3.
7. Financial Accountability Office of Ontario, *supra* note 6; Blackwell, *supra* note 6; Sandie Rinaldo & Jonathan Forani "Provinces Begin to Address Backlog of Surgeries in Wake of COVID-19", *CTV News* (9 May 2020), online: <www.ctvnews.ca/health/coronavirus/provinces-begin-to-address-backlog-of-surgeries-in-wake-of-covid-19-1.4932424>.
8. See Anne Levesque & Sophie Thériault, this volume, Chapter D-6; Aimée Craft, Deborah McGregor & Jeffery Hewitt, this volume, Chapter A-2; "Assembly of First Nations Declares State of Emergency on COVID-19 Pandemic" (24 March 2020), online: *Assembly of First Nations* <www.afn.ca/assembly-of-first-nations-declares-state-of-emergency-on-covid-19-pandemic/>; Teresa Wright, "First Nations Health Authorities Tell Commons Committee They Need More PPE" (24 May 2020), online: *Times Colonist* <www.timescolonist.com/first-nations-health-authorities-tell-commons-committee-they-need-more-ppe-1.24140363>.
9. "COVID-19 Status Update" (23 April 2020), online (pdf): *Office of the Correctional Investigator* <www.oci-bec.gc.ca/cnt/rpt/pdf/oth-aut/oth-aut20200423-eng.pdf>; "COVID-19 et prisons provinciales – Les données doivent être rendues publiques" (22 April 2020), online: *Ligue des droits et libertés* <liguedesdroits.ca/prison-covid19-transparence/>; Adelina Iftene, this volume, Chapter D-5.

abortion,[10] pharmaceuticals,[11] mental health care,[12] and substance dependence programs.[13] Perhaps most egregiously, the failed promise of equal access to care is reflected in the massive death toll in long-term care.[14] While we expect, and domestic and international human rights demand, that care be available based on need, COVID-19 has laid bare the reality that barriers continue to exist as a function of who patients are and where they are being treated. Focussing on the unfolding tragedy in long-term care, I will argue that governments and health care decision makers must recognize that access to a comprehensive range of care is a fundamental right, and that human rights-based accountability is urgently needed in the battle against COVID-19, and beyond.

COVID-19 and Long-term Care

In 2018–2019 there were 191,835 long-term care residents in 1,319 facilities in Canada, outside Quebec.[15] Their average age was 83, and over two thirds were women.[16] Over 70% had heart/circulation diseases; over half, musculoskeletal diseases; and over two thirds, neurological diseases, including dementia.[17] Like hospitals, long-term care facilities

10. Laura Osman, "Advocates Sound Alarm Over COVID-19 Limiting Access to Contraceptives, Abortion", *Globe and Mail* (2 April 2020), online: <www.theglobeandmail.com/canada/article-advocates-sound-alarm-over-covid-19-limiting-access-to-contraceptives/>.
11. Jan Malek, "COVID-19 Shows that Pharmacare is Needed Now" (24 April 2020), online: *Council of Canadians* <canadians.org/analysis/covid-19-shows-pharmacare-needed-now>.
12. Kathleen Finlay, "So Far, Canada's Answer to COVID-19 Mental Health Crisis Doesn't Measure up", *Ottawa Citizen* (30 April 2020), online: <ottawacitizen.com/opinion/finlay-so-far-canadas-answer-to-covid-19-mental-health-crisis-doesnt-measure-up/>.
13. Raina Delisle, "It's a Risky Time for People with Substance Use Issues", *The Tyee* (14 April 2020), online: <thetyee.ca/News/2020/04/14/How-A-Pandemic-Affects-Substance-Use/>; Jeff Turnbull, Vern White & Mathieu Fleury, "Treat Drug Addiction Through Safe Supply", *Ottawa Citizen* (25 May 2020) A7.
14. Tonda MacCharles, "82% of Canada's COVID-19 Deaths Have Been in Long-term Care, New Data Reveals", *Toronto Star* (7 May 2020), online: <www.thestar.com/politics/federal/2020/05/07/82-of-canadas-covid-19-deaths-have-been-in-long-term-care.html>.
15. "Quick Stats: Profile of Residents in Residential and Hospital-Based Continuing Care, 2018–2019" at Table 1, online: *Canadian Institute for Health Information* <www.cihi.ca/en/quick-stats>.
16. *Ibid* at Table 3.
17. *Ibid* at Table 6. See eg "British Columbia Residential Care Facilities Quick Facts Directory 2018 Summary" (2018) at 1, online (pdf): *Office of the Seniors Advocate*

are regulated at the provincial/territorial level. But although governments provide over 70% of funding, long-term care falls outside the framework of the *Canada Health Act* and the single-payer system.[18] As a result, levels of public investment and ownership vary greatly across the country, and no national standards or uniform conditions exist.[19]

There is wide agreement that "funding and services have not kept pace with increasing needs of residents."[20] Over the past 20 years, health care and seniors' advocacy groups, labour unions, public interest and human rights organizations, researchers, ombudspersons, and governments themselves, have criticized the substandard condition of many facilities, the insufficient level of public funding, the undue financial burden placed on low-income seniors, wait times, and the lack of oversight and failure to enforce existing health, safety and other regulations.[21] Poor wages and working conditions, as Pat Armstrong,

---

<www.seniorsadvocatebc.ca/app/uploads/sites/4/2018/01/QuickFacts2018-Summary.pdf>; "This is Long-Term Care 2019" (2019) at 3, online (pdf): *Ontario Long-term Care Association* <www.oltca.com/OLTCA/Documents/Reports/TILTC2019web.pdf>.

18. "Health Spending—Nursing Homes" (last visited 29 May 2020) online (pdf): *Canadian Institute for Health Information* <secure.cihi.ca/free_products/infosheet_Residential_LTC_Financial_EN.pdf>; Steven Lewis, "The Pandemic and the Politics of Long-term Care in Canada", *Policy Options* (11 May 2020), online: <policyoptions.irpp.org/magazines/may-2020/the-pandemic-and-the-politics-of-long-term-care-in-canada/>. In Ontario, for example, provincial funding in 2018 was $4.28 billion or 7% of the overall provincial health budget; "About Long-term Care in Ontario: Facts and Figures" (last visited 29 May 2020), online: *Ontario Long Term Care Association* <www.oltca.com/oltca/OLTCA/Public/LongTermCare/FactsFigures.aspx>.

19. "Ensuring Quality Care for All Seniors" (November 2018) 5-11, online (pdf): *Canadian Health Coalition* <www.healthcoalition.ca/wp-content/uploads/2019/12/Seniors-care-policy-paper-FINAL-Version-Dec-2019.pdf>; "Seniors in Transition: Exploring Pathways Across the Care Continuum" (2017), online (pdf): *Canadian Institute for Health Information* <www.cihi.ca/sites/default/files/document/seniors-transition-methodology-notes-2017-en-web.pdf>; "Dignity Denied: Long-term Care and Canada's Elderly" (February 2007) at 7, online (pdf): *National Union of Public and General Employees* <nupge.ca/sites/default/files/publications/Medicare/Dignity_Denied.pdf>.

20. "This is Long-Term Care 2016" (2016) at 8, online (pdf): *Ontario Long-term Care Association* <www.oltca.com/OLTCA/Documents/Reports/TILTC2016.pdf>.

21. See e.g. National Union of Public and General Employees, *supra* note 19; Canadian Health Coalition, *supra* note 19; Andrew Longhurst, *"Privatization and Declining Access to Seniors' Care: An Urgent Call for Policy Change"* (March 2017), online (pdf): *BC Office of the Canadian Centre for Policy Alternatives* <www.policyalternatives.ca/sites/default/files/uploads/publications/BC%20Office/2017/03/access_to_seniors_care_report_170327%20FINAL.pdf>; "Situation Critical: Planning, Access, Levels of Care and Violence in Ontario's Long-Term Care" (21 January 2019), online (pdf):

Hugh Armstrong, and Ivy Bourgeault outline in Chapter E-1 of this book, have been a long-standing issue for staff—also predominantly women.[22]

In this context, the impact on long-term care residents of COVID-19 and government decisions around how to manage it were catastrophic. While "horror stories from Italy convinced authorities they had to free up room on [hospital] wards and in intensive care units for potential COVID-19 sufferers,"[23] the obvious threat the virus posed in long-term care facilities did not seem to register. In Quebec, like elsewhere:

> The focus was on ensuring hospitals could manage their COVID-19 caseloads… Officials opened as many hospital beds as possible by postponing elective surgeries and relocating patients to hotels or elder-care facilities. Instead, the virus struck hardest in those very facilities for seniors. The ensuing devastation came in a part of the system that had long been underfunded, understaffed, and packed with vulnerable people.[24]

Reports from across Canada suggest that, even as patients were being moved from hospitals to long-term care facilities without prior testing, long-term care residents infected with COVID-19 were being denied transfer to hospitals for treatment.[25] Personal protective equipment and

---

Ontario Health Coalition <www.ontariohealthcoalition.ca/wp-content/uploads/FINAL-LTC-REPORT.pdf>; Québec, Protecteur du citoyen, *Mémoire du Protecteur du citoyen présenté à la Commission de la santé et des services sociaux* (Québec: Protecteur du citoyen, 2013).

22. Pat Armstrong, Hugh Armstrong and Ivy Bourgeault, this volume, Chapter E-1; Canadian Health Coalition, *supra* note 19 at 11.

23. Blackwell, *supra* note 6 at A3; Grant & Ha, *supra* note 5.

24. Tu Thanh Ha, "How Quebec's Long-term Care Homes Became Hotbeds for the COVID-19 Pandemic", *Globe and Mail* (7 May 2020), online: <www.theglobeandmail.com/canada/article-how-quebecs-long-term-care-homes-became-hotbeds-for-the-covid-1/>; Grant & Ha, *supra* note 5; Andrew MacLeod, "BC Seniors' Homes Problems Aren't New: The Virus Showed They Could be Deadly", *The Tyee* (27 April 2020), online: <thetyee.ca/News/2020/04/27/BC-Seniors-Homes-Problems-Arent-New/>.

25. Elizabeth Payne & Andrew Duffy, "No-transfer Practice at Some Long-term Care Homes Denies Residents Rights During Pandemic, Say Advocates", *Ottawa Citizen* (14 April 2020), online: <ottawacitizen.com/news/local-news/no-transfer-policy-at-some-long-term-care-homes-denies-residents-rights-during-pandemic-say-advocates/>; Terry Reith, "'No Benefit' to Sending Seniors ill with COVID-19 to Hospital, Some Nursing Homes Tell Loved Ones", *CBC News* (3 April 2020), online: <www.cbc.ca/news/health/covid-19-long-term-care-1.5519657>; Editorial, "How Canada Gave a Pandemic Key to the Country's

COVID-19 testing were heavily rationed and, in some cases unavailable, allowing the virus to spread rapidly among patients and staff, and leading to deadly outbreaks in almost every province.[26] As workers fell ill or were quarantined, conditions for remaining staff and residents deteriorated further.[27] Reports emerged of nurses caring for 20 to 30 residents without assistance, staff working back-to-back 12- and 16-hour shifts; and infected and non-infected residents sharing rooms. By the time health authorities intervened in one Montréal home, "residents were found … unclothed, severely malnourished, dehydrated, without their medication and left in their feces and urine…"[28]

Patient transfers from hospitals to long-term care facilities did not end in Ontario until a month after the province declared a state of emergency, with "hospital occupancy rates at a historic low … 69%, down from 96% before the pandemic."[29] Only then did the province

---

Nursing Homes", *Globe and Mail* (14 April 2020), online: <www.theglobeandmail.com/opinion/editorials/article-how-canada-gave-a-pandemic-the-key-to-the-countrys-nursing-homes/>. For instance, as of April 17, 2020, only 22 of 899 nursing and retirement home residents with COVID-19 in Toronto were being treated in hospital and, as of May 12, only 24 of 364 cases of COVID-19 in long-term care in Alberta had been hospitalized; Grant & Ha, *supra* note 5.

26. Kathy Tomlinson & Grant Robertson, "It Took a Pandemic: Why Systemic Deficiencies in Long-term Care Facilities Pose such a Danger to our Seniors", *Globe and Mail* (27 April 2020), online: <www.theglobeandmail.com/canada/article-it-took-a-pandemic-why-systemic-deficiencies-in-long-term-care/>; Rachel D'Amore, "Coronavirus: Hospital cleaners, admin workers need PPE too, unions say", *Global News* (7 April 2020), online: <globalnews.ca/news/6787770/coronavirus-canada-protective-equipment-cleaners-admin-workers/>.

27. Grant & Ha, *supra* note 5; Murray Brewster & Vassy Kapelos, "Military Alleges Horrific Conditions, Abuse in Pandemic-hit Ontario Nursing Homes", *CBC News* (26 May 2020), online: <www.cbc.ca/news/politics/long-term-care-pandemic-covid-coronavirus-trudeau-1.5584960>.

28. Jillian Kestler-D'Amours, "Canada: How Quebec Elder Care Homes Became Coronavirus Hotspots", *Al Jazeera* (24 April 2020), online: <www.aljazeera.com/indepth/features/canada-quebec-elder-care-homes-coronavirus-hotspots-200423214537289.html>; Lorian Hardcastle, "Opinion: COVID-19 Lays Bare Poor Conditions in Long-term Care Homes", *Edmonton Journal* (24 April 2020), online: <edmontonjournal.com/opinion/columnists/opinion-covid-19-lays-bare-poor-conditions-in-long-term-care-homes/>; Ha, *supra* note 24; Andrew Rankin, "Nova Scotia Delayed Implementing Federal COVID-19 Guidelines for Long-term Care Homes", *The Chronicle Herald* (1 May 2020), online: <www.thechronicleherald.ca/news/provincial/ns-government-delayed-implementing-federal-covid-19-guidelines-for-long-term-care-homes-444709/>; Elizabeth Payne, "Nurses Raise Concerns About Care Home", *Ottawa Citizen* (8 May 2020) A4.

29. Ha, *supra* note 24; Laura Stone, Karen Howlett & Les Perreaux, "Ontario Places Pause on Transfers from Hospitals to Seniors' Facilities; Quebec Issues Third Plea for Military Aid", *Globe and Mail* (16 April 2020), online: <www.theglobeandmail.

announce a plan to increase testing of staff and residents, restrict staff from working in more than one facility, and redeploy health care staff into long-term care homes.[30] A week later, Ontario and Quebec called on the federal government for aid from the Canadian military.[31]

COVID-19, the *Charter*, and Access to Care

By mid-April, governments across Canada recognized that long-term care homes were "facing unprecedented tragedy."[32] Ontario Premier Doug Ford admitted: "I know the system … is absolutely broken."[33] In Quebec, Premier François Legault asked: "How could we have gotten into the situation we're in, where we didn't take care of our elders, the most vulnerable?" Prime Minister Justin Trudeau confessed: "We are failing our parents, our grandparents, our elders."[34] What governments and health officials have not yet acknowledged is that this public health failure is an equally inexcusable violation of *Charter* and international human rights.

Article 12 of the *International Covenant on Economic, Social and Cultural Rights* recognizes the right of everyone in Canada "to the enjoyment of the highest attainable standard of physical and mental health,"[35] including to "medical service and medical attention in the event of sickness,"[36] "without discrimination of any kind."[37] Although the Canadian *Charter* does not contain an explicit right to health care,

com/canada/article-ontario-places-pause-on-transfers-from-hospitals-to-seniors/>.

30. Financial Accountability Office of Ontario, *supra* note 6 at 9, 20.
31. Lee Berthiaume, "Trudeau Says Military Is Short-Term Solution to Caring for Seniors", *CTV News* (23 April 2020), online: <www.ctvnews.ca/health/coronavirus/trudeau-says-military-is-short-term-solution-to-caring-for-seniors-1.4908602>.
32. "COVID-19 Action Plan: Long-term Care Homes—Version 1" (15 April 2020), online: *Ontario Ministry of Long-term Care* <www.ontario.ca/page/covid-19-action-plan-long-term-care-homes>.
33. Antonella Artuso, "Ford Vows to Fix Broken Long-term Care System", *Toronto Sun* (6 May 2020), online: <torontosun.com/news/provincial/ford-vows-to-fix-broken-long-term-care-system>.
34. Berthiaume, *supra* note 31.
35. *International Covenant on Economic, Social and Cultural Rights*, 16 December 1966, Can TS 1976 No 46 at art 12(1) (entered into force 3 January 1976, accession by Canada 19 May 1976).
36. *Ibid* art 12(2)(d).
37. *Ibid* art 2(2). See generally Bruce Porter, "International Human Rights in Anti-Poverty and Housing Strategies: Making the Connection" in Martha Jackman & Bruce Porter, eds, *Advancing Social Rights in Canada* (Toronto: Irwin Law, 2014) 33.

s. 7 protects "the right to life, liberty and security of the person and the right not to be deprived thereof except in accordance with the principles of fundamental justice."[38] Section 15 guarantees "equal protection and equal benefit of the law without discrimination and, in particular, without discrimination on the basis of race, national or ethnic origin, colour, religion, sex, age or mental or physical disability."[39]

The Supreme Court of Canada has affirmed that the *Charter* applies not only to governments, but to hospitals and other private entities when they are delivering publicly funded health care.[40] The Court has been more ambivalent about the *Charter* as a source of positive obligations to ensure access to such care.[41] In *Eldridge v British Columbia (Attorney General)*, the Court held that failure to provide interpretation services for the Deaf within the public system violated the *Charter*'s equality guarantees.[42] In contrast, in *Auton (Guardian ad litem of) v British Columbia (Attorney General)*, the Court ruled that lack of funding for autism treatment did not violate s. 15, because a finding of discrimination "would effectively amend the medicare scheme and extend benefits beyond what it envisions—core physician-provided benefits plus non-core benefits at the discretion of the province."[43] In *Chaoulli v Québec (Attorney General)*, striking down Quebec's ban on private health insurance, Chief Justice McLachlin opined that, "The *Charter* does not confer a freestanding constitutional right to health care. However, where the government puts in place a scheme to provide health care, that scheme must comply with the *Charter*."[44] Six years later, in *Canada (Attorney General) v. PHS Community Services Society*, the Court found that, by depriving the Insite supervised injection facility's clients of "potentially lifesaving medical care … and health-protecting services," the federal government had violated their rights to life and security of the person.[45]

38. *Charter*, *supra* note 3 at s 7.
39. *Ibid*, s 15.
40. [1997] 3 SCR 624, [*Eldridge*]. See Martha Jackman, "The Application of the Canadian *Charter* in the Health Care Context" (2001) 9 Health L Rev 22.
41. See Jackman, *supra* note 4; Martha Jackman, "Health Care and Equality: Is There a Cure?" (2007) 15 Health LJ 87.
42. *Eldridge*, *supra* note 40 at para 80.
43. 2004 SCC 78 at para 44.
44. 2005 SCC 35 at para 104.
45. 2011 SCC 44 [*Insite*] at paras 91-92. In the Chief Justice's words, at para 93: "Where a law creates a risk to health by preventing access to health care, a deprivation of the right to security of the person is made out… Where the law creates a risk not just to the health but also to the lives of the claimants, the deprivation is even clearer."

Given these inconsistencies in the case law, it is unclear to what extent pandemic-related inaction by health care decision makers within and outside the long-term care system, including the failure to provide sufficient COVID-19 testing or personal protective equipment, to adopt adequate containment measures, or to effectively regulate care and working conditions, might be subject to *Charter* review.[46] While *Chaoulli* and *Auton* have been heavily criticized, both decisions present significant hurdles for *Charter* claimants seeking positive rights to care under s. 7, or arguing s. 15 demands more than equal access to existing services.[47] But even a narrow reading of the current jurisprudence leaves little doubt that decisions to move patients from hospitals to long-term care, and not to transport long-term care residents to hospitals if they fell ill with COVID-19, raise serious *Charter* concerns.

In terms of s. 7, these transfer decisions severely compromised long-term care residents' physical and mental health, security, and autonomy. They increased not just the risk of death, but of dying in "horrific conditions."[48] These decisions did not, by any measure, comply with principles of fundamental justice. They were made without "effective participation" by those affected;[49] they undermined their own public health objectives,[50] and they caused grossly disproportionate harm.[51] As one adult son described his mother's experience—after being hospitalized for a fall that left her incapable of returning home—of being moved to a long-term care facility where she died of COVID-19 three weeks later: "When I talked to her at the hospital, she

46. In *Ontario Nurses Association v Eatonville/Henley Place*, 2020 ONSC 2467, nurses working in four Ontario long-term care facilities obtained an injunction, based in part on s. 7 of the *Charter*, forcing their employers to provide them with adequate personal protective equipment; Katherine Lippel, this volume, Chapter E-3; Vanessa Gruben & Louise Bélanger-Hardy, this volume, Chapter E-4.

47. See e.g. Marie-Claude Prémont, "L'affaire *Chaoulli* et le système de santé du Québec : cherchez l'erreur, cherchez la raison" (2006) 51:1 McGill LJ 167; Martha Jackman, "'The Last Line of Defence for [Which?] Citizens': Accountability, Equality and the Right to Health in *Chaoulli*" (2006) 44:2 Osgoode Hall LJ 349; Colleen M Flood, Kent Roach & Lorne Sossin, eds, *Access to Care, Access to Justice: The Legal Debate Over Private Health Insurance in Canada* (Toronto: University of Toronto Press, 2005); Jackman, "Health Care and Equality", *supra* note 41; Natasha Bakht, "Furthering an Economic/Social Right to Healthcare: The Failure of *Auton v British Columbia*" (2005) 4:2 JL and Equality 241; Jackman, *supra* note 4.

48. Brewster & Kapelos, *supra* note 27; *Insite*, *supra* note 45 at paras 91-93.

49. *New Brunswick (Minister of Health and Community Services) v G(J)*, [1999] 3 SCR 46 at paras 73, 119.

50. *Insite*, *supra* note 45 at paras 129-32.

51. *Ibid* at para 133.

told me she didn't want to go there... But they were telling her that was the only option she had."[52]

The violations of long-term care residents' s. 7 rights can be ascribed to *where* they receive care. As the *Globe and Mail* averred: "If COVID-19 has shown us anything, it's that whatever is done to protect hospitals during pandemics also needs to be done for seniors' facilities."[53] The infringement of long-term care residents' s. 15 rights are, on the other hand, a consequence of *who* they are. More than anywhere else, long-term care residents in Canada bore a disparate and unfair share of the cost of pandemic preparedness.[54] Unlike other Canadians, they did not receive the "equal protection and equal benefit" of that pandemic planning, or of the publicly funded health and hospital system it was trying to defend.[55] Instead, "most of the nursing—and retirement home residents who have succumbed to COVID-19 in Canada died inside the virus-stricken understaffed facilities, while many of the hospital beds opened up for coronavirus patients sat empty."[56]

Whether intentional or not, governments' pandemic-related actions and inaction amounted to differential, adverse, treatment that perpetuated disadvantage on a number of prohibited grounds of discrimination—most obviously on the basis of age. As Martine Lagacé, Linda Garcia, and Louise Bélanger-Hardy contend in Chapter D-2 of this book,[57] the role of ageism cannot be overstated: "The COVID-19 pandemic may be unprecedented in recent times, but its impacts are being felt in [long-term care facilities] because of the way seniors' care has been undervalued, underfunded, and privatized."[58] Carole Estabrooks summarizes a more insidious dynamic: "About 95 per cent

52. Grant & Ha, *supra* note 5. The facility in question was one singled out in the Canadian Military's damning report on conditions in five Ontario nursing homes the military was called in to support; Brewster & Kapelos, *supra* note 27.
53. Globe and Mail, *supra* note 25.
54. Adelina Comas-Herrera et al, *Mortality Associated with COVID-19 Outbreaks in Care Homes: Early International Evidence* (last modified 21 May 2020), online (pdf): *International Long Term Care Policy Network* <ltccovid.org/wp-content/uploads/2020/05/Mortality-associated-with-COVID-21-May-6.pdf>.
55. *Eldridge*, *supra* note 40; *Quebec (Attorney General) v A*, 2013 SCC 5 at para 332.
56. Brewster & Kapelos, *supra* note 27.
57. Martine Lagacé, Linda Garcia & Louise Bélanger-Hardy, this volume, Chapter D-2.
58. Andrew Longhurst & Kendra Strauss, "Time to End Profit-making in Seniors' Care" (22 April 2020), online: *Policynote* <www.policynote.ca/seniors-care-profit/>; Susan Bradley, "Our Long-term Care System is Failing Because we are Ageist", *Ottawa Citizen* (26 May 2020) A9; Susan Mintzberg, "Long-Term Care: Please Let Families Back In", *Ottawa Citizen* (15 May 2020) A7.

of the paid workers are women, 75 per cent of unpaid caregivers are women, two thirds of people with dementia are women and two thirds of people in nursing home are women. This is a highly gendered environment and we cannot ignore that."[59] Coupled with age and sex, social condition is, as Steven Lewis underscores, also a salient factor: "Less prosperous seniors who far outnumber those able to afford upscale alternatives are left to take their chances in the nursing home lottery."[60] Finally, a large majority of long-term care residents have physical and cognitive illnesses and impairments. The multiple failures that contributed to COVID-19 deaths and other harms in long-term care are, as Tess Sheldon and Ravi Malhotra's chapter (Chapter D-9 in this volume) explains, manifestations of systemic discrimination based on physical and mental disability that s. 15 prohibits.[61]

Charter rights are not absolute. Section 1 permits, "such reasonable limits prescribed by law as can be demonstrably justified in a free and democratic society."[62] Intensive hospital care or ventilation is not the appropriate treatment in every COVID-19 case.[63] Most long-term care residents have pre-existing medical conditions, and many are in their final years of life.[64] In one Nova Scotia facility experiencing one of Canada's worst COVID-19 outbreaks, only 20 of almost 500 residents had not signed do-not-resuscitate orders.[65] It is likely that only a small minority of residents would opt for aggressive COVID-19 hospital treatment, were it offered. But it is virtually certain that no one would have chosen to be needlessly exposed to the virus, to receive little or no palliative or comfort care, and to die in forced isolation, leaving family and loved ones to cope with anger as well as grief.[66]

59. Michael Brown, "How COVID-19 Overwhelmed Canada's Long-term Care System" (22 April 2020), online: *Folio* <www.folio.ca/how-covid-19-overwhelmed-canadas-long-term-care-system/>; Pat Armstrong et al, *Re-imagining Long-term Residential Care in the COVID-19 Crisis* (April 2020) at 7-8, online (pdf): *Canadian Centre for Policy Alternatives* <www.policyalternatives.ca/sites/default/files/uploads/publications/National%20Office/2020/04/Reimagining%20residential%20care%20COVID%20crisis.pdf>.
60. Lewis, *supra* note 18; *Canadian Health Coalition, supra* note 19; *National Union of Public and General Employees, supra* note 19.
61. Tess Sheldon & Ravi Malhotra, this volume, Chapter D-9.
62. Colleen M Flood, Bryan Thomas and Kumanan Wilson, this volume, Chapter C-1.
63. Amina Zafar, "What Is a Ventilator and Who Gets One If COVID-19 Turns Catastrophic in Canada?" *CBC News* (31 March 2020), online: <www.cbc.ca/news/health/covid19-ventilators-1.5515550>; Payne & Duffy, *supra* note 25.
64. *Canadian Institute for Health Information, supra* note 15.
65. Rankin, *supra* note 28.
66. Grant & Ha, *supra* note 5; Reith, *supra* note 25; Payne & Duffy, *supra* note 25.

In the face of COVID-19, governments and health authorities were forced to make difficult decisions and trade-offs, in a very short time, often with incomplete and inadequate information.[67] As Colleen M. Flood, Bryan Flood and Kumanan Wilson discuss, the courts will undoubtedly exercise considerable deference towards those choices.[68] Containing the pandemic and ensuring hospitals and the health care system could manage the projected surge of COVID-19 patients were critical objectives. There were, however, long-standing warnings about the danger of viral outbreaks in long-term care facilities. Recommendations made by the Federal SARS Commission to mitigate this risk were disregarded, even as measures were implemented in hospitals.[69] With few exceptions,[70] the threat to long-term care residents was not seriously considered in most parts of the country. Inattention to the vulnerability of the long-term care system and to the particular risks created by COVID-19 transfers was not a rational means of achieving public health objectives and, in fact, undermined them. In sum, the failure to take into account, much less adopt proactive measures to protect, the life, security, and equality of long-term care residents, cannot be justified under s. 1.

The Way Forward: Comprehensiveness and Accountability

With long-term care residents representing only 1% of the Canadian population, but over 80% of COVID-19 deaths,[71] political leaders have expressed sadness and shame; governments have committed to conducting post-pandemic reviews; health profession regulatory bodies have signalled their intention to investigate; criminal inquiries have been called for, and lawsuits have been launched.[72]

67. Flood, Thomas & Wilson, this volume, Chapter C-1.
68. *Ibid*; Paola Loriggio, "Proposed Lawsuits Raise Questions on 'Reasonable Care'" *Ottawa Citizen* (4 May 2020) NP3.
69. Tomlinson & Robertson, *supra* note 26; *Globe and Mail*, *supra* note 25.
70. Howlett, *supra* note 5; Hina Alan, "Vancouver Care Homes Cast a Wide Net in Testing", *Ottawa Citizen* (11 May 2020) NP4.
71. MacCharles, *supra* note 14.
72. Nick Boisvert, "Ontario Long-Term Care Homes in Scathing Report Could Face Charges, Says Ford", *CBC News* (26 May 2020), online: <www.cbc.ca/news/canada/toronto/ontario-military-ltc-report-1.5585131>; Christopher Guly, "I Know How Precious It Is to Say Goodbye to a Parent Dying In Care", *The Tyee* (12 May 2020), online: <thetyee.ca/Analysis/2020/05/12/Precious-Goodbye-Parent-Dying-In-Care/?utm_source=daily&utm_medium=email&utm_campaign=130520>; Béatrice Roy-Brunet, "CHSLD : deux organisations veulent que

Whatever answers are ultimately found, the devastation caused by the pandemic has exposed two significant fault lines that must be addressed.

The lack of comprehensiveness of the single-payer system is the first and most obvious barrier to equal access to care for long-term care residents, like for those seeking home care, mental health, substance abuse, pharmaceutical, dental, and other crucial services that are excluded from the *Canada Health Act*.[73] The prioritization of hospitals in governments' pandemic preparedness is a reflection of the privileged status of acute care delivered by physicians and hospitals within the public system.[74] William Lahey observes that:

> [The] compartmentalization of our health care system obscures the nature of the premises and assumptions on which we implicitly rely when we make choices about ... funding... These include a premise that ... curing is more important than caring (as well as prevention), that dealing with the episodic illness of the healthy is more important than dealing with chronic illness and disability, and that physical health takes priority over other dimensions of health, including mental health.[75]

Expansion of the *Canada Health Act* to include long-term care has been identified as a major step towards resolving underfunding, lack of uniform standards, and other systemic problems within the current "mashup of systems" as the National Institute on Aging has described it.[76] Whether through the *Canada Health Act* or new federal/provincial/territorial framework legislation, the full integration of long-term care

le gouvernement brasse la cage", *Journal de Montréal* (13 April 2020), online: <www.journaldemontreal.com/2020/04/13/chsld--deux-organisations-veulent-que-le-gouvernement-brasse-la-cage>; Loriggio, *supra* note 68.

73. Jackman, "Health Care and Equality", *supra* note 41.
74. Lewis, *supra* note 18; Colleen M Flood, Bryan Thomas & David Rodriguez, "The Role of Law in the Rise and Fall of Canadian Medicare" in Joanna Erdman, Vanessa Gruben & Erin Nelson, eds., *Canadian Health Law and Policy*, 5th ed (Toronto: LexisNexis Canada, 2017) 51.
75. William Lahey, "The Legal Framework of Canada's Health Care System" in Jocelyn Downie, Karen McEwen & William MacInnis, eds, *Dental Law in Canada* (Markham: Lexis/Nexis Butterworths, 2004) 29 at 79-80.
76. MacCharles, *supra* note 14; Armstrong, *supra* note 59; *National Union of Public and General Employees*, *supra* note 19; "Mark Hancock Calls on Trudeau to Fix Long-term Care Now" (21 May 2020), online: *Canadian Union of Public Employees* <cupe.ca/mark-hancock-calls-trudeau-fix-long-term-care-now>.

into a comprehensive, properly funded, public health care system is long overdue.[77]

The tragic experience of COVID-19 in long-term care highlights a second barrier to equal access to care for disadvantaged groups: the absence of human rights-based accountability for health care decision-making.[78] The interdependence between human rights and accountability is well understood internationally, and UN treaty monitoring bodies have criticized Canada for failing to meet its obligations in both areas.[79] Paul Hunt explains:

> Because of the complexity, sensitivity and importance of many health policy issues, it is vitally important that effective, accessible and independent mechanisms of accountability are in place to ensure that reasonable balances are struck by way of fair processes that take into account all relevant considerations, including the interests of disadvantaged individuals, communities, and populations.[80]

The life, security of the person, and equality rights of long-term care residents were directly implicated in choices made by governments and health and hospital authorities in relation to the pandemic—most especially by COVID-19 transfer decisions. Yet no accountability mechanisms were in place to ensure that the rights and interests of this vulnerable group were taken into account in early pandemic planning, or that long-term care residents or those advocating on their behalf were included or even consulted, until the rising death count became a national disgrace. Over and above public expressions "of anger … sadness … frustration [and] grief,"[81] federal and provincial/territorial governments must accept and affirm that access to care is a

77. Lewis, *supra* note 18; *Canadian Health Coalition*, *supra* note 19.
78. See generally Martha Jackman, "The Future of Health Care Accountability: A Human Rights Approach" (2016) 47:2 Ottawa L Rev 437; Colleen M Flood & Sujit Choudhry, *Strengthening the Foundations: Modernizing the Canada Health Act, Discussion Paper No 13* (Saskatoon: Royal Commission on the Future of Health Care in Canada, 2002).
79. Paul Hunt, *Promotion and Protection of All Human Rights, Civil, Political, Economic, Social and Cultural Rights: Report of the Special Rapporteur on the Right of Everyone to the Enjoyment of the Highest Attainable Standard of Physical and Mental Health*, UNHRC, 7th Sess, Un Doc A/HRC/7/11 (2008) at paras 51, 65; Porter, *supra* note 37.
80. Hunt, *supra* note 79 at para 64.
81. Brewster & Kapelos, *supra* note 27.

human right. And they must establish effective mechanisms, capable of preventing and providing meaningful accountability and remedies for violations of that right.

There is a growing understanding in Canada that "the pandemic did not cause the crisis; it came along and caused a massive shock to the long-term care system, shining a harsh light on fractures in a system that was ripe for catastrophe."[82] The lack of comprehensiveness and the absence of effective human rights accountability mechanisms within our publicly funded system, have created and reinforced discriminatory barriers to care for many disadvantaged groups. For residents in long-term care, caught in the battle against COVID-19, these fault lines have proven fatal. Moving forward, "The hope is that the deaths of so many people will not be in vain, and governments will finally take serious action."[83]

82. Brown, *supra* note 59.

83. Mohammed Adam, "Long-term Care: Military Support is a Short-term Solution Only", *Ottawa Citizen* (1 May 2020) A7.

CHAPTER D-4

The Front Line Defence: Housing and Human Rights in the Time of COVID-19

Leilani Farha* and Kaitlin Schwan**

Abstract

COVID-19 has laid bare the failure of Canadian governments to effectively implement the right to housing. In this chapter, we argue the pandemic presents Canada with the opportunity to correct the structural weaknesses of our housing system to ensure housing for all and reposition housing as a social good rather than a commodity. We explore how housing status has been determinative of outcomes for three vulnerable populations during the pandemic—people experiencing homelessness, survivors of intimate partner violence, and low-income renters. Their experiences demonstrate the urgent need for a rights-based approach to housing, highlighting the importance of breathing life into the *National Housing Strategy* and the *National Housing Strategy Act*. We argue that Canadian governments must act before this opportunity passes them by; otherwise they will find that though the pandemic itself is over, housing inequality has only worsened.

* Former United Nations Special Rapporteur on the Right to Housing and Global Director of The Shift.

** Director of Research at The Shift.

Résumé
Défense de première ligne : logement et droits de la personne au temps de la COVID-19

La COVID-19 a mis en évidence l'échec des gouvernements canadiens à mettre en œuvre de manière effective le droit au logement. Dans ce chapitre, nous soutenons que la pandémie offre au Canada une occasion de corriger les faiblesses structurelles de notre système afin de garantir un logement pour tous et de repositionner le logement comme un bien social plutôt qu'une marchandise. Nous examinons comment la situation du logement a été déterminante pour trois populations vulnérables pendant la pandémie : les sans-abri, les victimes de violence conjugale et les locataires à faible revenu. Leurs expériences démontrent le besoin urgent d'adopter une approche fondée sur les droits des personnes, en soulignant l'importance de donner un nouveau souffle à la Stratégie nationale sur le logement et à la *Loi sur la stratégie nationale sur le logement*. Nous soutenons que les gouvernements, au Canada, doivent agir sans attendre, sans quoi ils ne pourront que constater, une fois la pandémie terminée, que les inégalités en matière de logement n'ont fait que s'aggraver.

Governments around the world have invoked "stay home" policies as central to flattening the pandemic curve and reducing SARS-CoV-2 infection rates. In Canada and many other countries, housing, therefore, has become the front line of defence against the virus. If the centrality of housing to human life were ever in doubt, COVID-19 has powerfully illuminated that having a home is a matter of life or death. It has also illuminated that a one-size health policy does not fit all.

As Canada struggles with homelessness, high rates of core housing need, and a severe lack of affordable housing,[1] compliance with these policies is impossible for hundreds of thousands of people. While public health orders like "stay at home," "wash your hands," and "physically distance" are seemingly neutral, they have a disproportionate impact on people who are unsheltered or living

1. Stephen Gaetz et al, "The State of Homelessness in Canada 2016" (2016), online (pdf): *Canadian Observatory on Homelessness* <www.homelesshub.ca/sites/default/files/attachments/SOHC16_final_20Oct2016.pdf>.

in inadequate housing. It is impossible to physically distance while sleeping on a mat in a homeless shelter. It is difficult to properly wash your hands if you live under a water boil advisory on a First Nations reserve. How can you "stay home" if you haven't got one or if you have aged out of your foster-care home? For these populations, absent state intervention and support, the mantra of "stay home" serves as a mockery more than a life-saving measure.

COVID-19 has laid bare the failure of Canadian governments to effectively implement the right to housing. In this chapter, we argue the pandemic presents Canada with the opportunity to revisit our housing system to ensure housing for all, establish housing as a human right, and reposition housing as a social good rather than an asset or commodity. We explore how housing status has been determinative of outcomes for three vulnerable populations during the pandemic—people experiencing homelessness, survivors of intimate partner violence (IPV), and low-income renters. The experiences of these populations demonstrate the urgent need for a rights-based approach to housing in Canada.

An Uneven Burden: Housing Status as Determinative of Outcomes During COVID-19

Scholars, activists, and community leaders around the world have emphasized that COVID-19 has illuminated and exacerbated pre-existing inequities. This is vividly true with respect to housing, with emerging evidence that those residing in poor neighbourhoods, over-crowded or inadequate housing, or experiencing homelessness, are more likely to contract COVID-19 and experience worse health outcomes, including death.[2] While many media campaigns have centred on the message that "we're all in this together," it is clear that the burden of COVID-19 is not shared evenly.

Thus the importance of the human right to adequate housing becomes starkly visible. This right is codified in Article 11.1 of the *International Covenant on Economic, Social, and Cultural Rights*, defined as "the right of everyone to an adequate standard of living for himself

2. See e.g. Dennis Culhane, et al, "Estimated Emergency and Observational/ Quarantine Capacity Need for the U.S. Homeless Population Related to COVID-19 Exposure by County; Projected Hospitalizations, Intensive Care Units, and Mortality" (27 March 2020), online (pdf): <endhomelessness.org/wp-content/ uploads/2020/03/COVID-paper_clean-636pm.pdf>.

and his family, including adequate food, clothing and housing, and to the continuous improvement of living conditions."[3] To understand housing as a right is to understand it as a *social good*. This means recognizing housing as more than mere physical shelter, but as foundational to safety, security, and dignity.[4] In the wake of COVID-19, those without access to adequate housing face profound and complex barriers to staying safe or protecting themselves—in some cases threatening their very survival.

Despite Canadian governments' acknowledgement that COVID-19 presents disproportionate risks and burdens for some groups, policies have not been responsive enough to the distinct needs and human rights of vulnerable groups. Emerging evidence suggests the enforcement of universal public health orders has had detrimental effects on some of the most marginalized people in society and that targeted interventions for vulnerable groups have not always been rights-compliant or improved outcomes.[5] People experiencing homelessness, survivors of IPV, and low-income renters are three such groups whose housing status has powerfully shaped their pandemic experiences.

People Experiencing Homelessness

Despite being one of the wealthiest countries in the world, homelessness is commonplace in most Canadian communities. Policy responses to homelessness have historically been emergency-focused, with many cities failing to see significant reductions in homelessness year after year.[6] As a result, COVID-19 has emerged when hundreds of thousands of people live unsheltered on the streets, trying to survive through a patchwork of shelters, drop-ins, and social services.

For those trapped in situations of homelessness, COVID-19 presents a severe threat to life, security, and dignity. Those on the streets

3. *International Covenant on Economic, Social and Cultural Rights*, 16 December 1966, 993 UNTS 3 art 11 (entered into force 3 January 1976).
4. *Report of the Special Rapporteur on Adequate Housing as a Component of the Right to an Adequate Standard of Living, and on the Right to Non-discrimination in This Context*, UNHRC, 43rd Sess., Annex, Agenda Item 3, UN Doc A/HRC/43/43/Add.1 (2020).
5. "Statement–Inequality Amplified by COVID-19 Crisis" (2020), online: *Canadian Human Rights Commission* <www.chrc-ccdp.gc.ca/eng/content/statement-inequality-amplified-covid-19-crisis>. See also Alex Neve & Isabelle Langlois, "Canada's COVID-19 Response Demands Human-Rights Oversight", *Globe and Mail* (15 April 2020), online: <www.theglobeandmail.com/opinion/article-canadas-covid-19-response-demands-human-rights-oversight/>.
6. Gaetz, *supra* note 1.

face significant health challenges, including high rates of respiratory illnesses, putting them at greater risk of contracting COVID-19.[7] This population often lacks access to clean water and sanitation facilities, and available homeless shelters often operate at or over capacity,[8] making it impossible to physically distance.

Given that the Government of Canada's primary public health directive in response to COVID-19 was to "stay home," the policy response should have been the immediate elimination of street homelessness. Other cities have implemented urgent efforts to transition people off the streets in the wake of COVID-19, including Belfast (Ireland)[9] and London (U.K.).[10] Such a response would have been in keeping with the *National Housing Strategy Act* (NHSA), which stipulates that the housing policy of the Government of Canada recognizes that the right to adequate housing is a fundamental human right affirmed in international law. Under international human rights law, homelessness is understood as a *prima facie* violation of the right to housing, and requires immediate steps be taken to eliminate it. Instead of implementing a national rights-based response to homelessness and housing need during COVID-19, the federal government has largely left it to provinces/territories and municipalities to develop their own approaches.[11] As a result, policy responses to homelessness have primarily taken four forms: (i) *abandonment*, (ii) *emergency relief*, (iii) *heightened law enforcement*, and (iv) *housing-led responses*.

Abandonment

In some Canadian communities, people experiencing homelessness have been left to fend for themselves in the wake of COVID-19. With

7. Robert W Aldridge et al, "Morbidity and Mortality in Homeless Individuals, Prisoners, Sex Workers, and Individuals with Substance Use Disorders in High-Income Countries: A Systematic Review and Meta-Analysis", The Lancet (2018) 391:10117 241.
8. "Shelter Capacity Report 2018" (2018), online: *Employment and Social Development Canada* <www.canada.ca/en/employment-social-development/programs/homelessness/publications-bulletins/shelter-capacity-2018.html>.
9. See e.g. Shauna Corr, "Coronavirus Pandemic Sees Homeless People in Belfast All Get a Place to Stay", *Belfast Live* (30 March 2020), online: <www.belfastlive.co.uk/news/belfast-news/coronavirus-pandemic-sees-homeless-people-18009375>.
10. See e.g. "Coronavirus: Rough Sleepers in London Given Hotel Rooms", *BBC News* (21 March 2020), <www.bbc.com/news/uk-england-london-51987345>.
11. David Hulchanski at al, "Finding Room: Policy Options for a Canadian Rental Housing Strategy" (2005) 92:10 Urban Studies 1881.

limited access to personal protective equipment (PPE), dwindling staff, and insufficient facilities to enable physical distancing, many shelters and drop-ins have had little choice but to reduce services or close entirely (despite best efforts).[12] While some communities have replaced or adapted services, advocates report significant gaps across the country.

Emergency Relief

Some cities have chosen to create new temporary shelters in existing public or private buildings (e.g., convention centres), seeking to enable physical distancing (e.g., through positioning floor mats six feet apart). While these facilities have been welcomed in some communities, they have also been criticized for failing to comply with public health measures and displacing people from existing support systems.[13]

Heightened Law Enforcement

Many cities have heightened law enforcement to control the spread of COVID-19 among people experiencing homelessness and the general public. In cities such as Hamilton and Vancouver, people experiencing homelessness report being ticketed $880 for failing to physically distance.[14] Tent encampments have increasingly been forcibly evicted under the mantle of COVID-19, often in ways that are contrary to international human rights law.[15]

---

12. See e.g. Al Donato "Homeless Canadians Face Increasing Danger Because Of COVID-19 Lockdowns", *Huffington Post* (last updated 18 April 2020), online: <www.huffingtonpost.ca/entry/homeless-canadians-danger-coronavirus_ca_5e83665fc5b62dd9f5d6a72d>.
13. See e.g. Cathy Crowe, "Fifty Days into the COVID-19 Pandemic, and Homeless People Are Still in a Desperate Situation" (28 April 2020), online (blog): *Rabble* <rabble.ca/blogs/bloggers/cathy-crowes-blog/2020/04/fifty-days-covid-19-pandemic-and-homeless-people-are-still>.
14. See e.g. Matthew Van Dongen, "'I Can't Pay It Anyway': Why Are Hamilton Police Ticketing The Homeless During The Covid-19 Pandemic?" *Toronto Star* (21 April 2020), online: <www.thestar.com/news/gta/2020/04/21/i-cant-pay-it-anyway-why-are-hamilton-police-ticketing-the-homeless-during-the-covid-19-pandemic.html>.
15. Leilani Farha & Kaitlin Schwan, "A National Protocol for Homeless Encampments in Canada: A Human Rights Approach" (30 April 2020), online (pdf): *United Nations Special Rapporteur on the Right to Adequate Housing* <www.unhousingrapp.org/user/pages/07.press-room/A%20National%20Protocol%20for%20Homeless%20Encampments%20in%20Canada.pdf>.

Housing-led Responses

Some communities have focused on transitioning people experiencing homelessness into temporary housing, such as hotel rooms. While some communities have provided access to housing for those on the streets, in many cases the provision of housing or hotel rooms has been temporary (e.g., three to six months) and is often not accompanied by a commitment to permanent housing post-pandemic.

***

While the landscape continues to shift, it is not clear that these current policies will result in permanent housing for people who are homeless. To comply with domestic and international human rights housing obligations, all levels of government must immediately focus on adopting housing-led responses that result in access to permanent housing for those who are homeless. If not, the lessons learned from this pandemic will not result in greater safety for all when the next pandemic hits, and "staying home" will continue to be a privilege, not a right.

Survivors of Intimate Partner Violence

Intimate partner violence (IPV) was already a crisis in Canada prior to the arrival of COVID-19. IPV accounts for one of every four violent crimes reported to police in Canada, with research consistently indicating widespread underreporting.[16] Despite the prevalence of this violence, national data indicates that violence against women (VAW) shelters have been systematically operating at or over capacity for years.[17]

The emergence of COVID-19 has exacerbated IPV globally, and Canada is no exception. Evidence indicates public health orders to "stay home" have contributed to IPV that is more violent, more frequent, and more dangerous, with United Nations Population Fund suggesting three months of quarantine will result in a 20% increase in IPV around the world.[18] For many women, staying home means being

16. Statistics Canada, *Family Violence in Canada: A Statistical Profile, 2011*, by Marie Sinha, Catalogue No 85-002-X (Ottawa: Statistics Canada, 25 June 2013).
17. Statistics Canada, *Canadian Residential Facilities for Victims of Abuse, 2017/2018*, Catalogue No 11-001-X (Ottawa: Statistics Canada, 17 April 2019).
18. "Impact of the COVID-19 Pandemic on Family Planning and Ending Gender-Based Violence, Female Genital Mutilation and Child Marriage" (27 April 2020),

trapped with abusive partners while also being cut off from social supports and avenues for access to justice.[19] Alarmingly, gender-based violence against Indigenous women and girls has increased steeply in Canada during COVID-19.[20] Given these realities, the United Nations Secretary-General has called on all States to urgently address the "horrifying global surge" of domestic violence.[21] Importantly, the increase in IPV domestically and globally has been accompanied by significant concerns that child abuse is also increasing but going unreported.[22]

The ability to escape IPV is tied to women's ability to access adequate housing, which is structurally undermined by the feminization of poverty and the reality women are more likely to work poorer-paying jobs, head single-parent households, and assume responsibility for caregiving and childcare.[23] These factors contribute to higher levels of core housing need for women in Canada, and untold levels of homelessness.[24] In the face of COVID-19, these inequities mean that women are more likely to be laid off, face eviction or other housing challenges, and experience food insecurity—particularly if they are experiencing multiple forms of marginalization.

COVID-19 has thus deepened the housing and safety challenges many women and their children in Canada were facing prior to the

---

online (pdf): *United Nations Population Fund* <www.unfpa.org/sites/default/files/resource-pdf/COVID-19_impact_brief_for_UNFPA_24_April_2020_1.pdf>. See also Amanda Taub, "A New Covid-19 Crisis: Domestic Abuse Rises Worldwide", *The New York Times* (14 April 2020), online: <www.nytimes.com/2020/04/06/world/coronavirus-domestic-violence.html>.

19. "COVID-19 and Violence Against Women–What the Health Sector/System Can Do" (7 April 2020), online (pdf): *World Health Organization* <apps.who.int/iris/bitstream/handle/10665/331699/WHO-SRH-20.04-eng.pdf>.
20. Teresa Wright, "Violence Against Indigenous Women During Covid-19 Sparks Calls for MMIWG Plan", *CBC Manitoba* (10 May 2020), online: <www.cbc.ca/news/canada/manitoba/violence-against-indigenous-women-action-plan-covid-19-mmiwg-1.5563528>.
21. "UN Chief Calls for Domestic Violence 'Ceasefire' Amid 'Horrifying Global Surge'", *UN News* (6 April 2020), online: <news.un.org/en/story/2020/04/1061052>.
22. See e.g. Michelle Ward, "Increase in Child Abuse a Big Concern during COVID-19 Pandemic", *Globe and Mail* (20 March 2020), <www.theglobeandmail.com/canada/article-increase-in-child-abuse-a-big-concern-during-covid-19-pandemic/>.
23. Amy Van Berkum & Abe Oudshoorn, "Best Practice Guideline for Ending Women's and Girl's Homelessness" (2015), online (pdf): *London Homelessness* <londonhomeless.ca/wp-content/uploads/2012/12/Best-Practice-Guideline-for-Ending-Womens-and-Girls-Homelessness.pdf>.
24. "Core Housing Need Data–By the Numbers" (2019), online: *Canada Mortgage and Housing Corporation* <www.cmhc-schl.gc.ca/en/data-and-research/core-housing-need/core-housing-need-data-by-the-numbers>.

pandemic. Most critically, it has illuminated the ways IPV is directly linked to the housing crisis that Canada has failed to address for decades. These realities demonstrate the urgent need for a gendered analysis of housing policy in Canada and a need to ensure the right to housing is actualized for women and their children.

Low-Income Renters

The Canadian housing system is characterized by a severe lack of affordable housing. Since the over-emphasis on a market-driven housing system from the mid-1980s onward, Canadian governments have overseen massive decreases in social housing stock, weaker tenant protections, and huge increases in housing need and homelessness.[25] More broadly, Canadian cities are increasingly shaped by the "financialization of housing," characterized by the expanded role and unprecedented dominance of financial markets and corporations in the housing sector.[26]

The pandemic has further exacerbated the pre-existing housing challenges faced by those living on low incomes. Low-income renters are more likely to be working low-paying service jobs, and national data indicates since the emergence of COVID-19, half of those making under $16 an hour in Canada have either lost their jobs or a majority of their hours since February 2020.[27] Just two months into the pandemic, national data indicated that one in three Canadians feared they would miss rent or mortgage payments.[28]

To date, Canadian governments have provided limited rent relief during the pandemic. Instead, they have focused on replacing income, but in light of the pre-pandemic housing affordability issues, an income-only approach is proving insufficient. Recognizing the widespread employment challenges faced during the pandemic, a majority of Canadian provinces and territories have adopted moratoriums on

25. John R Graham, Karen Swift & Roger Delaney, *Canadian Social Policy: An Introduction*, 4th ed, (Toronto: Pearson Canada, 2012).
26. *Report of the Special Rapporteur on Adequate Housing as a Component of the Right to an Aequate Standard of Living, and on the Right to Non-Discrimination in this Context*, UNHRC, 34th Sess, Annexe, Agenda Item 3, UN Doc A/HRC/34/51 (2017).
27. David Macdonald, "Early Warning: Who's Bearing the Brunt of COVID19's Labour Market Impacts?" (9 April 2020), online: *Behind the Numbers* <behindthe-numbers.ca/2020/04/09/early-warning-covid19-labour-market-impacts/>.
28. "State of Renters During COVID-19: Survey Report" (2020), online: *Acorn Canada* <acorncanada.org/resource/state-renters-during-covid-19-survey-report>.

evictions.[29] However, neither the federal government nor most provincial/territorial governments have provided protection from eviction for tenants post-pandemic. This means Canada may see a wave of mass evictions when public health orders are lifted and landlords demand back pay for rent arrears.[30] When asked whether the federal government would provide rent relief to tenants, Prime Minister Justin Trudeau responded, "If provinces, in whom the relationship between renters and landlords is their jurisdiction, want to move forward with more help for residential rent, they can of course do that."[31]

In contrast to the challenges low-income renters currently face, COVID-19 is presenting financial actors with further opportunities to cannibalize the Canadian housing market for profit. By spring 2020, the Bank of Canada had already brought in BlackRock (the world's largest asset manager) to assist in developing an economic recovery plan, with direct bearing on Canada's housing market.[32] Like the financial crisis of 2008, COVID-19 provides real estate investment trusts (REITS) and private equity firms the opportunity to capitalize on distressed assets in the housing market by purchasing cheap debt (foreclosed mortgages) from banks and other lenders. Speaking to this opportunity in the American context, David Schechtman of the Meridian Capital Group stated: "Our thoughts and prayers are with all of our fellow Americans and nobody wants to capitalize on anybody's misfortune. But I will tell you, real-estate investors—when you take the emotion out of it—many of them have been waiting for this for a decade."[33]

---

29. "COVID-19: Eviction Bans and Suspensions to Support Renters" (25 March 2020), online: *Canadian Housing and Mortgage Corporation* <www.cmhc-schl.gc.ca/en/rental-housing/covid-19-eviction-bans-and-suspensions-to-support-renters>.
30. See e.g. Alastair Sharp, "Toronto Renters in for a 'Bloodbath' of Evictions after Pandemic Ends, Advocate Warns", *Toronto Star* (22 May 2020), online: <www.thestar.com/news/canada/2020/05/22/toronto-renters-in-for-terrifying-bloodbath-of-evictions-after-pandemic-ends.html>.
31. See Trudeau quoted in Jennifer Pagliaro, "Nearly Half of Canadian Tenants Fear They Can't Pay Rent on May 1—and Provinces, Feds Can't Agree on Where Relief Will Come From", *Toronto Star* (29 April 2020), online: <www.thestar.com/news/city_hall/2020/04/28/as-may-1-nears-tenants-and-landlords-worry-about-lack-of-rent-relief-from-queens-park-ottawa.html>.
32. Kevin Carmichael, "Why the Bank of Canada Needs BlackRock's Help While Fighting the Coronavirus Downturn", *Financial Post* (1 April 2020), online: <business.financialpost.com/news/economy/why-the-bank-of-canada-needs-blackrocks-help-while-fighting-the-coronavirus-downturn>.
33. Konrad Putzier & Peter Grant, "Real-Estate Investors Eye Potential Bonanza in Distressed Sales", *Wall Street Journal* (7 April 2020), online: <www.wsj.com/articles/real-estate-investors-eye-potential-bonanza-in-distressed-sales-11586260801>.

Without significant state investment and strong regulation of financial actors, COVID-19 will result in a deepening of the housing crisis the country was in prior to the pandemic. This will likely hit low-income renters the hardest, and for many the Canada Emergency Response Benefit will be inaccessible, insufficient, or too short-term to prevent eviction or the worsening of housing need.

Realizing the Right to Housing in a Post-Pandemic Canada

COVID-19 has exposed the way governments in Canada have failed to effectively implement the right to housing. As such, the pandemic has provided governments with an opportunity to correct the structural weaknesses of the Canadian housing system by breathing life into the *National Housing Strategy* and the *National Housing Strategy Act*. Opportunities of this nature do not often arise. Governments must act before it passes them by, otherwise they will find that though the pandemic itself is over, housing inequality has only worsened.

The Canadian government therefore must:

- Ensure access to safe and long-term adequate housing for people experiencing homelessness, including through the acquisition of hotels/motels, office spaces, or other properties. In the short term, these might act as emergency respite centres. These should be repurposed as expeditiously as possible into social, deeply affordable housing.
- Adopt a nationwide prohibition on all evictions (except in cases where a resident is harming others) and foreclosures during the pandemic and for a reasonable time thereafter, ensuring renters have adequate legislative protections and resources to prevent mass evictions post-pandemic.
- Establish an independent national human rights body responsible for providing oversight on federal expenditures in response to COVID-19, to ensure government investments advance all human rights. This national body should seek to advance the right to housing across Canada, in concert with the Department of Justice and the Canadian Human Rights Commission.
- Adopt a rights-based approach to homeless encampments,[34] upholding the human rights and dignity of encampment

34. Farha & Schwan, *supra* note 15.

residents while they wait for adequate, affordable housing solutions.

- Ensure no one in Canada is rendered homeless or heavily indebted as a result of the pandemic, providing people experiencing housing needs with reasonable financial support to ensure that COVID-19 does not worsen their housing status, poverty, or level of debt.
- Immediately appoint, and robustly fund, the Federal Housing Advocate and the National Housing Council to act as government accountability mechanisms and to ensure emergent issues are brought to the attention of government.
- Ensure any approach to economic recovery includes a commitment to realizing the right to housing for all people in Canada, prioritizing the housing needs of those who are most marginalized, including women and Indigenous Peoples.

CHAPTER D-5

COVID-19 in Canadian Prisons: Policies, Practices and Concerns*

Adelina Iftene**

Abstract

Correctional Service of Canada and the provincial prison systems have a duty to provide incarcerated individuals with health services that are comparable to those in the community, but they have failed to do so during the COVID-19 pandemic. There are inherent practical difficulties to implementing health care in prisons. In addition, prison demographics include a higher proportion of populations that are vulnerable to disease. These factors together mean that the prison response to COVID-19 must involve depopulation and the implementation of guidelines provided by public health agencies in all institutions. So far, the measures taken have been insufficient, as is evidenced by the rapid rates of spread of COVID-19 within prisons compared to the community. An overreliance on segregation of incarcerated individuals as a preventive measure raises concerns under s. 7 of the *Charter of Rights and Freedoms* (the *Charter*) and international human rights. There are also equality concerns under s. 15 of the *Charter*, given the high proportion of Indigenous people in prison. Ultimately, some prison systems'

* I am very grateful to Anthony Doob, Constance MacIntosh, Andrew Martin, Martha Paynter, Sophie Theriault, and the anonymous peer reviewer for their thoughtful comments and suggestions on earlier drafts. I am also thankful to Maggie McCann (JD'21) for her outstanding research assistance.

** Assistant Professor at Schulich School of Law, Dalhousie University and incoming Associate Director of the Health Law Institute at Dalhousie.

failure to respond adequately to the pandemic impedes the successful flattening of the curve and will likely prolong the life of COVID-19 in the community. Such failure highlights the urgency of the much-needed prison reforms that have been overlooked for decades.

Résumé
La COVID-19 dans les prisons canadiennes : politiques, pratiques et inquiétudes

Le Service correctionnel du Canada et les systèmes carcéraux provinciaux ont le devoir de fournir aux personnes incarcérées des services de santé comparables à ceux qui sont offerts dans la communauté, mais ils ont failli à cette tâche pendant la pandémie de COVID-19. La mise en œuvre des services de santé en milieu carcéral comporte des difficultés pratiques inhérentes. En outre, la population carcérale comprend une proportion plus élevée d'individus vulnérables aux maladies. En raison de ces facteurs, la réponse des prisons à la COVID-19 doit passer par le dépeuplement et la mise en œuvre dans tous les établissements des directives fournies par les agences de santé publique. Jusqu'à présent, les mesures prises ont été insuffisantes, comme en témoigne la vitesse de propagation du virus dans les prisons par rapport à celle dans les collectivités. Le recours excessif à la ségrégation des personnes incarcérées comme mesure préventive soulève des inquiétudes au regard de l'article 7 de la *Charte des droits et libertés* et des normes internationales relatives aux droits de la personne. Il existe aussi des préoccupations sur le plan de l'égalité en vertu de l'article 15 de la *Charte*, étant donné la forte proportion d'Autochtones en prison. En fin de compte, l'incapacité de certains systèmes carcéraux à répondre adéquatement à la pandémie entrave l'aplatissement de la courbe et prolongera probablement la durée de vie de la COVID-19 dans la communauté. Cette incapacité souligne l'urgence de procéder à des réformes indispensables dans les prisons, que l'on a négligées pendant des décennies.

On any given day, about 40,000 people are incarcerated in a Canadian prison,[1] either in a provincial institution (where

1. Public Safety Canada, *Corrections and Conditional Release Statistical Overview* (2018 Annual Report), (Ottawa: Public Works and Government Services Canada, August 2019) at 47.

people who await trial or serve short sentences are placed) or a federal penitentiary (where people serve sentences of two years or more). Correctional Service Canada (CSC), the governmental agency responsible for the management of the federal prisons, and the provincial prison systems have a duty under international standards and national laws to provide incarcerated individuals with health services comparable to those in the community.[2] The *Corrections and Conditional Release Act (CCRA)*, which governs the federal correctional system, states that an individual must have access to essential health care and reasonable access to non-essential health care, both of which are to be provided at "professionally accepted standards."[3] The Office of the Correctional Investigator (OCI), the federal prison ombudsperson, has interpreted the *CCRA*[4] to implicitly impose an obligation on CSC to seek alternatives to incarceration for those whose health becomes incompatible with imprisonment.[5] Similarly, most provincial correctional systems contain statutory duties owed to incarcerated people, particularly as they relate to health care.[6]

The COVID-19 pandemic has exposed limitations to the governments' ability or willingness to discharge these duties and to ensure the safety of those in custody. Given the background of the enhanced vulnerabilities of prisoners and of the risks posed by congregated living spaces generally, and prisons in particular, the response needed to protect those in custody in times of crisis must be principled, immediate, and multifaceted. First, as also discussed by Jennifer A Chandler et al, in Chapter D-10 of this volume, it is difficult, if not impossible, to implement necessary preventive measures (particularly physical distancing and cleanliness)[7] in congregate living spaces, including

---

2. *The United Nations Standard for Minimum Rules for the Treatment of Prisoners (the Nelson Mandela Rules)*, GA Res 70/175, UNGAOR, 70th Sess, UN Doc A/RES/70/175 (2015) at Rules 24–35.
3. *Corrections and Conditional Release Act*, SC 1992, c 20, s 86 [*CCRA*].
4. *Ibid*, s 121.
5. Canada, Office of the Correctional Investigator, *An Investigation of the Correctional Service's Mortality Review Process*, (Ottawa: Office of the Correctional Investigator, December 2018) at 7.
6. See e.g. *Correctional Services Act*, SNS 2005, c 37, s 25; *Correctional Services Regulations*, NS Reg 99/2006, s 45(2)(b); *Ministry of Correctional Services Act*, RSO 1990, c M 22, s 24(1); *The Correctional Services Act*, 1998 CCSM c C 230, s 37.
7. On public health measures see "Infection Prevention and Control During Health Care When Novel Coronavirus (nCoV) Infection is Suspected" (19 March 2020), online (pdf): *World Health Organization Publications* <perma.cc/5WNC-7URB>.

prisons, without first depopulating to the extent possible.[8] Second, depopulation must be done safely, while providing individuals with adequate community supports upon release. Third, prevention protocols following the public health agencies' guidelines must be adopted and implemented in all institutions.[9]

Some prison systems in Canada failed to respond adequately to the pandemic, leading to serious consequences for incarcerated people and the community. In the next sections, after providing a brief overview of the heightened vulnerability of prisoners to COVID-19, I will critique the prison responses to the pandemic, both from a rights and public health perspective. I will conclude with a set of recommendations that should be considered to avoid future crises in prisons.

Demographic and Institutional Risk Factors

Prison populations are at higher risk of contracting COVID-19 and of developing severe complications. The prison environment heightens these risks and prisons are ill prepared to prevent or address infections among those in custody.[10]

Most of the marginalized groups discussed in this book are overrepresented in prisons: individuals with serious health issues, including physical and mental disability, people living in poverty, Indigenous people and other racial minorities, and homeless people.[11] Due to their pre-existing social marginalization, in addition to

8. See e.g. Sean Fine, "Calls to Release Some Prisoners Intensify as First Known Coronavirus Outbreak Announced in Canadian Prison", *The Globe and Mail* (30 March 2020), online: <perma.cc/J57V-EUQ3>; Jane Philpott & Kim Pate, "Time Running out to Protect Prisoners and Prison Staff from Calamity", *Policy Options* (31 March 2020), online: <perma.cc/675U-GTJL>; "UNODC, WHO, UNAIDS and OHCHR Joint Statement on COVID-19 in Prisons and Other Closed Settings", (13 May 2020), online: *World Health Organization* <perma.cc/S4KM-H7E7> [WHO].
9. "Interim Guidance on Management of Coronavirus Disease 2019 (COVID-19) in Correctional and Detention Facilities" (23 March 2020), online (pdf): *Centers for Disease Control and Prevention* <perma.cc/GR4Q-N7UB>; WHO, *supra* note 8.
10. Talka Burki, "Prisons Are 'in no Way Equipped' to Deal with COVID-19" (2020) 395:10234 Lancet at 1411; Laura Hawks et al, "COVID-19 in Prisons and Jails in the United States" [2020] JAMA Intern Medicine.
11. Law Council of Australia, *Prisoners and Detainees*, Final Report Part 1 (Canberra: Law Council of Australia, August 2018) at 6; Canada, Office of the Correctional Investigator, *Aging and Dying in Prison: An Investigation into the Experiences of Older Individuals in Federal Custody*, (Ottawa: Office of the Correctional Investigator, 2019) at 20, 27; Senate Committee on Human Rights, *Interim Report–Study on the Human Rights of Federally-Sentenced Persons: The Most Basic Human Right Is to Be*

the risks posed to health by prison environments, incarcerated individuals have higher rates than those in the community for most of the illnesses identified by preliminary studies as COVID-19 risk factors.[12] These include cardiovascular disease, cancer, diabetes, asthma, other respiratory diseases, HIV, hepatitis C, tuberculosis,[13] and mental illnesses.[14] Substance use and addiction rates are also high, while harm reduction measures remain limited in prisons.[15] Moreover, the prison demographic in Canada has been aging over the last decade. Currently, in federal prisons, 25% of people are considered elderly,[16] which has also been deemed a risk factor for COVID-19.[17]

In addition, there are barriers to accessing satisfactory health care in custody. In federal prisons, for instance, these include a lack of adequate training for first responders (generally correctional officers) for identifying and managing health crisis, overcrowding, a lack of escorting officers (resulting in difficulties taking people to community

---

Treated as a Human Being, (Ottawa: Senate Committee on Human Rights, February 2019) (Chair: The Honourable Wanda Elaine Thomas Bernard); Office of the Correctional Investigator, News Release, "Indigenous People in Federal Custody Surpasses 30%" (21 January 2020), online: *Office of the Correctional Investigator* <perma.cc/48HK-TDP2>; Canada, Office of the Correctional Investigator, *A Case Study of Diversity in Corrections: The Black Inmate Experience in Federal Penitentiaries*, (Ottawa: Office of the Correctional Investigator, 2013) at 22.

12. Nancy Chow et al, "Preliminary Estimates of the Prevalence of Selected Underlying Health Conditions Among Patients with Coronavirus Disease 2019" (2020) 69:13 MMWR 382 at 382 [Chow et al]. For a list of peer-reviewed papers that detail the interactions of these risk factors with COVID-19, see "COVID-19 Risk Factors" (last visited May 28 2020), online: *Nature* <perma.cc/B8AA-T6H2>.
13. See e.g. Fiona Kouyoumdjian et al, "Health Status of Prisoners" (2016) 62 Can Family Physician 215 at 216 [Kouyoummjian]; Adelina Iftene, *Punished for Aging: Vulnerability, Rights and Access to Justice in Canadian Penitentiaries*, (Toronto: University of Toronto Press, 2019) at 34–77; Correctional Service Canada, *Summary of Emerging Findings from the 2007 National Inmate Infectious Diseases and Risk-Behaviours Survey*, by Dianne Zakaria et al, Research Report, R-211 (Ottawa: Correctional Service Canada, March 2010) at iii.
14. Correctional Service Canada, *National Prevalence of Mental Disorders among Incoming Federally-Sentenced Men*, by JN Beaudette et al, Research Report, R-357 (Ottawa: Correctional Service Canada, February 2015).
15. Senate Committee on Human Rights, *supra* note 11; Emily van der Meulen et al, "On Point: Recommendations for Prison-Based Needle and Syringe Programs in Canada" (January 2016), online: <perma.cc/YWT5-7P4N>.
16. Public Safety Canada, *Corrections and Conditional Release Statistical Overview*, (2018 Annual Report), (Ottawa: Public Works and Government Services Canada, August 2019) at 47.
17. Stephanie Bialek et al, "Severe Outcomes Among Patients with Coronavirus Disease 2019 (COVID-19)" (2020) 69:12 MMWR 343 at 344 [Bialek et al].

medical specialists), and a chronic shortage of health professionals.[18] Issues with untimely or inaccurate diagnosis, at times leading to death, have been reported with some regularity.[19] The availability and distribution of medication are both issues.[20]

COVID-19 Prison Policies, Practices, and Rates of Infection

Federal and provincial responses to COVID-19 have been variable, with some key measures having been taken in some instances, but overall there are serious deficits. For example, most provincial systems,[21] have taken steps, to various degrees, to release individuals serving intermittent sentences (weekends) or who had little time left on their sentences.[22] Based on these criteria, Nova Scotia reduced their incarcerated numbers by half,[23] while Ontario released over 2,000 people.[24] Some provinces have been providing released individuals with

18. Adelina Iftene, *supra* note 13.
19. Canada, Office of the Correctional Investigator, *supra* note 5 at 9.
20. Canada, Office of the Correctional Investigator, *National Drug Formulary Investigation: Summary of Findings and Recommendations*, (Ottawa: Office of the Correctional Investigator, January 2015), online: *Office of the Correctional Investigator* <perma.cc/ZJF6-TD3R>.
21. Tracking the Politics of Criminalization and Punishment in Canada, "Carceral Depopulation Measures to Prevent COVID-19 Transmission in Canada" (April 9, 2020), online (blog): *TPCP-Canada* <perma.cc/2XQ3-6XSX>.
22. NL Newfoundland and Labrador, Justice and Public Safety, *COVID-19 and the Department of Justice and Public Safety*, (St John's: Justice and Public Safety, May 1, 2020), online: *Justice and Public Safety* <perma.cc/74LH-Q8CN>; New Brunswick, Office of the Premier, *Update on COVID-19*, (Fredericton: Office of the Premier, 17 March 2020), online: *Office of the Premier* <perma.cc/V42Z-WCCE>; Alberta, Correctional Services, *Adult Correctional and Remand Centres*, (Calgary: Correctional Services), online: *Correctional Services* <perma.cc/78TG-6QHB>; British Columbia, Corrections, *BC Corrections Response to COVID-19*, (Vancouver: Corrections), online: *Corrections* <www2.gov.bc.ca/gov/content/justice/criminal-justice/corrections>; Ontario, Ministry of the Solicitor General, *Correctional Services Update on COVID-19*, (Toronto: Ministry of the Solicitor General, 9 April 2020), online: *Ministry of the Solicitor General* <perma.cc/DB5G-5G3G>; Saskatchewan Government News and Media, "Update On COVID-19 Measures Being Taken In Correctional Facilities" (27 March 2020), online: *Government News and Media* <perma.cc/KK5A-HG76#utm_campaign=q2_2015&utm_medium=short&utm_source=%2Fgovernment%2Fnews-and-media%2F2020%2Fmarch%2F27%2Fcovid-19-update-correctional-facilities>; Letter from Minister of Justice Cliff Cullen to Canadian Prison Law Association (27 April 2020).
23. Haley Ryan, "Nova Scotia Jail Population Almost Cut in Half Under COVID-19 Measures", *CBC News* (22 April 2020), online: <perma.cc/7885-MCMV>.
24. CBC News, "More than 2,000 Inmates Released, 6 COVID-19 Cases Confirmed Inside Ontario Jails", *CBC News* (9 April 2020), online: <perma.cc/8UKW-P5TZ>.

additional medication in anticipation of the possible challenges they may face in accessing health care in the community during the pandemic.[25] It is unclear what other governmental supports, if any, have been in place for those transitioned to the community.[26]

The information on institutional measures taken and prevention protocols adopted in provincial prisons to protect the remaining incarcerated population is inconsistent and vague. In some provinces, the measures listed on their websites are minimal, such as suspending visits from the outside.[27] Other provinces noted their efforts to secure cleaning supplies and personal protective equipment (PPE) for staff.[28] The little information available, generally from Ontario, on how measures are being implemented suggests that there is a lack of testing, a failure to treat flu-like symptoms, and a failure to implement physical distancing measures (with as many as 30 people bunked in the same dorm) in some provincial institutions.[29]

Federally, CSC has resisted calls to consider federal prison depopulation.[30] Not only have no release strategies been made public, but the Minister of Public Safety (responsible for federal corrections) has also made misleading statements regarding the release of individuals

25. Ontario, Ministry of the Solicitor General, *Correctional Services Update on COVID-19* (Toronto: Ministry of the Solicitor General, 9 April 2020), online: *Ministry of the Solicitor General* <perma.cc/73PL-SQ6D>; Saskatchewan, Government News and Media, *supra* note 22; Letter from Minister of Justice Cliff Cullen, *supra* note 22.

26. For a criticism of the lack of governmental release support and community-led initiatives see e.g. Nova Scotia Advocate, News Release, "Emergency Housing Project Launched for People Exiting Jail During COVID-19" (13 May 2020), online: *Nova Scotia Advocate* <perma.cc/Y8B8-H5DN>.

27. See Newfoundland and Labrador, Justice and Public Safety, *supra* note 22; New Brunswick, Office of the Premier, *supra* note 22; Alberta, Correctional Services, *supra* note 22; British Columbia, Corrections, *supra* note 22.

28. Ontario, Ministry of the Solicitor General, *supra* note 22; Saskatchewan, Government News and Media, *supra* note 22; Letter from Minister of Justice Cliff Cullen, *supra* note 22.

29. Jorge Barrera, "Tension, Fear Rising inside Dorm 3 of Ottawa Jail over COVID-19", *CBC News* (19 March 2020), online: <perma.cc/6CTQ-8XP8>; Liam Casey, "Guards at Ottawa Jail Refuse to Work over Lack of COVID-19 Screening Protocols", *Global News* (1 April 2020), online: <perma.cc/8FAL-HQNG>; Alyshah Hasham & Jim Rankin, "Eight Staff, 60 Inmates Test Positive for COVID-19 at Brampton Jail. Inmates Transferred to Toronto South Detention Centre", *The Star* (20 April 2020), online: <perma.cc/VH3F-NZVN>.

30. Karen Harris, "Bill Blair Asks Prison, Parole Heads to Consider Releasing Some Inmates to Stop Spread of COVID-19", *CBC News* (31 March 2020), online: <perma.cc/RUV6-RUAJ>; Terry Haig, "Corrections Canada Keeping Very Mum About COVID-19 Early Releases", *Radio Canada International* (22 April 2020), online: <perma.cc/LNK6-AEC5>.

on account of the pandemic.[31] In fact, there has been only one sick person released due to COVID-19 and that release was secured under threat of legal action.[32] Hundreds of people listed by CSC as having a low risk of reoffending, who are weeks or months away from their release date, who are old and sick, or who have already been granted a form of release, are still in prison.[33] At the same time, overcrowding (known as double-bunking, or placing two people in a cell made for one) remains prevalent in penitentiaries,[34] in shocking disregard for the most basic physical distancing rules.

The institutional preventive measures made public by CSC include expanding urgent health care while suspending other kinds of health care; providing relevant health information to medical personnel; implementing their "well-established" existing prevention protocols; enhancing cleaning practices; securing more medication and other health supplies; distributing additional soap and hand sanitizer; and prisoner testing.[35] However, emerging evidence shows that these have been poorly implemented.[36]

The Correctional Investigator noted that PPE and hand sanitizer are only available to staff and not to incarcerated people.[37] Physical distancing has generally not been possible. Communal eating, food serving, and group activities have not been suspended in all institutions.[38] While CSC has worked towards hiring more health care personnel,

31. Kathleen Harris, "Prisons Watchdog in the Dark on Inmate Early Release Plan to Limit Spread of COVID-19", *CBC News* (22 April 2020), online: <perma.cc/VN6W-UXFD>.
32. Samantha Beattie, "Inmate With Cancer Wins Prison Release During Pandemic. This Is His Story", *Huffington Post* (24 April 2020), online: <perma.cc/2J5W-BEND>.
33. Anthony Doob, *Understanding Imprisonment in the Time of COVID-19, Report* [unpublished], (Toronto: University of Toronto, 11 May 2020) at 11–17; Justin Ling, "The Government Said It's Releasing Many Inmates to Combat COVID-19. It's Not", *Vice News* (1 May 2020), online: <perma.cc/9GTC-A4J5>.
34. Correctional Service Canada, *Double-Bunking in Canadian Federal Corrections*, Research in Brief, RIB-18-12 (Ottawa: Correctional Service Canada, October 2018), online: *Correctional Service Canada* <perma.cc/F6UN-KWYB>.
35. Correctional Service Canada, *COVID-19 Preparedness and Plans*, (Ottawa: Correctional Service Canada, 30 March 2020), online: *Correctional Service Canada* <perma.cc/2P82-2HQN>.
36. Canada, Office of the Correctional Investigator, *COVID-19 Status Update*, (Ottawa: Office of the Correctional Investigator, 23 April 2020) at 3, online: *Office of the Correctional Investigator* <perma.cc/DT46-PADV>.
37. *Ibid.*
38. *Snow v Canada*, [2020] FC file number T-464-20 (Affidavit, Paul Robert Quick) at 23–37, online: <documentcloud.adobe.com/link/review/?uri=urn%3Aaaid%3Ascds%3AUS%3Aa0dfe49f-3668-42bb-9e54-88efa9f1bdc1&pageNum=1>.

there is still such a shortage that, for example, one institution dealing with an outbreak has only two nurses available (one more than pre-pandemic), and one part-time physician, for nearly 200 people.[39] The Public Health Agency of Canada has not performed any external audits of the implementation of the protocols and measures adopted by CSC.[40]

Extensive segregation with little to no stimuli or family contact has been the most common response to the pandemic in federal penitentiaries. Infected or presumptively infected people are locked up in medical isolation, or on "infected ranges."[41] In the institutions where there are active outbreaks, even individuals who are not presumed infected are held for up to 24 hours in their cells. When permitted to go outside their cell for 20 minutes each day, they have to choose whether they will call their family, or their lawyer, or take a shower.[42] In some institutions without outbreaks, individuals who are not presumptive COVID-19 cases are allowed outside between two and four hours daily. This regime is, at least at times, in breach of international norms and human rights,[43] according to which, in all circumstances, prolonged isolation (more than 14 days of being locked up for 22 hours or longer in a cell) and indefinite isolation (without a clear end) constitute torture.[44]

Decarceration efforts in provincial prisons have had some success in most provinces. As of May 15, 2020, there have been 168 confirmed cases of infection[45] in provincial custody, and one death in Quebec.[46] Nearly all of these cases came from the same two jails in Ontario[47] and Quebec.[48] This is likely correlated with the reported

39. Canada, Office of the Correctional Investigator, *supra* note 36 at 7.
40. *Ibid* at 8.
41. *Ibid*. See also Justin Ling, "Inmates With Coronavirus Are Being Thrown Into 'Extremely Difficult' Confinement: Prison Watchdog", *Vice News* (27 April 2020), online: <perma.cc/DZ2K-6PQE>. .
42. *Ibid* at 4–6.
43. Canada, Office of the Correctional Investigator, *supra* note 36 at 5.
44. United Nations, *supra* note 2 at Rule 44 and 43(a).
45. Tracking the Politics of Criminalization and Punishment in Canada, "Confirmed COVID-19 Cases Linked to Canadian Carceral Institutions" (April 26, 2020), online (blog): *TPCP-Canada* <perma.cc/R2L8-ZLAB>.
46. Paul Cherry, "Inmate at Bordeaux Jail Dies of COVID-19", *Montreal Gazette* (21 May 2020), online: <perma.cc/T8U9-2WTA>; Daniel Renaud, "Le détenu de Bordeaux hospitalisé est décédé", *La Presse* (20 May 2020), online: <www.lapresse.ca/covid-19/202005/20/01-5274256-le-detenu-de-bordeaux-hospitalise-est-decede.php>.
47. Alyshah Hasham & Jim Rankin, *supra* note 29.
48. CBC News, "Civil Rights Groups Call for Action After Bordeaux Jail Inmate Dies from COVID-19", *CBC News Montreal* (20 May 2020), online: <perma.cc/CP88-4MAV>.

challenges Ontario encountered in implementing adequate institutional prevention measures, and with the fact that Quebec is one of the few provinces where depopulation measures were not taken.[49]

In federal prisons, the failure to depopulate and the shortcomings of the prevention measures taken have likely contributed to the 333 infected people reported on May 15, 2020,[50] and the two deaths.[51] This means that the rate of infection among this population is over 13 times higher than in the community (13.16 vs. 0.99 cases per 1000).[52] Federally incarcerated women have been the most affected by the infection. The rate of infection in women's penitentiaries was 77 times higher than among women in the community.[53] The inadequacy of some of the prison responses to COVID-19 raises significant legal and ethical issues; I will now turn to those issues.

Legal and Ethical Concerns Regarding Prison Responses to COVID-19

Given the historic failures to ensure the health of prisoners,[54] there is reason to be concerned about the dearth of information on the protocols adopted by any of the prison systems across the country and about the lack of oversight of the implementation of those protocols by public health and human rights agencies. Additionally, the high rates of infection and the inadequate implementation of preventive measures and treatment in some prisons suggest that at least some prison systems may be in breach of the international and statutory duties owed to incarcerated people.

---

49. *Ibid.*
50. Anthony Doob, *supra* note 33, at 10; Correctional Service Canada, *Inmate COVID-19 Testing in Federal Correctional Institutions (May 10, 2020)*, (Ottawa: Correctional Service Canada, 10 May 2020), online: *Correctional Service Canada* <www.csc-scc.gc.ca/001/006/001006-1014-en.shtml>.
51. "Inmate at Mission Institution Dies of COVID-19 Complications", *CBC News* (16 April 2020), online: <perma.cc/TS44-DAV6>; Selena Ross, "A Second Inmate in a Canadian Federal Prison has Died of COVID-19", *CTV News Montreal* (5 May 2020), online: <perma.cc/FR8N-X9Q6>.
52. *Ibid.*
53. Anthony Doob, *supra* note 33, at 10.
54. See e.g. Adelina Iftene, *supra* note 13; Adam Miller, "Prison Health Care Inequality", CMAJ 2013 185(6), 249; Adelina Iftene and Allan Manson, "Recent Crime Legislation: The Challenge for Prison Health Care" (9 July 2013) 185:10 CMAJ 886; Ontario, Ministry of the Solicitor General, *Corrections in Ontario: Directions for Reform*, Independent Review, (Toronto: Ministry of the Solicitor General, September 2017) at 216.

Moreover, there may be concerns arising from how prisoners' rights under the *Charter of Rights and Freedoms* (the *Charter)* and human rights statutes are being upheld during the pandemic.[55] First, as mentioned, incarcerated individuals often belong to communities impacted by social inequality and thus are already at a higher risk and in need of enhanced protection during a pandemic. Not only does state custody not offer that protection, but it heightens the risks to their health and lives. In the words of Professor Anthony Doob, a leading Canadian criminologist and statistician, "We currently have a situation, then, that suggests quite strongly that being in a CSC penitentiary has the effect of putting a prisoner at a much higher risk of a very serious disease with a non-trivial mortality rate."[56]

Second, the insufficient prison responses to the pandemic have, percentage-wise, disproportionately impacted women[57] and individuals with underlying health conditions. Third, Indigenous people are overrepresented in prisons, as they make up over 30% of federally incarcerated people.[58] Thus, the pandemic disproportionately affects Indigenous incarcerated individuals, especially Indigenous women. In this context, as also exemplified by Aimée Craft, Deborah McGregor and Jeffery Hewitt, this volume, Chapter A-2, and by Anne Levesque & Sophie Thériault, in Chapter D-6 of this volume, the government's inaction is reminiscent of historic harms against Indigenous people and communities, which can be considered another form of colonial violence—something the Canadian criminal justice system has regularly been accused of perpetuating.[59] Equality issues (under s. 15 of

55. On the need for human rights oversight of pandemic responses generally, and for prisons specifically, see "Canada's COVID-19 Response Needs Human Rights Oversight, says Amnesty International" (March 25, 2020), online: *Amnesty International* <perma.cc/RK94-2UND>; Canada, Office of the Correctional Investigator, *supra* note 36.
56. Anthony Doob, *supra* note 33, at 10.
57. *Ibid.*
58. Office of the Correctional Investigator, *supra* note 11.
59. See e.g. Elspeth Kaiser-Derrick, *Implicating the System: Judicial Discourses in the Sentencing of Indigenous Women*, (Winnipeg: University of Manitoba Press, 2019); Gillian Balfour, "Do Law Reforms Matter? Exploring the Victimization-Criminalization Continuum in the Sentencing of Aboriginal Women in Canada" (2013) 19:1 Int Rev Vict 85; Kent Roach, *Canadian Justice, Indigenous Injustice,* (Montreal, Kingston: McGill-Queen's University Press, 2019); David Milward, "Locking up Those Dangerous Indians for Good: An Examination of Canadian Dangerous Offender Legislation as Applied to Aboriginal Persons" (2013) 51:3 Alta Law Rev 619.

the *Charter*[60] and *Canadian Human Rights Act*[61]) stand out as a significant concern.

In addition, the exposure of incarcerated people to a high risk of infection, as well as the prolonged isolation in a cell with no mental stimulation, may violate s. 7 (the right to life, liberty, and security of the person in accordance with the principles of fundamental justice)[62] and s. 12 (right to be free from cruel and unusual punishment)[63] *Charter* rights. At least two class actions have been filed by prisoners against the federal government so far, as well as a human rights lawsuit.[64]

From a public health perspective, the government's failure is devastating. First, allowing hot spots of infection to grow impedes the successful flattening of the curve and will likely prolong the life of the pandemic in the community.[65] Second, incarcerated people are more likely to have severe complications from COVID-19 due to their pre-existing conditions, which in turn will be taxing on the health care systems. Third, the measures taken, in particular lockdowns and lack of communication with families, will negatively affect the mental health of incarcerated individuals, increasing the chances of a substance overdose and the frequency of self-harm incidents.[66] This could bring about increased unrest in prisons, stretching health care resources, and negatively affecting prisoner health. Finally, COVID-19 may have severe and long-lasting consequences on health, especially

60. *Charter of Human Rights and Freedoms*, s 7, Part I of the *Constitution Act, 1982*, being Schedule B to the *Canada Act 1982* (UK), 1982, c 11 [*Charter*].
61. *Canadian Human Rights Act*, RSC 1985, c H-6, s 15.
62. *Charter*, *supra* note 60, s 7.
63. *Ibid*, s 12.
64. Kim Bolan, "COVID-19: Inmate Suit Filed Against Federal Government over Mission Outbreak", *Vancouver Sun* (24 April 2020), online: <perma.cc/MKS6-J7RY>; The Canadian Press, "Quebec Federal Inmate Files Application for COVID-19 Class Action", *The Star* (21 April 2020), online: <perma.cc/5URR-JVVH>; Canadian Civil Liberties Association, Canadian Prison Law Association, "HIV & AIDS Legal Clinic Ontario, HIV Legal Network, and Sean Johnston v The Attorney General of Canada, Notice of Application" (12 May 2020), online: <documentcloud.adobe.com/link/review/?uri=urn%3Aaaid%3Ascds%3AUS%3A191a51df-8da6-4757-a9ee-f1dca94f255e&pageNum=1>.
65. On hot spots of infection in other congregated living spaces and their consequences, see Martine Lagacé, Linda Garcia & Louise Bélanger-Hardy, Chapter D-2, this volume; Tess Sheldon & Ravi Malhotra, Chapter D-9, this volume; Chandler et al, Chapter D-10, this volume.
66. Evidence is starting to emerge. See Canada, Office of the Correctional Investigator, *supra* note 36 at 4–5.

for those at higher risk. Thus, there are heightened concerns regarding the higher rates of infection in people who will ultimately return to marginalized communities in a more fragile state of health than when they entered prison.

Concluding Thoughts

For those conducting prison work, the impacts of COVID-19 on prison populations come as no surprise. The overreliance on incarceration, inadequate health care, and the general disregard for prisoner well-being and prisoner rights, have been an overlooked reality for decades. In many ways, the pandemic was a disaster waiting to happen.[67]

The lack of transparency regarding the measures taken to protect incarcerated people, the failure of some prison systems to have emergency strategies and support for release of those in custody, as well as the insufficient institutional preparedness for the pandemic, are by-products of the pre-COVID-19 shortcomings of the correctional systems and of the broader criminal and social justice practices that have perpetuated equity gaps in the society. Canada's carceral practices are linked to its ongoing failure to respond to the needs of other marginalized groups discussed in this book.

As discussed in other chapters, the pandemic has revealed just how big Canada's social and health inequities are. These inequities have long been feeding the prison systems. In turn, prisons are now cracking under the pressure of the pandemic, and the spill-outs will impact all of society. The current crisis has shown how connected prison and social justice issues are to public health. Returning to "normal" should not be an option; instead, sweeping reforms that ensure Canada's ability to equitably protect everyone in the case of a public health crisis are needed.

Some of the much needed long-term reforms, intrinsically connected to imprisonment and well-being of criminalized people, include a universal basic income, better health care, better child support and other community supports for marginalized people, as well as sentencing reforms (such as the abolition of mandatory minimum sentences) that will effectively reduce the over-reliance on incarceration and increase diversion and community sentences.

67. Adelina Iftene, "We Must Decarcerate Across the Country, then Fix the Prison System", *Policy Options* (20 April 2020), online: <perma.cc/7KVB-SUAU>.

In the short term, during a pandemic wave, the government should use the tools available to them to identify low-risk incarcerated individuals that have high health needs, and to release them while providing community support. There are numerous options available for releasing different eligible individuals (none of which had been used during the first wave of COVID-19 to release federally incarcerated people), including parole, parole by exception, statutory release, s. 81 releases for Indigenous individuals (through which CSC may release an individual into the custody and care of an Indigenous authority, with the consent of that authority and of the individual), temporary absence passes,[68] and the royal prerogative of mercy.[69] Finally, all correctional systems should have some general pandemic protocols, reviewed and approved by public health agencies, that can be swiftly implemented when the need arises.

68. Temporary absences have been used during the first COVID-19 wave by some provincial correctional systems, such as Nova Scotia, to release individuals.

69. *CCRA*, *supra* note 3, ss 81, 115, 119, 121, 127; *Criminal Code*, RSC 1985, c C-46, s 748.

CHAPTER D-6

Systemic Discrimination in Government Services and Programs and Its Impact on First Nations Peoples During the COVID-19 Pandemic*

Anne Levesque** and Sophie Thériault***

Abstract

Historic and contemporary forms of colonialism predispose First Nations peoples to higher risk for COVID-19. This chapter argues that the health disparities faced by First Nations communities are directly attributable to the underfunding and discrimination in public services, especially on reserves. The first part of the chapter canvasses the inequities in government services and programs that impede the capacity of First Nations communities to effectively prevent and manage public health crises, such as the COVID-19 pandemic, in accordance with their own priorities, circumstances, and needs. The second part proposes *Caring Society v Canada,* a precedent-setting decision of the Canadian Human Rights Tribunal (CHRT), as establishing the legal standard for Canada when designing and funding its response to the COVID-19 pandemic for First Nations communities. We argue

* The authors would like to thank the anonymous reviewers and Dr. Cindy Blackstock for their insightful suggestions and thoughtful comments, as well as our talented research assistants Jennifer Linde and Laurie-Anne Mercier for their invaluable support in drafting this chapter. Any errors are our own. Anne Levesque is one of the lawyers representing the First Nations Child and Family Caring Society in its litigation against Canada discussed in this chapter.

** Assistant Professor in the French Common Law Program in the Faculty of Law at the University of Ottawa.

*** Full Professor and Vice-Dean (Academic) in the Faculty of Law (Civil Law Section), University of Ottawa.

that if the Government of Canada does not immediately and comprehensively address the systemic inequities in its services and programs to First Nations peoples, as required under the *Canadian Human Rights Act*, measures aimed at managing the COVID-19 pandemic and potential future health crises will inevitably fail to produce equitable outcomes in these communities.

Résumé

La discrimination systémique dans les services et programmes gouvernementaux et ses conséquences sur les Premières Nations pendant la pandémie de COVID-19

Les formes historiques et contemporaines de colonialisme prédisposent les peuples des Premières Nations à un risque plus élevé de contracter la COVID-19. Ce chapitre avance que les disparités en matière de santé auxquelles sont confrontées les communautés des Premières Nations sont directement attribuables au sous-financement et à la discrimination dans les services publics, en particulier dans les réserves. La première partie du chapitre examine les inégalités dans les services et les programmes gouvernementaux qui entravent la capacité des Premières Nations à prévenir et à gérer efficacement les crises de santé publique, comme la pandémie de COVID-19, conformément à leurs propres priorités, circonstances et besoins. La deuxième partie propose que l'affaire *Société de soutien c. Canada*, une décision du Tribunal canadien des droits de la personne (TCDP) qui fait jurisprudence, établisse la norme juridique pour le Canada lorsqu'il s'agit de planifier et de financer sa réponse à la pandémie de COVID-19 pour les communautés des Premières Nations. Nous soutenons que si le gouvernement du Canada ne s'attaque pas immédiatement et de manière exhaustive aux inégalités systémiques qui existent dans ses services et programmes destinés aux Premières Nations, comme l'exige la *Loi canadienne sur les droits de la personne*, les mesures visant à gérer la pandémie de COVID-19 et les crises sanitaires futures n'obtiendront forcément pas de résultats équitables pour ces communautés.

The most jarring manifestation of these human rights problems is the distressing socio-economic conditions of indigenous peoples in a highly developed country.[1]

Historic and contemporary forms of colonialism predispose First Nations peoples to higher risk for COVID-19. This chapter argues that health disparities observed amongst First Nations communities in Canada are related to the underfunding and discrimination in public services, especially on reserves.[2] The first part of the chapter outlines the inequities in government services and programs that impede the capacity of First Nations communities to effectively prevent and manage public health crises—such as the COVID-19 pandemic—in accordance with their own priorities, circumstances, and needs. The second part proposes that *Caring Society v Canada,* a precedent-setting decision of the Canadian Human Rights Tribunal, establishes the legal standard for Canada when funding its response to public health crises for First Nations communities.[3] The decision requires Canada to consider the distinct cultural, historical, and geographical needs and circumstances of First Nations communities in the funding and provision of their services and programs.[4] We argue that if the Government of Canada does not immediately and comprehensively address the systemic inequities in its services and programs to First Nations peoples as required under the *Canadian Human Rights Act*[5], measures aimed at managing the COVID-19 pandemic and future health crises will inevitably fail to produce equitable outcomes in these communities.

1. *Report of the Special Rapporteur on the rights of indigenous peoples, James Anaya. The situation of indigenous peoples in Canada,* UNHRC, 27th Sess., Annex, Agenda item 3, UN Doc A/HRC/27/52/Add.2 (2014) at 7 [*UNHRC*].
2. See note 1 in Craft, McGregor & Hewitt, Chapter A-2, this volume, for an explanation of the terminology and language surrounding Indigenous identity. As this chapter focuses primarily on the situation on reserves, we use the term First Nations.
3. *First Nations Child and Family Caring Society of Canada et al v Attorney General of Canada (for the Minister of Indian and Northern Affairs Canada),* 2016 CHRT 2 at para 465 [*Caring Society 2016*].
4. *Ibid.*
5. *Canadian Human Rights Act,* RSC 1985, c H-6.

Canada's Racial Discrimination against First Nations Peoples in Public Services and Programs

The November 15, 1907, headline of the *Evening Citizen* newspaper in Ottawa read "Schools Aid White Plague: Startling Death Rolls Revealed Among Indians—Absolute Inattention to Bare Necessities of Health."[6] The article described the findings of Indian Affairs Health Officer, Dr. Peter Bryce, linking inequalities in "Indian" health care funding and poor health practises in the schools with the overwhelming death rates of residential school students. The federal government took note of the inequality but did not fix it.[7] The Truth and Reconciliation Commission of Canada identified 3,200 deaths of students in residential schools and the Chief Commissioners estimates that up to 6,000 children may have lost their lives due to preventable disease and maltreatment.[8] Overall, children in residential schools had the same odds of dying as a soldier in the Second World War.[9]

Many other credible voices have chronicled the inequalities in First Nations public services, and proposed solutions to remedy them, including the Office of the Auditor General of Canada,[10] the National Inquiry into Missing and Murdered Indigenous Women,[11] and the Truth and Reconciliation Commission of Canada,[12] as well as

6. "Schools Aid White Plague" *The Evening Citizen*, 1907, cited in Travis Hay, Cindy Blackstock & Michael Kirlew, "Dr. Peter Bryce (1853–1932): whistleblower on residential schools" (2020) 192:9 CMJA 223 at 224.
7. *Ibid* at 224.
8. Truth and Reconciliation Commission of Canada, *Canada's Residential Schools: Missing Children and Unmarked Burials*, vol 4 (Winnipeg: Truth and Reconciliation Commission of Canada, 2015) at 1; Chinta Puxley, "How many First Nations kids died in residential schools? Justice Murray Sinclair says Canada needs answers", *Toronto Star* (31 May 2015), online: <www.thestar.com/news/canada/2015/05/31/how-many-first-nations-kids-died-in-residential-schools-justice-murray-sinclair-says-canada-needs-answers.html>.
9. Daniel Schwartz, "Truth and Reconciliation Commission: By the numbers", *CBC News* (2 June 2015), online: <www.cbc.ca/news/indigenous/truth-and-reconciliation-commission-by-the-numbers-1.3096185>.
10. Canada, Office of the Auditor General of Canada, *Access to Health Services for Remote First Nations Communities* (Report to Parliament), (Ottawa: OAG, Spring 2015) [*OAG 2015*]; Canada, Office of the Auditor General of Canada, *2011 June Status Report, Programs for First Nations on Reserves* (Report to Parliament), (Ottawa: OAG, June 2011) at chapter 4 [*OAG 2011*].
11. See Canada, *Reclaiming Power and Place: the Final Report of the National Inquiry into Missing and Murdered Indigenous Women and Girls*, vol 1a (Ottawa: MMIWG, 2019) and vol 1b (Ottawa: MMIWG, 2019), [*MMIWG*].
12. "Our Mandate" (last visited 12 May 2020), online: *Truth and Reconciliation Commission of Canada* <www.trc.ca/about-us/our-mandate.html>.

the Royal Commission on Aboriginal Peoples over two decades ago.[13] Canada's failure to take adequate action has resulted in disparities in access to housing, health care, clean water, and food, among other necessities, that predispose First Nations to public health crises such as the COVID-19 pandemic and undermine their ability to respond effectively in accordance with their specific needs and priorities.[14]

For instance, while public health authorities consider physical distancing, hand-washing, and the cleaning of potentially infected surfaces as the most effective means of reducing the transmission of SARS-CoV-2, many First Nations communities do not have access to clean and safe tap water.[15] Despite recent efforts to provide access to safe and clean water to First Nations communities, at least 61 long-term drinking water advisories are currently in effect, some having lasted several decades, in addition to several other short-term advisories.[16] These figures reveal that some First Nations communities not only lack the resources to implement basic hygiene measures to prevent the spread of SARS-CoV-2, but also are at heightened risk of contracting water-borne diseases from using potentially contaminated water.

In addition to lack of access to clean water, overcrowded housing and the poor condition of many homes make physical distancing nearly impossible. According to recent statistical data, nearly

13. Royal Commission on Aboriginal Peoples, *Report of the Royal Commission on Aboriginal Peoples* (Report to Parliament), (Ottawa: RCAP, October 1996).
14. Shiri Pasternak & Robert Houle, "No Such Thing As Natural Disasters: Infrastructure and the First Nation Fight Against COVID-19", *Yellowhead Institute* (9 April 2020), online: <yellowheadinstitute.org/2020/04/09/no-such-thing-as-natural-disasters-infrastructure-and-the-first-nation-fight-against-covid-19/>; Shirley Thompson, Marleny Bonycastle & Stewart Hill, "COVID-19, First Nations and Poor Housing" (24 May 2020), online: *Canadian Centre for Policy Alternatives* <www.policyalternatives.ca/sites/default/files/uploads/publications/Manitoba%20Office/2020/05/COVID%20FN%20Poor%20Housing.pdf>.
15. David R Boyd, "No Taps, No Toilets: First Nations and the Constitutional Right to Water in Canada" (2011) 57:1 McGill LJ 81; Nathalie J Chalifour, "Environmental Discrimination and the *Charter*'s Equality Guarantee: Is Section 15 an Avenue for Environmental Justice? The Case of Drinking Water for First Nations Living on Reserves" (2018) 43 RGD 183; Pamela Palmater, "First Nations Water Problems a Crisis of Canada's Own Making", Policy Options (6 February 2019), online: <policyoptions.irpp.org/magazines/february-2019/first-nations-water-problems-crisis-canadas-making/>.
16. "Ending long-term drinking water advisories" (last modified 17 February 2020), online: *Indigenous Services Canada* <www.sac-isc.gc.ca/eng/1506514143353/1533317130660>; "Short-term drinking water advisories" (last modified 15 May 2020), online: *Indigenous Services Canada* <www.sac-isc.gc.ca/eng/1562856509704/1562856530304>.

one-quarter (23.1%) of First Nations peoples on reserves live in crowded housing, and 44.2% live in houses needing major repairs.[17] It is well established that overcrowding and substandard housing lead to poor health outcomes.[18] In the context of the COVID-19 pandemic, crowded housing with poor air circulation would facilitate the transmission of the virus and prevent First Nations families from complying with physical distancing recommendations.[19]

Moreover, housing shortages on and off reserves for low income First Nations families, combined with public health directives on confinement, increase the risk faced by First Nations women and children, who are disproportionately affected by domestic, physical, and sexual violence, notably as a result of the intergenerational trauma induced by sexist and patriarchal colonial laws and policies.[20] The harm for women and children is heightened by the dire lack of safe houses and shelters on reserves[21] and long-standing inequities in the funding of child welfare services.[22]

Furthermore, First Nations peoples are more likely to develop complications from COVID-19 due to the prevalence within their communities of chronic diseases considered as risk factors, including diabetes and severe asthma. Yet the capacity of First Nations communities to prevent SARS-CoV-2 infections and address related complications are considerably reduced by unequal access to health care services.[23] Many First Nations communities lack access to health

---

17. Statistics Canada, *Census in Brief. The Housing Conditions of Aboriginal people in Canada*, Catalogue No 98-200-X2016021 (Ottawa: Statistics Canada, 25 October 2017); OAG 2011, *supra* note 10 at paras 4.35-4.45.
18. *UNHRC, supra* note 1 at 1.
19. *Ibid.*
20. MMIWG, *supra* note 11 at vol. 1a, 229-307, 319; Native Women's Association of Canada (NWAC), "NWAC President Says COVID-19 is Increasing Violence Against Indigenous Women, Says Government Must Release an Action Plan", *NWAC News & Press Releases* (7 May 2020), online: *NWAC* <www.nwac.ca/nwac-president-says-covid-19-is-increasing-violence-against-indigenous-women-says-government-must-release-an-action-plan/>; Teresa Wright, "Violence against Indigenous Women during COVID-19 Sparks Calls for MMIWG Plan", *CTV News* (10 May 2020), online: <www.ctvnews.ca/canada/violence-against-indigenous-women-during-covid-19-sparks-calls-for-mmiwg-plan-1.4932833>.
21. *MMIWG, supra* note 11 at vol 1b, 149.
22. Marina Sistovaris et al, *Child Welfare and Pandemics: Literature Scan* (Toronto: Policy Bench, Fraser Mustard Institute for Human Development, University of Toronto, 2020).
23. Canada, House of Commons, *The Challenges of Delivering Continuing Care in First Nations Communities: Report of the Standing Committee on Indigenous and Northern*

professionals, adequate health facilities, and emergency ambulatory services. While these issues can in part be attributed to the barriers created by the complex shared jurisdiction over First Nations' health care, the lack of consideration for the specific health needs of First Nations in the allocation of resources is a leading cause of health inequities.[24] Moreover, experiences of racism and prejudice in health care delivery can have grave consequences during an ongoing pandemic, such as deprivation from exams and tests, and delayed diagnosis and treatment.[25]

Other long-standing inequities in access to essential goods and services increase the risk presented by SARS-CoV-2 to First Nations communities. Lack of consistent access to sufficient and affordable healthy foods will be compounded by potential disruptions in the food supply chain.[26] Unreliable internet connections make distance education impossible in many First Nations communities, with adverse consequences for the dissemination of public health information, in severing of social relationships among families with members on and off reserve, and for the educational progress of First Nations learners.[27]

These structural inequities pose distinct challenges for First Nations communities in the context of the COVID-19 pandemic. Yet there are valuable lessons to be learned from past experiences in the design and funding of services and programs when confronting these new circumstances.

Affairs, Chair: Honourable MaryAnn Mihychuk (Ottawa: House of Commons, December 2018) at 42-1; OAG 2015, *supra* note 10.

24. Colleen M Flood, William Lahey & Bryan Thomas, "Federalism and Health Care in Canada. A Troubled Romance?" in Peter Oliver, Patrick Macklem & Nathalie Des Rosiers, eds, *The Oxford Handbook of the Canadian Constitution* (Oxford: Oxford University Press, 2017) at 459-63; OAG 2015, *supra* note 10 at 4.92-4.96.

25. Commission on relations between Indigenous Peoples and certain public services in Québec, *Final Report of the Public Inquiry Commission on relations between Indigenous Peoples and certain public services in Québec: Listening, reconciliation and progress*, Chair: Honourable Jacques Viens (Québec, Commission on relations between Indigenous Peoples and certain public services in Québec, 2019) at 367.

26. Elisa Levi & Tabitha Robin, "COVID-19 Did Not Cause Food Insecurity in Indigenous Communities But It Will Make It Worse", *Yellowhead Institute* (29 April 2020), online: <yellowhead institute.org/2020/04/29/covid19-food-insecurity/>.

27. Cindy Blackstock & Isadore Day, "History will repeat itself if First Nations remain underfunded in the fight against COVID-19", *Globe and Mail* (8 April 2020), online: <www.theglobeandmail.com/opinion/article-history-will-repeat-itself-if-first-nations-remain-underfunded-in-the/>.

Canada's Statutory Human Rights Obligations Towards First Nations Peoples When Responding to Public Health Crises

Canada's approach to the provision of services to First Nations children and their families is a chilling reminder of the harmful impacts of inequities in government services. The decision and remedial orders of the Canadian Human Rights Tribunal ("CHRT") regarding Canada's inequitable funding of children's services for First Nations families provide a comprehensive roadmap of the federal government's legal obligations for the funding and provision of measures designed to prevent and respond to health crises.

For decades, the Government of Canada was well aware of the inequities in its First Nations Child and Family Services Program ("FNCFSP"). It failed to act, despite its knowledge that its inequitable program caused children to be taken from their families and communities at alarming rates. In 2007, the First Nations Children and Family Caring Society of Canada ("Caring Society") and the Assembly of First Nations ("AFN") lodged a complaint against the Government of Canada under the *Canadian Human Rights Act* ("*CHRA*"), alleging discrimination on the basis of race and/or national or ethnic origin in the provision of child and family services to First Nations children and their families and in the failure to implement Jordan's Principle.[28] After nearly a decade of procedural tactics by government lawyers to have the case dismissed on technicalities, the CHRT began a hearing relating to the complaint.

In January 2016, the CHRT released its long-awaited decision on the merits of the complaint and upheld all of the allegations of discrimination. In particular, the CHRT found that First Nations children and their families were adversely impacted by Canada's provision of child services and its failure to implement Jordan's Principle, a child-first principle that helps to ensure that all First Nations children living on and off reserve have access to the government-funded products, services, and supports they need when they need them. According to the CHRT, Canada's conduct was contrary to s. 5 of the *CHRA*. Based on these findings of systemic discrimination, the CHRT ruled that in order to comply with its domestic and international human rights law obligations, Canada must "consider the distinct

28. See *First Nations Child & Family Caring Society of Canada et al v Attorney General of Canada (representing the Minister of Indigenous and Northern Affairs Canada)*, 2017 CHRT 14 at para 135.

needs and circumstances of First Nations children and families living on reserve—including their cultural, historical and geographical needs and circumstances." According to the CHRT panel, substantive equality in services for First Nations children could not be achieved through applying ad hoc and piecemeal measures to the funding. It analogized:

> It is like adding support pillars to a house that has a weak foundation in an attempt to straighten and support the house. At some point, the foundation needs to be fixed or, ultimately, the house will fall down. Similarly, a *REFORM* of the FNCFS Program is needed in order to build a solid foundation for the program to address the real needs of First Nations children and families living on reserve.[29]

In retrospect, the CHRT's conclusion that the Government of Canada had been aware for many years of the harmful impact of its discriminatory behaviour on First Nations children, but nevertheless did not act, foreshadowed its inability or unwillingness to immediately cease its unlawful conduct. Faced with Canada's inaction following its decision on the merit of the complaint, the CHRT was required to issue nine further remedial orders in which it specified with precision the measures the federal government needed to take to comply with its legal obligations under the *CHRA*. Of most relevance to the current situation, Canada was ordered to cease unnecessarily reallocating funds from other social programs, especially housing, to compensate for shortfalls or increased costs in its FNCFSP;[30] to fund requests for services to First Nations children that are culturally appropriate and necessary to safeguard their best interests, and to fund certain services and programs for First Nations children based on their actual costs.[31]

While the CHRT's ruling and remedial orders relate specifically to FNCFSP and Jordan's Principle, the decision clarifies the legal standard with which Canada must comply to satisfy its obligations under the *CHRA* in the provision and funding of all services and programs to

---

29. *Caring Society 2016, supra* note 3 at para 463.
30. *First Nations Child & Family Caring Society of Canada et al v Attorney General of Canada (representing the Minister of Indigenous and Northern Affairs Canada)*, 2018 CHRT 4 at para 422.
31. *Ibid* at para 462.

First Nations peoples in Canada. Firstly, measures taken in response to public health crises, such as the COVID-19 pandemic, must reflect their cultural, historical, and geographical needs and circumstances. Secondly, the additional costs associated with responding to new public health crises cannot be offset by cutting into existing services and programs geared toward First Nations peoples. Put more simply, the Government of Canada must allocate new money to fund these services. Thirdly, care must be taken to ensure that services and programs for children are culturally appropriate and safeguard their best interests. Finally, it must be recognized that any measures taken in the context of the pandemic will inevitably be futile if they are not coupled with swift and effective strategies to comprehensively and holistically address all inequities in government services and programs for First Nations peoples. To borrow the analogy of the CHRT, the house will fall down if Canada does not fix the foundation.

The COVID-19 pandemic has cast in the starkest light the urgency of comprehensively addressing the inequities in government services for First Nations peoples. Fortunately, a roadmap for doing this already exists. Knowing that the discrimination identified by the CHRT in Canada's child services was just the tip of the iceberg, the Caring Society and the AFN have proposed a plan to Canada to end all of the inequalities in public services for First Nations children, youth, and families. The "Spirit Bear Plan" calls on the Government of Canada to proactively identify inequities in all services offered to children of First Nations, such as preschool, elementary, and secondary education, health, and water, and to address them comprehensively and holistically. As Canada has refused to implement the Spirit Bear Plan, the long-standing inequities in government services continue to harm First Nations peoples. The failure to implement the Spirit Bear Plan during the pandemic will further aggravate these harms.

Conclusion

At the time of writing, the Government of Canada had begun rolling out measures aimed specifically at limiting the spread of SARS-CoV-2 in First Nations communities across Canada. For example, as detailed by Aimée Craft, Deborah McGregor and Jeffery Hewitt in Chapter A-2 of this volume, Canada has provided portable and temporary shelter solutions for health services, reminders to self-isolate for 14 days after travel outside of Canada, and the stockpiling of bottled water, hand sanitizer, and personal protective equipment. As pointed out by experts, however, these investments represent less than 1% of the federal government's COVID-19 funding, although First Nations Peoples account for nearly 5% of the population of Canada.[32] Put more simply, the measures fail to achieve even the modest standard of formal equality. While Canada has yet to reveal any specific plan of action for responding to the threat of COVID-19 on reserves, the approach it has adopted thus far has generally been to replicate measures put in place elsewhere in the country.[33] Currently, the federal government has yet to take any measure aimed at addressing the systemic inequalities that cause First Nations communities to be disproportionately impacted by SARS-CoV-2. As Dr. Bryce pointed out 113 years ago, effective public health care responses for First Nations must include remedial measures and substantive equality in the provision of public services. One without the other will fail.

For decades, Canada has known about the inequities in the funding of services and programs for First Nations peoples, but has failed to act. Instead, it has repeated the same refrain: addressing these inequities will take time. It has implored First Nations peoples to be patient as incremental changes are made to the inequitable funding formulas of the services they receive from government. In *Caring Society v Canada*, the CHRT has ruled that it is unlawful for Canada to put financial considerations ahead of the best interests of First Nations children. The decision echoed what First Nations peoples had been saying for a long time: that discrimination as a fiscal policy is the manifestation of embedded racism and colonialism in Canadian society.[34] The Government of Canada's same old assertion that it cannot afford substantive equality for First Nations Peoples is particularly unconscionable in these circumstances. If there is one thing we have learned from Canada's response to this crisis, it is that various levels of government can act swiftly to deliver billions of dollars' worth of social

32. See Blackstock and Day, *supra* note 27; Pasternak and Houle, *supra* note 14.

33. "Indigenous Services Canada's preparedness and response to COVID-19" (last visited 16 May 2020), online: *Indigenous Services Canada* <www.sac-isc.gc.ca/eng/1584456952392/1584456999460>.

34. Anna Stanley, "Indigenous children and racial discrimination as fiscal policy" (25 May 2016), online (blog): *Broadbent Institute* <www.broadbentinstitute.ca/annastanley/indigenous_children_racial_discrimination_fiscal_policy>; Pamela Palmater, *Indigenous Nationhood: Empowering Grassroots Citizens* (Halifax: Fernwood Publishing, 2015); Shiri Pasternak, "The Fiscal Body of Sovereignty: To 'Make Live' in Indian Country" (2015) 6:4 Settler Colonial Studies 317.

programs and economic support when that is prioritized. If substantive equality is not set as an immediate policy objective in government programs and services, Canada's colonialist policies will once again have foreseeable and fatal consequences for First Nations peoples.

CHAPTER D-7

Spread of Anti-Asian Racism: Prevention and Critical Race Analysis in Pandemic Planning

Jamie Chai Yun Liew*

Abstract

The racist discourse and attacks on Asian Canadians in the COVID-19 outbreak has illustrated the differentiated risks, vulnerability, and marginalization of racialized persons. A race-based analysis is essential in public health policy. First, public health responses may reinforce long-standing racist narratives of how a virus is transmitted. Second, the "viralizing" of persons may lead to unfair blame on a racialized community for an outbreak, taking focus away from structural problems in particular environments, as for example in the case of Filipino migrant workers in meat-packing plants who have no control over their working conditions. Finally, there is now data showing that, accounting for other factors, some racialized groups of people, including Black and South Asian people, may be succumbing to COVID-19 more than others. Focusing on the partial border closure as a case study, this chapter looks at how historical and contemporary selective but simultaneous inclusion and exclusion at the border has constructed social ideas of foreigners. The border measures reflect an ongoing tension to admit cheap labour for essential services while pacifying public fear of the Asian person as a vector of the virus. Critical race analysis should be employed when evaluating public

* Immigration and refugee lawyer and Associate Professor in the Faculty of Law, University of Ottawa.

health responses to ensure that differential experiences of racialized communities are considered during a pandemic.

Résumé

Prévenir la propagation du racisme contre les Asiatiques : inclure l'analyse raciale critique dans un plan de lutte contre la pandémie

Le discours raciste et les attaques contre des Canadiens d'origine asiatique dans la foulée de la pandémie de COVID-19 ont illustré les risques différenciés, la vulnérabilité et la marginalisation des personnes racisées. Une analyse fondée sur la race est essentielle dans le cadre de la politique de santé publique. D'abord, les initiatives de santé publique peuvent renforcer les discours racistes persistants sur la façon dont un virus se transmet. Ensuite, la « viralisation » des personnes peut mener à blâmer injustement une communauté racisée pour une épidémie, tout en détournant l'attention des problèmes structurels dans des environnements particuliers, comme dans le cas des travailleurs migrants philippins employés dans les abattoirs, qui n'ont aucun contrôle sur leurs conditions de travail. Enfin, il existe maintenant des données qui prouvent que, compte tenu d'autres facteurs, certains groupes de personnes racisées, notamment les Noirs et les Asiatiques du Sud, pourraient succomber à la COVID-19 plus que d'autres. Ce chapitre, qui se penche sur la fermeture partielle de la frontière à titre d'étude de cas, examine la manière dont l'inclusion et l'exclusion historiques et contemporaines sélectives, mais simultanées, à la frontière ont construit les idées sociales à propos des étrangers. Les mesures frontalières reflètent une tension permanente : laisser entrer une main-d'œuvre bon marché pour assurer les services essentiels tout en apaisant la peur du public à l'égard de l'Asiatique comme vecteur du virus. Il conviendrait de recourir à une analyse raciale critique au moment d'évaluer les mesures de santé publique afin de s'assurer que les diverses expériences des communautés racisées sont prises en compte durant une pandémie.

Fear of the "yellow peril," a colour metaphor that refers to Asians as a threat to the West, has shaped and been shaped by Canada's response to the COVID-19 pandemic. Diminishing that fear and discrimination against persons perceived to be vectors of an infectious disease is an important strategy in controlling transmission.[1] As public health researchers have stated, "Persons who are feared and stigmatized may delay seeking care and remain in the community undetected."[2]

The experiences of Asian Canadians in the COVID-19 outbreak have brought into sharp focus the differentiated risks, vulnerability, and marginalization of racialized persons, both generally and in a health crisis. Before implementing measures to control the spread of emerging infectious diseases, public health officials must contemplate how those responses may be experienced differently by racialized persons. Part of this evaluation includes considering how law, policy, and discourse may racialize a disease and conversely, how people may be "treated as pathogens."[3] Further, in seeking to address public fear about the spread of disease, decision makers should evaluate to what extent strategies address the aim of reducing transmission or appease and/or promote public perceptions (sometimes racist perceptions) of how diseases spread.

This chapter provides a preliminary account of the racism experienced by Asian Canadians and calls for a robust race-based analysis of public health measures. While this chapter focuses on the partial border closure as a case study, I invite others to apply a critical race analysis to Canada's other responses to the pandemic.

The selective but simultaneous inclusion and exclusion of persons at the border has constructed social ideas of a foreign or Asian virus and affected how Canadians perceive the spread of the virus and the valid ways to limit its transmission. The federal government's border measures "selectively include" some persons, including temporary foreign workers to work in essential services, while "selectively excluding" others. This chapter posits that this partial border closure somewhat serves to pacify the wider public's fears and anxiety regarding Asian people as vectors of the virus, and raises questions about not only the efficacy of border restrictions but how it may perpetuate racist discourse in Canada.

It is too early to fully assess the extent to which border restrictions were and are effective in stemming the spread of COVID-19.

1. Bobbie Person et al, "Fear and Stigma: The Epidemic within the SARS Outbreak" (2004) 10:2 Emerging Infections Diseases 358 at 358 [Person et al].
2. *Ibid.*
3. Gerald Chan, "The Virus of Anti-Asian Prejudice", *The Star* (13 April 2020), online: <www.thestar.com/opinion/contributors/2020/04/13/the-virus-of-anti-asian-prejudice.html>.

There is debate among scientists[4], and I leave it to my colleagues to discuss this, including Steven J. Hoffman and Patrick Fafard in Chapter F-4 of this volume. This chapter addresses the way in which government responses can inform and shape the fear that people will have regarding a novel disease, and how this may fuel racist and harmful behaviour.

Anti-Asian Racism in Canada During the Pandemic

Racism, xenophobia and violence against Asian Canadians, including Chinese, Korean, Filipino, and Vietnamese people, among others, has intensified during the COVID-19 pandemic. While racism against Asians in Canada is not new,[5] anxiety associated with COVID-19 has increased the virulence of anti-Asian sentiment. Fear has manifested in the decline of visitors to Chinatowns and Asian restaurants,[6] the vandalization of Asian businesses,[7] the perpetuation of myths that Chinese people eat bats,[8] the use of the term "Chinese virus,"[9] and the

4. Marta Paterlini, "'Closing Borders Is Ridiculous': The Epidemiologist Behind Sweden's Controversial Coronavirus Strategy" (21 April 2020), online: *Nature* <www.nature.com/articles/d41586-020-01098-x>.
5. For example Joanna Chiu, "House-Hunting as an Asian Immigrant in Vancouver Means Navigating Racism", *The Star* (3 November 2019), online: <www.thestar.com/vancouver/2019/11/03/corrupt-immigrants-serve-as-real-estate-scapegoats-in-vancouvers-tight-market.html>; Kimberley Molina, "Vandals Target Chinese-Language Street Signs", *CBC News* (17 September 2019), online: <www.cbc.ca/news/canada/ottawa/street-sign-vandalized-ottawa-chinatown-1.5287001>; Melody Ma, "I've Lived the Racism Seen in that Viral Vancouver Parking Lot Video – Many Asians Have", *Welland Tribune* (29 August 2019), online: <www.wellandtribune.ca/opinion-story/9572052-i-ve-lived-the-racism-seen-in-that-viral-vancouver-parking-lot-video-many-asians-have/>.
6. Colette Derworiz, "'Support Them or Lose Them': Chinatowns Across Canada Grapple with Coronavirus Fears", *Global News* (27 February 2020), online: <globalnews.ca/news/6602754/coronavirus-chinatown-canada-business/>; Megan Shaw, "Watson and Public Health Team Visit Chinatown to Allay COVID-19 Fears", *CTV News* (6 March 2020), online: <ottawa.ctvnews.ca/watson-and-public-health-team-visit-chinatown-to-allay-covid-19-fears-1.4842445?cache=yes%3FclipId%3D89619%3FautoPlay%3Dtrue%3FautoPlay%3Dtrue>.
7. Diona Macalinga, "Rise in Asian Hate Crimes as COVID-19 Pandemic Grows", *The Link* (7 April 2020), online: <thelinknewspaper.ca/article/rise-in-asian-hate-crimes-as-covid-19-pandemic-grows_>.
8. Eleanor Cummins, "The New Coronavirus is not an Excuse to be Racist", *The Verge* (4 February 2020), online: <www.theverge.com/2020/2/4/21121358/coronavirus-racism-social-media-east-asian-chinese-xenophobia>.
9. Eren Orbey, "Trump's 'Chinese Virus' and What's at Stake in the Coronavirus's Name", *The New Yorker* (25 March 2020), online: <www.newyorker.com/culture/cultural-comment/whats-at-stake-in-a-viruss-name>.

revival of the derogatory slur, "Chink."[10] People of Filipino descent, blamed for the spread COVID-19 in meat-packing plants, are subject to racist comments, and are being barred from entering grocery stores and banks.[11] The pandemic has also brought awareness of the risks migrant workers take in working in Canada and the abusive treatment they are subject to.[12]

Since the virus emerged, there has been an increasing number of assaults of Asian people in Canada. For example, in Toronto, an Asian Canadian emergency room nurse was spat on, attacked with an umbrella, and told to "go home."[13] Toronto police decided not to treat this as a hate crime.[14] In another example, in Vancouver, a white male yelled racist comments and shoved an elderly Asian man with dementia out of a store.[15] A recent poll revealed that one in five Canadians think it is not safe to sit beside an Asian person on the bus.[16] Even Canada's Chief Public Health Officer, Dr. Tam, has not escaped racist abuse. Member of Parliament and Conservative leadership candidate

10. Rob Buscher, "'Reality is Hitting Me in the Face': Asian Americans Grapple with Racism Due to COVID-19" (21 April 2020), online: *Whyy* <whyy.org/articles/reality-is-hitting-me-in-the-face-asian-americans-grapple-with-racism-due-to-covid-19/>.
11. Stephanie Babych, "Filipino Workers Face Backlash in Towns over COVID-19 Outbreaks at Packing Plants", *Calgary Herald* (29 April 2020), online: <calgaryherald.com/news/filipino-employees-not-to-blame-for-meat-packing-plant-outbreaks-that-have-surpassed-1000-cases/>; Joel Dryden, "Filipino Workers at Meatpacking Plant Feel Unfairly Blamed for Canada's Biggest COVID-19 Outbreak", *CBC News* (26 April 2020), online: <www.cbc.ca/news/canada/calgary/cargill-high-river-jbs-brooks-deena-hinshaw-1.5545113>.
12. Max Martin, "COVID-19: Southwestern Ontario Outbreak Puts Migrant Farm Workers in Spotlight" (28 April 2020), online: *Woodstock Sentinel-Review* <www.woodstocksentinelreview.com/news/local-news/covid-19-southwestern-ontario-outbreak-puts-migrant-farm-workers-in-spotlight/wcm/543d7fab-57d0-4aab-9d39-094fbbd28f8a>; see also Babych and Dryden, *ibid.*
13. Phil Tsekouras, "'It Happened Because I'm Asian': Toronto ER Nurse Says She Was Spit on, Verbally Assaulted", *CTV News* (9 April 2020), online: <toronto.ctvnews.ca/it-happened-because-i-m-asian-toronto-er-nurse-says-she-was-spit-on-verbally-assaulted-1.4890363>.
14. *Ibid.*
15. "Vancouver Police ID Suspect in Alleged Racially Motivated Attack Against Elderly Asian Man with Dementia", *CBC News* (23 April 2020), online: <www.cbc.ca/news/canada/british-columbia/vancouver-police-id-suspect-racially-motivated-attack-elderly-asian-man-dementia-1.5542763>.
16. Wanyee Li, "One in 5 Canadians Think It's not Safe to Sit Beside an Asian Person on the Bus, According to Recent Poll", *The Star* (27 April 2020), online: <www.thestar.com/news/canada/2020/04/27/one-in-5-canadians-think-its-not-safe-to-sit-beside-an-asian-person-on-the-bus-according-to-recent-poll.html>.

Derek Sloan questioned Dr. Tam's loyalty, accusing her of working for the government of China.[17]

All of these racist incidents happened in a span of eight weeks. This racist hostility has affected how Asian Canadians cope with the pandemic. Some make efforts to demonstrate they are taking greater than necessary precautions. But when Asian Canadians were among the first in Canada to wear masks in public, these precautions were vilified and misunderstood as evidence Asian Canadians were the primary source of the virus.[18] For others, the pandemic has meant more intense, remote, and lonely isolation to avoid confrontations and violence.[19]

Canada's Pandemic Border Inclusions and Exclusions

On March 16, 2020, Prime Minister Justin Trudeau announced the Canadian border was closed to all persons showing symptoms of COVID-19 and foreign nationals, with some exceptions that included U.S. citizens.[20] The government soon had to walk this back. A few days later, the government stated that temporary foreign workers and international students would also be exempted, but that refugee claimants at the Canada-U.S. border would be turned away.[21] Since

17. Kathleen Harris, "Conservatives Blast MP Who Asked Whether Top Pandemic Doctor 'Works for China' as Scheer Steers Clear", *CBC News* (23 April 2020), online: <www.cbc.ca/news/politics/sloan-tam-china-coronavirus-pandemic-1.5542497>.
18. Jonathan Hayward, "Cultures Clash over Wearing Masks Amid Virus", The Globe and Mail (29 March 2020), online: <www.theglobeandmail.com/canada/british-columbia/article-cultures-clash-over-wearing-masks-amid-virus/>; Tony Lin, "Want to hear something f***ed-up? While the entire dining industry is suffering from COVID, Chinese restaurants across US took the earliest hit months b4 the local outbreak, yet they were actually the most cautious & prepared, many were buying masks and sanitizers way earlier." (29 April 2020 at 11:30), online: Twitter <twitter.com/tony_zy/status/1255519790950690826>.
19. Carol Liao, "This is why I've told my parents they aren't to go out at all & my white husband is the only one going out to get groceries for both households. It's COVID19 but also threat of racist acts. Not worth the risk. Sometimes this city really breaks my heart." (23 April 2020 at 12:43), online: Twitter <twitter.com/carolmliao/status/1253363805309898752>.
20. Maclean's, "Justin Trudeau's Address to the Nation on Border Restrictions: Full Transcript", *Maclean's* (16 March 2020), online: <www.macleans.ca/news/canada/justin-trudeaus-address-to-the-nation-on-border-restrictions-full-transcript/>. See *Minimizing the Risk of Exposure to COVID-19 Coronavirus Disease in Canada Order (Prohibition of Entry into Canada)*, PC 2020-0157.
21. Global News, "Temporary Foreign Workers Exempt from Some COVID-19 Travel Restrictions", *Global News* (20 March 2020), online: <globalnews.ca/

then, restrictions have both increased and loosened for various persons travelling from the United States.[22]

Déjà vu: Restrictions Based on Fear

The racist reaction to the pandemic is not surprising. Public health researchers have noted, "During the SARS outbreak, some persons became fearful or suspicious of all people who looked Asian, regardless of their nationality or actual risk factors for SARS, and expected them to be quarantined."[23] Further, "[o]ther infectious disease epidemics have been associated with specific ethnic groups," such as the bubonic plague and the Chinese community in 1900, and the hantavirus infection dubbed the "Navajo disease" in 1993.[24]

Historically, immigration law in both Canada and the U.S. used public health reasons to restrict immigration of Asians.[25] The listing of contagious diseases alongside requirements for detailed reports of passengers on ships not only acted to exclude racialized migrants, but contributed to the conflation of racialized persons with disease. Racism has led to, and has been encouraged by, a number of exclusionary policies toward racialized persons in Canada.[26] The first example is the tragedy of the Komagata Maru in 1914, a ship carrying 376 Sikh passengers fleeing India.[27] Canada refused entry of the passengers on the ship and when the Komagata Maru returned to India, 19 persons

---

news/6711597/temporary-foreign-workers-travel-rules/>; see *Minimizing the Risk of Exposure to COVID-19 in Canada Order (Prohibition of Entry into Canada from the United States)*, PC 2020-0161; *Minimizing the Risk of Exposure to COVID-19 in Canada Order (Prohibition of Entry into Canada from Any Country Other Than the United States)*, PC 2020-0162.

22. See *Minimizing the Risk of Exposure to COVID-19 in Canada Order (Prohibition of Entry into Canada from the United States)*, PC 2020-0185, which imposed greater restrictions on persons coming from the U.S. in general, including refugee claimants; *Minimizing the Risk of Exposure to COVID-19 in Canada Order (Prohibition of Entry into Canada from the United States)*, PC 2020-0263, which loosened restrictions so that some persons coming from the U.S. can make refugee claims.
23. Person et al, *supra* note 1 at 358-59.
24. *Ibid* at 361-62.
25. Erika Lee, "The 'Yellow Peril' and Asian Exclusion in the Americas" (2007) 76:4 Pacific Historical Rev 537.
26. This essay acknowledges there are many other examples, including the internment of Ukrainian and Japanese people, and the refusal to allow the St Louis to dock, a ship carrying Jewish refugees.
27. "The Incident" (last visited 29 May 2020), online: *Komagata Maru: Continuing the Journey* <komagatamarujourney.ca/incident>.

were killed.[28] Hugh Johnston wrote of the "fear that Asian immigration might overwhelm white British Columbian society"[29] and how Sikhs already in Canada, "were well aware of Canadian hostility" since they "heard it openly and rudely on the streets, and they saw it in the immigration law that prevented their friends and relatives from entering the country."[30]

The second example is the head tax imposed on Chinese persons immigrating to Canada.[31] As Lily Cho explains, the head tax was a policy response to allow some form of cheap labour to enter Canada, while "pacifying fear and anxiety in Western Canada."[32] Cho writes that the head tax permitted selective inclusion to allow for the economic exploitation of Chinese persons while "appeasing an increasingly angry BC population."[33]

The research of both Johnston and Cho discuss the tension the Sikh and Chinese figure raised: the need to import cheap labour while addressing the fear in the white settler public of the Asian other.[34] In these and other examples, racialized migrants are constructed as foreign, contributing to the perception that they are disloyal and threaten not only national security and public health but also cultural and economic life in Western democracies.[35] Labelling persons as foreign permitted exploitative and abusive labour practices, while generating the idea that migrant workers were disposable. It is the stickiness of the label of foreignness that allows Asian Canadians to slip between identities of the model minority and yellow peril, always pitting Asian Canadians either against other racialized persons or against white persons.

---

28. *Ibid.*
29. Hugh Johnston, *The Voyage of the Komagata Maru: The Sikh Challenge to Canada's Colour Bar* (Vancouver: University of British Columbia Press, 1989) at 90. See also Rita Dhamoon et al, *Unmooring the Komagata Maru* (Vancouver: University of British Columbia Press, 2020).
30. *Ibid* at 20.
31. Andrea Yu, "The Enduring Legacy of Canada's Racist Head Tax on Chinese-Canadians", *Maclean's* (1 March 2019), online: <www.macleans.ca/society/the-enduring-legacy-of-canadas-racist-head-tax-on-chinese-canadians/>.
32. Lily Cho, "Rereading Chinese Head Tax Racism: Redress, Stereotype, and Antiracist Critical Practice" (2002) 75 Essays on Can Writing 62 at 67.
33. *Ibid.*
34. Johnston, *supra* note 29; Cho, *supra* note 32.
35. Natsu Taylor Saito, "Model Minority, Yellow Peril: Functions of 'Foreignness' in the Construction of Asian American Legal Identity" (1997) 4 Asian LJ 71.

Keeping out the Yellow Peril

As Canada's Chief Public Health Officer, Dr. Tam, has explained, shutting the border to persons coming from China may not have solved the problem because the virus, "had already travelled somewhere else" by the time cases manifested in Canada, and those cases were linked to countries that were not reporting significant numbers of COVID-19 cases, such as Iran and some European countries.[36]

It is early days and statistics provided by the Canadian government may not have been collected in an optimal manner, but data disclosed thus far reveal interesting trends. As of April 7, 2020, 26% of COVID-19 cases have been related to travel exposure.[37] In March 2020, 42% of all non-resident travellers who had COVID-19 were from Europe, 35% were from Asia, and 10% were from North America, Central America, and the Caribbean.[38] By early March, only 10 cases in Canada could be traced back to travel from China.[39]

In another set of government data, as of April 27, 2020, 20% of persons with COVID-19 in Canada were exposed while travelling or exposed to a traveller coming to Canada, while 80% had no known contact with a travel-related case and had not travelled outside of Canada in the 14 days prior to illness onset.[40] It is difficult to assess whether the partial border closure is effective, given that some restrictions were placed starting March 18, 2020, and considering that people continue to cross our borders. It is unclear whether the rate of testing may have changed this data and to what extent non-Asian permanent residents or citizens were travelling from Asia.

Dr. Tam admitted, "The idea of shutting Canada's borders to international travel wasn't in the playbook of most health experts."[41] Despite this, Canada initially moved to close the border to everyone

---

36. Peter Zimonjic, Rosemary Barton & Philip Ling, "'Was It Perfect? No': Theresa Tam Discusses Canada's Early Pandemic Response", *CBC News* (27 April 2020), online: <www.cbc.ca/news/politics/theresa-tam-could-have-acted-sooner-1.5546819>.
37. Statistics Canada, *Travel-Related Exposure to COVID-19* (Ottawa: Statistics Canada, 8 April 2020), online: *Statistics Canada* <www150.statcan.gc.ca/n1/pub/89-28-0001/2018001/article/00018-eng.htm>.
38. *Ibid.*
39. Zimonjic et al, *supra* note 36.
40. Government of Canada, *Epidemiological Summary of COVID-19 Cases in Canada* (Ottawa: Government of Canada, last updated 27 April 2020), online: *Government of Canada* <health-infobase.canada.ca/covid-19/epidemiological-summary-covid-19-cases.html>.
41. Zimonjic et al, *supra* note 36.

except U.S. citizens, even though data now shows a large number of travellers infected with COVID-19 were American as opposed to Asian.[42]

Did Canada contemplate the effect border closures would have on the public's fears? Public health researchers recognize that "[f]ear is further fuelled when infection control techniques and restrictive practices such as quarantine and isolation are employed to protect the public's health."[43] The partial closure of the border is a continuation of the practice of "selective inclusion," allowing racialized labour to work in essential services (albeit in problematic conditions) while calming the fears and anxiety of a public that views Asians as a disease.

While there is not a complete border shutdown and the measures do not directly prohibit the entry of Asians, the exclusions still may serve no other function but to pacify fear and anxiety of people in Canada while allowing useful Asians in. By closing off the border to the non-essential, the government may have reinforced narratives that foreigners, specifically Asians, are the source of the virus and that we should keep them out.

Essential Migrant Labour in a Pandemic

What is striking is that essential work in health care, food processing, and agriculture is largely being done by racialized migrant workers, including asylum seekers.[44] Outbreaks in these environments have been blamed on them: for example, Filipino workers in meat-packing plants and long-term care facilities. In both of these examples, Asian migrant workers are cast as carriers of the disease, further perpetuating narratives of the yellow peril. Some news coverage has pointed to crowded living and working conditions, the lack of safety equipment, and the fact that health care workers in long-term care facilities

42. Ryan Tumility, "Canada's Early COVID-19 Cases from the U.S. not China, Provincial Data Shows", *National Post* (30 April 2020), online: <nationalpost.com/news/politics/canadas-early-covid-19-cases-came-from-the-u-s-not-china-provincial-data-shows>.
43. Person et al, *supra* note 1 at 358.
44. Verity Stevenson & Benjamin Shingler, "Quebec Relies on Hundreds of Asylum Seekers in Long-Term Care Battle Against COVID-19", *CBC News* (8 May 2020), online: <www.cbc.ca/news/canada/montreal/quebec-chsld-asylum-seekers-1.5559354?__vfz=medium%3Dsharebar>; Yves Boisvert, "Il s'appelait Marcelin Francois", *La Presse* (8 May 2020), online: <plus.lapresse.ca/screens/3c5f9503-455d-479e-9b25-72fa1b1944c8__7C___0.html?utm_medium=Twitter&utm_campaign=Microsite+Share&utm_content=Screen>.

are forced to work in part-time positions in multiple facilities to survive economically. What is often overlooked, however, is that these conditions are not those constructed by the migrant worker but by the industry or employers paying low wages or ignoring basic living, employment, and labour rights.[45] Y. Y. Chen and Sarah Berger Richardson in Chapters D-8 and E-5 of this volume write about how working conditions for migrant workers make them vulnerable to infection.

The pandemic has amplified the vulnerabilities of those with temporary immigration status in Canada. While migrant workers are among those exempted from the restrictions at the border, their temporary immigration status is the very reason they may be seen as carriers of COVID-19, even though the conditions that promote the spread are not under their control. The precarity of migrant workers' immigration status has contributed to the exploitative and abusive conditions[46] (including the inability to be physically distant, lack of proper safety equipment, low pay, part-time nature of the job, and fear of reprisals or loss of the job) which potentially allow the virus to spread. Their experience during the pandemic raises questions about why these workers don't have immediate pathways to permanent residence in Canada, especially because it is the temporality of their immigration status that allows exploitative conditions to exist. The fact that some of the migrant workers are racialized fuels public discourse that the spread of the virus at these workplaces is due to their presence there, and not the conditions of their employment.

Including Race-Based Analysis in a Pandemic Plan

Policy-makers have many factors to consider. It is an unenviable position to be dealing with a new, unknown, and unpredictable harm. Public health officials should consider, when evaluating the need to protect the public with restrictive practices, how those measures affect racialized persons. There is emerging data showing racialized persons, like Black, Latinx, and South Asian persons, are more likely

45. Ethel Tungohan, "Filipino Healthcare Workers During COVID-19 and the Importance of Race-Based Analysis" (1 May 2020), online (blog): *The Broadbent Blog* <www.broadbentinstitute.ca/filipino_healthcare_workers_during_covid19_and_the_importance_of_race_based_analysis>.

46. Amrita Hari, "Temporariness, Rights and Citizenship: The Latest Chapter in Canada's Exclusionary Migration and Refugee History" (2014) 30:2 Refuge 35.

to die from COVID-19 than white people. This increased risk of death has been attributed in the U.S. to "[s]tructural factors including health care access, density of households, unemployment, pervasive discrimination and others"[47] but data in the U.K. also show that the difference may not be caused by pre-existing differences in wealth, health, education or living arrangements.[48] Responses to the pandemic must consider how racialized communities experience the pandemic differently, whether they are Asian, Black, Indigenous, or Latinx. Further, pandemic plans should include strategies to reduce the fear that necessarily comes with the virus, which can stimulate racism, xenophobia, stereotyping, and stigmatization.

While partial border closures are one line of defence, policymakers should contemplate the impact this and other kinds of restrictions will have on certain populations. A gender-based plus analysis, including a race-based analysis, needs to be undertaken when a particular measure is being considered, especially given the history of how infectious diseases have stigmatized racialized persons and how historical border restrictions can shape racist narratives. While there has been a condemnation of racist attacks,[49] a more systemic strategy to combat racism is needed.

Many racialized persons are putting their lives at risk serving on the front lines in health care, and ensuring our food supply is stable. One serves as Canada's top doctor. Being the "model minority" is not a good strategy, because in times of crisis, Asian Canadians are constructed as instant outsiders, regardless of whether we are temporary foreign workers, naturalized immigrants, or have spent generations here. Belonging in Canada is complicated by immigration and public health policies which imply that some are transmitters of disease and some are "essential." The normative discourse born of long-held immigration policies and more recent pandemic responses is, in part, responsible for reifying foreignness on racialized bodies.

---

47. Shelby Lin Erdman, "Black Communities Account for Disproportionate Number of COVID-19 Deaths in the US, Study Finds", *CNN* (6 May 2020), online: <www.cnn.com/2020/05/05/health/coronavirus-african-americans-study/index.html>.
48. Robert Booth & Cailainn Barr, "Black People Four Times More Likely to Die from COVID-19, ONS Finds", *The Guardian* (7 May 2020), online: <www.theguardian.com/world/2020/may/07/black-people-four-times-more-likely-to-die-from-covid-19-ons-finds?CMP=share_btn_tw>.
49. Kathleen Harris, "Canada's Chief Public Health Officer Condemns Racist Acts Linked to Coronavirus Outbreak", *CBC News* (30 January 2020), online: <www.cbc.ca/news/politics/tam-public-health-coronavirus-racism-1.5445713>.

While the government is starting to acknowledge how the spread of a novel virus can differentially affect racialized persons by gathering data during the pandemic,[50] in the long term, what we consider to be health-relevant data should include race and immigration profiles.[51] Further, Canada should be creating permanent residence programs for essential foreign workers. As well, pandemic plans must address racist misinformation by anticipating and actively reacting to public discourse. Most of all, while public health officials should recognize that an outbreak will be accompanied with fear, our responses should not be driven by fear.

---

50. Johanna Weidner, "Ontario Will Soon Gather Race, Income-Related COVID Data", *The Record* (7 May 2020), online: <www.therecord.com/news/waterloo-region/2020/05/07/ontario-will-soon-gather-race-income-related-covid-data.html>.
51. Aimée-Angélique Bouka & Yolande Bouka, "Over the Long Term, Canada Should Collect Better Health Data that Looks Closely at the Intersecting Issues of Race and Immigration", *Policy Options* (19 May 2020), online: <policyoptions.irpp.org/magazines/may-2020/canadas-covid-19-blind-spots-on-race-immigration-and-labour/>.

CHAPTER D-8

Migrant Health in a Time of Pandemic: Fallacies of Us-Versus-Them

Y.Y. Brandon Chen*

Abstract

International migrants—including, among others, immigrants, refugees, asylum seekers, foreign workers, and international students—are at greater risk of being affected by COVID-19. However, following the onset of the pandemic, many of them continue to be denied publicly funded health care and income supports in Canada. For migrants who are granted entitlement to these government programs, significant access barriers exist. These exclusionary policies underscore a dynamic of us-versus-them, in which migrants are portrayed as a threat to public health and undeserving of the Canadian society's help. This process of "othering" fails to adequately appreciate migrants' belonging in and contributions to Canada. It runs counter to the principles of equality and reciprocity that are central to our legal order, and it also risks compromising our collective pursuit of public health. An effective response to the current pandemic requires solidarity among all members of society instead of insistent line drawing between citizens and migrants who are similarly situated.

* Assistant Professor in the University of Ottawa's Faculty of Law (Common Law Section).

Résumé
La santé des migrants en période de pandémie : les erreurs du « nous contre eux »

Les migrants internationaux, notamment les immigrants, les réfugiés, les demandeurs d'asile, les travailleurs étrangers et les étudiants internationaux, sont plus susceptibles d'être touchés par la COVID-19. Cependant, depuis le début de la pandémie, nombre d'entre eux continuent de se voir refuser l'accès aux soins de santé et aux programmes de soutien du revenu financés par l'État au Canada. Pour les migrants qui ont droit à ces programmes gouvernementaux, les obstacles sont considérables. Ces politiques d'exclusion témoignent d'une dynamique du « nous contre eux », dans laquelle les migrants sont présentés comme une menace pour la santé publique et comme des personnes qui ne méritent pas l'aide de la société canadienne. Cette discrimination envers « l'autre » ne permet pas d'apprécier à leur juste valeur l'appartenance et la contribution des migrants au Canada. Elle va à l'encontre des principes d'égalité et de réciprocité qui sont au cœur de notre système de droit, et risque de compromettre notre quête collective de santé publique. Pour réagir efficacement à la pandémie actuelle, tous les membres de la société doivent faire preuve de solidarité plutôt que d'insister pour établir une distinction entre les citoyens et les migrants qui se trouvent dans une situation similaire.

Research has repeatedly confirmed that, upon arrival in Canada, international migrants on average exhibit equal if not better health than their native-born counterparts.[1] But this relative health advantage dissipates over time, in part due to migrants' encounter with discrimination in receiving communities.[2] Notwithstanding this reality, public policy and discourse in Canada regularly conjure up images of migrants as diseased and dangerous rather than as a population vulnerable to the adverse effects of ill health.[3] Canada's responses to the COVID-19 pandemic to date have proven to be no different. So far as

1. Zoua M Vang et al, "Are Immigrants Healthier Than Native-Born Canadians? A Systemic Review of the Healthy Immigrant Effect in Canada" (2017) 22:3 Ethnicity & Health 209.
2. Fernando G De Maio & Eagan Kemp, "The Deterioration of Health Status Among Immigrants to Canada" (2010) 5:5 Global Public Health 462.
3. See Jamie Liew, this volume, Chapter D-7.

these government measures are directed at migrants, they have been primarily aimed at regulating migrants' admission into the country, as opposed to safeguarding migrants' health and well-being.[4]

The suggestion that migrants are "of risk," despite their being "at risk" in actuality, both reflects and reinforces the "othering" of migrants in receiving societies.[5] Through the process of othering, an in-group exploits its privilege to define who belongs and rationalize the status loss of those deemed deviant.[6] With regard to migrants, this process is advanced by the narrative of public health threat, which pits them against the native-born: allegedly, *their* exotic diseases endanger *our* health. This notion of us-versus-them in turn dulls receiving societies' sense of responsibility for the protection *of* migrants and instead steers public health policies toward the protection of society *from* migrants.

In this essay, I set out to problematize the othering of migrants amid Canada's COVID-19 responses. I begin by offering a counter-narrative to the typical portrayal of migrants as a threat, in which I lay bare migrants' heightened risk of COVID-19 infection in Canada. Next, I show that irrespective of migrants' vulnerability, many continue to be excluded from government health care and income support programs in the wake of the pandemic. Even when migrants do qualify for these programs, there remain concerns about accessibility because of the government's insufficient assurance that service utilization will not negatively affect migrants' ability to stay in the country. Such an insistent divide between citizens and migrants as us and them, I argue, is especially problematic in a time of a pandemic. Not only does it disregard migrants' belonging in Canadian society, but it also undermines the pursuit of public health.

Migrants as a Vulnerable Population

Canada has long relied on migrants, including an increasing number of temporary foreign workers, to alleviate its labour shortages.[7]

4. See e.g. *Minimizing the Risk of Exposure to COVID-19 Coronavirus Disease in Canada Order (Prohibition of Entry into Canada)*, PC 2020-0157.
5. Natalie J Grove and Anthony B Zwi, "Our Health and Theirs: Forced Migration, Othering, and Public Health" (2006) 62 Social Science & Medicine 1931.
6. *Ibid* at 1933.
7. Alan G Green & David A Green, "The Economic Goals of Canada's Immigration Policy: Past and Present" (1999) 25:4 Can Public Policy 425; Myer Siemiatycki, "Marginalizing Migrants: Canada's Rising Reliance on Temporary Foreign Workers" (2010) Can Issues 60.

During the COVID-19 pandemic, many migrant workers have come to shoulder the responsibility of providing essential goods and services to Canadians, ranging from maintaining the food supply to caregiving.[8] This puts them and their families at greater risk of being exposed to the virus. Above all, farms and food-processing facilities have emerged as hotbeds of COVID-19 transmission for migrants.[9] Cargill's meat plant in Alberta alone, where a majority of the employees were foreign-born, was linked to over 1,500 COVID-19 cases, making it the largest outbreak to date in North America attributable to a workplace.[10]

To the extent that the danger of working during the pandemic can be mitigated by taking appropriate protective measures, migrants' ability to do so is significantly curtailed. In many industries with a concentration of migrant workers, physical distancing is not readily observable: migrants frequently work in cramped space, and some must live in close quarters provided by employers.[11] Inadequate screening protocols and a lack of personal protective equipment at these workplaces further enable the virus's spread.[12] Compounding

8. Zhenzhen Ye, "Maintaining Food Security During the Coronavirus Pandemic Means Looking After the Health of Migrant Workers", *National Post* (7 April 2020), online: <nationalpost.com/opinion/zhenzhen-ye-on-covid-19-maintaining-food-security-during-the-coronavirus-pandemic-means-looking-after-the-health-of-migrant-workers>; Verity Stevenson & Benjamin Shingler, "Quebec Relies on Hundreds of Asylum Seekers in Long-Term Care's Battle Against COVID-19", *CBC News* (8 May 2020), online: <www.cbc.ca/news/canada/montreal/quebec-chsld-asylum-seekers-1.5559354>.

9. See Sarah Berger Richardson, this volume, Chapter E-5; see also Jenna Hennebry, "Canada Jeopardizes Migrant Workers Amid Pandemic", *Cornwall Standard Freeholder* (6 June 2020) A7; Omar Mosleh, "Dealing With a Precarious Present for a Stable Future: Despite Virus's Looming Threat, Immigrants Say They Must Keep Working to Support Their Families", *Toronto Star* (5 May 2020) B1.

10. Joel Dryden & Sarah Rieger, "Inside the Slaughterhouse", *CBC News* (6 May 2020), online: <newsinteractives.cbc.ca/longform/cargill-covid19-outbreak>.

11. See e.g. Mosleh, *supra* note 9; Sara Mojtehedzadeh, "Migrant Farm Workers from Jamaica Are Being Forced to Sign COVID-19 Waivers", *Toronto Star* (13 April 2020), online: <www.thestar.com/business/2020/04/13/migrant-farm-workers-fear-exposure-to-covid-19.html>.

12. Carrie Tait, Kathryn Blaze Baum & Tavia Grant, "Unions Question Worker Safety as Cargill Reopens Plant at Centre of COVID-19 Outbreak", *The Globe and Mail* (5 May 2020), online: <www.theglobeandmail.com/canada/article-union-questions-worker-safety-as-cargill-reopens-plant-at-centre-of/>; Ethel Tungohan, "Filipino Healthcare Workers During COVID-19 and the Importance of Race-Based Analysis" (1 May 2020), online (blog): *The Broadbent Blog* <www.broadbentinstitute.ca/filipino_healthcare_workers_during_covid19_and_the_importance_of_race_based_analysis>.

the problem is the acute power imbalance between many migrant workers and their employers. Migrants with precarious legal status are often fearful of deportation, and they depend heavily on employers to help them maintain and renew their immigration authorization.[13] Even for migrants whose legal status is more secure, many find themselves trapped in their existing jobs because the prospects of obtaining alternative employment are hampered by their limited official language proficiency and formal education.[14] Such a power differential, coupled with the necessity to make ends meet, exerts considerable pressure on migrants to accept unsafe working conditions, including the need to keep working while ill, and it deters migrants from speaking out against employers' non-compliance with public health directives.[15]

Employment-related risk factors aside, migrants' vulnerability to contracting COVID-19 is exacerbated by their relative economic insecurity. Migrants, especially those who have been in the country for less than five years, are much more likely than their Canadian-born counterparts to live in poverty.[16] In 2010, nearly one in three newcomers to Canada struggled with low income.[17] Such financial insecurity causes many migrants to resort to living in overcrowded, substandard housing, which is known to facilitate the transmission of pathogens.[18] One refugee shelter in Toronto, for example, was home to a COVID-19 outbreak involving 88 of its residents.[19] Additionally, low income puts migrants in peril of experiencing malnutrition and

13. Sarah Marsden, "Silence Means Yes Here in Canada: Precarious Migrants, Work and the Law" (2014) 18 CLELJ 1.
14. Mosleh, *supra* note 9.
15. Max Martin, "Outbreak Puts Migrant Farm Workers in Spotlight", *Brantford Expositor* (29 April 2020) A5; Lorian Hardcastle, "COVID-19 Lays Bare Poor Conditions in Long-Term Care Homes", *Edmonton Journal* (24 April 2020), online: <edmontonjournal.com/opinion/columnists/opinion-covid-19-lays-bare-poor-conditions-in-long-term-care-homes/>.
16. Garnett Picot & Feng Hou, "Immigration, Poverty and Income Inequality in Canada" in David A Green, W Craig Riddell & France St-Hilaire, eds, *Income Inequality: The Canadian Story*, (Montreal: Institute for Research on Public Policy, 2016) 175.
17. *Ibid*.
18. Ian Wanyeki et al, "Dwellings, Crowding, and Tuberculosis in Montreal" (2006) 63:2 Social Science & Medicine 501.
19. Liam Casey, "COVID-19 Outbreak Surges Among Homeless in Toronto with 135 Cases", *CTV News* (25 April 2020), online: <toronto.ctvnews.ca/covid-19-outbreak-surges-among-homeless-in-toronto-with-135-cases-1.4911670?cache=esoj ovbbggirjp>.

chronic stress, thus compromising their immunity and making them more susceptible to infection.[20] Indeed, preliminary data from Canada and abroad indicate that the current pandemic disproportionately impacts low-income, racialized neighbourhoods.[21]

Othering of Migrants in Canada's COVID-19 Responses

Despite being subjected to an elevated risk of infection, many migrants in Canada remain left out of government programs that are key to preventing and alleviating the deleterious impact of COVID-19, including health care and income support.

Prior to the pandemic, migrants' entitlement to publicly funded health care in Canada depended on their immigration and resident statuses, and it sometimes varied from one province/territory to another.[22] Broadly speaking, provincial and territorial health care plans covered all permanent residents. Some jurisdictions also extended coverage to both migrant workers and international students, while others only the former; in approximately half of the provinces and territories, these temporary residents must possess a permit valid for at least six months to qualify, whereas in the other half their permit must be good for one year or longer. In Quebec, Ontario, and British Columbia, eligible migrants generally had to wait for up to three months before their health care coverage would take effect. Some refugees and asylum seekers received health care from a federal program instead, but undocumented migrants were excluded from all government health care benefits.

Following the onset of the COVID-19 outbreaks, several provinces have decided to expand migrants' entitlement under their

20. Sylvia Reitmanova & Diana Gustafson, "Rethinking Immigrant Tuberculosis Control in Canada: From Medical Surveillance to Tackling Social Determinants of Health" (2012) 14 J Immigrant & Minority Health 6.
21. See e.g. Hannah Chung et al, *COVID-19 Laboratory Testing in Ontario: Patterns of Testing and Characteristics of Individuals Tested, as of April 30, 2020*, (Toronto: ICES, 2020) at 14, online: <ices.on.ca/Publications/Atlases-and-Reports/2020/COVID-19-Laboratory-Testing-in-Ontario>; Jarvis T Chen & Nancy Krieger, "Revealing the Unequal Burden of COVID-19 by Income, Race/Ethnicity, and Household Crowding: US County vs. ZIP Code Analyses" (2020) Harvard Center for Population and Development Studies Working Paper 19:1, online: <tinyurl.com/ya44we2r>.
22. YY Brandon Chen, "Social Determinants & Marginalized Populations" in Joanna Erdman, Vanessa Gruben & Erin Nelson, eds, *Canadian Health Law and Policy*, 5th ed (Toronto: LexisNexis, 2017) 527.

respective health insurance programs in an effort to stem the spread of the virus. Most notably, Ontario has temporarily extended coverage for medically necessary health care to all previously uninsured people in the province, and the three-month waiting period it typically imposed on new and returning residents has been suspended for the time being.[23] British Columbia has adopted similar policy changes. However, its broadening of essential health care coverage to formerly uninsured individuals is restricted to foreign workers with a permit of less than six months, as well as temporary residents who remain in the province on lapsed work or study permits—many of whom are facing administrative delays in renewing their immigration documents or are stranded by pandemic-related border closures and flight cancellations.[24] For other uninsured migrants such as undocumented persons, only health care services "related to suspected or confirmed cases of infection with COVID-19" will be publicly covered.[25]

Comparatively, other provinces and territories, as well as the federal government, have been much less responsive to migrants' health care needs during the pandemic. They have either not expanded migrants' health care entitlement at all within their jurisdictions, or only introduced what may at best be described as half measures. For instance, Alberta has extended health care coverage to foreign workers with expired permits for the duration of the province's pandemic-triggered state of emergency.[26] But unlike British Columbia, it has made no effort to provide publicly funded health care to other uninsured residents, not even services required to assess, test, or treat COVID-19.

In contrast, Newfoundland and Labrador, Quebec, and Manitoba have announced that they would cover the cost of COVID-19 testing and treatment for all residents regardless of their health insurance

23. Ontario Health Insurance Plan Bulletin, 4749, "COVID-19 Expanding Access to OHIP Coverage and Funding Physician and Hospital Services for Uninsured Patients" (25 March 2020), online: *Ontario Ministry of Health* <health.gov.on.ca/en/pro/programs/ohip/bulletins/4000/bul4749.aspx>.
24. "Medical Services Plan Response to COVID-19" (last modified 9 April 2020), online: *British Columbia* <gov.bc.ca/gov/content/health/health-drug-coverage/msp/bc-residents/msp-covid-19-response>.
25. *Ibid.*
26. Rachel Ward, "Alberta Extends Health Care to Uninsured Foreigners With Lapsed Work Permits During Pandemic", *CBC News* (23 April 2020), online: <cbc.ca/news/canada/calgary/alberta-health-care-extension-expired-work-permits-1.5543174?__vfz=medium%3Dsharebar>.

status.[27] In Quebec, such public coverage would also be given to people who are in the three-month waiting period.[28] However, policies concerning coverage for other health care services remain unchanged in these provinces. This dichotomy between health care for COVID-19 and that for other medical conditions raises practical challenges. Do screening and treatment for suspected COVID-19 patients who subsequently test negative for the virus count as COVID-19-related? Likewise, when COVID-19 patients' symptoms are intensified by underlying medical conditions such as hypertension and diabetes, would the cost of treating such comorbidities be paid by the government? No provincial authorities have provided ready answers to these questions.

Uncertainty also abounds for previously uninsured migrants when seeking to exercise their newly acquired health care entitlement. Reportedly, not all health care facilities in relevant provinces are aware of the policy changes, and some have continued to demand payment from migrant patients for services that are supposed to be free.[29] For undocumented migrants, this disjunction between entitlement and access is aggravated by their fear of detection and deportation. Although Canada has temporarily halted almost all deportations in the wake of the pandemic,[30] collection of personal data by the law enforcement persists. In particular, as a part of its emergency measures during the pandemic, Ontario has granted its first responders access to the personal information of individuals who test positive

27. "COVID-19 MCP Updates" (last modified 6 May 2020), online: *Newfoundland and Labrador Health and Community Services* <health.gov.nl.ca/health/mcp/covid-19-mcp-updates.html>; "Questions and Answers About Our Services During the Pandemic" (last visited 9 May 2020), online: *Régie de l'assurance maladie* <ramq.gouv.qc.ca/en/regie/press-room/Pages/questions-answers-services-during-pandemic.aspx> [RAMQ Policy]; Rachel Bergen, "Though Few are Aware, Newcomers in Manitoba Without Health Coverage Can Access COVID-19 Testing, Treatment", *CBC News* (19 April 2020), online: <cbc.ca/news/canada/manitoba/newcomers-manitoba-health-covid-19-1.5532114>.

28. RAMQ Policy, *supra* note 27.

29. See e.g. Emma Paling, "Migrants in Ontario Aren't Getting the Free Health Care They were Promised", *Huffington Post* (22 April 2020), online: <huffingtonpost.ca/entry/migrants-ontario-coronavirus-free-health-care_ca_5ea062eec5b69150246c07f7>; Lisa-Marie Gervais, "Des soins liés à la COVID-19 facturés à des sans-papiers", *Le Devoir* (27 April 2020), online: <ledevoir.com/societe/sante/577784/des-soins-factures-a-des-sans-papiers>.

30. Rachel Ward, "Canadian Border Officials Halt Most Deportations in Face of COVID-19", *CBC News* (18 March 2020), online: <cbc.ca/news/canada/calgary/cbsa-refugees-immigrants-deportations-1.5501334>.

for COVID-19.[31] Public interest organizations have warned of the possibility of such information being shared and used beyond its intended purposes.[32] Even if this threat does not ultimately materialize, the worry that seeking health care could make them known to law enforcement and jeopardize their ability to stay in the country serves as a strong deterrent in and of itself for undocumented migrants considering health care utilization.

In short, Canada's health care policies in response to COVID-19 have largely maintained the fault line between citizens and migrants, as us and them. Most jurisdictions in the country have not broadened their health care programs to help protect all migrants' health. To the extent that certain provinces have bucked the trend, the insistence of some to only cover the cost of COVID-19-related services insidiously links migrants' health care deservingness to the perceived threat *they* pose to *our* well-being. Meanwhile, ongoing immigration enforcement not only deters migrants from accessing health care, but also accentuates migrants' standing as outsiders.

The same dynamics of us-versus-them pervade the federal government's approach to emergency income assistance during the pandemic as well. While numerous migrant workers have continued to perform essential services following the COVID-19 outbreak, many have been laid off or become unable to work because they are ill or quarantined.[33] The consequent loss of income has caused many migrants' already-precarious financial situation to worsen. And yet, not all migrant workers who otherwise meet the eligibility criteria will qualify for Employment Insurance (EI). Undocumented migrants and seasonal agricultural workers, for example, are excluded by reason of their legal status, although many have paid into the EI program.[34] Some of these migrants again fell through the cracks when the Canada Emergency Response Benefit was introduced by the

31. Betsy Powell, "COVID-19 Database 'Extraordinary' Privacy Invasion: Civil Liberties Group", *Toronto Star* (24 April 2020), online: <thestar.com/news/gta/2020/04/24/covid-19-database-extraordinary-privacy-invasion-civil-liberties-group.html>.
32. *Ibid.*
33. Carl Meyer, "Migrant and Undocumented Workers Plead for Help During COVID-19", *National Observer* (17 April 2020), online: <nationalobserver.com/2020/04/17/news/migrant-and-undocumented-workers-plead-help-during-covid-19>.
34. See generally United Food and Commercial Workers Canada & the Agricultural Workers' Alliance, "The Great Canadian Rip-Off! An Economic Case for Restoring Full EI Special Benefits Access to SAWP Workers" (2014) at 6, online (pdf): *UFCW Canada* <ufcw.ca/templates/ufcwcanada/images/directions14/

government to fill the gaps in EI during the pandemic. Anyone without a valid Social Insurance Number, including undocumented migrants and foreign workers with expired permits, is ineligible for the new benefit.[35] Apparently, these migrants lack the right documentation to make them part of us and to deserve our aid.

Problems With a Us-Versus-Them Approach

People who embrace a cosmopolitan worldview often find it morally problematic to distinguish individuals based on citizenship and immigration statuses.[36] Many of them have pointed to international law's guarantee of universal human rights to demand the provision of health and social care by governments to everyone within their respective jurisdiction.[37] Others, by contrast, have defended the right of national communities to define who they are and whom they allow to join them.[38] From such a perspective, some degree of us-versus-them in public policy making is said to help bind a community together and facilitate resource sharing among community members.[39] It is not my intention to resolve this long-standing debate here. Instead, I argue that even without resorting to cosmopolitan ethics, the line drawing between citizens and migrants embedded in Canada's pandemic responses falls short, as it contravenes the dictates of equality and reciprocity, as well as public health objectives.

Citizenship as a legal regime recognizes and protects the interests of individuals who belong to a specific community on such bases as their personal ties and social participation.[40] As made plain by the pandemic, many migrants who are currently denied health care and income supports in fact closely resemble their citizen counterparts in terms of their belonging to the Canadian society. Far from strangers to us, they are our coworkers, caregivers, families, neighbours, and

march/1420/The-Great-Canadian-Rip-Off-An-Economic-Case-for-Restoring-Full-EI-Special-Benefits-Access-to-SAWP-Workers.pdf>.

35. Meyer, *supra* note 33.
36. Thomas W Pogge, "Cosmopolitanism and Sovereignty" (1992) 103:1 Ethics 48 at 48–49.
37. See e.g. Cécile Rousseau et al, "Health Care Access for Refugees and Immigrants With Precarious Status" (2008) 99:4 Can J Public Health 290.
38. See e.g. Michael Walzer, *Spheres of Justice: A Defense of Pluralism and Equality*, (New York: Basic Books, 1983).
39. David Miller, "In What Sense Must Socialism Be Communitarian?" (1989) 6:2 Social Philosophy & Policy 51.
40. Joseph Carens, *The Ethics of Immigration*, (Oxford: Oxford University Press, 2013).

more. They perform crucial tasks that keep our society functioning, and they follow the same laws as we do, including the various liberty-constraining public health orders now imposed. For all intents and purposes—and even more so in times of international border closures—Canada is their home. Treating them differently in our responses to the pandemic, notwithstanding their same if not greater risk of ill health and financial hardship, is arguably arbitrary and runs counter to the value of equality that permeates our legal system.[41]

Moreover, as seen, migrants make important contributions to society that render our health care and social programs possible. They are integral to all sectors of our economy, including health and social care provision, and they pay into these government programs through taxes and payroll deductions. Excluding migrants from health and social care, therefore, violates the principle of reciprocity: people are *prima facie* entitled to reap what they sow.[42]

From a policy standpoint, leaving migrants out of government health care and income support programs during the pandemic also puts public health at risk. Past experience demonstrates that when diagnosis and treatment of infectious diseases are delayed, the likelihood of the diseases spreading in the community rises.[43] It is reasonable to expect the same possibility to ensue when migrants with COVID-19 are forced to put off seeking medical attention because they lack public health care coverage or they are afraid of revealing themselves to the authorities following service access. What is more, the concern about community transmission is potentially made worse by the government's exclusion of migrants from income assistance. Doing so puts pressure on migrants to work even when feeling unwell, which increases their risk of being exposed to the virus and exposing others to the virus.

Migrants in Canada have had to shoulder a disproportionate burden of the pandemic's negative effects as a result of their living and working environments. Denying migrants health care coverage and income supports adds insults to injury and is both unprincipled and irrational. To protect the health of migrants and the general public, at

41. See generally The Honorable Claire L'Heureux-Dubé, "It Takes a Vision: The Constitutionalization of Equality in Canada" (2002) 14 Yale JL & Feminism 363.
42. John Rawls, *A Theory of Justice*, (Cambridge, MA: Harvard University Press, 1971).
43. See generally Patrick J Glen, "Health Care and the Illegal Immigrant" (2012) 23 Health Matrix 197 at 225.

least during the pandemic, governments across Canada must work together to ensure migrants' timely and effective access to medically necessary health care and sufficient income assistance, akin to what is promised to citizens. This must be accompanied by the assurance that accessing benefits will not jeopardize migrants' ability to remain in and/or return to Canada. Solidarity, as opposed to a mentality of us-versus-them, will be our key to success in weathering this pandemic.

CHAPTER D-9

Not All in This Together: Disability Rights and COVID-19*

Tess Sheldon** and Ravi Malhotra***

Abstract

Persons with disabilities are significantly and disproportionately impacted by COVID-19. In this paper, we address the accessibility of emergency preparedness and the failure of governments to consistently include people with disabilities in their response strategies, even when statutes mandate inclusions and accessibility. In particular, persons with disabilities have not consistently been included in COVID-19 communication strategies, and may encounter barriers to accessing vital information and advice about the pandemic. We also highlight the implications of the economic marginalization of people with disabilities during a pandemic. The economic disruption caused by COVID-19 particularly undermines the income security of persons with disabilities. People with disabilities largely live in poverty and yet their concerns have largely been ignored by pandemic stimulus funding. Finally, we explore how institutionalization in this brave new world has grave consequences for people with disabilities. The institutions, where many people with disabilities

* Special thanks to Arfi Hagi-Yusuf (2L Windsor Law) for her expert research assistance.

** Assistant Professor in the Faculty of Law at the University of Windsor.

*** Full Professor in the Faculty of Law (Common Law Section), cross-appointed to the School of Rehabilitation Sciences, University of Ottawa.

live, are quickly becoming epicentres of SARS-Cov-2 transmission. COVID-19 calls into question the utility of their confinement in general terms and magnifies the concerns that pre-existed the pandemic.

Résumé

Pas tous dans le même bateau : droits des personnes handicapées et COVID-19

Les personnes handicapées sont touchées de manière considérable et disproportionnée par la COVID-19. Dans ce chapitre, nous abordons l'accessibilité de la préparation aux situations d'urgence et l'incapacité des gouvernements à inclure systématiquement les personnes handicapées dans leurs stratégies d'intervention, même lorsque les lois commandent l'inclusion et l'accessibilité. En particulier, les personnes handicapées n'ont pas été prises en compte à tous coups dans les stratégies de communication relatives à la COVID-19, et peuvent donc se heurter à des obstacles lorsqu'elles souhaitent obtenir des renseignements et des conseils essentiels sur la pandémie. Nous abordons également les conséquences de la marginalisation économique des personnes handicapées durant une pandémie. Les bouleversements économiques provoqués par la COVID-19 fragilisent particulièrement la sécurité de revenu des personnes handicapées. Plusieurs d'entre elles vivent en situation de pauvreté, et pourtant, leurs inquiétudes ont été largement ignorées dans le cadre des fonds de relance pour lutter contre la pandémie. Enfin, nous examinons les conséquences sérieuses de l'institutionnalisation sur les personnes handicapées. Les établissements où vivent nombre d'entre elles sont rapidement devenus l'épicentre de la transmission du SRAS-CoV-2. La pandémie actuelle remet en question l'utilité de leur confinement en termes généraux et amplifie les craintes qui existaient avant la pandémie.

COVID-19 is a profound human rights crisis that has exposed the persistent ableism that infects our communities. Ableism has deadly effects for people with disabilities, but especially during a pandemic. Persons with disabilities face unique and increased economic risks during disasters.[1] Their vulnerability is heightened when they live in congregate and communal and often forced living environments, including large group homes, long-term care, jails, shelters, forensic hospitals, and psychiatric facilities. Women and racialized people with disabilities face greater marginalization at the best of times, including higher levels of poverty and unemployment. This economic marginalization is typically magnified during times of crisis. Violence against women rises during times of crisis and compulsory isolation,[2] particularly for women with disabilities.[3]

Only some persons with some kinds of disability-related needs are vulnerable to the virus itself, including if they are immune-compromised, have respiratory conditions, or are prescribed antipsychotic medications associated with diabetes, a risk factor for COVID-19 complications. Many more persons with disabilities are vulnerable to other effects of COVID-19: poverty, barriers to access to employment and income supports, inaccessibility of information and communications about disaster planning, transportation barriers when COVID-19 testing sites encourage the use of private vehicles to reduce transmission, and inequality of access to health care and supports.

COVID-19 lays bare society's responsibility for the disablement of others.[4] The social model of disability proposes that factors external to a person's actual limitations determine that person's ability to function within society. A person may have no functional limitations other than those created by prejudice, stigma, and stereotype.[5] A political response to addressing ableism may be formulated through the

1. United Nations, "Preventing Discrimination Against People with Disabilities in COVID-19 Response", *UN News* (19 March 2020), online: <news.un.org/en/story/2020/03/1059762>.
2. See Leilani Farha & Kaitlin Schwan, this volume, Chapter D-4.
3. Special Envoy of the Secretary-General on Disability and Accessibility, "Joint Statement Women and Girls with Disabilities and Older Women in Relation to the COVID-19 Pandemic" (28 April 2020), online (pdf): *United Nations* <www.un.org/development/desa/disabilities/wp-content/uploads/sites/15/2020/04/covid19-joint-statement-women-girls-disabilities-olderwomen-covid19.pdf>.
4. Nancy Doyle, "We Have Been Disabled: How The Pandemic Has Proven The Social Model Of Disability", *Forbes* (29 April 2020), online: <www.forbes.com/sites/drnancydoyle/2020/04/29/we-have-been-disabled-how-the-pandemic-has-proven-the-social-model-of-disability/#40ec9ef72b1d>.
5. Ena Chadha, "The Social Phenomenon of Handicapping" in Elizabeth Sheehy, ed, *Adding Feminism to Law: The Contributions of Justice Claire L'Heureux-Dubé*, (Toronto: Irwin Law, 2004) 209.

articulation of legal reform projects, or it may encompass grassroots disability rights organizing.[6]

In bold relief, COVID-19 has revealed the financial, social, and political structures that exclude persons with disabilities. That exclusion is predictable and reminiscent of historical eugenic strategies to ration access to scarce resources, reproduction, and immigration.[7] At the heart of those utilitarian decisions are systematically biased quality of life assessments that are predicated on the inherently discriminatory notion that disabled lives are not worth living. In Part I, we explore the accessibility of emergency preparedness. In Part II, we turn to a discussion of the economic implications of COVID-19. In Part III, we discuss institutionalization and its relation to COVID-19.

Accessibility of Emergency Preparedness

The *Accessibility for Ontarians with Disabilities Act* (the AODA)[8] and its associated Accessibility Standards[9] were adopted over a staggered period of years after 2005 and set out guidelines for people with disabilities, but largely have no coherent enforcement mechanism. Similar legislation has been more recently adopted in a few other provinces, such as British Columbia, Manitoba, and Nova Scotia, culminating in the passage of the federal *Accessible Canada Act*.[10] Section 13 of the Integrated Accessibility Standards requires the Government of Ontario and other obligated organizations to, upon request, provide emergency procedures, plans, and public safety information in an accessible format or with appropriate communication.[11] Article 11 of the *Convention on the Rights of Persons with Disabilities* (CRPD), to

6. See Ravi Malhotra, ed, *Disability Politics in a Global Economy: Essays in Honour of Marta Russell*, (New York: Routledge, 2016).
7. Geoffrey Reaume, "Eugenics Incarceration and Expulsion: Daniel G. and Andrew T.'s Deportation from 1928 Toronto, Canada" in Liat Ben-Moshe, Chris Chapman & Allison Carey, eds, *Disability Incarcerated: Imprisonment and Disability in the United States and Canada*, (New York: Palgrave Macmillan, 2014) at 63; Ena Chadha, "'Mentally Defectives' Not Welcome: Mental Disability in Canadian Immigration Law, 1859–1927" (2008) 28:1 Disability Studies Quarterly 1.
8. RSO 2005, c 11.
9. O Reg 191/11 [*Integrated Accessibility Standards*].
10. Bill M-219, *British Columbia Accessibility Act*, 3rd Sess, 41st Parl, British Columbia, 2018; Bill 26, *The Accessibility for Manitobans Act*, 2nd Sess, 4th Leg, Manitoba, 2013; *An Act Respecting Accessibility in Nova Scotia*; 3rd Sess, 62nd Leg, Nova Scotia, 2017.
11. *Integrated Accessibility Standards*, *supra* note 9, s 13.

which Canada is a signatory, requires State Parties to take necessary measures to protect people with disabilities in humanitarian emergencies and would likely be applicable in this context.[12]

Yet barriers, such as COVID-19 websites operated by the Ontario government, which are inaccessible to blind users, and addresses by the Prime Minister without sign language interpretation, have already been reported.[13] Barrier removal will be of key importance as the COVID-19 crisis continues to ensure Deaf people and others with communication needs obtain timely information in an accessible manner.

The issue of access to lifesaving ventilators also raises important human rights questions. A discussion paper produced by the AODA Alliance boldly insists that medical triage not discriminate against people with disabilities. This might occur by inappropriately considering impairments in evaluating future quality of life or determining that reliance on publicly funded attendant services ought to be a factor deprioritizing a disabled person for a ventilator. Disability rights activists have also raised concerns that people who have always used ventilators for pre-existing conditions may have them confiscated by hospital staff should they end up getting COVID-19.[14] American disability rights activists have engaged in legal action under the *Americans with Disabilities Act* to challenge discriminatory triage policies. In Alabama, a complaint by disability rights organizations and noted

12. UN General Assembly, *Convention on the Rights of Persons with Disabilities: Resolution/Adopted by the General Assembly*, A/RES/61/106 (24 January 2007) at art 11 [*CRPD*].
13. Michelle McQuigge, "Disabled Canadians Feel Excluded from Covid-19 Messaging", *CTV News* (18 March 2020), online: <www.ctvnews.ca/health/coronavirus/disabled-canadians-feel-excluded-from-covid-19-messaging-1.4857691>.
14. "A Discussion Paper on Ensuring that Medical Triage of Health Services During the Covid-19 Crisis Does Not Discriminate Against Patients with Disabilities" (14 April 2020), online: *AODA Alliance* <www.aodaalliance.org/whats-new/a-discussion-paper-on-ensuring-that-medical-triage-or-rationing-of-health-care-services-during-the-covid-19-crisis-does-not-discriminate-against-patients-with-disabilities/>; "Disability Community Wins Interim Step Forward–Ford Government Backs Down on Its Controversial Secret Protocol for Rationing Critical Medical Care During the COVID Crisis and Agrees to Consult Human Rights and Community Experts" (21 April 2020), online: *AODA Alliance* <www.aodaalliance.org/whats-new/disability-community-wins-interim-step-forward-ford-government-backs-down-on-its-controversial-secret-protocol-for-rationing-critical-medical-care-during-the-covid-crisis-and-agrees-to-consult-human/>.

law professor Samuel Bagenstos led to the government withdrawing a ventilator rationing policy that discriminated against people with intellectual disabilities, dementia, and severe traumatic brain injury.[15]

Intersections: Income Security, Poverty, and Disability

COVID-19 highlights stark and persistent financial inequalities that have plagued the disability community long before the current virus.[16] Compared to people without disabilities, they are far more likely to experience poverty, have lower levels of education, and be un- or underemployed, and are less likely to live in adequate, safe, and affordable housing.[17] Even before the pandemic, social assistance rates for persons with disabilities in Ontario were far below the poverty line,[18] insufficient for coping with additional needs and increased cost of living while in quarantine, including transportation costs as a result of the suspension of transit services. Federal income support strategies, like the Canada Emergency Response Benefit (CERB), exclude persons with disabilities who are not able to meet the minimum income thresholds. In Ontario, the rates for persons with disabilities receiving benefits under the Ontario Disability Support Program (ODSP) are far below the rates offered to workers laid off during the pandemic.

The economic disruption caused by COVID-19 particularly undermines the income security of persons with disabilities and is the product of unconscious biases or injurious stereotypes about the value of their labour. As Marta Russell and others have shown, disabled people have been devalued by prioritizing conventional neoliberal understandings of productivity, which link a person's value to

15. "Alabama Withdraws Discriminatory Ventilator Rationing Policy and Issues Directive About Non-Discrimination in Accessing Life-Saving Treatment" (8 April 2020), online (pdf): *Center for Public Representation* <www.centerforpublicrep.org/wp-content/uploads/2020/04/AL-OCR-press-release_4.8.20.pdf>. See also Samuel R. Bagenstos, "May Hospitals Withhold Ventilators from COVID-19 Patients with Pre-Existing Disabilities? Notes on the Law and Ethics of Disability-Based Medical Rationing" 130 Yale LJ Forum (Forthcoming in 2020).
16. *Eldridge v British Columbia (Attorney General)*, [1997] 3 SCR 624 at para 56, 151 DLR (4th) 577.
17. "As a Matter of Fact: Poverty and Disability in Canada" (23 September 2009), online: *Council of Canadians with Disabilities* <www.ccdonline.ca/en/socialpolicy/poverty-citizenship/poverty-disability-canada>.
18. "Accessing Income Support in Wake of COVID-19" (26 March 2020), online: *Income Security Advocacy Center* <incomesecurity.org/public-education/accessing-income-support-in-the-wake-of-covid-19-updated-march-26/>.

their ability to generate profits.[19] People with disabilities experience complex forms of discrimination: their claims often involve intersecting and multiple grounds, which are compounded by COVID-19. Disability injustice amplifies gender and racial injustices, as illustrated by the particular risk the virus poses to Black women with disabilities.[20]

The needs of persons with disabilities, including persons labelled with intellectual disabilities and consumers/survivors of the psychiatric system, have not consistently been considered a priority. Disability services have generally closed from face-to-face contact, including Service Canada's locations that administer the Canada Pension Plan Disability Benefit (CPP-D). There have been delays in processing payments through Ontario's Passport Program, which provides essential funding to adults labelled with intellectual disabilities,[21] and the Alberta Assured Income for the Severely Handicapped program (AISH). Other critical services have closed altogether, such as Ontario's Assistive Devices Program (ADP) which funds mobility devices, communication aids, and prostheses.[22] These closures compound the isolation of those who rely on these essential supports to participate in our communities, leaving people without mobility devices altogether and more vulnerable to the physical, social, and economic impacts of the virus. Media reports described the shocking case of Michael Wilson, a Kitchener man with cerebral palsy, whose wheelchair broke down during the COVID-19 pandemic. With the closure of the ADP office, he was unable to get a wheelchair vendor to provide a replacement. He has consequently been unable to leave his apartment and forced to survive on delivery pizza. Interestingly, he had initially been denied funding for a replacement wheelchair prior to the onset of the pandemic, leaving him no choice but to file an appeal, illustrating how the impact of routine—but devastating—neoliberal cuts to the provision

19. Marta Russell, *Beyond Ramps: Disability at the End of the Social Contract*, (Monroe, Maine: Common Courage Press, 1998).

20. Treva Lindsey, "Why COVID-19 Is Hitting Black Women so Hard", *Women's Media Center* (17 April 2020), online: <womensmediacenter.com/news-features/why-covid-19-is-hitting-black-women-so-hard>; see Jamie Liew, this volume, Chapter D-7.

21. "ARCH Bulletin on COVID-19: Ontario Temporarily Increases Eligible Expenses under the Passport Program" (29 April 2020), online: *ARCH Disability Law Center* <archdisabilitylaw.ca/resource/arch-bulletin-on-covid-19-passport-program/>.

22. "ARCH Bulletin on COVID-19: Ontario's Assistive Devices Program No Longer Available" (22 April 2020), online: *ARCH Disability Law Center* <archdisabilitylaw.ca/resource/arch-bulletin-on-covid-19-ontario-assistive-devices-program/>.

of assistive devices were compounded by the dislocations caused by COVID-19.[23] Other reports document how people with disabilities who require attendant services for activities of daily living such as meal preparation and personal care to live independently in the community have been forced to rely on family members, as personal support workers are redeployed to work in long-term homes.[24]

A human rights lens ensures that COVID-19 is not used as a pretext to adopt repressive measures to expand the authority of guardianship. Persons with disabilities, whose lives are already overregulated, may be subject to additional surveillance during COVID-19.[25] Historically, the privatization and deregulation of disability services are driven by cost-cutting agendas.[26] Austerity measures have accompanied neoliberal politics, along with the reduction of government inspections in congregate settings, understaffing, and reliance on part-time, precarious labour.[27]

"Think prison is bad, try a nursing home!":[28] Disability Detention in Canada

The segregation of persons with disabilities in large institutions was based on violent stereotypes about their capacity to live independently and being in need of coerced care.[29] Residents were subject to horrific

23. Paula Duhatschek, "Man Stuck Hours Daily on Floor While Province Closes Assistive Devices Office", *CBC News* (22 April 2020), online: <www.cbc.ca/news/canada/kitchener-waterloo/man-stuck-hours-daily-on-floor-while-province-closes-assistive-devices-office-1.5540041>.
24. Omar Dabaghi-Pacheco, "People with Disabilities Forced to Rely on Family as PSW Options Dwindle", *CBC News* (5 May 2020), online: <www.cbc.ca/amp/1.5554052>.
25. "HALCO Raises Serious Concern with Ontario Decision to Share COVID-19 Test Results with Police and Others" (24 April 2020), online: *HIV and AIDS Legal Clinic Ontario* <www.halco.org/2020/news/halco-raises-serious-concern-with-ontario-decision-to-share-covid-19-test-results-with-police-and-others>.
26. Vera Chouinard & Valorie A Crooks, "Negotiating Neoliberal Environments in British Columbia and Ontario, Canada: Restructuring of State–Voluntary Sector Relations and Disability Organizations' Struggles to Survive" (2008) 26:1 Environment & Planning C: Government & Policy 173.
27. Mary Jean Hande & Christine Kelly "Organizing Survival and Resistance in Austere Times: Shifting Disability Activism and Care Politics in Ontario, Canada" (2015) 3:7 Disability & Society 961.
28. Eli Clare, *Exile and Pride: Disability, Queerness, and Liberation*, (Cambridge, MA: SouthEnd Press, 1999) at xxii.
29. Canadian Association for Community Living (CACL), "Deinstitutionalization: A Call to Action" (2019), online: *Institution Watch* <www.institutionwatch.ca/

neglect and abuse. Many of those major institutions were closed in the 1970s, and residents were discharged to community settings.

Despite the promise of deinstitutionalization, community-based services remain underfunded and over-subscribed.[30] Many fell into crisis after being discharged from large congregate living facilities, revolving between other institutions like prisons, homeless shelters, hospitals and large group homes.[31] While Ontario formally shuttered the institutions that warehoused persons labelled with intellectual disabilities, some community placements remain unsafe,[32] without adequate oversight,[33] and resemble "present-day versions of the moribund institutions from a century ago."[34] People with disabilities continue to face barriers accessing community-based services,[35] and have been institutionalized in inappropriate custodial settings such as long-term care,[36] facilities not suited to their needs,[37] raising significant human rights and liberty concerns.[38] COVID-19 is an opportunity

---

wp-content/uploads/2019/10/a-call-to-action.pdf>.

30. Daniel Yohanna, "Deinstitutionalization of People with Mental Illness: Causes and Consequences" (2013) 15:10 Virtual Mentor 886, online: <journalofethics.ama-assn.org/article/deinstitutionalization-people-mental-illness-causes-and-consequences/2013-10>.
31. Ted Frankel, "Exodus: 40 Years of Deinstitutionalization and the Failed Promise of Community-Based Care" (2003) 12 Dal J Leg Stud 1.
32. See e.g. Community Living Ontario, "Preventing the neglect of vulnerable victims: Jamie Hawley's death by neglect", *Cision* (30 August 2013), online: <www.newswire.ca/news-releases/preventing-the-neglect-of-vulnerable-victims-jamie-hawleys-death-by-neglect-512863751.html>.
33. See e.g. Office of the Chief Coroner, "Verdict of Coroner's Jury at the Inquest into the death of: Guy Mitchell" (24 July 2015), online: *Ontario Ministry of the Solicitor General* <www.mcscs.jus.gov.on.ca/english/Deathinvestigations/Inquests/Verdictsandrecommendations/OCCInquestMitchell2015.html>.
34. Megan Linton, "Institutional Legacies of Violence: Neoliberalism and Custodial Care in Ontario", *Canadian Dimension* (12 April 2020), online: <canadiandimension.com/articles/view/institutional-legacies-of-violence-of-custodial-care-in-ontario>.
35. Natalie Spagnuolo, "Building Backwards in a 'Post' Institutional Era: Hospital Confinement, Group Home Eviction, and Ontario's Treatment of People Labelled with Intellectual Disabilities" (2016) 36:4 Disability Studies Quarterly 1.
36. "Intellectually disabled Canadians are dying in residential institutions: What's happening & what can be done" (17 April 2020), online: *Autistics for Autistics* <a4aontario.com/2020/04/17/intellectually-disabled-canadians-are-dying-in-residential-institutions-whats-happening-what-can-be-done>.
37. "Nowhere to Turn: Investigation into the Ministry of Community and Social Services' Response to Situations of Crisis involving Adults with Developmental Disabilities" (24 August 2016), online: *Ontario Ombudsman* <www.ombudsman.on.ca/resources/reports-and-case-summaries/reports-on-investigations/2016/nowhere-to-turn>.
38. *MacLean v Nova Scotia (Attorney General)*, 2019 CanLII 115231 (NSHRC).

to remedy the failed promise of the last century's deinstitutionalization movement.

The institutional and custodial sites that continue to warehouse persons with disabilities have become infectious hotspots.[39] Preventing new outbreaks in those congregate settings must be an urgent priority for any strategy intending to flatten the curve. Viruses spread rapidly in these confined spaces. Cleaning of surfaces in both public rooms and living quarters may not meet public health standards. Physical distancing is impossible, and " … unlike cruise ships, people in congregate living settings including the staff who work there transfer disease into the general population."[40]

Monitoring, prevention and treatment of COVID-19 in congregate settings must be narrowly tailored, non-intrusive and least restrictive of human rights. Restrictions to personal liberty—including through the inappropriate deployment of mental health legislation[41]—are not a substitute for adequate prevention and raise serious equality and liberty considerations. Once the virus is inside an institution, staff may be tempted to use heavy-handed, dangerous, and correctional-inspired responses, including seclusion and lockdowns.

Even if intended to protect vulnerable persons from transmission, visitor restrictions can be experienced as punitive, limit oversight, and expose vulnerable persons to additional abuse or neglect. They impair access to family members,[42] substitute decision makers, or counsel. Other disability institutions have expanded bans to include communication devices, such as iPads.[43] A recent judi-

39. Danny Hakim, "'It's Hit Our Front Door': Homes for the Disabled See a Surge of Covid-19", *New York Times* (8 April 2020), online: <www.nytimes.com/2020/04/08/nyregion/coronavirus-disabilities-group-homes.html>; Richard Warnica, "Jane Philpott on Life Inside the Care Home Where 95% of the Residents Have COVID-19", *National Post* (1 May 2020), online: <nationalpost.com/news/jane-philpott-on-life-inside-the-care-home-where-95-per-cent-of-the-residents-have-covid-19>.

40. *R v JR*, 2020 ONSC 1938 at para 29.

41. Brendan D Kelly, "Emergency Mental Health Legislation in Response to the Covid-19 (Coronavirus) Pandemic in Ireland: Urgency, Necessity and Proportionality" (2020) 70 Intl JL & Psychiatry.

42. Talia Ricci, "'He Can't Understand Why He's not Seeing His Family': Mother of Non-Verbal Son Begs for Visitor Exemption", *CBC News* (4 May 2020), online: <www.cbc.ca/news/canada/toronto/mother-of-disabled-son-begs-for-visitor-exception-1.55\1544>.

43. Sue Ann Levy, "Hospital Bans Disabled Patient from Using iPad Calling it 'Surveillance Tool'", *Toronto Sun* (1 May 2020), online: <torontosun.com/news/local-news/levy-hospital-bans-disabled-patient-from-using-ipad-calling-it-sur-

cial review of a hospital's COVID-19 "no visitor" policy challenged its disproportionate impact on older residents incapable of making treatment decisions.[44] In *Sprague v Her Majesty the Queen in Right of Ontario*, the Ontario Court of Justice dismissed an application for judicial review, alleging that the Chief Medical Officer of Health for Ontario violated the s. 15 equality rights of a 77-year-old man when it recommended that hospitals adopt a "no visitor" policy to stem the tide of COVID-19. The Court held that there was in fact no statutory duty for hospitals to provide unimpeded access by visitors to its premises. The Court went on to conclude that there was no breach of the equality provision because the visitor policy was based on epidemiological evidence intended to protect elderly patients.[45] Jeff Preston, a disabled academic, in testimony to the House of Commons Standing Committee on Human Resources, Skills and Social Development and the Status of Persons with Disabilities, emphasized how family members and in-home caregivers need to be regarded, not as visitors, but as part of a disabled person's care team that can work in tandem with hospital staff.[46] Visitor restrictions particularly threaten the safety of residents who require support persons to interpret or communicate with staff.[47] This was poignantly illustrated by the tragic case of a 40-year-old nonverbal British Columbia woman with cerebral palsy, Ariis Knight, who died due to reasons unrelated to COVID-19 alone after her support workers were not permitted to accompany her in hospital. As the Council of Canadians with Disabilities has demanded, such restrictive policies must end.[48] The disability legal clinic ARCH has also cor-

veillance-tool>.

44. *Sprague v Her Majesty the Queen in Right of Ontario*, 2020 ONSC 2335. See also *BP v Surrey County Council & Anor*, [2020] EWCOP 17, online: *England and Wales Court of Protection Decisions* <www.bailii.org/ew/cases/EWCOP/2020/17.html>.

45. *Ibid* at paras 32-38.

46. "Covid-19 and Disability in Canada" (5 May 2020), online: *Jeff Preston* <www.jeffpreston.ca/2020/05/05/opening-remarks-to-huma-committee/>

47. Sean Boynton, "Disability Advocates Say B.C.'s Woman's Death Shows Need for Clearer COVID-19 Policy", *Global News* (26 April 2020), online: <globalnews.ca/news/6869079/coronavirus-bc-disability-death-reaction/>.

48. Council of Canadians with Disabilities, "Disability Advocates Call for Immediate Change to Hospital Policies Designating 'Essential' Supports/Visitors Following the Death of Ariis Knight" (7 May 2020), posted on *Council of Canadians with Disabilities*, online: *Facebook* <www.facebook.com/ccdonline/posts/1624724117687878?__tn__=K-R>; The Canadian Press Staff, "Covid-19 Highlights Existing Barriers for Canadians with Communication Disabilities", *CTV News* (7 May 2020), online: <www.ctvnews.ca/health/coronavirus/covid-19-highlights-existing-barriers-for-canadians-with-communication-disabilities-1.4929736>.

rectly pointed out the need for flexibility in allowing visitors to group homes for people with intellectual disabilities.[49] As this chapter was being finalized, the British Columbia government announced a revision to its visitor policy, allowing designated representatives to assist people with disabilities to eat, communicate, and make decisions.[50]

Others, including Adelina Iftene, Chapter D-5 in this volume, have written persuasively about the urgent need to reduce the number of persons detained in prisons. COVID-19 has also confirmed the urgent need to release people with disabilities from institutional and congregate settings into community settings.[51] Preventative deinstitutionalization protects their health, as well as the health of staff and the public.[52] Reducing the number of admissions and accelerating discharges frees up valuable health care resources.[53] Depopulation also reduces overcrowding so those remaining can practise physical distancing.

Institutional release may raise other issues for residents unable to return to accessible, private, or safe homes in the community. Preventative deinstitutionalization raises the same issues that deinstitutionalization raised about the lack of community support for people being released into the community that pre-existed COVID-19. Emergency funding must be directed to municipalities and social

---

49. "People Living in Developmental Services Group Homes Need Access to Essential Support Persons" (7 May 2020), online: *ARCH Disability Law Centre* <CTVarchdisabilitylaw.ca/resource/arch-bulletin-on-covid-19-people-living-in-developmental-services-group-homes-need-access-to-essential-support-persons/>.
50. "B.C. Updates Policy on Hospital Visitors After Outcry Over Disabled Woman's Death", *CBC News* (19 May 2020), online: <www.cbc.ca/news/canada/british-columbia/b-c-updates-policy-on-hospital-visitors-after-outcry-over-disabled-woman-s-death-1.5576316>.
51. Tess Sheldon, Karen Spector & Sheila Wildeman, "Viruses Feed on Exclusion: Psychiatric Detention and the Need for Preventative Deinstitutionalization", *Ricochet Media* (12 April 2020), online: <ricochet.media/en/3038/viruses-feed-on-exclusion-psychiatric-detention-and-the-need- for-preventative-deinstitutionalization>.
52. Oliver Lewis, "Why Social Workers Should be Aiming to Get Residents Out of Care Homes During the Pandemic", *Community Care* (21 April 2020), online: <www.communitycare.co.uk/2020/04/21/social-workers-aiming-get-residents-care-homes-pandemic/>.
53. Bazelon Centre for Mental Health Law, "During the Pandemic, States and Localities Must Decrease the Number of Individuals in Psychiatric Hospitals, by Reducing Admissions and Accelerating Discharges" (15 April 2020), online (pdf): *Bazelon Centre for Mental Health Law* <www.bazelon.org/wp-content/uploads/2020/04/4-15-20-BC-psych-hospitals-statement-FINAL.pdf>.

service providers such as shelters, supportive housing, food banks, and emergency services. On an urgent basis, municipalities have repurposed hotels, community centres, and schools, and other spaces that are empty. COVID-19 has called into question the utility of institutionalization in unsafe congregate settings, and magnified decades-old calls for appropriate, safe, and accessible community support.

Conclusion

COVID-19 is both a disaster and an opportunity for people with disabilities. Another world of accessibility is possible, and COVID-19 is the perfect time to reimagine our relationships to society and to each other. From online learning to working at home and the establishment of more creative income support programs, there is endless potential for people with disabilities to thrive with the right accommodations in place. In a time of tragedy, a world of inclusion and disability empowerment can be built from the ashes of COVID-19. This is not an opportunity to be missed.

CHAPTER D-10

Weighing Public Health and Mental Health Responses to Non-Compliance with Public Health Directives in the Context of Mental Illness

Jennifer A. Chandler,* Yasmin Khaliq,** Mona Gupta,*** Kwame McKenzie,**** Simon Hatcher,***** and Olivia Lee******

Abstract

COVID-19 has highlighted and reinforced the vulnerability of multiple populations, including people who live with mental illness. Challenges are posed by the requirements for physical distancing and self-isolation. Mental illness does not automatically render a person incapable of adopting such measures or their decisions not to do so suspect. People with mental illnesses may decide not to follow public health directives just as other people without mental illness may choose to do, and public health enforcement measures would apply. In some cases, symptoms of mental illness do affect a person's

* Full Professor of Law and holder of the Bertram Loeb Research Chair at the University of Ottawa.

** Currently studying in the Programme de common law en français at the University of Ottawa.

*** Psychiatrist at the Centre Hospitalier de l'Université de Montréal (CHUM) and Clinician-Investigator at the Centre de recherche du CHUM; Associate Clinical Professor in the Department of Psychiatry and Addictions of the Université de Montréal.

**** CEO of Wellesley Institute and an international expert on the social causes of mental illness, suicide, and the development of effective, equitable health systems; Director of Health Equity at the Centre for Addiction and Mental Health (CAMH), and Professor in the Department of Psychiatry at the University of Toronto.

***** Full Professor of Psychiatry at the University of Ottawa.

****** Resident physician, University of Ottawa, Department of Psychiatry.

adherence to public health directives by undermining the abilities to understand, to exercise appropriate judgment, and to evaluate risk. Should a person whose ability to follow directives is compromised by mental illness face the sanctions and enforcement procedures under public health laws, or should a mental health intervention such as involuntary hospitalization be pursued to protect both the person concerned and others, as well as the community in general? In this chapter, we consider the interplay of these two legislative regimes, recognizing that the balance may change with the evolution of the pandemic, shifting information, risk trade-offs, and social attitudes.

Résumé
Évaluation des mesures de santé publique et de santé mentale en cas de non-respect des directives de santé publique dans le contexte de la maladie mentale

La COVID-19 a mis en évidence et renforcé la vulnérabilité de plusieurs populations, y compris les personnes atteintes d'une maladie mentale. Les exigences en matière de distanciation physique et d'auto-isolement posent certains défis. Une personne ayant des problèmes de santé mentale n'est pas forcément incapable de se conformer à de telles contraintes, tout comme sa décision de ne pas le faire ne doit pas être automatiquement considérée comme suspecte. En fait, elle peut décider de ne pas suivre les directives de santé publique tout comme n'importe qui d'autre peut choisir de le faire, et dans tous les cas, les mesures d'application de ces directives pourront s'imposer. Dans certains cas toutefois, les symptômes de la maladie mentale influent sur la capacité d'une personne à respecter les directives de santé publique en altérant sa compréhension, son jugement et son évaluation des risques. Un individu dont l'aptitude à suivre les directives est compromise par une maladie mentale doit-il être soumis aux sanctions et aux procédures d'exécution prévues par les lois sur la santé publique, ou doit-on plutôt procéder à une intervention en santé mentale telle que l'hospitalisation involontaire pour protéger à la fois la personne concernée et la communauté en général ? Dans ce chapitre, nous examinons l'interaction de ces deux régimes législatifs, tout en reconnaissant que l'équilibre peut changer avec l'évolution de la pandémie et de l'information disponible, et en fonction des risques et des attitudes sociales.

The outbreak of COVID-19 has highlighted and reinforced the vulnerability of multiple populations, including people who live with mental illness. Among the many challenges are the requirements for physical distancing, and in the case of symptomatic persons or suspected or positive cases, self-isolation. Mental illness does not automatically render a person incapable of adopting such measures or their decisions not to do so suspect. People with mental illnesses may decide not to follow public health directives related to physical distancing, hygiene, and self-isolation, just as other people without mental illness may choose to do, and public health enforcement measures would apply. Here we consider how best to respond in those cases where the symptoms of mental illness do affect a person's adherence to public health directives by undermining the abilities to understand, to exercise appropriate judgment, and to evaluate risk, among other things. Should a person whose ability to follow directives is compromised by mental illness face the sanctions and enforcement procedures under public health laws? Or should a mental health intervention such as involuntary hospitalization be pursued to protect both the person concerned and others, as well as the community in general? At the same time, involuntary hospitalization is an exceptional measure that may come with its own risks of infection, and it is evidently a much greater deprivation of liberty than a monetary fine for refusing to follow public health orders in the community. In this chapter, we consider the interplay of these two legislative regimes, recognizing that the balance may change with the evolution of the pandemic, shifting information, risk trade-offs, and social attitudes.

Mental health legislation varies among the provinces, although the basic underlying objectives are similar. We base our analysis on the Ontario *Mental Health Act*.[1] The objectives of Ontario's law are to protect the person with mental illness from serious bodily harm or physical impairment; to protect others where a person poses a risk of serious bodily harm to other people; and to facilitate treatment where a person is incapable and is at risk of deterioration.[2] Public health legislation, on the other hand, aims to protect the collective health and safety of the community as a whole. Both laws embody a trade-off between the legislative objectives and the liberty interests of those subject to the rules and restrictions adopted to promote these objectives.

1. *Mental Health Act*, RSO 1990 c M.7 [*MHA*].
2. *Thompson v Ontario (Attorney General)*, 2016 ONCA 676 [*Thompson*].

In the context of COVID-19, orders are currently in place under public health and emergency legislation to close certain public spaces, require physical distancing, and enforce self-isolation in the case of known or suspected infections.[3] The most frequent penalties employed so far have been monetary fines,[4] although court orders, police involvement, enforced isolation, and detention are also possible in more serious cases.[5] Although the health risk to the majority of infected non-elderly individuals, particularly those in good health, may be relatively low, the needs to safeguard the community and to maintain a functioning health care system have been judged to be important objectives that justify restriction on the civil liberties of the whole community.

One of the challenges that has emerged is the proper response in the case of people whose behaviour suggests that their failure to comply with public health orders is because of mental illness. Some of the ways this question arises are illustrated by the following scenarios:

- A person known by the staff of a homeless shelter to have a chronic psychotic disorder is refusing to follow hygiene and distancing directives. The person is barred from the shelter to protect other residents and staff.
- A person who is known to have a serious mental illness is showing signs of infection. The person denies their evident symptoms and refuses mental health treatment, as well as testing and self-isolation.
- A person with depression and a serious substance use disorder is awaiting test results for suspected infection but does not self-isolate.

---

3. *Emergency Management and Civil Protection Act*, RSO 1990, c E.9; *Organized Public Events, Certain Gatherings*, O Reg 52/20; *Closure of Outdoor Recreational Amenities*, O Reg 104/20.
4. Josh Pringle "43 tickets issued to people in closed Ottawa parks, non-essential businesses over the weekend", *CTV News* (6 April 2020), online: <ottawa.ctvnews.ca/43-tickets-issued-to-people-in-closed-ottawa-parks-non-essential-businesses-over-the-weekend-1.4884703>.
5. Holly Mckenzie-Sutter "Mounties could enter homes to enforce Quarantine Act orders if Canadians don't self-isolate", *Globe and Mail* (10 April 2020), online: <www.theglobeandmail.com/canada/article-rcmp-warns-it-will-enforce-the-quarantine-act-if-canadians-dont-self/>; Isaac Olson, "Québec City police arrest COVID-19 patient for defying quarantine", *CBC News* (20 March 2020), online: <www.cbc.ca/news/canada/montreal/quebec-city-police-arrest-covid-19-1.5505349>.

- A person is showing unusual behaviour suggestive of psychosis, and is refusing to leave a public park, which has been closed pursuant to a public health directive.
- A person is approaching strangers in the community and spitting or coughing on them without apparent reason or provocation.

Could such situations lead to serious bodily harm to the person or others or to serious physical impairment of the person? We explore this possibility below.

Vulnerability of Persons Who Have a Mental Illness in the Context of COVID-19

As a group, people with mental illnesses are vulnerable in the face of COVID-19 and the associated public health precautions because of risk factors that are correlated with mental illness. They may be at greater risk of infection and severe course of disease, their underlying psychiatric condition can be exacerbated by the public health precautions, and they may face greater barriers to accessing care for their psychiatric condition or for COVID-19 or both.

The risk of contracting or transmitting COVID-19 may be increased for multiple reasons when a person has mental illness, trauma, or substance use disorders. Some people with mental illnesses may have trouble understanding and responding to public health directives.[6] Homelessness and mental illness are both associated with worse baseline health and medical comorbidities compared to the general population, which increase the risk of developing a complicated course of illness if a person becomes infected.[7] Furthermore, some homeless shelters and community resources are refusing access to people who do not abide by precautions in order to protect other clients and staff, leaving them with reduced access to vital community-based resources. Since self-isolation can exacerbate some mental

6. J Clapton et al, "Precarious social inclusion: chronic homelessness and impaired decision-making capacity" (2014) 23:1 J of Social Distress and Homelessness 32.
7. A Chevance et al, "Assurer les soins aux patients souffrant de troubles psychiques en France pendant l'épidémie à SARS-CoV 2 ; Ensuring mental health care during the SARS-CoV-2 epidemic in France: A narrative review" (2020), online: *L'Encephale* <doi.org/10.1016/j.encep.2020.03.001>; SW Hwang et al, "Mortality among residents of shelters, rooming houses, and hotels in Canada: 11 year follow-up study" (2009) 339 BMJ b4036.

illnesses and trigger distress,[8] people may leave mandatory isolation and risk infecting others. People with substance use problems may put themselves at risk of infection in order to access the substances upon which they depend.[9]

Some have expressed concern that triage policies that make prognosis a key factor would mean that people with pre-existing comorbidities would fare less well under these policies should they become infected and require intensive care support, and it became necessary to triage. People who have mental illnesses, particularly those who are also homeless, are among those groups that tend to have medical comorbidities at higher rates, and this might affect prognosis and triage decision-making.[10] Another suggestion is that unless appropriate procedural safeguards are in place, subconscious stigma toward this group—for example, with respect to perceptions of their quality of life—might affect triage decisions made under pressure, further disadvantaging the population with mental illness.[11]

There are other kinds of possible vulnerabilities that people with mental illnesses may face during the pandemic. One potential risk is hostility from members of the public. In some cases, people with mental illness may behave in ways that do not comply with evolving community norms about personal distancing and social interaction. Members of the public may perceive this as unpredictable or threatening, and it may provoke hostile responses. Harassment, aggression, and vigilantism toward people perceived as posing a risk of infection to others is already being documented around the world during this

8. A Fiorillo & P Gorwood, "The consequences of COVID-19 pandemic on mental health and implications for clinical practice" (2020) 63:1 European Psychiatry e32 at 1–2.
9. A Guirguis, "There is a vulnerable group we must not leave behind in our response to COVID-19: people who are dependent on illicit drugs" (28 April 2020), online: *Pharmaceutical Journal* <www.pharmaceutical-journal.com/news-and-analysis/opinion/comment/there-is-a-vulnerable-group-we-must-not-leave-behind-in-our-response-to-covid-19-people-who-are-dependent-on-illicit-drugs/20207926.article?firstPass=false>.
10. Katie Savin & Laura Guidry-Grimes, "Confronting Disability Discrimination During the Pandemic" (2 April 2020), online: *The Hastings Center Bioethics Forum* <www.thehastingscenter.org/confronting-disability-discrimination-during-the-pandemic/?fbclid=IwAR2ssY8aVhxj5284prI9S2WqZUM3VZvtSzJGQ6DeX4cB_FhqmZ7vOv90msk>; Sean Fine, Mike Hager & Tom Cardoso, "Ontario draws up health-care plan in event hospitals become overcrowded", *Globe and Mail* (3 April 2020), online: <www.theglobeandmail.com/canada/article-ontario-hospitals-instructed-to-prioritize-life-saving-coronavirus/>.
11. Savin and Guidry-Grimes, *supra* note 10; Fine, Hager & Cardoso, *supra* note 10.

pandemic.[12] While these reports do not involve people with mental illness, they do reflect an environment of heightened stress and intolerance of perceived risk and norm-breaking behaviour. Behaviour that appears unpredictable or aggressive may also increase the risk of conflict with law enforcement during the pandemic.[13]

Thus, in light of the vulnerabilities they face as a group, along with current public health requirements, people with mental illness may be at increased risk of experiencing or causing novel forms of harm during the pandemic. The risks will differ based on the person's individual mental and physical health, whether he or she is infected with the coronavirus or not, and the specific nature of his or her behaviour.

How Does the *Mental Health Act* Apply to These Risks?

We now consider how Ontario's mental health legislation would respond to the kinds of harms and scenarios described above, involving a failure to follow public health directives. Public health authorities have determined that the coronavirus poses a serious threat to public health, but would the risk of contracting or transmitting it fit within the types of risks to which the mental health legislation seeks to respond by involuntary hospitalization?

The mental health law attempts to strike a balance between the civil liberties of people with mental illnesses and the use of state power to forcibly intervene to protect them and others from risk of harm resulting from their mental illness. Ontario's *Mental Health Act* allows involuntary hospitalization against a person's will in one of two types of situations:

---

12. Lucy Quaggin, "Coronavirus update: NSW Health Minister announces massive fine for those abusing frontline workers", *7 News* (9 April 2020), online: <7news.com.au/lifestyle/health-wellbeing/coronavirus-update-nsw-health-minister-announces-massive-fine-for-those-abusing-frontline-workers-c-967171>; Matt Loffman, "Asian Americans describe 'gut punch' of racist attacks during coronavirus pandemic", *PBS* (7 April 2020), online: <www.pbs.org/newshour/nation/asian-americans-describe-gut-punch-of-racist-attacks-during-coronavirus-pandemic>; Lily Kuo & Helen Davidson, "'They see my blue eyes then jump back'–China sees new wave of xenophobia", *The Guardian* (29 March 2020), online: <www.theguardian.com/world/2020/mar/29/china-coronavirus-anti-foreigner-feeling-imported-cases>; Jacquie Miller, "Virus vigilantes: 'My neighbour isn't self-isolating'", *Ottawa Citizen* (2 April 2020), online: <ottawacitizen.com/news/local-news/virus-vigilantes-my-neighbour-isnt-self-isolating/>.
13. Pringle, *supra* note 4.

> Where a person has a mental disorder that is "likely" to result in "serious bodily harm" to the person or to others, or "serious physical impairment" to the person. Lack of decision-making capacity is not a requirement for hospitalization in this kind of situation in Ontario (although incapacity is a hospitalization criterion in some Canadian jurisdictions).[14]
>
> Where a person is incapable and has a known history of mental disorder that is "likely" to result in "substantial mental or physical deterioration" (or one of the above kinds of risks) unless treated, the person has improved with treatment in the past, and substitute consent has been given to administer treatment.[15]

The risk of "serious bodily harm" criterion is unlikely to be met in the case of a person who does not follow public health directives, as this criterion is usually interpreted to mean a risk of violence to oneself or others. However, behaviour that poses a risk of transmitting a serious infection to others has occasionally been found to meet the criteria of posing a likely risk of serious bodily harm to another person. For example, in *Re MC*,[16] a hospitalized patient who was infected with two contagious treatment-resistant bacteria was found to pose such a risk because of spitting and throwing urine at hospital staff. In the context of COVID-19, an infected person who refuses, due to mental illness, to self-isolate would pose a risk of transmitting the virus to the public, although the risk of transmission may be lower than in the case of an assault, as was the case in *Re MC*. Furthermore, risk of infection with the coronavirus may not meet the threshold of likely serious bodily harm to others, given that the course of illness is usually mild. The risk might, however, be sufficient depending on the specific situation—for example, if the person was living with an elderly person.

As for "serious physical impairment" of the person with a mental illness, the criterion might be met where the mental disorder leads to behaviour that is likely to result in a serious infection,[17] or to provocative behaviour that is likely to result in violent retaliation by others.[18]

14. *MHA*, *supra* note 1, s 20(5)(a).
15. *MHA*, *supra* note 1, s 20(1.1).
16. *MC (Re)*, 2010 CanLII 68898 (ONCCB).
17. See e.g. *CL (Re)*, 2017 CanLII 92634 (ONCCB);) *JF (Re)*, 2011 CanLII 71439 (ONCCB); *AD (Re)*, 2011 CanLII 85307 (ONCCB); *DC (Re)*, 2003 CanLII 54111(ONCCB).
18. See e.g. *DA (Re)*, 2016 CanLII 88909 (ONCCB); *IM (Re)*, 2006 CanLII 52776 (ONCCB).

The harm feared must be likely to occur; it does not need to be certain, but it must be probable rather than merely possible.[19] When a person who is uninfected fails to comply with public health directives related to COVID-19 as a result of mental illness, it seems unlikely that their risk of infection would be sufficiently likely in most cases to meet the standard for involuntary hospitalization. Even if a person is homeless and faces expulsion from a shelter for failure to comply with public health measures, that factor alone is unlikely to meet the standard of likely serious physical impairment, particularly if the person has managed on the streets in the past. The standard might be met, however, where a person is elderly or has major medical comorbidities.

Another relevant example is offered by the case of *Re KP*, which involved a woman who was involved in risky work (such as sex work) and held delusional beliefs that she could put curses on people and that she had the power to cure and cause plagues like SARS and West Nile Virus. The Board evaluating her case concluded that serious physical impairment was likely on the basis of her provocative behaviour and because "her belief that she has special powers could likely lead her to behave dangerously."[20] Other more general delusions regarding invulnerability have been accepted as posing a risk of serious physical impairment because of the high probability of risky behaviour.[21] So it is possible—depending upon the specific behaviour—that delusions related to invulnerability to infection might also impair a person's ability to respond properly to public health advice about COVID-19, and could meet the criteria of likelihood of serious physical impairment if that person was at risk of serious illness.

The criterion of "substantial mental or physical deterioration" allows for earlier intervention before a person has deteriorated to the point where serious bodily harm or physical impairment is likely. This criterion applies only to the subset of people who are incapable, who have a history of treatable mental disorder, and for whom substitute consent to treatment has been given.[22] It is possible that the risk of infection with the virus might, together with other factors, satisfy the lower threshold of "substantial deterioration" and allow for the hospitalization and treatment of the incapable person with a treatable condition who is not following public health directives.

19. See e.g. *DE (Re)*, 2003 CanLII 54880 (ONCCB).
20. *KP (Re)*, 2003 CanLII 28021 (ONCCB).
21. *KR (Re)*, 2013 CanLII 86463 (ONCCB).
22. *Thompson*, *supra* note 2 at para 35.

Is a Mental Health or a Public Health Approach Preferable in the Case of People Who Do Not Follow Public Health Measures Due to Mental Illness?

Under current interpretations of Ontario's mental health legislation, it appears that the failure, due to mental illness, of an uninfected person to follow public health advice would only rarely be sufficient on its own to satisfy the criteria for involuntary hospitalization. However, from the public health perspective, the failure to follow preventive measures or to self-isolate where infection is known or suspected poses risks that justify enforceable restrictions on the liberties of the general population.

The question we raise here is whether the interpretation of the hospitalization criteria ought to be different during a public health emergency. Should the risk to public health—and the need for a preventive approach to be taken by all—be factored into the interpretation of when a person poses a serious risk to others due to mental illness? It is true that the marginal risk to the public health effort posed by any one non-compliant individual is small, but the success of the effort to contain the virus depends upon the small contributions of everyone.

One of the arguments against applying the mental health legislation to uninfected people with mental illnesses is that the degree of the restriction on liberty posed by involuntary hospitalization dwarfs that posed by preventative public health measures being applied to the general uninfected population. Public health restrictions on gathering in groups and entering certain public spaces are being enforced at least initially by fines, although serious repeat offenders might be subject to a court order or larger penalties. It would be disproportionately severe to involuntarily hospitalize people with mental illnesses when enforcement against other members of the public who behave in similar ways remains relatively lenient.

If there are outbreaks of the virus in a psychiatric hospital, another strong argument against taking a mental health response to the public health risk is that it is unfair to expose people with mental illness to the risk of infection in hospital when non-compliant members of the public are simply receiving fines. The risk of infection is elevated within hospitals and other institutions and with congregate living environments, and there have been some outbreaks in Canadian psychiatric hospitals.[23]

---

23. Bryan Passifiume, "CAMH patient dies from COVID-19", *Toronto Sun* (23 April 2020), online: <torontosun.com/news/local-news/camh-patient-dies-

All who are at risk of likely serious bodily harm or physical impairment due to mental illness have an equal claim on the resources of psychiatric hospitals. However, in some cases the risk may be more likely or imminent, such as with an acutely suicidal person. Another consideration is that the use of involuntary hospitalization to protect a person from contracting or transmitting the virus could consume psychiatric hospital resources needed for such emergencies.

In the case of known or suspected infection, people who disregard public health directives may face harsher penalties such as detention, court orders, contempt of court proceedings, or potential imprisonment for offences under public health legislation. Would it be appropriate to use these kinds of enforcement measures in the case of people whose abilities to understand, to exercise appropriate judgment, and/or to evaluate risk, are affected by mental illness? During a pandemic, perhaps a broader concept of risk should be employed to permit a mental health response rather than a public health response where these harsher public health measures would be applicable. It is true that mechanisms exist to divert a person with mental illness from prosecution to treatment, such as specialized mental health courts. This might be an alternative means to address the issue other than proceeding initially with involuntary hospitalization.

The intersection of mental health and public health laws brings tensions to the fore between protecting the health, liberty, and equality interests of people whose ability to protect themselves from infection is affected by mental illness, protecting other vulnerable people from infection, and pursuing the public health goal of containing the virus. Not all people will agree on how best to address these risks. A woman with lived experience of schizophrenia recently expressed her concern about how she might have fared during the current pandemic while homeless and unwell.[24] She indicated that, in the past, she had been unwilling while ill to accept help, and wished that intervention had come earlier in her case. Others may disagree.

---

from-covid-19>; Lisa-Marie Gervais & Marco Bélair-Cirino, "Éclosion de cas de COVID-19 à l'Institut psychiatrique Douglas", *Le Devoir* (30 April 2020), online: <www.ledevoir.com/societe/sante/577982/eclosion-de-covid-19-a-l-institut-psychiatrique-douglas>.

24. Bethany Yeiser, "Homeless with COVID-19: What will happen to the homeless during this pandemic?" *Psychology Today* (11 April 2020), online: <www.psychologytoday.com/ca/blog/recovery-road/202004/homeless-covid-19>.

At a minimum, pandemic response and preparedness should endeavour to ensure that the structures and resources that assist mentally ill persons to follow public health directives are in place. Although better attention to the needs of this vulnerable group will not avoid all of the challenging cases and tensions identified in this chapter, it will certainly help and should be pursued now and after the pandemic.

SECTION E

THIS JOB IS GONNA KILL ME: WORKING AND COVID-19

CHAPTER E-1

Privatization and COVID-19: A Deadly Combination for Nursing Homes

Pat Armstrong,* Hugh Armstrong,** and Ivy Bourgeault***

Abstract

In this chapter, we make visible the different forms of privatization of nursing homes to help understand how it has made residents and workers so highly susceptible to the deadliest aspects of the COVID-19 pandemic. Privatization includes the move to private (often for-profit) delivery of services, managerial practices, and responsibilization of individuals and their families. All these forms are evident in nursing homes, exacerbated by austerity measures. The conditions of work in nursing homes intensified with increasing privatization, decreased staffing, and increased resident acuity before the pandemic, but deteriorated dramatically when it began to hit home after home. The extent to which this deterioration can be directly linked to privatization is difficult to determine, but there are clear indications that privatization set the stage. Bold responses are needed to correct this course, not just during the current emergency, but going forward, to ensure that the many deaths in this sector have come with important lessons learned.

* Distinguished Research Professor in Sociology at Toronto's York University and a Fellow of the Royal Society of Canada.

** Distinguished Research Professor and Professor Emeritus of Social Work, Political Economy, and Sociology at Carleton University.

*** Professor in the School of Sociological and Anthropological Studies at the University of Ottawa, and holder of a University Research Chair in Gender, Diversity and the Professions.

Résumé
Privatisation et COVID-19 : une combinaison fatale pour les maisons de retraite

Dans ce chapitre, nous exposons les différentes formes de privatisation des centres d'hébergement et de soins de longue durée afin de mieux comprendre comment elles ont rendu les résidents et les travailleurs si vulnérables aux aspects les plus meurtriers de la pandémie de COVID-19. La privatisation suppose le transfert à l'entreprise privée (souvent à but lucratif) de la prestation des services et des pratiques de gestion, ainsi que la responsabilisation des individus et de leur famille. Toutes ces formes sont bien présentes dans les maisons de retraite, où elles sont exacerbées par les mesures d'austérité. Les conditions de travail dans les maisons de retraite s'étaient déjà détériorées avant la pandémie, avec la privatisation croissante, la diminution du personnel et l'augmentation du niveau d'intensité des services nécessaires pour fournir des soins aux résidents, mais elles se sont considérablement aggravées lorsque la COVID-19 a commencé à frapper ces établissements les uns après les autres. Il est difficile de déterminer dans quelle mesure cette détérioration peut être directement liée à la privatisation, mais il y a des indications claires que le passage au privé a préparé le terrain. Il faut réagir avec courage pour rectifier le tir, non seulement dans la situation d'urgence actuelle, mais aussi à l'avenir, afin que l'on puisse tirer des enseignements des nombreux décès survenus dans ce secteur.

The combined exposure of increased privatization and COVID-19 for those living and caring in nursing homes has emerged as a toxic cocktail with enormous consequences. In this chapter, we make visible the different forms of privatization of these homes to help understand how it has made residents and workers so highly susceptible to the deadliest aspects of the COVID-19 pandemic.

Forms of Privatization

Privatization takes many forms.[1] It can involve any or all of moving away not only from public delivery and public payment for health

1. Pat Armstrong & Hugh Armstrong, eds, *The Privatization of Care: The Case of Nursing Homes* (New York: Routledge, 2020); Pat Armstrong et al, eds, *Exposing*

services, but also from a commitment to shared responsibility, democratic decision-making, and the idea that the public sector operates according to a logic of service to all.

The most obvious form of privatization is the move to *for-profit delivery* of all or part of a health care service. Canada has a history of private, non-profit delivery of many services, but the considerable expansion of for-profit delivery for publicly funded services is a relatively new development. This shift has been promoted on the assumption that for-profit provision is more efficient and provides better quality, primarily as a result of competition, and can provide the necessary capital without requiring public investment. These same assumptions provide the basis for privatization through the promotion of *for-profit managerial practices* within the not-for-profit and public services that remain.

The *shift of payment from the public to families and individuals* is less obvious. Services are quietly removed from public coverage and charges raised. Care deficits that remain push Canadians to seek privately paid options. As Macarov explains, privatization "is sometimes attained not by outright sales but by deliberately allowing services to run down, by erecting barriers to access, by withholding information and by making receiving benefits so difficult and demeaning that the public has little alternative but to turn to the private sector."[2]

It is not only the *costs* that are shifted, but also the *work* of providing care when public options are not available or at least available in forms that provide adequate care. Over the last three decades there has been a growing emphasis on what has been called *responsibilization,*[3] a transfer of responsibility for health and care to individuals and sometimes their families, often ironically under the guise of "choice."

Along with these processes comes the *privatization of decision-making*. For-profit corporations are allowed a considerable degree of

---

Privatization: Women and Health Care Reform in Canada (Toronto: University of Toronto Press Higher Education, Broadview Press, 2001); Hugh Armstrong, Pat Armstrong & M Patricia Connelly, "The Many Forms of Privatization" (1997) 53:1 Studies in Political Economy 3.

2. David Macarov, *What the Market Does to People: Privatization, Globalization and Poverty* (Atlanta: Clarity Press, 2003) at 7.

3. See, for example, Mike Dent, "Patient Choice and Medicine in Health Care: Responsibilization, Governance and Proto-Professionalization" (2006) 8:3 Public Management Review 449, DOI: <10.1080/14719030600853360>; Gary C Gray, "The Responsibilization Strategy of Health and Safety: Neo-liberalism and the Reconfiguration of Individual Responsibility for Risk" (2009) 49:3 British Journal of Criminology 326.

secrecy on the grounds that a competitive environment protects corporate rights to trade secrecy, including over exactly how profits are made.

All these forms are evident in nursing homes, residential facilities that receive considerable public funding to provide 24-hour nursing care.

Nursing Home Privatization

Labelled by several different names, what are most commonly called nursing homes are primarily a provincial/territorial responsibility. They are not explicitly named under the *Canada Health Act*, the legislation that establishes principles for federal funding. As a result, there is considerable variation among jurisdictions in relation to funding, regulation, and policy.

Nevertheless, as McDonald[4] explains, there are five common funding patterns across jurisdictions:

- health care costs are publicly covered;
- residents bear some responsibility for accommodation costs;
- public subsidies of accommodation costs are targeted based on residents' ability to pay;
- residents' payments should not take all of their income;
- residents' payments should take into account the needs of other family members.

Another commonality has been the closure of chronic care and psychiatric hospitals, a narrowing of the definition of acute care, and the dramatic shortening of hospital stays in the name of health care reform. Policy increasingly emphasizes *aging in place*, which primarily means looking after yourself (i.e., *responsibilization*) or having—usually female—relatives look after you, with some support from government-funded home care. Homecare provides some services previously available in hospitals and nursing homes, but many do not have private homes, or homes organized in a way that can safely accommodate their needs, or relatives with the time, skill, or other capacities to provide the required care. The complexity of the care and equipment required means that much

4. Martha MacDonald, "Regulating Individual Charges for Long-Term Residential Care In Canada" (2015) 95:1 Studies in Political Economy 83 at 89.

of the care once provided in hospitals must now be provided in nursing homes.

Paralleling these reforms is population aging. Although most older people are in reasonable health and can continue to live at home, a significant proportion are surviving with multiple, severe chronic conditions that require skilled support of the kind provided in nursing homes. The number of beds available has not kept up with the verified need. One indicator is wait times for admission. For example, once a person qualifies as needing 24-hour care, the median wait time for being offered a place in Ontario is over 150 days.[5]

The care deficits that remain cause many to seek private care. Not only does homecare shift significant costs and work to individuals and families, those who cannot get into a nursing home have to pay a retirement home anywhere "... from $3,000 to roughly $7,000 a month for basic care. These numbers can easily climb another $1,000 to $3,000 a month as extra care is required."[6] Within nursing homes residents are paying for more of their services, such as physiotherapy and foot care,[7] and a growing number of families are paying for private companions for their relatives in order to make up for care gaps.[8]

For-Profit Privatization in Nursing Home Care

The shifts in responsibility, costs, and care work in nursing homes have been accompanied by a troubling trend towards for-profit chain ownership, especially in the big provinces. For example, between 2010 and 2016, Alberta lost 335 beds in public facilities while 3,255 were added in for-profit ones. By 2016, 43% of the beds were in for-profit facilities.[9]

5. Health Quality Ontario, *Long-Term Care Home Wait Times in Ontario* (Ottawa: Health Quality Ontario, last visited 28 April 2020), online: *Health Quality Ontario* <https://www.hqontario.ca/System-Performance/Long-Term-Care-Home-Performance/Wait-Times>.
6. Ted Rechtshaffen, "Here's What it Costs to Live in a Retirement Home — And the Bottom Line is Less Than You Might Think", *Financial Post* (13 March 2019), online: <https://business.financialpost.com/personal-finance/retirement/heres-what-it-costs-to-live-in-a-retirement-home-and-the-bottom-line-is-less-than-you-might-think>.
7. MacDonald, *supra* note 4.
8. Tamara Daly, Pat Armstrong & Ruth Lowndes, "Liminality in Ontario's Long-Term Care Facilities: Private Companions' Care Work in the Space 'Betwixt and Between'" (2015) 19:3 Competition & Change 246.
9. David Campanella, *Losing Ground: Alberta's Residential Elder Care Crisis* (Edmonton: Parkland Institute, 2016) at 11.

In BC, between 2001 and 2016, the number of beds in for-profit homes increased by 2,621, while those in non-profit homes declined by 2,082.[10] Currently, 58% of Ontario homes are for-profit, compared with 24% non-profit and 16% publicly owned by municipalities.[11]

For-profit ownership is further complicated by the contracting out of services within non-profit and government-owned homes, blurring the lines among the various forms of ownership.[12] The outsourcing may involve hiring individuals, often through agencies that take a proportion of the pay. Instead of hiring their own therapists and other professionals or expanding their nursing staff, homes contract for individuals to provide these services through private agencies. Similarly, homes fill gaps in their nursing and other staff by using temporary help agencies. This form of contracting out may be based on the argument that the home does not need these individuals full-time and thus paying by day or by service is a more efficient way of hiring.

Another growing form of contracting involves handing over entire services to a for-profit company. This has become common for cleaning, dietary, laundry, and security services, most often provided by international corporations that also deliver services to other organizations, such as hotels and universities. This kind of contracting is based on the argument that these are ancillary services rather than health care services, and that they are more efficiently and effectively undertaken by corporations with experience to achieve economies of scale. But research demonstrates that these services are critical to care.[13] Perhaps the most surprising kind of contracting out involves management services. As Daly[14] shows, a growing number of non-profit and publicly owned homes contract out their management to

10. Andrew Longhurst, "Privatization & Declining Access to BC Seniors' Care" (2017) at 14, online (pdf): *Canadian Centre for Policy Alternatives* <https://www.policyalternatives.ca/sites/default/files/uploads/publications/BC%20Office/2017/03/access_to_seniors_care_report_170327%20FINAL.pdf>.

11. Ontario Long-Term Care Association, "This Is Long-Term Care 2019" (2019) at 13, online (pdf): *Ontario Long-Term Care Association* <https://www.oltca.com/OLTCA/Documents/Reports/TILTC2019web.pdf>, citing Ontario Ministry of Health and Long-Term Care, *Long-Term Care Homes System Report 2018* (Ottawa: Ontario Ministry of Health and Long-Term Care, 2018).

12. Pat Armstrong & Hugh Armstrong, "Contracting Out Care" in Fran Collyer & Karen Willis, eds, *Navigating Private and Public Healthcare: Experiences of Patients, Doctors and Policy-Makers* (London: Palgrave Macmillan, 2020) 87.

13. Pat Armstrong, Hugh Armstrong & Krista Scott-Dixon, *Critical to Care: The Invisible Women in Health Services* (Toronto: University of Toronto Press, 2008).

14. Tamara Daly, "Dancing The Two-Step in Ontario's Long-Term Care Sector: Deterrence Regulation = Consolidation" (2015) 95:1 Studies in Political Economy 29.

for-profit chains, further blurring the lines between for-profit and non-profit homes.

While there are for-profit facilities that provide quality care, there are clear patterns of lower staffing contributing to lower quality care in for-profit homes.[15] For-profit staffing strategies are not only about fewer staff but also about a different mix of staff, with more having fewer formal qualifications, who in turn are paid less. There is evidence that this kind of staff mix also has an impact on the quality of care, demonstrating the importance of a mix that includes staff with more formal qualifications. For-profit strategies also encourage more precarity: hiring more casual and part-time staff and failing to replace staff absent for leaves or other reasons in order to reduce costs related to benefits, such as sick leave and pensions, union pay rates, and other job protections related to unionization.[16] These strategies reduce hours to the absolute minimum. Precarity not only leaves workers without any form of security, it makes it more difficult to have continuity in care and the development of relationship-based care with residents, essential for good quality.

Other indications that quality tends to be lower in for-profit homes include higher morbidity and hospitalization rates in for-profit chains.[17] Hospitalization suggests that problems with the care received in the nursing home may put residents at risk.[18] Verified complaints are also higher.[19] That the public also judge non-profit and public homes as having higher quality is indicated by their relative preference: in Ontario, 67% of the first choices for nursing home admission in 2010 were to non-profit and public homes although they accounted for only 46% of the province's beds.[20] This is the case

15. Charlene Harrington, Allyson M Pollock & Shailen Sutaria, "Privatization of Nursing Homes in the United Kingdom and the United States" in Pat Armstrong & Hugh Armstrong, eds, *The Privatization of Care: The Case of Nursing Homes* (New York: Routledge, 2020) 51.
16. David Harvey, *A Brief History of Neoliberalism* (Oxford: Oxford University Press, 2005) at 167.
17. Peter Tanuseputro et al, "Hospitalization and Mortality Rates in Long-Term Care Facilities: Does For-Profit Status Matter?" (2015) 16:10 Journal of the American Medical Directors Association 874.
18. Gudmund Ågotnes et al, "A Critical Review of Research on Hospitalization from Nursing Homes; What is Missing?" (2016) 41:1 Ageing International 3.
19. Margaret J McGregor et al, "Complaints in For-Profit, Non-Profit and Public Nursing Homes in Two Canadian Provinces" (2011) 5:4 Open Medicine 183.
20. Dan Buchanan, "The Not-For-Profit Contribution and Issues from the Provider Perspective" (Presentation delivered at Reimagining Long-Term Residential Care Annual Meeting, Toronto, 2011) [unpublished].

even though the residents' fees are the same in both public and private homes.

It has become harder and harder to track for-profit ownership and its consequences, largely because of the lack of transparency concerning complex financing structures.[21] Complex ownership structures contribute to the efforts to reduce taxes, litigation actions, and regulatory oversight.[22] As a result, it is not easy to have democratic control, and residents, families, and staff may find it more difficult to engage with major corporations than they would with local government or not-for-profit owners. The attempts to provide alternative forms of accountability have resulted in the requirement for increasing documentation that focuses on counting what can easily be counted. Staff are required to do a growing amount of reporting on residents and their care, time that takes them away from applying their skills to care. More regulations have also been introduced, with the purported purpose of addressing quality care, that here too have a paradoxical effect. Research shows that scandals publicized in the media have resulted in more regulations, and this is particularly the case in the jurisdictions where for-profit ownership is highest.[23] The regulations, however, tend to focus on the workers rather than on the owners, ownership, and management.[24]

For-profit ownership is also harder to track because many non-profit homes have for-profit services within them, but also because austerity measures adopted by governments across Canada promoted market methods and for-profit managerial strategies within all homes.[25] Public funding cuts add pressure to keep or reduce the labour force to a minimum, and to rely both on more part-time and

21. Daly, *supra* note 14.
22. Charlene Harrington et al, "Ownership, Financing, and Management Strategies of the Ten Largest For-Profit Nursing Home Chains in the United States" (2011) 41:4 International Journal of Health Services 725; Jordan Rau, "Care Suffers as More Nursing Homes Feed Money Into Corporate Webs", *The New York Times* (2 January 2018), online: <https://www.nytimes.com/2018/01/02/business/nursing-homes-care-corporate.html>.
23. Liz Lloyd et al, "It's a Scandal! Comparing the Causes and Consequences of Nursing Home Media Scandals in Five Countries" (2014) 34:1/2 International Journal of Sociology and Social Policy 2.
24. Albert Banerjee & Pat Armstrong, "Centring Care: Explaining Regulatory Tensions in Residential Care for Older Persons" (2015) 95 Studies in Political Economy 7.
25. Eleanor D Glor, "Has Canada Adopted the New Public Management?" (2001) 3:1 Public Management Review 121.

casual staff and on the workers with less formal credentials. This is particularly the case for those called personal support workers or care aides.[26] These trends result in particularly dire consequences when residents and workers are exposed to COVID-19.

The Nature of Nursing Home Work

To understand the impact of COVID-19 on nursing homes, it is necessary to understand the nature of the work, and how it has intensified with increasing privatization, decreased staffing, and increased resident acuity.

According to the Canadian Institute for Health Information, 62% of residents have dementia, with a third experiencing severe cognitive impairment. Three quarters have some bladder incontinence and over half have bowel incontinence, while 40% exhibit some aggressive behaviour.[27] The Ontario Long Term Care Association[28] reports that the actual severity is much higher, with significant overlaps in these categories:

- 90% have some form of cognitive impairment
- 86% need extensive help with activities such as eating or using the washroom
- 80% have neurological diseases
- 76% have heart/circulation diseases
- 64% have a diagnosis of dementia
- 62% have musculoskeletal diseases such as arthritis and osteoporosis
- 40% need monitoring for an acute medical condition
- 21% have experienced a stroke
- 61% take 10 or more prescription medications.

26. Katherine Zagrodney & Mike Saks, "Personal Support Workers in Canada: The New Precariat?" (2017) 13:2 Healthcare Policy 31, DOI: <10.12927/hcpol.2017.25324.>.
27. Canadian Institute for Health Information, "Profile of Residents in Residential and Hospital-Based Continuing Care, 2018-2019" (2020), online (pdf): *Canadian Institute for Health Information* <https://www.cihi.ca/en/access-data-reports/results?f%5B0%5D=field_primary_theme%3A2054&f%5B1%5D=field_primary_theme%3A2061&f%5B2%5D=field_content_format%3A2166>.
28. Ontario Long-Term Care Association, "This Is Long-Term Care 2019" (2019) at 3, online (pdf): *Ontario Long-Term Care Association* <https://www.oltca.com/OLTCA/Documents/Reports/TILTC2019web.pdf>.

The average age of nursing home residents is 83,[29] and most are female. The predominance of women in part reflects their greater longevity combined with more disabilities, and in part the pattern of women taking responsibility for the care of their male partners at home. Nevertheless, compared to the past, more are male. Men tend to be heavier and more prone to violence. More of the residents are under the age 65, and there is increasing diversity among both staff and residents.

The majority of residents must be assisted to get out of bed, use the toilet, dress, bathe, and eat, all tasks that require attending to frailty, medical equipment, personal preferences, and resistance. The majority use incontinence products. Many spend most of their time in bed, and thus need to be constantly repositioned to prevent ulcers and to be bathed in bed. Many require specialized medical care, and not just assistance with activities of daily living, as this nurse explains:

> Anyone who tells you long-term care is easy is lying. Or they haven't worked in long-term care. … I have a guy who's having a heart attack over there, a stroke over there, this one's got a pic line, this one's got this … like all sorts of complex [care] … so I'm running my own blood work, X-rays and everything else … so I'm actually operating in a sense at a higher level than you would as a hospital nurse.[30]

All this work requires a high level of technical skill, as well as the social, psychological, and emotional skills that require familiarity with both residents and other staff. It also takes staff into direct and close contact with residents. That almost all the residents have some form of cognitive impairment complicates any intervention, especially if the care provider is not known to or recognized by the resident.

Close, regular, personal contact is an essential part of this skilled work. Administering medications, for example, means knowing who can swallow the medication, how to convince them to take it, and who usually spits it out or is at risk of choking. This may involve touching the resident's face and mouth to assist or ensure the resident swallows. Similarly, treating pressure ulcers requires technical skills that not only includes close personal contact but also working in close

29. *Ibid.*
30. Pat Armstrong et al, "RNs in Long-Term Care: A Portrait" (2019) at 12, online: *Ontario Nurses Association* <https://www.ona.org/carenow/>.

proximity to other health care workers to turn and position the resident. There is no way this can be done from two metres away.

Much of the work of bathing, dressing, changing briefs, and assisting residents to the toilet and the shower is carried out by those variously called personal support workers, health care aides, or care aides, and the like. To supervise them, nurses must know how to do this work and be prepared to assist, especially in these times of very short staffing. Residents regularly cough, spit, and dribble, risking the spread of the virus. There is no guarantee that residents will remember to cough into their arms, blow their nose into a Kleenex, or wash their hands, let alone do it to singing "Happy Birthday" twice. Even if they are able to take these precautions in the morning, they may not remember to do so in the afternoon.

Dressing and undressing, and especially changing diapers, exposes workers to physical risks, both because such intimate work can prompt resistance and because workers are so close to the residents. Residents may lash out when dressing or clinical tasks are underway. Exposed to frequent scratching, kicking, punching, spitting, and biting, the skilled work of staff is difficult. The work becomes more difficult and skilled under COVID-19 conditions. With many residents upset and confused by today's changed conditions, the work becomes even more risky. Resistance and violence are increased, and workers must call on a wide range of skills to calm and reassure residents.

Dietary workers, laundry workers, and housekeeping staff also require specialized skills for operating in this care environment. They, too, frequently interact with residents and need to know about their capacities. The need for special cleaning has become more obvious during the pandemic, as it did during SARS, but cleaning is always a critical factor in care for this vulnerable population. Urine and feces, for example, are frequently found on seats, floors, and beds, carrying risks. Laundry too can spread infection and requires careful and knowledgeable handling.[31] Moreover, it is essential to coordinate these workers with those who provide nursing care.

All these workers frequently encounter families seeking information and help. Moreover, many families provide a considerable amount of care, especially in terms of assistance in eating, dressing, walking, comforting, and advocating, and many receive training to do

31. Pat Armstrong & Suzanne Day, *Wash, Wear, and Care: Clothing and Laundry in Long-Term Residential Care* (Montréal & Kingston: McGill-Queen's University Press, 2017) [Armstrong & Day].

so. Volunteers also assist in care work and receive training, but this requires additional supervision and integration work for staff. This is also the case with privately paid companions. The coordination and search for information are more complicated during a pandemic, especially when family, volunteers, and paid companions are locked out.

Nursing homes are often called long-term residential care because, even with stricter admission criteria, residents spend a long time in the home. Staff get to know them, and often their families, well. When death happens, staff must deal with their own grief, with that of families, and with that of other staff. Multiple deaths and threatened deaths during this time multiply the grief and dealing with the dead necessarily involves not only additional work with families and staff but also touching the dead, creating new risks.

The growing complexity of resident care needs means there is a growing demand for more and different skills, skills specific to the variety of physical conditions that are combined with cognitive demands particular to nursing home care. The overwhelming majority of nursing home workers are women. Their different skills are often assumed to be work that any woman can do. That these places are usually called homes encourages the association of the work with what most women do in the home, too often rendering the skills invisible and undervalued.[32]

In sum, nursing home work is physically and emotionally demanding and requires a range of skills in all job categories, skills that are often undervalued and low-paid. Instead of supporting a skilled and resourced labour force, privatization has been undermining and intensifying it. This created a powder keg when COVID-19 hit.

Privatization and the Conditions of Care during COVID-19

The conditions of work are the conditions of care.[33] Care can only be as good as the conditions that allow care providers to do their work. The same conditions shape the health of those who provide and those who need care. The conditions of work in nursing homes had already

32. Pat Armstrong, "Puzzling Skills: Feminist Political Economy Approaches" (2013) 50:3 Canadian Review of Sociology 256.
33. See Re-imagining Long-term Residential Care Project, "Re-imagining Long-term Residential Care: An International Study of Promising Practices" (last visited 14 May 2020), online: *Re-imagining Long-term Residential Care* <https://reltc.apps01.yorku.ca/>.

intensified before the pandemic, but deteriorated dramatically when the disease began to hit home after home. The extent to which this deterioration can be directly linked to privatization is difficult to determine, but there are clear indications that privatization set the stage.

Adequate staffing levels are a necessary condition for quality care or even minimal care. As the recent Gillese inquiry in Ontario made clear, the "vulnerability of residents in LTC homes is not only a function of their physical and mental states. It also stems from the shortage of staff—particularly nurses—in the home."[34] While most Canadian jurisdictions require an RN on site at all times, only a few set out minimum staffing levels, and none are set at the 4.1 hours of direct nursing hours per resident per day that research indicated was necessary[35] before their needs spiked with the pandemic. According to AdvantAge Ontario calculations, Ontario residents receive 3.45 hours of care per resident per day.[36] This calculation may be generous, because the data are based on staffing on the books rather than who is actually present for care. Many staff are regularly off work due to illness, injury, or other leaves, and the data often include those not involved in providing direct care. Indeed, our research indicates that staff regularly work short.[37] The low staffing levels can be linked to privatization, both in the sense that for-profit homes have lower staffing levels than do the others, and that public funding has not kept up with need as governments have promoted for-profit managerial strategies for the non-profit homes that remain. Profits must come from somewhere and, in a labour-intensive sector, that is typically from labour costs.

These trends existed before the pandemic, and now the workload and stress have grown significantly. So has the need for more staff, with the care required per resident doubling. Putting on and taking

---

34. The Honourable Eileen E Gillese, *Public Inquiry into the Safety and Security of Residents in the Long-Term Care Homes System,* (Toronto: Ministry of the Attorney General, 2019) at 87, online (pdf): *Ministry of the Attorney General* <https://www.attorneygeneral.jus.gov.on.ca/english/about/pubs/ltc-review/>.
35. Charlene Harrington et al, "The Need for Higher Minimum Staffing Standards in U.S. Nursing Homes" (2016) 9 Health Services Insights 13.
36. AdvantAge Ontario, "The Way Forward: Next Steps to Meet the Needs of Ontario's Seniors" (2020), online (pdf): *AdvantAge Ontario* <http://www.advantageontario.ca/AAO/Content/Resources/Advantage_Ontario/2020-Pre-Budget.aspx>.
37. Pat Armstrong et al, "Long-Term Care Home Wait Times in Ontario" (2009), online: *Health Quality Ontario* <https://www.hqontario.ca/System-Performance/Long-Term-Care-Home-Performance/Wait-Times>.

off personal protective equipment (PPE)—if available, which it often has not been—alone increases the workload substantially. Changes to workflow are also required during an outbreak, such as ensuring medication administration and clinical assessments are consolidated to optimize PPE conservation. Residents are confined to their rooms, so all medications and meals must be administered in each room, rather than more efficiently in the dining room, for example.

In addition, gaps in care created by low staffing levels had often been filled by family members and volunteers, the same families and volunteers now barred from entering due to infection control. Families also create more work as a result of their understandable demands for information. Similarly, volunteers had taken on some of the work involved in keeping residents active, also as a result of low staffing levels. These people too have been removed from the homes, leaving residents without activities. The result can be increased stress, agitation, and violence.

While adequate staffing levels are a necessary condition for quality care, they are not the only one. Training for the specific and changing needs of residents in long-term care, especially during a pandemic, is also required. In these times, this includes the use of new equipment and protection for everyone who enters the home. Anyone new to the home also needs information on particular residents in order to protect both the person providing and the person needing care. The work is more complicated if workers without specific training in nursing home care are brought in. Workload is further increased during an outbreak when staff are unfamiliar with the residents, the home, or with other workers as a result of relying on part-time or agency staff. Moreover, part-time staff not only move from home to home, as has become obvious during this pandemic, but they are often without the benefits that would enable them to stay home when sick. Coordination and teamwork are essential in these times of extra work and rising fear. Both are made more complicated by workers unfamiliar with the place and people.

Physical environments also matter.[38] Austerity has meant that many homes have not been redeveloped to meet current health needs. The problem of wards that house up to four residents separated by little more than a sheet has become obvious. Crowded rooms force

38. Pat Armstrong & Susan Braedley, eds, "Physical Environments for Long-term Care" (2016), online: *Canadian Centre for Policy Alternatives* <https://www.policyalternatives.ca/publications/reports/physical-environments-long-term-care>.

workers to move in close to residents and to each other, whether or not they are providing personal care. Curtains do not protect residents from witnessing the death of others sharing their room. Spaces to accommodate and commemorate death are critical but mostly non-existent.

Shared washrooms, especially down the hall, put an extra burden and risk on staff. Many homes have no extra room for quarantine in light of admission policies that push homes to fill all rooms as quickly as possible, in hours rather than days. Dining rooms are often crowded, leaving very little space among residents and staff or between tables. Outdoor spaces are often locked, in part because there is not enough staff to keep watch. The only TVs and computers are often in shared spaces. Many homes have only small, cramped spaces for staff to get away for the respite that is especially necessary now. Sharing these spaces translates into close contact among workers.

Similarly, the way laundry is physically located, shared, and organized has an impact on infection and other risks for both residents and workers.[39] If it is collected in hallways before being shipped out to a service, it can constitute a particular risk of transmission, especially in these times. Food services that are contracted out, with the workers and the food itself imported from outside the home, may involve workers moving from floor to floor. These workers may not have special infection training or PPE.

Another obvious working condition is access to equipment, including but not limited to PPE. Those working in long-term care have the highest rates of absences due to illness and injury of any industry, in part because the equipment needed for lifts and transfers is not accessible or because they do not have the time to use it as prescribed. Here, too, space is important. Many rooms make it difficult to move equipment into place without close personal contact, or to even use the equipment required. Then there is the lack of time necessary to sanitize equipment to prevent spread. Legal cases recently taken against for-profit homes by unions speak to their failure to provide the needed equipment, not the least of which is PPE.[40]

39. Armstrong & Day, *supra* note 31.
40. Ontario Labour Relations Board, OLRB Case No: 0091-20-HS, OLRB Case No 0092-20-HS, OLRB Case No 0093-20-HS; *Ontario Nurses' Association v Participating Nursing Homes*, 2019 ONSC 2168, Divisional Court File NO.: 362/16 and 364/16. See also Katherine Lippel, this volume, Chapter E-3.

Concluding Remarks

Privatization has permeated nursing homes in a variety of visible and invisible ways, creating living and working conditions that have proven deadly for residents and staff during this pandemic. Bold responses are needed to correct this course, not just during the current emergency, but going forward, to ensure that the many deaths in this sector have come with important lessons learned. What is needed is a comprehensive, evidence-informed strategy, not only as a short-term response to the pandemic, but as a longer-term approach to create safer and more equitable environments for all who live, work, and visit long-term residential care. We must enforce evidence-informed minimum care standards, stockpile sufficient PPE, create sufficient surge capacity to cope with the next pandemic, and end the siphoning-off of care resources to profit. Our elders, and those who care for them, deserve better.

CHAPTER E-2

A View from the Front Lines of a COVID-19 Outbreak

Jane Philpott*

Abstract

This chapter offers a narrative of a COVID-19 outbreak at Participation House Markham. It is a not-for-profit group home for adults with disabilities, established in 1972 by the Cerebral Palsy Parent Council of Toronto. With this outbreak, 95% of the home's residents were infected. Six of them died. Fifty-seven workers were infected. The story illustrates themes discussed elsewhere in this book, but focuses particularly on the role of the labour force in a care home. It notes the pre-pandemic vulnerability of any congregate setting without a full staffing complement. In any group home or long-term care facility, an infectious outbreak exacerbates workforce challenges, as workers may be exposed to the virus; become ill; or become restricted to a single place of employment. By describing the clinical cases of three residents in one group home, this chapter demonstrates why the shortage of nurses, personal support workers, kitchen staff, and others, would trigger a crisis in this institution or others like it. The chapter includes policy recommendations that are amplified elsewhere in this section. These could contribute to a national review of how to provide residential care for people living with disabilities in a manner that is safe, healthy, and dignified.

* Dean of the Faculty of Health Sciences (Queen's University), and former Minister of Health (Canada).

Résumé
En première ligne d'une éclosion de COVID-19

Ce chapitre propose le récit d'une une éclosion de COVID-19 telle que vécue à la Participation House de Markham. Il s'agit d'un foyer de groupe à but non lucratif pour adultes handicapés, fondé en 1972 par le Cerebral Palsy Parent Council of Toronto. La COVID-19 a frappé 95 % des résidents de ce foyer. Six d'entre eux sont décédés. Cinquante-sept membres du personnel ont été infectés. Cette histoire illustre certains thèmes abordés ailleurs dans cet ouvrage, mais se concentre particulièrement sur le rôle de la main-d'œuvre dans une maison de soins. Elle souligne la vulnérabilité prépandémique de tout établissement de soins qui ne dispose pas d'un effectif complet. Dans n'importe quel foyer de groupe ou centre de soins de longue durée, une épidémie infectieuse exacerbe les défis auxquels est confronté le personnel, qui peut être exposé au virus, tomber malade ou être confiné à un seul lieu de travail. En présentant les cas cliniques de trois résidents d'un foyer de groupe, ce chapitre montre pourquoi la pénurie d'infirmières, de personnel de soutien, de personnel de cuisine et autres allait entraîner une crise dans cet établissement et dans d'autres semblables. Je propose en outre des orientations politiques qui sont reprises ailleurs dans cette section, et qui pourraient contribuer à un examen national sur la prestation de soins résidentiels aux personnes vivant avec un handicap d'une manière qui soit sûre, saine et digne.

It was Easter Sunday morning, April 12, at 7:42 a.m. when I received a text from my friend Leea: "Hi there. Sorry to be texting so early, but the Executive Director of Participation House asked me to see if you can help. They are desperate for staff and she is getting frantic."

Thus began my involvement with the terrible COVID-19 outbreak at the Butternut Lane site of Participation House Markham (PHM) in Ontario, Canada, in April 2020.

PHM is a group home for 42 adults with a range of physical, intellectual, and developmental disabilities. The primary diagnoses of residents include conditions like cerebral palsy, Down syndrome, Angelman syndrome, and Rett syndrome.

PHM's first case of COVID-19 was confirmed on April 6, 2020. Three days later, tests on people with symptoms showed ten residents and four staff were COVID-19 positive. On Saturday, April 11, all residents were swabbed. Definitive results showed 40 out of 42 residents had been infected. Tragically, six of them died. Fifty-seven workers were also infected.

I am a family doctor. Cancellations caused by the pandemic left me with some availability, so I didn't hesitate to assist at PHM, thankful for an opportunity to be useful. This chapter is my account of the COVID-19 outbreak in that location, but it reveals public policy challenges with broad implications.[1] For it is on the front lines of care that health policy finds both inspiration and a testing ground.

A major problem for facilities like PHM was severe personnel shortages. Even before COVID-19, PHM was short of staff. Most residents need assistance for feeding, bathing, and toileting. Most need to be moved by mechanical lift from bed to wheelchair and back. As described in the opening chapter of this section, providing appropriate care at PHM requires a high degree of human touch, making public health measures such as physical distancing almost impossible. The personal care needs of residents put them and their caregivers at heightened risk of transmitting infections. The complex medical conditions of residents also put them at increased risk of severe illness with COVID-19.[2]

With news of the outbreak, many staff were unable to continue working. Some needed to self-isolate because they'd had contact with positive cases before full personal protective equipment (PPE) was introduced. Others had symptoms of COVID-19. They needed to be tested and sent home. Those who worked in multiple institutions had to select one location only, and several decided to leave PHM.

My first step that Sunday was to connect with Shelley, the Executive Director of PHM. I arranged to go see how I could help. The crisis was evident immediately. The site had 98 people listed on staff. Full function required about 35 staff members in any 24-hour period. That morning they were down to about 10 regular staff, management included. There was a serious need for help to ensure

1. Elizabeth Lin et al, *Addressing Gaps in the Health Care Services Used by Adults with Developmental Disabilities in Ontario* (Toronto: ICES, 2019).
2. Dalton Stevens & Scott D Landes, "Potential Impacts of COVID-19 on Individuals with Intellectual and Developmental Disability: A Call for Accurate Cause of Death Reporting" (2020), online (pdf): *Syracuse University Lerner Center for Public Health Promotion* <https://lernercenter.syr.edu/wp-content/uploads/2020/04/Stevens_Landes.pdf>.

infection prevention and control, not to mention the residents' regular care needs.[3]

I went to the resident rooms that morning and saw those who were the sickest. Jeanette, who manages the Personal Support Worker (PSW) staff, identified whom she was most concerned about. They had fever, fatigue, and coughing. There were so few workers to provide care.

PHM was never designed nor intended to be a medical facility. It is a home for 42 adults. The only way we could support them properly was to rapidly acquire new caregivers and ensure the home could provide high-quality, home-based care. That's what we did. We contacted every possible organization or agency in a hunt for health professionals. We put out an SOS for more PPE. We ordered oxygen tanks and Symptom Relief Kits.

The first few days are now a blur. Some memories stick in my mind, including the first Tuesday night. I had returned after dinner to check the sicker residents. I assessed six people that night. What I remember is not the clinical examinations, but the sense of despair I felt looking at unfinished meals and beverage trays outside the residents' rooms. Night had fallen and many were asleep, but they had not been fed. I was unsure if this was because people had lost their appetite and thirst or because there simply weren't enough PSWs to feed the residents. From agitated behaviours and comments of those who could talk, we knew the residents were upset about how the place had been turned upside down. Familiar faces were gone. Strangers were providing care. Someone new every day, every shift. Caregivers were wearing masks, gloves, and plastic face shields. It's hard to see a smile behind a mask. It's hard to hear words of kindness spoken through a plastic shield. The glasses of unfinished drinks were a symbol of anguish. How would people survive if we couldn't keep them hydrated and fed?

It was the residents who gave us hope. I met Billy[4] Wednesday morning. I wanted to check in with him because the night before his temperature had spiked to 40 °C. I walked into his room expecting to see someone looking ill. Not Billy. He was sitting up with a smile a

3. Elizabeth Grier et al, "Health Care of Adults with Intellectual and Developmental Disabilities in a Time of COVID-19" (2020), online: *Canadian Family Physician* <https://www.cfp.ca/news/2020/04/09/04-09-02>.

4. Names and identifying details about residents have been changed to protect privacy.

mile wide. He greeted me cheerfully, told me he felt fine, and wanted a coffee. Billy makes friends instantly with everyone. He remembered the fever but now felt as good as ever. On Wednesday night he had a fever again and became short of breath, with low oxygen saturation in his blood. We started him on oxygen. But Thursday morning he looked good again. He wanted to get rid of those annoying nasal prongs. This would become a pattern. High temperatures and shortness of breath in the evenings—then perking up in the morning to charm us as we made rounds. He was the definition of resilience. I felt confident that Billy was going to make it through this infection—and he did.

Wednesday evening, I had at least four phone calls with the nurse on duty. He was worried about Helen. She was short of breath and couldn't stop coughing. They were struggling to keep her oxygen saturation near 90%. On top of COVID-19 infection, Helen had heart failure. She was on a high dose of diuretics. Neither she nor her family wanted her to go to the hospital. She hated hospitals. The family wanted her kept comfortable. I decided to prescribe hydromorphone to help the laboured breathing and settle the agitation. But I discovered there were no narcotics on site. It was almost midnight. We opted to try lorazepam to settle her. I reviewed what I would need to do if Helen died in the home. I slept lightly, worried I would be heading back to PHM at some point in the night to pronounce a death. To my surprise and relief that call never came. Somehow Helen made it through the night.

Thursday would be the worst day of the first week. I was pulling into the parking lot at PHM when I received a couple of texts from Jen who was the charge nurse that day: "Helen is on 6L and sats are 84–88%. We don't have a plan for air hunger. I don't know that we have meds for it either."

Then a minute later: "Can you come see Stuart right away?"

There were two residents with severe shortness of breath. Each was getting 6 litres per minute of oxygen. We hadn't yet acquired oxygen concentrators, so we were using small mobile tanks. Jen calculated, at that rate, each of them would use a tank an hour. I walked into the building, ready to kick into action, determined to procure medications to help with the agitation and shortness of breath.

I went directly to the purple pod where Nurse Jen was watching over Stuart. I donned personal protective gear and went in. I'd been checking Stuart every day. He sat in his wheelchair, coughing frequently. His condition was declining. Thursday morning, he looked exhausted and uncomfortable. Stuart had big brown eyes. That morning there was fear in them. We needed narcotics to settle his breathing. I called a local pharmacy. They were extremely helpful and had injectable hydromorphone. They didn't have subcutaneous sets, but they had needles and syringes that would work. I wrote a script and our nurse practitioner dashed over to pick up the supplies.

Now we could provide symptomatic relief to Helen and Stuart, the sickest residents. But I saw how unstable things were. Nurse Jen needed to run back and forth between these two—changing PPE each time because they were in different pods. The other nurse was giving medications and checking the other residents on site, many of whom were also exhibiting symptoms from their COVID-19 infection.

Despite all efforts to keep these two patients in their home, surrounded by a few people who knew them, I could see that the situation was unsustainable. In those early days, we barely had assurance from one shift to the next that there would be a nurse on site. PSWs were still coming mostly from agencies. So, they were often new people every shift who needed to be oriented in their role and instructed in proper PPE use. The small core team of regular PHM staff was getting smaller by the day, as more workers became sick and had to stay home.

When the crisis started, PHM made the bold decision to offer double wages for the duration of the outbreak to PSWs who would stay and new ones who would come on board. Looking back, that was one of the keys to stabilization. About two weeks after the PHM outbreak was declared, the Ontario government announced a policy to increase pay for many front line health workers during this period.[5]

Still, it was distressingly difficult to meet the staffing needs. Shelley and her team were using multiple job portals, agencies, and regional health resources. The Ministry of Children, Community and Social Services was trying to recruit help. Markham Stouffville Hospital made their human resources team available to assist. I made calls and sent emails to professional nursing organizations. Here's what I learned: In the context of a pandemic, particularly in the setting of an outbreak, it's a massive undertaking to hire and train a brand-new team of nurses and PSWs in a matter of days.

5. Office of the Premier, News Release, "Ontario Supporting Frontline Heroes of COVID-19 with Pandemic Pay" (25 April 2020), online: *News Ontario* <https://news.ontario.ca/opo/en/2020/04/ontario-supporting-frontline-heroes-of-covid-19-with-pandemic-pay.html>.

The crisis reached its worst that Thursday morning—about a week after the outbreak came to light. Two of the residents were struggling for their lives. We were endeavouring to provide the supportive care they deserved. Two residents had already died after being transferred to hospital. Four others had been admitted. I had no idea when one of the other 34 residents could take a turn for the worse. We had more COVID-19 positive cases in our building than most Ontario hospitals were caring for at that time—and we had two nurses on duty.

From the start, we had daily calls with the Vice-President of Markham Stouffville Hospital. They were tremendously helpful in ensuring we had adequate supplies of PPE. They made hospital food services available to deliver purées and other meals for residents because PHM had lost their kitchen staff.

That Thursday morning, the daily call with the hospital was a cry for help. I described our situation as a war zone. Perhaps that was a bit dramatic. But we felt fragile. If the families wanted them to be cared for at home, we were prepared to offer palliative care for residents who might not survive. But it wasn't right to do so without the people in place to make it possible.

We decided to transfer both Helen and Stuart to the hospital. It was the most compassionate option. With sadness, I watched the reaction of one long-time staff member as the paramedics rolled each gurney out the doors. She couldn't say a proper goodbye. She had cared for one of those two residents for over thirty years. They were her family. Would she see them again? Would the hospital staff understand the best way to feed and comfort them?

The look of heartache in the eyes of that health worker is etched in my mind, along with the faces of all six residents of PHM who died. My grief is small compared to that of their families and the long-time caregivers. It's a special person who works for decades in a place like PHM. The nurses and PSWs who make this care possible don't do it because it pays well. It doesn't. They do it because they are people of compassion. They immerse themselves in the vulnerabilities of humanity. Dutch writer and theologian Henri Nouwen, who served at L'Arche Daybreak community near Toronto, describes it this way:

> Compassion asks us to go where it hurts, to enter into the places of pain, to share in brokenness, fear, confusion, and anguish. Compassion challenges us to cry out with those in misery, to

> mourn with those who are lonely, to weep with those in tears. Compassion requires us to be weak with the weak, vulnerable with the vulnerable, and powerless with the powerless. Compassion means full immersion in the condition of being human.[6]

Much has been written about health workers in the COVID-19 pandemic, noting that they, "unlike ventilators or wards, cannot be urgently manufactured or run at 100% occupancy for long periods. It is vital that governments see workers not simply as pawns to be deployed, but as human individuals."[7]

A strong, dynamic health workforce is crucial to managing any pandemic. These workers put their lives on the line in the short term. They remain at risk of the long-term psychological effects of enduring trauma and loss.[8] It will take some time to tally the full impact on the health workforce. It will be extensive. For example, the toll this virus has taken must include the risks that caregivers accept not just for themselves, but those they extend to their loved ones as well.[9]

This book is intended to influence policymakers' responses to the pandemic and help frame public and scholarly conversations around COVID-19. This includes ideas about how to strengthen public health legislation; how we could bring pandemic surveillance into the modern age; and other topics.

One focus for policy improvement that cannot be excluded is about caring for the caregivers.[10] PSWs, for example, are the backbone of the care a home like PHM provides. Other chapters in this section propose some immediate policy improvements. PSWs should be trained properly and remunerated fairly. They should be offered full-time hours and secure contracts with benefits. There should be regulations, including limitations on the pattern of working in multiple facilities. Front line workers should never have to worry about whether they will have the right PPE to do their job safely.[11]

6. Donald P McNeill, Douglas A Morrison & Henri J M Nouwen, *Compassion: A Reflection on the Christian Life* (Garden City, New York: Image Books, 1983) at 4.
7. The Lancet, "COVID-19: Protecting Health-Care Workers" (2020) 395:10228 The Lancet 922.
8. Peter E Wu, Rima Styra & Wayne L Gold, "Mitigating the Psychological Effects of COVID-19 on Health Care Workers" (2020) 192:17 CMAJ E459.
9. James G Adams & Ron M Walls, "Supporting the Health Care Workforce During the COVID-19 Global Epidemic" (2020) 323:15 JAMA 1439.
10. Nathan Stall, "We Should Care More About Caregivers" (2019) 191:9 CMAJ E245.
11. Pat Armstrong et al, "Re-imagining Long-term Residential Care in the COVID-19

Despite the tragedy endured by PHM, this experience will leave the home stronger because of the resilience of its residents and the healing power of skilled, sensitive caregivers. Pandemic or not, we must never forget our duty to protect and support health workers who put themselves on the front line.

Crisis" (24 April 2020), online: *Canadian Centre for Policy Alternatives* <https://www.policyalternatives.ca/publications/reports/re-imagining-long-term-residential-care-covid-19-crisis>.

CHAPTER E-3

Occupational Health and Safety and COVID-19: Whose Rights Come First in a Pandemic?

Katherine Lippel*

Abstract

This chapter explores the occupational health and safety of Canadian workers during the COVID-19 pandemic. Analysis of information in the media shows that workers in various sectors, including health care, meat packing, warehousing, and other essential services, have contracted COVID-19 at work. Many were denied protections required by the occupational health and safety regulatory frameworks governing the prevention of occupational illness and disease. Benefits under workers' compensation legislation are theoretically available for those who contract the illness out of and in the course of their employment, but preliminary figures from Ontario and Quebec suggest that under-reporting of work-related COVID-19 is prevalent and that access to compensation is not provided in a timely manner to those affected. The chapter sheds light on violations of the right to personal protective equipment and on transmission of the virus attributable to extensive use of workers employed by temporary employment agencies. It finds that unions and professional associations have contributed to improvement of the effectiveness of OHS legislation by accessing the media and the courts. It also provides suggestions for policy going into the deconfinement period in order to ensure that the most vulnerable to COVID-19 are not forced to return to work against their will.

* Full Professor of Law in the Faculty of Law (Civil Law Section) at the University of Ottawa and Distinguished Research Chair in Occupational Health and Safety Law since March 2020.

Résumé
Santé et sécurité au travail et COVID-19 : quels droits sont prioritaires en cas de pandémie ?

Ce chapitre explore la santé et la sécurité au travail de la main-d'œuvre canadienne durant la pandémie de COVID-19. L'analyse des informations diffusées dans les médias montre que des travailleurs de divers secteurs, y compris les soins de santé, le conditionnement des viandes, l'entreposage et d'autres services essentiels, ont contracté la COVID-19 au travail. Plusieurs se sont vu refuser les mesures de protection exigées par les cadres réglementaires en matière de santé et sécurité au travail régissant la prévention des maladies professionnelles. Les indemnités pour accident de travail prévues par la loi sont théoriquement accessibles aux personnes qui contractent la maladie dans le cadre de leur emploi, mais les chiffres préliminaires de l'Ontario et du Québec suggèrent que la déclaration des cas de COVID-19 liés au travail est insuffisante et que les personnes concernées ne sont pas indemnisées en temps opportun. Ce chapitre fait la lumière sur les violations du droit à l'équipement de protection individuelle et sur la transmission du virus attribuable à l'utilisation massive de personnel employé par des agences de travail temporaire. On constate que les syndicats et les associations professionnelles ont contribué à améliorer l'efficacité de la législation en matière de santé et sécurité au travail en étant présents dans les médias et en ayant accès aux tribunaux. Ce chapitre propose également des politiques à adopter pendant la période de déconfinement afin de veiller à ce que les personnes les plus vulnérables à la COVID-19 ne soient pas contraintes de retourner au travail contre leur gré.

The health and safety of health care workers have been the focus of much media attention and for just cause. Worker deaths in both Ontario[1] and Quebec[2] are the most visible indicators of the dangerous working conditions prevailing in many health care settings.

1. Bryann Aguilar, "Fifth Ontario Personal Support Worker Dies After Contacting COVID-19", *CTV News* (7 May 2020), online: <https://toronto.ctvnews.ca/fifth-ontario-personal-support-worker-dies-after-contracting-covid-19-1.4930176>.
2. Améli Pineda & Guillaume Lepage, "Une autre préposée tombe au combat", *Le Devoir* (1 May 2020), online: <https://www.ledevoir.com/societe/sante/578006/covid-19-deces-d-une-troisieme-preposee-aux-beneficiaires>.

Yet thousands of workers in transport,[3] meat processing,[4] and warehouses[5] have fallen ill and hundreds have died from COVID-19 in Canada and the U.S. The Collegium Ramazzini, an international body of occupational physicians, published guidance materials that divide the most vulnerable workers in the pandemic into three categories: those at "very high risk," a category that includes those working in health care, transport, sales and cleaning; at "high risk," including those working in security, hotel and food services, and the cruise industry; and, finally, those at "significantly increased risk," including workers in meat packing, manufacturing, construction, and mining.[6]

To examine the regulatory protections governing health and safety, this chapter focuses on COVID-19 as an occupational health and safety (OHS) hazard, looking specifically at the hazard represented by the illness itself. The mental health consequences of working in the pandemic are huge, but beyond the scope of this chapter,[7]

3. Barbara Neis, Kerri Neil & Katherine Lippel, "Mobility in a Pandemic: Covid-19 and the Mobile Labour Force" (21 April 2020) On the Move Partnership Working Paper at 37, online: *On the Move* <https://www.onthemovepartnership.ca/>; Chris Fox, "Six Taxi and Limo Drivers Working Out of Toronto Pearson Airport Have Died of Covid-19", *CTV News* (6 May 2020 Chapter E-4020), online: <https://toronto.ctvnews.ca/six-taxi-and-limo-drivers-working-out-of-toronto-pearson-airport-have-died-of-covid-19-1.4927304>.
4. Joel Dryden & Sarah Rieger, "Inside the Slaughterhouse: North America's Largest Single Coronavirus Outbreak Started at this Alberta Meat-Packing Plant", CBC News (6 May 2020), online: <https://newsinteractives.cbc.ca/longform/cargill-covid19-outbreak>; Daphné Cameron, "Les leçons de Yamachiche", *La Presse* (1 May 2020), online: <https://www.lapresse.ca/covid-19/202004/30/01-5271642-les-lecons-de-yamachiche-.php>; Andrew Russell, "After Failing to Publicly Reveal Covid-19 Outbreak Ontario Meat Plant Now Has 24 confirmed Cases", *Global News* (6 May 2020), online: <https://globalnews.ca/news/6913049/coronavirus-ontario-meat-packing-plant/l>; Collin Harris, "Cargill Meat-Processing Plant South of Montreal Says 64 Workers Infected with COVID-19", *CBC News* (20 May 2020), online: <https://www.cbc.ca/news/canada/montreal/cargill-chambly-covid-19-shut-down-1.5563539>; Sarah Berger Richardson, this volume, Chapter E-5.
5. Sara Mojtehedzadeh, "Amazon Worker at GTA Warehouse Tests Positive for COVID-19", *The Star* (23 April 2020), online: <https://www.thestar.com/business/2020/04/23/amazon-worker-at-gta-warehouse-tests-positive-for-covid-19.html>; Joel Dryden, "Alberta Declares COVID-19 Outbreak at Amazon Warehouse Near Calgary", *CBC News* (1 May 2020), online: <https://www.cbc.ca/news/canada/calgary/calgary-amazon-covid-warehouse-outbreak-1.5553126>.
6. "Prevention of Work-Related Infection in the Covid-19 Pandemic" (5 May 2020), online: *The Collegium Ramazzini*, <http://www.collegiumramazzini.org/≥.
7. Ali Watkins et al, "Top E.R. Doctor Who Treated Virus Patients Dies by Suicide", *New York Times* (27 April 2020), online: <https://www.nytimes.com/2020/04/27/nyregion/new-york-city-doctor-suicide-coronavirus.html>.

as are the regulatory ramifications of indirect OHS issues that arise because of home-based work.[8] Aside from a small percentage of federally regulated industries, laws governing the prevention of occupational injuries and disease and workers' compensation fall under provincial jurisdiction[9]; here we focus primarily on Ontario and Quebec.

What Are the Relevant Regulatory Issues Relating to OHS in a Pandemic?

Protection of workers' health is governed by OHS legislation, while access to compensation for disability arising out of and in the course of employment is governed by workers' compensation. The federal government temporarily provides the Canada Emergency Response Benefit[10] which, as we shall see, is of relevance to the understanding of workers' options to protect their own health and that of their families during the pandemic.

OHS legislation throughout Canada provides that employers have a general duty to protect workers' health[11] and workers have the duty to protect their own health and that of others in the workplace (OHSQ, s. 49; OHSO, s. 28). The key foundation of Quebec legislation (OHSQ, s. 2) is the elimination of the hazard at source; workers have the right to information and training and the right to refuse hazardous work, and the employer is obliged to provide personal protective equipment (PPE) in the event that hazards cannot be eliminated at source. In Ontario, three basic health and safety rights include the right to know, the right to participate, and the right to refuse unsafe work.

Based on dozens of pages of information summarized in a Superior Court injunction,[12] a decision of the Ontario Labour Relations Board

8. Sylvie Montreuil & Katherine Lippel, "Telework and Occupational Health: Overview and Reflections Based on Empirical Research Conducted in Québec" (2003) 41 Safety Science 331.
9. Katherine Lippel, "The Future of Workplace Health and Safety Law in the Context of Globalisation" (2016) 47:2 Ottawa L Rev 535.
10. "Canada Emergency Response Benefit" (last visited 8 May 2020), online: *Government of Canada* <https://www.canada.ca/en/services/benefits/ei/cerb-application.html> [Government of Canada].
11. In Ontario, *Occupational Health and Safety Act*, RSO 1990, c O-1, [OHSO] s 25; in Quebec, *An Act Respecting Occupational Health and Safety*, RSQ c S-2.1, [OHSQ] s 51.
12. *Re Ontario Nurses' Association et al and Eatonville Care Centre Facility Inc et al*, 2020 ONSC 2647 [*Eatonville*].

(OLRB),[13] and an order rendered by an arbitrator,[14] since the outset of the pandemic, all of these rights have been violated in many workplaces. Workers are not provided with adequate protective equipment, they are not consistently informed of the hazards, and they are not told who among their colleagues or patients has COVID-19. OHS inspections in Ontario were the subject of a court order to ensure that inspections actually happened. The OLRB (paragraph 5) required that an inspector "shall physically attend the Respondents' workplaces to meet with the workplace parties and conduct inspections under the OHSA on a weekly basis for a two-month period." These judgments show that access to appropriate masks and gowns was denied to front line workers, and workers' rights to participate have been stymied by a lack of transparency, a finding acknowledged by the arbitrator's order to involve and inform joint health and safety committees on issues relating to COVID-19 in the respondent facilities in a decision rendered in expedited arbitration involving the Ontario Nurses Association and dozens of nursing homes. *The Star* quoted the president of the Ontario Public Service Employees' Union that represents Ministry inspectors as saying "inspectors are being told to send their reports and orders to lawyers and managers within the Ministry" and he added, "inspectors are telling us they can't do their jobs." The same article noted that across all occupational sectors, none of the over 200 work refusals had been upheld.[15]

***

In Quebec, while some work refusals have been upheld, there appears to have been little litigation, although dialogue between

13. Ontario Labour Relations Board, OLRB Case No: 0091-20-HS; 0092-20-HS; 0093-20-HS, decision rendered on April 24, 2020; Sara Mojtehedzadeh, "Ontario Labour Board Orders Weekly Safety Inspections at Three Nursing Homes After COVID-19 Deaths", *The Star* (24 April 2020), online: <https://www.thestar.com/news/canada/2020/04/24/ontario-labour-board-orders-weekly-safety-inspections-at-three-nursing-homes-after-covid-19-deaths.html?fbclid=IwAR2t7bAsDGvn3TK7clzSDm4107LAxxBm30q2JADAi5_tBDS7zXHSz8syc8A>.
14. *Participating Nursing Homes v Ontario Nurses' Association* (2020), online (pdf): *Hicks Morley* <https://hicksmorley.com/wp-content/uploads/2020/05/ONA-and-Participating-Homes-May-4-2020-Award.pdf>.
15. Sara Mojtehedzadeh, "Many Ontario Workers Are Trying to Refuse Work Due to COVID-19 Fears—But the Government Isn't Letting Them", *The Star* (27 April 2020), online: <https://www.thestar.com/business/2020/04/27/many-ontario-workers-are-trying-to-refuse-work-due-to-covid-19-fears-but-the-government-isnt-letting-them.html>.

unions and employers is reported to have continued in several sectoral associations legally empowered to provide OHS guidance applicable throughout their sectors (OHSQ, s. 101). Thousands of workers have fallen ill, leading to the closure of essential services such as abattoirs, and leaving residents of long-term care facilities without adequate care. A criminal inquiry is underway, in a case where 31 residents from the Herron private care home were found dead, some suspected to have died from lack of care.[16] It is reported that workers are being prevented from leaving the workplace at the end of their shifts.[17]

Workers' compensation legislation provides economic support for workers who are unable to work because of illness or injury. Funded by employers' premiums, legislation protects employers from lawsuits filed by their employees,[18] but also protects them from lawsuits filed by employees of others (AIAOD, s. 441; WSIA s. 28). To access benefits or to receive protection from lawsuits, the industrial sector of the workplace must have coverage under the *Act*. In Quebec, 93.17% of the workforce has coverage;[19] in Ontario, only industries explicitly mentioned in policy have coverage, 74.48%.[20] Significantly, public long-term care homes are mandatorily covered under WSIA, but coverage of private care homes is not mandatory.[21] This leaves many Ontario workers at the heart of the pandemic without workers' compensation and those employers vulnerable to lawsuits.

***

16. Morgan Lowrie, "Quebec Coroner to Investigate 31 Deaths at Seniors' Home in Montreal", *Global News* (12 April 2020), online: <https://globalnews.ca/news/6810089/quebec-coroner-to-investigate-31-deaths-at-seniors-home-in-montreal/>.
17. Angela MacKenzie & Adam Kovac, "Staff at Verdun Seniors' Residence Were Locked in to Prevent Them from Leaving", *CTV News* (14 April 2020), online: <https://montreal.ctvnews.ca/staff-at-verdun-seniors-residence-were-locked-in-to-prevent-them-from-leaving-1.4894875?cache=%3FclipId%3D89750>.
18. *An Act Respecting Industrial Accidents and Occupational Diseases*, RSQ c A-3.001, s 438; *Workplace Safety and Insurance Act 1997*, SO 1997, c 16, Sch A, s 26(2).
19. "Workers Compensation Legislation & Policy" (last visited 10 May 2020), online: Association of Workers' Compensation Boards <http://awcbc.org/?page_id=79>.
20. *Ibid.*
21. "Employer Classification Manual: 623310 Community Care Facilities for the Elderly" (last visited 12 May 2020), online: *Workplace Safety and Insurance Board* <https://safetycheck.onlineservices.wsib.on.ca/safetycheck/ecm/naics/623310?lang=en>.

Although compensation boards provide guidance online,[22] proving that COVID-19 was contracted at work is difficult in a pandemic. The Ontario Federation of Labour has asked for the creation of a presumption that will facilitate compensation;[23] WorkSafe BC is currently studying this option,[24] but nothing has been mentioned by the Ontario authorities to date and acceptance rates seem lower than those in Quebec, with only 513 accepted claims, 164 denied, and 2,807 pending as of May 11, 2020, statistics representing all sectors.[25] In Quebec, a key informant from a union in the health care sector reported that as of May 3, 2020, regarding compensation claims from that sector, 1,007 had been accepted, 15 had been denied, and 730 were pending. Yet she also shared that in just two of the 18 regional health care authorities there had been 1,562 cases of COVID-19, suggesting that underreporting was rampant. On April 23, the Premier reported that over 9,500 health care providers were absent, 4,000 because of a COVID-19 diagnosis; those absent because of mental health diagnoses were left unmentioned by the authorities when they requested that those not suffering from COVID-19 come back to work.[26]

Structural gaps become evident in a pandemic. Workers are at risk when getting to work by public transport, but injury occurring while the worker travels to work is not compensable in any Canadian jurisdiction.[27] Workers with health conditions found to increase the likelihood of dying from COVID-19 are not eligible for workers'

22. "Novel Coronavirus (COVID-19) Update" (last visited 10 May 2020), online: *Workplace Safety and Insurance Board* <https://www.wsib.ca/en/novel-coronavirus-covid-19-update> [Workplace Safety and Insurance Board 2020]; "Questions et réponses-COVID-19" (last visited 23 May 2020), online: *Commission des normes, de l'équité de la santé et de la sécurité du travail* <https://www.cnesst.gouv.qc.ca/salle-de-presse/covid-19/Pages/coronavirus.aspx?oft_id=3363899&oft_k=2UCJpvJj&oft_lk=IgNHUU&oft_d=637243765664600000#question-retour-malade>.
23. Sara Mojtehedzadeh, "Province Urged to Make Workers' Compensation Automatic for Essential Employees Diagnosed with COVID-19", *The Star* (6 April 2020), online: <https://www.thestar.com/news/canada/2020/04/06/province-urged-to-make-workers-compensation-automatic-for-essential-employees-diagnosed-with-covid-19.html>.
24. "WorkSafe BC Looking at Presumption for COVID-19 Claims" (30 April 2020), online: *WorkSafe BC* <https://www.worksafebc.com/en/about-us/news-events/news-releases/2020/April/worksafebc-looking-at-presumption-for-covid-19-claims>.
25. Workplace Safety and Insurance Board 2020, *supra* note 22.
26. Hugo Pilon-Larose, "9500 personnes absentes du réseau de la santé Québécois", *La Presse* (23 April 2020), online: <https://www.lapresse.ca/covid-19/202004/23/01-5270584-9500-personnes-absentes-du-reseau-de-la-sante-quebecois.php>.
27. Katherine Lippel & David Walters, "Regulating Health and Safety and Workers' Compensation in Canada for the Mobile Workforce: Now You See Them, Now

compensation unless they are actually ill. The federal Emergency Response Benefit can provide income if they stay at home because of the hazards involved in going to work, but if they quit their jobs they are not eligible,[28] and it is legally unclear whether they would remain eligible if they were fired for failing to return to work during the deconfinement period, despite verbal assurances from Minister Freeland.[29]

Stories from the Trenches

In both Ontario and Quebec it has become abundantly clear that adequate supplies of PPE, including appropriate respiratory protections and gowns, were not available.[30] Although priority was given to the acute care hospitals in Quebec, supplies were insufficient and sometimes obsolete,[31] and workers in long-term care facilities were denied supplies,[32] which, if available, were sometimes kept under lock and key.[33] Workers and residents paid the price.[34] By mid-April, so many workers were absent in the health care sector that Quebec officials, empowered by a decree that overrode collective agreements,[35] ordered

---

You Don't" (2019) 29:3 New Solutions: A J Occupational & Environmental Health Policy 317.

28. Government of Canada, *supra* note 10.
29. Mark Gollom, "Anxious About COVID-19 and Returning to Work? Here's What You Need to Know", *CBC News* (6 May 2020), online: <https://www.cbc.ca/news/business/work-return-coronavirus-employers-employees-1.5555593>.
30. Nicolas Bérubé, "Manque de masques: des médecins lancent un cri d'alarme aux entreprises", *La Presse* (26 March 2020), online: <https://www.lapresse.ca/covid-19/202003/26/01-5266541-manque-de-masques-des-medecins-lancent-un-cri-dalarme-aux-entreprises.php>.
31. Thomas Gerbet, "Des masques périmés depuis 11 ans qui craquent sur le visage des infirmières", *Ici Radio Canada* (28 April 2020), online: <https://ici.radio-canada.ca/nouvelle/1697940/masques-perimes-covid-n95-elastique-hopital-lakeshore>.
32. Patrick Lagacé, "Chronique Covid-19 : Les vieux, les malades les plus contagieux", *La Presse+* (23 April 2020), online: <https://www.lapresse.ca/covid-19/202004/22/01-5270512-les-vieux-les-malades-les-plus-contagieux.php>; Isabelle Hachey, "Cinq jours en zone rouge", *La Presse* (3 May 2020), online: <https://www.lapresse.ca/covid-19/202005/02/01-5271901-cinq-jours-en-zone-rouge.php>.
33. Patrick Martin et al, "De la reconnaissance dans les soins", *Le Devoir* (24 April 2020), online: <https://www.ledevoir.com/opinion/idees/577628/de-la-reconnaissance-dans-les-soins>.
34. Alexis Riopel, "Une hécatombe hors norme dans les CHSLD du Québec", *Le Devoir* (25 April 2020), online: <https://www.ledevoir.com/societe/577716/une-hecatombe-hors-norme>.
35. Gouvernement du Québec, *L'arrêté numéro 2020-007 de la ministre de la Santé et des Services sociaux en date du 21 mars 2020* (Québec: Gouvernement du Québec, 21 March 2020).

social workers and speech therapists, after two hours training, to work in seniors' homes where COVID-19 was raging. If they refused, they were threatened with dismissal.[36] Workers who accepted jobs in the hot spots were often the most vulnerable; unsurprisingly, the community spread is greatest in the poorest neighbourhoods, where precarious migrants are recruited as personal support workers (PSWs), often by temporary employment agencies (TEAs), to work in long-term care facilities where COVID-19 is rampant.[37]

Who Gets the Equipment When There Isn't Enough to Go Around?

We hear of workplaces where supervisors[38] or doctors[39] wear the protective equipment to which the nurses and PSWs don't have access, although they are the ones in closest proximity to the residents suffering from COVID-19. Evidence provided in the Eatonville injunction proceedings showed that N-95 respirators were kept under lock and key and that employers refused to rely on nurses' professional judgment as to the need for equipment, forcing them to comply with complex procedures to obtain permission to access a mask, a process that precluded effective access in a timely manner.

The day after a clear statement was issued by Quebec professional associations representing doctors, nurses, respiratory therapists, and nurses' aides, demonstrating that they were not legally obliged to care for a patient suffering from COVID-19 without the

36. Kate McKenna, "Montreal Speech Therapists, Social Workers Threatened with Firing if They Refuse to Work in Seniors' Homes", *CBC News* (25 April 2020), online: <https://www.cbc.ca/news/canada/montreal/physios-social-workers-redeployed-montreal-1.5545292>.
37. Émilie Dubreuil & Romain Schué, "Covid-19: 'C'est un peu hors de contrôle' à Montréal-Nord", *Radio Canada: Ici Grand Montréal* (28 April 2020), online: <https://ici.radio-canada.ca/nouvelle/1698270/coronavirus-cas-montreal-nord-quebec-covid-tests>; Agnès Gruda, "Préposées aux bénéficiaires : la filière Roxham", *La Presse* (2 May 2020), online: <https://www.lapresse.ca/debats/editoriaux/202005/01/01-5271799-preposees-aux-beneficiaires-la-filiere-roxham.php>.
38. Sara Mojtehedzadeh, "'Frontline Workers Do Not Have N95s but Supervisors are Wearing Them': Troubling Allegations Emerge at Care Homes Hit by COVID-19", *The Star* (22 April 2020), online: <https://www.thestar.com/business/2020/04/22/frontline-workers-do-not-have-n95s-but-supervisors-are-wearing-them-labour-board-documents-allege-shortages-exhaustion-and-fear-amongst-nursing-home-staff.html>.
39. Hachey, *supra* note 32.

necessary PPE,[40] it was reported that ambulance technicians and first responders were targeted by a new directive of the Ministry of Health and Social Services to the effect that it was no longer necessary for them to wear an N95 respirator when dealing with a patient diagnosed with COVID-19: unless the patient had "serious respiratory problems" and required procedures such as intubation, a simple surgical mask, gloves, and a gown were henceforth deemed to be sufficient.[41] Their union alerted the press, as is the case in most of the articles shedding light on working conditions during the pandemic.

Agencies and Subcontracting

TEAs supply workers to multiple client employers and, when workers are potentially sent to different facilities every day, this may contribute to the spread of the virus between institutions. Analysis of a major outbreak in a meat-packing plant in Quebec led public health officials to suspect that the regular workforce was first contaminated by one of the workers bused in by a TEA, although they admitted that it was difficult to trace contacts of employees of agencies because they return to their communities in another region and sometimes don't speak French, which makes tracking more difficult.[42] A TEA employee was found to be the source of a cluster of cases in a long-term care facility in Quebec City[43]; another, who was placed by his agency in a long-term care facility on weekends as a PSW, was the fifth front-line health care worker to die of COVID-19.[44] TEAs have been under scrutiny by the Ministry of Health in Quebec for price gouging.[45]

40. Janie Gosselin, "Les soignants pas tenus d'intervenir sans matériel de protection, disent différents ordres", *La Presse* (23 April 2020), online: <https://www.lapresse.ca/covid-19/202004/23/01-5270639-les-soignants-pas-tenus-dintervenir-sans-materiel-de-protection-disent-differents-ordres.php>.
41. Ariane Lacoursière, "Les ambulanciers inquiets par une nouvelle directive sur les masques N95", *La Press* (24 April 2020), online: <https://www.lapresse.ca/covid-19/202004/23/01-5270688-les-ambulanciers-inquiets-par-une-nouvelle-directive-sur-les-masques-n95.php>.
42. Cameron, *supra* note 4.
43. Louis Gagné, "Un employé externe infecte six personnes dans une résidence pour aînés de Québec", *Radio Canada* (1 May 2020), online: <https://ici.radio-canada.ca/nouvelle/1698967/employe-agence-externe-infecte-covid-19-manoir-cours-atrium-residence-aines-quebec>.
44. Yves Boisvert, "Il s'appelait Marcelin François", *La Presse* (8 May 2020), online: <https://www.lapresse.ca/covid-19/202005/07/01-5272693-il-sappelait-marcelin-francois.php>.
45. Tommy Chouinard, "Agences de placement : des pratiques abusives inquiètent Québec", *La Presse* (24 April 2020), online: <https://www.lapresse.ca/covid-

Denounced by the Premier during a daily briefing for charging $50 an hour for a PSW and $90 for a nurse, a spokesperson for the TEA industry said it was Quebec's fault for agreeing to pay these amounts in their tenders deployed during COVID-19, which led to a ministerial response.[46] Faced with mounting evidence of the transmission attributable to the use of TEA workers, it is surprising to see the *Conseil du Patronat*, the Quebec organization representing corporate employers, promote increased flexibility to facilitate their use by recommending a two-year suspension of the recently adopted provisions in the *Labour Standards Act* designed to improve the working conditions of workers recruited by these agencies.[47] The difficulties inherent to the application of OHS protections in situations involving TEAs had been well documented in Quebec[48] and Ontario[49] prior to COVID-19.

In summary, thousands of people across Canada working in multiple sectors have contracted COVID-19 because of their work; many have been seriously ill, several have died. In theory the legal frameworks governing OHS should have protected them. Despite lessons learned from the SARS epidemic, which included recommendations requiring that sufficient protective equipment for health care workers be available at all times,[50] and as shown by Pat Armstrong,

---

19/202004/24/01-5270723-agences-de-placement-des-pratiques-abusives-inquietent-quebec.php>.

46. Jean-Nicolas Blanchet, "Québec blâmé pour les tarifs abusifs des agences de placement", *Le Journal de Québec* (26 April 2020), online: <https://www.journaldequebec.com/2020/04/26/quebec-blame-pour-les-tarifs-abusifs-des-agences-de-placement>; Tommy Chouinard, "Québec serre la vis aux agences de placement", *La Presse* (19 May 2020), online: <https://www.lapresse.ca/covid-19/202005/19/01-5274108-quebec-serre-la-vis-aux-agences-de-placement.php>.

47. "Feuille de route pour une relance économique sécuritaire et durable" (20 April 2020) at 21, online (pdf): *Conseil du Patronat du Québec* <https://conseiltaq.com/wp-content/uploads/2020/04/feuille_de_route_pour_une_relance_economique2020.pdf>.

48. Direction régionale de santé publique, *Invisible Workers: Health Risks for Temporary Agency Workers: 2016 Report of the Director of Public Health for Montreal, Québec* (Montréal: Direction régionale de santé publique, 2016), online (pdf): *Santé Montréal* <https://santemontreal.qc.ca/fileadmin/fichiers/professionnels/DRSP/Directeur/Rapports/Rap_Travailleurs_Invisibles_2016_ANG.pdf>.

49. Katherine Lippel et al, "Legal Protections Governing Occupational Health and Safety and Workers' Compensation of Temporary Employment Agency Workers in Canada: Reflections on Regulatory Effectiveness" (2011) 9:2 Policy & Practice in Health & Safety 69; Ellen MacEachen et al, "Workers' Compensation, Experience—Rating Rules and the Danger to Workers' Safety in the Temporary Work Sector" (2012) 10:1 Policy & Practice in Health & Safety 77.

50. Marieke Walsh, "Canada Cut Number of Stockpile Storage Locations for Critical Medical Supplies by One Third in Past Two Years", *The Globe and Mail*

Hugh Armstrong and Ivy Bourgeault in Chapter E-1 of this book, lean management practices have led to insufficient supplies of protective equipment, and insufficient staffing levels, in health care institutions that now rely on an increasingly precarious labour force that often moves between multiple workplaces, putting workers and patients at risk.

Conclusion: What Does the Situation Say About Regulatory Effectiveness?

OHS legislation exists throughout Canada requiring employers to ensure that workers are not exposed to hazardous situations that can lead to injury or death because of their work. The precautionary principle that provides that prevention measures be put in place when scientific uncertainty prevails is intrinsic to OHS law.[51] The violations described in this chapter go beyond failure to apply the precautionary principle: Evidence is abundant that workers were and are endangered because they are exposed to obvious hazards with insufficient protective equipment and with inadequate effort to eliminate the hazards at source. This is a clear demonstration of regulatory failure. Others, including residents of long-term care facilities and their survivors, have also been disproportionately affected by these breakdowns, and several have launched class action suits against the facilities that failed to provide adequate care;[52] those workers who are covered by workers' compensation can't sue their employers, so there is no potential economic incentive that lawsuits could provide with regard to Quebec workers and those working in publicly funded long-term care facilities in Ontario. Even in the private facilities in Ontario that do not have coverage, it is unlikely that workers would choose to sue their employers, as this would bring an end to their employment; in addition, civil remedies would be costly and beyond the means of most employees of long-term care facilities. Recourse for family members who contract the illness from workers is unclear.

(22 April 2020), online: <https://www.theglobeandmail.com/politics/article-canada-cut-number-of-stockpile-storage-locations-for-critical-medical/>.

51. *Bombardier Aéronautique Inc* v *TAT,* 2017 QCCS 5488, confirmed in results in *Bombardier Aéronautique* v *CNESST,* 2020 QCCA 315.

52. Mark Gollom, "Flood of COVID-19 Related Lawsuits Expected to Hit Courts", *CBC News* (8 May 2020), online: *<https://www.cbc.ca/news/coronavirus-lawsuits-insurance-nursing-homes-1.5559520>.*

Whose rights come first in a pandemic? Without media reports, employers would have the last word, and the public would know nothing of current conditions; those reports are in large part dependent on information provided by unions, and it is unions that have taken legal action to access enforcement measures. Professional associations have also made clear statements requiring that their members have access to protective equipment. And then there are the others, more precarious workers whose stories may become public if they die.

In reaction to the *ONA* v. *Eatonville* court order [paragraph 96], to "provide nurses [...] with access to fitted N95 facial respirators and other appropriate PPE when assessed by a nurse at point of care to be appropriate and required," Eric Tucker asked, "In what world is a court order needed to require employers to provide front line health care workers with the personal protective equipment that they, in their professional judgment, relying on best practices and government directives, determine is needed to perform their jobs safely?"[53] I ask here, in such a world, what rights are needed to protect workers as we head into a period of deconfinement?

Public health authorities acknowledge the emerging scientific consensus that people with certain characteristics (including age and various chronic health problems[54]) are more likely to have serious adverse consequences if they contract COVID-19. If workers refuse to return to their employment because they or their family members are disproportionately vulnerable, it is currently highly uncertain whether they will be legally protected from job loss and economic deprivation. Ensuring their right to refuse to go back, if to do so puts them at serious risk, is a priority.[55] It is unlikely that employers will be in a posi-

53. Eric Tucker, "Court Orders Should Not be Required For Health Care Workers to Get PPEs", *The Star* (30 April 2020), online: <https://www.thestar.com/opinion/contributors/2020/04/30/court-orders-should-not-be-required-for-health-care-workers-to-get-ppes.html>.

54. Institut national de santé publique du Québec, *COVID-19: Recommandations intérimaires pour la protection des travailleurs avec maladies chroniques* (Québec: Institut national de santé publique du Québec, 10 May 2020), online: *INSPQ* <https://www.inspq.qc.ca/publications/2967-protection-travailleurs-maladies-chroniques-covid-19>; Institut national d'excellence de santé et en service sociaux, *COVID-19 et personnes immunosupprimées, Québec* (Québec: Institut national d'excellence de santé et en service sociaux, last visited 26 May 2020), online: *INESS* <https://www.inesss.qc.ca/covid-19/presentations-cliniques/personnes-immunosupprimees-mise-a-jour-completee-07-05-2020.html>.

55. Janet Cleveland et al, "Il faut protéger les plus vulnérables", *Le Devoir* (6 May 2020), online: <https://www.ledevoir.com/opinion/idees/578337/il-faut-proteger-les-plus-vulnerables>.

tion to assume the costs associated with better protections than those currently available, but collectively, as was done in response to needs created by the ice storm of 1998,[56] we should adopt measures that provide enforceable options for workers in a world that has been shown to have failed to protect workers' basic rights to health and safety in Canada, which is among the wealthiest countries in the world.

56. *An Act to Establish a Fund in Respect of the Ice Storm of 5 to 9 January 1998*, SQ 1998, c 9.

CHAPTER E-4

Risking It All: Providing Patient Care and Whistleblowing During a Pandemic

Vanessa Gruben* and Louise Bélanger-Hardy**

Abstract

In this chapter, we discuss the rights and responsibilities of health care workers during the COVID-19 pandemic, both as care providers (part I) and as whistleblowers (part II). Health care providers have a duty to provide care to patients during a pandemic. However, this duty may be limited by the type of practice, the implied consent to risks, the strength of competing duties such as family obligations, and the need to weigh benefits to patients and potential harm to caregivers. The duty to care of regulated health professionals such as doctors and nurses is framed by the standards of their respective professions. In contrast, personal care workers (PSWs) are not self-regulated. This group forms a large part of the workforce in long-term care homes where most deaths have occurred. We believe it may be time to consider whether PSWs should be self-regulating, as this could offer both greater clarity about the standard of care to be provided to patients during pandemics and clear disclosure standards to guide those who wish to denounce the practices they witness. As for health care

* Vice-Dean of the English Common Law Program and Associate Professor and a member of the Centre for Health Law, Policy and Ethics at the University of Ottawa.

** Full Professor in the Faculty of Law, University of Ottawa, where she has been Vice-Dean (1996–1999, 2013–2014, and 2020) and a member of the Centre for Health Law, Policy and Ethics at the University of Ottawa.

providers as whistleblowers, after noting that whistleblower protection across Canada is piecemeal at best, we recommend a comprehensive approach where statutory instruments would be complemented by professional guidelines and codes of ethics issued by regulatory bodies and by professional associations.

Résumé

Risquer gros : soigner et dénoncer en temps de pandémie

Dans ce chapitre, nous abordons les droits et les responsabilités des professionnels de la santé pendant la pandémie de COVID-19, à la fois en tant que prestataires de soins (partie I) et en tant que lanceurs d'alerte (partie II). Les prestataires de soins de santé ont le devoir de fournir des soins aux patients durant une pandémie. Toutefois, ce devoir peut être limité par le type de pratique, le consentement tacite face aux risques, la force des devoirs concurrents comme les obligations familiales, et la nécessité de soupeser les avantages pour les patients et les dangers potentiels pour les soignants. L'obligation de soigner des membres d'une profession de la santé réglementée, comme les médecins et les infirmières, est encadrée par les normes de leurs professions respectives. En revanche, les préposés aux soins personnels ne sont pas soumis à une autorégulation. Ce groupe représente une grande partie de la main-d'œuvre dans les établissements de soins de longue durée où la plupart des décès sont survenus. Nous estimons que le temps est peut-être venu d'examiner la possibilité de réglementer le travail des préposés aux soins personnels, puisque cela permettrait à la fois de clarifier les normes de soins à fournir aux patients en situation de pandémie et d'établir des normes de divulgation claires pour orienter les personnes qui souhaitent dénoncer les pratiques dont elles sont témoins. Quant aux prestataires de soins de santé qui veulent sonner l'alarme, après avoir constaté que la protection des lanceurs d'alerte au Canada est au mieux fragmentaire, nous recommandons une approche exhaustive dans laquelle les textes réglementaires seront assortis de directives professionnelles et de codes de déontologie émis par des organismes de réglementation et des associations professionnelles.

Thousands of health care providers around the world are working tirelessly on the front lines of the COVID-19 crisis. Their critical roles as care providers and as whistleblowers have dominated news headlines. Health care workers are being called upon to care for infected patients, to work outside their usual specialties,[1] and to make difficult decisions about patient care.[2] Many are placing their health and lives at risk to combat this pandemic. Health care workers make up nearly 16% of Ontario's COVID-19 cases.[3] Many of them have also played critical roles as whistleblowers—raising the alarm to the rapid spread of the virus and identifying unethical and illegal responses to the pandemic.

In this chapter, we briefly address the dual roles health care workers have played during the COVID-19 crisis. In the first part, we address the rights and responsibilities of health care providers who are on the front lines caring for patients. We also discuss the responsibilities that health care employers and governments owe to our health care providers. In the second part, we highlight the critical role these workers have played as whistleblowers during the pandemic and advocate for stronger whistleblower protection.

Ensuring Safe and High-Quality Patient Care

The Rights and Responsibilities of Health Care Providers to Provide Care

Health care providers are a diverse group and include a wide range of workers, including nurses, technicians, personal support workers (PSWs), and physicians. These workers differ in many ways. For example, they may be categorized as unionized or non-unionized; employees or independent contractors; full-time, part-time, or casual employees; and they may be members of a regulated health care profession or not.

1. Melanie Grayce West, "New York City Hospitals Face New Strain: Not Enough Workers", *The Wall Street Journal* (24 March 2020), online: <https://www.wsj.com/articles/new-york-city-hospitals-face-new-strain-not-enough-workers-11585059601>.
2. Peter Walker, "London Covid-19 Doctor Says Soon Staff Will Be Forced to Choose Whose Life to Save", *The Guardian* (23 March 2020), online: <https://www.theguardian.com/world/2020/mar/23/london-covid-19-doctor-staff-choose-whose-life-to-save>.
3. OCHU CUPE, "Ontario Health Care Worker Infections Jump 43.5 per cent in 8 days, COVID-19 Protections, Transmission Advice Inadequate: CUPE Media Release" (6 May 2020), online: *OCHU CUPE* <https://ochu.on.ca/2020/05/06/ontario-health-care-worker-infections-jump-43-5-per-cent-in-8-days-covid-19-protections-transmission-advice-inadequate-cupe/>.

Despite their differences, they face many similar challenges. Must a health care worker who is not trained to treat respiratory infections provide care to patients suffering from COVID-19? May health care providers be redeployed elsewhere when there is a shortage of staff? Are health care providers obliged to work in environments they perceive as threatening to their own health? It is important to acknowledge that health care providers often have competing interests and obligations to family members and others that could influence their decision-making at work.[4]

In this chapter, we compare the rights and responsibilities of health care workers who are members of a regulated health profession and those who do not enjoy this same status.

Regulated Health Care Providers[5]

In Canada, regulated health care providers are subject to specific education and registration requirements, as well as disciplinary and oversight processes, by their regulatory colleges. It is well established that they have a duty to care for patients during a pandemic. This duty is rooted in their professional and moral obligation to act in the best interests of their patients. Many professional policies[6] and codes of ethics[7] recognize a duty to care for patients during a pandemic, but they acknowledge there are limits on this duty, including an entitlement to safe working conditions.

The scope of a regulated health care provider's duty of care depends on several factors.[8] For example, regulated health care providers who have chosen to work in high-risk settings, such as an

4. Yu-Tao Xiang et al, "Timely Mental Health Care for the 2019 Novel Coronavirus Outbreak is Urgently Needed" (2020) 7:3 The Lancet 228.
5. Part of this section is taken from: Vanessa Gruben & Alicia Czarnowski, "What Can We Expect From Healthcare Workers Facing the Deadly Demands of COVID-19? What Can They Expect from Their Employers, Governments and Us?" *Policy Options* (1 April 2020), online: <https://policyoptions.irpp.org/magazines/april-2020/what-are-the-rights-and-responsibilities-of-healthcare-providers-in-a-pandemic/>.
6. CMA, "CMA Policy: Caring in a Crisis: The Ethical Obligations of Physicians and Society During a Pandemic" (2008), online: *CMA* <https://policybase.cma.ca/documents/policypdf/PD08-04.pdf>.
7. CNA, *Code of Ethics for Registered Nurses* (2017), online: *CNA* <https://www.cna-aiic.ca/~/media/cna/page-content/pdf-en/code-of-ethics-2017-edition-secure-interactive> [CNA, *Code of Ethics*].
8. Cara E Davies & Randi Zlotnik Shaul, "Physicians' Legal Duty of Care and Legal Right to Refuse to Work During a Pandemic" 182:2 CMAJ 167.

intensive care unit or emergency room, are considered to have greater obligations to provide patient care during pandemics than those who work in lower-risk settings, such as dermatology. This is because the former group is considered to be better trained to deal with these crises, and to have accepted a higher risk work environment.

Weighing the potential harm to a health care provider against the potential benefit to a patient is another important consideration.[9] Where the risk to the worker is low and the benefit to the patient is high, because the condition is quite treatable, the obligation increases. Conversely, where the risk to the worker is high and the benefit to the patient is low, the obligation to care for the patient decreases.

In addition to their obligation to provide care, regulated health care providers may also be called upon to make difficult decisions about who should receive care and who should not. In harder-hit jurisdictions, the number of COVID-19 patients needing ICU beds or ventilators have greatly exceeded the number of hospital resources. As a result, health care providers have been forced to make ethically and morally charged decisions about prioritizing patients with the best chance of survival.

Personal Support Workers

PSWs, who form the largest part of the health care workforce in Canada,[10] have been at the epicentre of some of the deadliest COVID-19 outbreaks in our country. Indeed, about 65% of PSWs work in long-term care (LTC), assisted living, and retirement homes[11] where, as is now well-known, the great majority of COVID-19 deaths have occurred.

Unlike nurses and physicians, PSWs are unregulated care providers who perform a range of duties that have traditionally included assistance with activities of daily living (ADL) and personal care. This role has evolved, however, and workers are increasingly asked to perform additional tasks, including controlled acts delegated by regulated health professionals.[12]

9. CNA, *Code of Ethics, supra* note 7 at 39.
10. Katherine Zagrodney & Mike Saks, "Personal Support Workers in Canada: The New Precariat?" (2017) 13:2 Healthcare Policy 31 at 32-33.
11. Christine Kelly, "Exploring Experiences of Personal Support Worker Education in Ontario, Canada" (2017) 25:4 Health and Social Care in the Community 1430 at 1431.
12. Arsalan Afza et al, "The Role of Unregulated Care Providers in Canada – A Scoping Review" (2018) 13:3 Int J Older People Nurs e12190 at 11; see for example: *Regulated Health Professions Act, 1991*, SO 1991, c 18, s 29(1)(e).

Because PSWs are unregulated, they have no legally defined scope of practice, no mandatory educational qualifications, no professional misconduct regulations or discipline process.[13] While the absence of an overarching regulatory framework outlining standards of practice makes it challenging to delineate precisely the nature of the workers' rights and obligations, it does not mean they are not required to practise safely and competently, including in the context of a pandemic.

For example, when tasks are delegated, regulated health professionals have a duty to make sure that PSWs are competent to perform the procedure and that they understand the extent of their responsibilities.[14] As well, facilities and agencies who employ PSWs provide some oversight through guidelines and in-house practices.[15] Further, enhanced education standards provide PSWs with more skills and better training.[16] Finally, some associations have developed codes of ethics outlining values such as competence, integrity, and respect of dignity.[17]

There has been considerable debate about whether these piecemeal interventions to oversee PSWs' practice are sufficient. The COVID-19 crisis has shone a light on existing problems, especially in the LTC context. There have been numerous reports of PSWs being denied the use of personal protective equipment (PPE) and having to work very long hours in extraordinarily stressful conditions. Because wages are low, many workers have been forced to work in multiple locations in order to make a decent living, thus increasing the risk of spreading the virus. By contrast, some front line staff have refused to work, leaving LTC residents to their own devices, often with catastrophic consequences.[18]

13. *Ibid* at 3.
14. See for example: CNO, *Practice Guideline: Working with Unregulated Healthcare Providers* (2013) at 3.
15. See for example: Saint Elizabeth, *A Practical Guide to Implementing Person-Centred Care Education for PSWs in the Home, Community and Long-Term Care Sectors* (October 2013), online: *Saint Elizabeth* <https://www.saintelizabeth.com/getmedia/3b053be0-3313-45e5-8aea-872781c0b76d/Practical-Guide-for-Implementing-PCC-Education-for-PSWs-October-2013.pdf.aspx>.
16. See for example: Ontario Ministry of Colleges and Universities, "Personal Support Worker Program Standard" (last visited 14 May 2020), online: *Ontario Ministry of Colleges and Universities* <http://www.tcu.gov.on.ca/pepg/audiences/colleges/progstan/health/supwork.html>.
17. See for example: The Ontario Personal Support Workers Association, *OPSWA's Code of Ethics* (last visited 14 May 2020), online: *OPSWA* <https://www.ontariopswassociation.com/code-of-ethics>.
18. Katie Pedersen & Melissa Mancini, "Ontario's long-term care workers still working at multiple facilities as B.C. clamps down", *CBC News* (8 April 2020), online: <https://www.cbc.ca/news/health/nursing-home-workers-1.5526076>

Do these problems warrant a second look at self-regulation for PSWs? The matter was last considered in 2006 by the Health Professions Regulatory Advisory Council (HPRAC). This body recommended against self-regulation for a number of reasons, including the absence of a defined body of knowledge for PSWs; the workers' apparent lack of widespread support for self-regulation; the vicarious liability of employers for acts of professional misconduct in the workplace; and the economic impact of regulation. Although there were efforts to form a PSW Register in Ontario, those attempts proved unsuccessful.[19]

In our view, a number of factors could justify reopening of this debate. First, more and more health care workers are self-regulated, including practitioners of traditional Chinese medicine and acupuncturists, naturopaths, and homeopaths. Second, as noted, the scope of practice of PSWs is expanding. Third, as Pat Armstrong, Hugh Armstrong and Ivy Bourgeault note in Chapter E-1 of this volume, the complexity of the care, especially in the LTC setting, is increasing. This points to a need to develop standards of care and a code of ethics that could guide PSWs.

We are mindful that self-regulation is not a panacea and there may be disincentives to this approach.[20] More generally, there are concerns about "bias, lack of transparency and regulatory capture" inherent in self-regulatory model.[21] But given the problems that have been exacerbated by the COVID-19 pandemic, we feel it is worth considering.

The Responsibilities of Health Care Employers

Governments and health care employers, such as hospitals, LTC facilities, and others, bear the responsibility to protect health care workers and to promote high quality and safe care.[22] This includes putting

---

19. Some years following the HPRAC report, in 2011 Ontario decided to create a PSW Registry, as exists in British Columbia and Nova Scotia. However, in Ontario, the registry was shut down in 2016: not all PSWs were registered and the information provided in the registry was unreliable.
20. Christine Kelly & Ivy Lynn Bourgeault, "The Personal Support Worker Program Standard in Ontario: An Alternative to Self-Regulation?" (2015) 11:2 Healthcare Policy 20 at 25.
21. Joanna Erdman, Vanessa Gruben & Erin Nelson, eds, *Canadian Health Law and Policy*, 5th ed (Toronto, LexisNexis Canada, 2017), chapter 6 at 172.
22. Katherine Lippel, this volume, Chapter E-3.

appropriate precautions in place for health care providers, regardless of their employment status and of whether they are members of a regulated health care profession. Throughout the pandemic, health care providers have repeatedly alleged that they do not have access to adequate PPE.[23] As well, some institutions did not have enough PPE, while others were stockpiling it.[24] Perhaps not surprisingly, there were many reports of health care workers who refused to work due to the unavailability of PPE.[25]

Governments and employers should also be prepared to put a range of other measures in place to protect those who are serving on the front lines. These measures include providing relevant, accessible, and up-to-date information to health care providers; creating stand-alone assessment and testing centres; introducing technologies that mitigate risks to health care providers, such as using telemedicine to assess and treat patients who are suffering from milder forms of the virus and to reduce the burden on the health care system; and ensuring that much-needed counselling and mental health supports are in place for health care providers.[26]

Promoting Disclosure of Important Health and Safety Risks

In addition to courageously providing care to patients, health care workers have raised the alarm about unsafe and illegal practices throughout the COVID-19 crisis. Whistleblowing plays an important role in protecting public health by ensuring timely investigation and appropriate response to a public health risk.

---

23. Ontario Nurses Association, "MEDIA STATEMENT: Health-Care Unions Call for Honest, Frank Collaboration from Ontario Government Regarding COVID-19 Protection for Health-Care Workers" (11 March 2020), online: *ONA* <https://www.ona.org/news-posts/20200311-covid19-joint-statement/>.
24. Andrew Russell, "At Least 2 Toronto Hospitals Begin Rationing Protective Gear as COVID-19 Crisis Deepens", *Global News* (25 March 2020), online: <https://globalnews.ca/news/6731507/coronavirus-ontario-hospitals-protective-gear-rationing-covid-19/>.
25. Tom Blackwell, "Canadian Nurses Treating COVID-19 Patients Cite Unsafe-Work Laws to Demand N95 Masks", *The National Post* (31 March 2020), online: <https://nationalpost.com/health/canadian-nurses-working-with-covid-19-patients-demand-legal-right-to-wear-n95-masks>.
26. The Lancet, "COVID-19: Protecting Health-Care Workers" (2020) 395:10228 The Lancet 922.

Health Care Providers as Whistleblowers

Many definitions of "whistleblowing" exist; we adopt Mannion and Davies' definition: "the disclosure to a person or public body, outside normal channels and management structures, of information concerning unsafe, unethical or illegal practices."[27] Throughout this pandemic many workers have provided vital information about the existence of the virus itself,[28] outbreaks at different facilities, and the failure of governments and institutions to adequately address the virus, for example, by failing to provide appropriate PPE.[29] Whistleblowers have been variably characterized as "heroes" and "snitches," despite criticisms of these polarizing characterizations.[30]

The decision to blow the whistle can have significant consequences. Most disturbing have been criminal penalties imposed by the state, including imprisonment and fines.[31] More commonly, we have witnessed a range of professional consequences, such as discipline or dismissal by the employer; disciplinary procedures for members of a regulated health profession; and retaliation by peers.[32] Health care providers may also suffer personal consequences, including physical and psychological harm.[33]

Whistleblowing by health care workers is not new. Most widely known in Canada are the health care workers who reported public

27. Russell Mannion & Huw TO Davies, "Cultures of Silence and Cultures of Voice: The Role of Whistleblowing in Healthcare Organisations" (2015) 4:8 Int J Health Policy Manag 503 at 503 [Mannion].
28. Ankita Rao, "Doctors Have Been Whistleblowers Throughout History. They've also Been Silenced", *The Guardian* (8 April 2020), online: <https://www.theguardian.com/education/2020/apr/08/coronavirus-doctors-whistleblowers-history-silenced> [Rao]; Hillary Leung, "'An Eternal Hero' Whistleblower Doctor Who Sounded Alarm on Coronavirus Dies in China", *Time* (7 February 2020), online: <https://time.com/5779678/li-wenliang-coronavirus-china-doctor-death/>.
29. Nicholas Kristof, "'I Do Fear for My Staff,' a Doctor Said. He Lost His Job", *The New York Times* (1 April 2020), online: <https://www.nytimes.com/2020/04/01/opinion/coronavirus-doctors-protective-equipment.html> [*Kristof*]; Avery Haines, "Whistleblower Says Workers at Nursing Homes Aren't Being Given Protective Gear", *CTV News* (31 March 2020), online: <https://www.ctvnews.ca/health/coronavirus/whistleblower-says-workers-at-nursing-homes-aren-t-being-given-protective-gear-1.4877005>.
30. Mannion, *supra* note 27 at 503-504; Marilou Gagnon & Amelie Perron, "Whistleblowing: A Concept Analysis" (2019) Nurs Health Sci 1 at 5-6 [*Gagnon*].
31. Rao, *supra* note 28.
32. Kristof, *supra* note 29.
33. Gagnon, *supra* note 30 at 6.

health risks during SARS,[34] the health care workers who blew the whistle on the Winnipeg Health Sciences Centre cardiac surgery program,[35] and Dr. Nancy Oliveri's disclosure, despite strong warnings from the manufacturer and others, of risks associated with the use of deferiprone to her patients.[36]

Not surprisingly, each of these incidents sparked calls for stronger whistleblowing protections.[37] Imposing effective regulations on employers and institutions fosters a workplace culture that promotes wider disclosure of risks to public health and patient safety.[38]

However, despite repeated calls for improvement, whistleblower protection across Canada is piecemeal at best.[39] Some provinces (for example, Ontario) have laws that protect whistleblowers, but their application is limited to certain types of activities or workers.[40] Most notable for broad protection is Manitoba, which enacted comprehensive legislation for health care workers following the Sinclair inquiry. The *Public Interest Disclosure (Whistleblower Protection) Act* and accompanying regulations protect health care workers who make a disclosure in good faith against reprisals.[41]

34. The SARS Commission, *SARS Commission Executive Summary* (Toronto: The SARS Commission, 2006) (Commissioner: The Honourable Justice Archie Campbell), online: *Archives of Ontario* <http://www.archives.gov.on.ca/en/e_records/sars/report/index.html> [Campbell]. The SARS Commission brought to light real fears of reprisals and retaliation among health care workers.
35. Justice Murray Sinclair, *The Report of the Manitoba Paediatric Cardiac Surgery Inquest* (Winnipeg: Provincial Court of Manitoba, 27 November 2000) [Sinclair].
36. Mariam Schuman, "The Drug Trial: Nancy Olivieri and the Scandal That Rocked the Hospital For Sick Children" (Toronto: Random House Canada, 2005).
37. Campbell, *supra* note 34; Sinclair, *supra* note 35; Jon Thompson, Patricia Baird & Jocelyn Downie, *Report of the Commission of Inquiry on the Case Involving Dr. Nancy Olivieri, the Hospital for Sick Children, the University of Toronto, and Apotex Inc.* (Ottawa: Canadian Association of University Teachers, 2001).
38. Aled Jones, "The Role of Employee Whistleblowing and Raising Concerns in an Organizational Learning Culture–Elusive and Laudable?" (2016) 5:1 Int J Health Policy Manag 67 at 67.
39. Miriam Shuman, "Medical Whistle-Blower Protection Lacking" 2008 CMAJ 178(12) 1529; Elise von Scheel, "'A Tissue Paper Shield': Expert Slams Canada's Lack of Protections for Whistleblowers", *CBC News* (16 November 2019), online: <https://www.cbc.ca/news/politics/whistleblower-trump-canada-laws-1.5360774>.
40. For example, in Ontario, the *Occupational Health and Safety Act*, RSO 1990, c O.1, s 50, includes whistleblower protection for workers who report on workplace safety as opposed to public health. See also: *Public Interest Disclosure (Whistleblower Protection) Act*, SA 2012, c P-39.5; *The Public Interest Disclosure Act*, SS 2011, c P-38.1.
41. CCSM c P217 [*Public Interest Disclosure (Whistleblower Protection) Act*]; *Public Interest Disclosure (Whistleblower Protection) Regulation*, Man Reg 64/2007.

Similarly, the policies, codes of ethics, and guidelines of regulatory colleges and professional associations vary widely. Only a few regulatory colleges have whistleblowing policies that impose consequences on members who engage in reprisals.[42] Certain professional associations have instilled a culture of support for whistleblowers in their codes of ethics.[43]

Stronger Protection for Whistleblowers

In our view, governments, regulatory bodies, professional associations, and health care institutions ought to support and encourage health care workers to disclose unsafe, unethical, and illegal practices and ought to address workers' fears and protect them against reprisals. Otherwise, health care workers will be discouraged from raising the alarm where they believe it is necessary to do so. Although a detailed analysis is beyond the scope of this chapter, there are advantages and disadvantages associated with the regulation-making by these various bodies.[44] For example, laws with strong enforcement provisions are often considered to be more effective than guidelines, which provide recommendations but do not enjoy the same level of enforceability.

We recommend a comprehensive framework to protect whistleblowers, one that includes statutory instruments, regulatory guidelines, and institutional policies. Statutory instruments should be complemented by professional guidelines and codes of ethics issued by regulatory bodies and professional associations. These instruments should address workers' need to balance disclosure with their responsibility to protect confidential patient information.[45] Professional guidelines and codes may be viewed with greater legitimacy by health care workers because they are created by individuals with expertise in their field. Indeed, this may lend further support to self-regulation

---

42. See for example: College of Dental Hygienists of Ontario, *Whistleblower Policy* (August 2017) [*CDHO Whistleblower Policy*].
43. For example, the CNA, *Code of Ethics*, *supra* note 7 at 16, provides that "[n]urses support a climate of trust that sponsors openness, encourages the act of questioning the status quo and supports those who speak out in good faith to address concerns (e.g. whistle-blowing). Nurses protect whistleblowers who have provided reasonable grounds for their concerns."
44. Joanna Erdman, Vanessa Gruben & Erin Nelson, eds, *Canadian Health Law and Policy*, 5th ed. (Toronto, LexisNexis Canada, 2017), chapter 6.
45. Gagnon, *supra* note 30 at 5.

for PSWs and the need to develop disclosure standards that could guide them. As is well known, a culture of open disclosure and a clear framework for whistleblowers will have a positive impact on some aspects of patient safety.[46] Finally, health care institutions must introduce processes for whistleblowing and should also create and foster a culture of disclosure.

The framework should include several features, many of which have been recommended by previous scholars and review bodies. First, a statute must apply to all health care workers, from physicians to cleaning staff, regardless of their employment status. Past inquiries have noted that concerns raised by nurses, as opposed to doctors, are not always treated with the "same respect or seriousness as those raised by doctors."[47] Second, these instruments must extend to all forms of reprisal, including threats of reprisal.[48] Third, these instruments should support disclosure by a health care worker in good faith. Fourth, the anonymity of a whistleblower must be protected where it is requested.[49] Fifth, there must be robust penalties where these provisions are breached.[50]

Conclusion

Health care workers have played two critical roles during the pandemic: as providers of patient care and as whistleblowers. The overwhelming majority of health care workers have discharged their duty to provide patients with care during the COVID-19 crisis. However,

46. Minsu Ock et al, "Frequency, Expected Effects, Obstacles, and Facilitators of Disclosure of Patient Safety Incidents: A Systematic Review" (2017) 50 J Prev Med Public Health 68.
47. Sinclair, *supra* note 325 chapter 10 at 1.
48. For example: under Manitoba's *Public Interest Disclosure (Whistleblower Protection) Act, supra* note 38, s 2: "reprisal" means any of the following measures taken against an employee because the employee has, in good faith, sought advice about making a disclosure, made a disclosure, or co-operated in an investigation under this *Act*:
(a) a disciplinary measure;
(b) a demotion;
(c) termination of employment;
(d) any measure that adversely affects his or her employment or working conditions;
(e) a threat to take any of the measures referred to in clauses (a) to (d)."
49. See for example: *CDHO Whistleblower Policy, supra* note 39 at 2; *Public Interest Disclosure (Whistleblower Protection) Act, supra* note 38, s 32.1(1).
50. *Public Interest Disclosure (Whistleblower Protection) Act, supra* note 38, s 33(4).

the duty to provide care to patients during a pandemic is not unlimited. Regulated health care professionals enjoy the benefit of seeking guidance from their professional bodies and associations regarding the scope of their duty. PSWs, by contrast, are unregulated health care providers. They have been impacted during the COVID-19 crisis because of the nature of their work in the LTC setting and the poor working conditions they have encountered. We believe it may be time to consider whether PSWs should be self-regulating, as this could offer greater clarity about the standard of care to be provided to patients during pandemics and otherwise. Given the significant risks health care workers face on the front lines, it has been deeply troubling to learn that governments and health care institutions have not always met their responsibilities to provide safe working conditions for health care workers.

Health care workers have also played a critical role as whistleblowers by disclosing unethical and illegal practices. Although this is not a new role, whistleblower protection for health care workers continues to be piecemeal at best. Given the importance of whistleblowing to patient safety and public health, we believe a comprehensive framework composed of legislation, professional guidance, and institutional processes is greatly needed.

CHAPTER E-5

Worked to the Bone: COVID-19, the Agrifood Labour Force, and the Need for More Compassionate Post-Pandemic Food Systems

Sarah Berger Richardson*

Abstract

The coronavirus pandemic has rendered visible the previously invisible labour that gets our food from farm to fork for minimal pay and at great personal risk to workers' health. From grocery clerks working on the front lines without protective equipment, to truckers denied entry to restrooms, to temporary foreign workers forced to sign liability release waivers, to disease transmission at meat processing facilities, the virus is revealing the frailties and the inequities of our food system. Although the coronavirus pandemic is unprecedented, the ways the global food supply chain has responded to the crisis were, in fact, predictable. For years, scientists and food policy experts have been warning that our food system is broken, and that policies geared towards efficiency and cheap food are exploitative of the agri-food labour force, the animals we raise and slaughter for food, and the ecosystems we inhabit. This chapter focuses on the impact of COVID-19 on labour, with particular emphasis on the meat processing industry. It also seeks to illustrate the interconnectedness of all actors across the supply chain and the need for greater compassion as we rebuild post-pandemic food systems.

* Assistant professor, Faculty of Law (Civil Law Section), University of Ottawa.
The author gratefully acknowledges the research assistance of Nicole Camacho.

Résumé

Travailler d'arrache-pied : la COVID-19, la main-d'œuvre agroalimentaire et la nécessité de disposer de systèmes alimentaires plus compatissants après la pandémie

La pandémie de COVID-19 a révélé le travail jusqu'alors invisible qui permet d'assurer le parcours de nos aliments de la ferme à la table, pour un salaire minime et en mettant en danger la santé des travailleurs. Des commis d'épicerie en première ligne sans équipement de protection aux camionneurs à qui l'on refuse l'accès aux toilettes, en passant par les travailleurs étrangers temporaires contraints de signer des décharges de responsabilité et la transmission de la maladie dans les usines de transformation de la viande, le virus a dévoilé les faiblesses et les inégalités de notre système alimentaire. Bien que la pandémie de COVID-19 soit sans précédent, la façon dont la chaîne d'approvisionnement alimentaire mondiale a réagi à la crise était en fait prévisible. Pendant des années, les scientifiques et les experts en politique alimentaire ont sonné l'alarme : notre système alimentaire est en péril et les politiques axées sur l'efficacité et les aliments pas chers exploitent la main-d'œuvre du secteur agroalimentaire, les animaux que nous élevons et abattons pour notre consommation ainsi que les écosystèmes que nous occupons. Ce chapitre aborde les conséquences de la COVID-19 sur le travail, en particulier dans l'industrie de la transformation de la viande. Il cherche aussi à illustrer l'interconnexion de tous les acteurs de la chaîne d'approvisionnement et la nécessité de faire preuve d'une plus grande compassion dans la reconstruction des systèmes alimentaires après la pandémie.

Over the past few months, the coronavirus pandemic has caused unprecedented disruptions across the global food supply chain. From food shortages to food dumping, COVID-19 is revealing the frailties of global food chains. We are now familiar with the images of empty shelves in grocery stores and the shortages of toilet paper, flour, yeast, eggs, and other staples. Confinement measures have changed consumption patterns, putting a strain on supermarkets' just-in-time inventory systems. Meanwhile, producers whose usual buyers were restaurants, hotels, schools, and other large institutions have struggled to redirect their products to retail markets. While farmers around the world are forced to leave crops to rot in the field and cull herds as both domestic and international markets collapse, the UN World Food Programme is warning that 130 million people will go hungry due to COVID-19.[1]

This chapter discusses the impact of the coronavirus on the agrifood labour force. Despite the industrialization of agricultural practices around the world, food production remains a labour-intensive industry. While public health directives instruct people to stay home to protect themselves and others from the virus, food production and distribution have been declared an essential service. Fears of food shortages have rendered visible the previously invisible labour that gets our food from farm to fork. These include, but are not limited to, the temporary foreign workers who harvest our crops, the employees at processing facilities who prepare and package our food, the truckers who transport it, the grocery store clerks who run the cash and stock shelves, and the couriers who deliver takeout meals.

Labour, Lockdowns, and Economic Lifelines

While people around the world bang on pots and applaud health care providers during the pandemic, employees in the agricultural sector are also being praised for their essential work ensuring that people have access to healthy and nutritious food. In recognition of the risks associated with frontline work, some grocery stores have been installing plexiglass screens and limiting store hours to protect their employees, and even raising salaries.[2] Protective measures and compensation are not, however, universal. In a powerful editorial published in *The Atlantic*, a grocery store clerk resists the label of "hero" that has been used to describe frontline workers in the food industry.[3] "Cashiers and shelf-stockers and delivery-truck drivers aren't heroes," she

1. World Food Programme, News Release, "WFP Chief Warns of Hunger Pandemic as COVID-19 Spreads (Statement to UN Security Council)" (21 April 2020), online: *World Food Programme* <https://www.wfp.org/news/wfp-chief-warns-hunger-pandemic-covid-19-spreads-statement-un-security-council>; David Yaffe-Bellany & Michael Corkery, "Dumped Milk, Smashed Eggs, Plowed Vegetables: Food Waste of the Pandemic", *New York Times* (11 April 2020), online: <https://www.nytimes.com/2020/04/11/business/coronavirus-destroying-food.html>.
2. Hayley Ryan, "4 Major Canadian Grocers Give Front-Line Workers a Raise During COVID-19 Pandemic", *CBC News* (23 March 2020), online: <cbc.ca/news/canada/nova-scotia/sobeys-grocery-loblaw-metro-wages-pay-raise-covid-19-1.5506935>.
3. Karleigh Frisbie Brogan, "Calling Me a Hero Only Makes You Feel Better", *The Atlantic* (18 April 2020), online: <theatlantic.com/ideas/archive/2020/04/i-work-grocery-store-dont-call-me-hero/610147/>.

writes, "[t]hey're victims."[4] With limited training and for minimal pay, grocery store clerks are quite literally putting their lives on the line so that we can put food on the table. Tragically, many workplace fatalities have been recorded.[5]

Inch by Inch, Row by Row: Exceptional Risks for Employees Working Elbow to Elbow

It should come as no surprise that meat processing facilities are at the epicentre of disease transmission in North America. Dangerous and exploitative working conditions are well documented in North American abattoirs, including injuries related to repetitive movements, holding awkward postures for extended periods, and working in extreme temperatures surrounded by fast-moving sharp instruments.[6] Despite strong union presence in abattoirs and advocacy for their members, many incidents go unreported due to the precarious immigration status of some workers, as well as language barriers, that discourage them from standing up for their rights on the job or seeking compensation if they are injured.[7]

With COVID-19, dangerous working conditions have become even worse. Employees work elbow-to-elbow on fast-moving assembly lines, making physical distancing difficult. Rather than acting swiftly to protect employees by slowing line speeds or halting operations

4. *Ibid.*
5. Abha Bhattarai, "'It Feels Like a War Zone': As More of Them Die, Grocery Workers Increasingly Fear Showing up at Work", *The Washington Post* (12 April 2020), online: <washingtonpost.com/business/2020/04/12/grocery-worker-fear-death-coronavirus/>.
6. Leonor Cedillo, Katherine Lippel & Delphine Nakache, "Factors Influencing the Health and Safety of Temporary Foreign Workers in Skilled and Low-Skilled Occupations in Canada" (2019) 29:3 New Solutions: A J Environmental & Occupational Health Policy at 422; Timothy Pachirat, *Every Twelve Seconds: Industrialized Slaughter and the Politics of Sight* (New Haven: Yale University Press, 2013) [*Pachirat*]; Jennifer Dillard, "A Slaughterhouse Nightmare: Psychological Harm Suffered by Slaughterhouse Employees and the Possibility of Redress through Legal Reform" (2008) 15:2 Geo J on Poverty L & Pol'y 391; Sally C Moyce & Marc Schenker, "Migrant Workers and Their Occupational Health and Safety" (2018) 39 Annual Rev Public Health at 351.
7. Pachirat, *supra* note 6; Verity Stevenson & Jaela Bernstien, "How a Haitian Asylum Seeker Was Swept Up in a Shadowy Industry of Temp Agency Work", *CBC News* (28 March 2018), online: <cbc.ca/news/canada/montreal/temp-worker-accident-1.4594744>; Grant Gerlock, "We Don't Know How Many Workers Are Injured At Slaughterhouses. Here's Why", *NPR* (25 May 2016), online: <npr.org/sections/thesalt/2016/05/25/479509221/we-dont-know-how-many-workers-are-injured-at-slaughterhouses-heres-why>.

altogether, many processing companies have been accused of ignoring physical distancing protocols, ramping up production, pressuring employees to return to work after they had contracted the disease, and even offering bonus compensation for not missing shifts.[8] As of May 18, it is estimated that at least 59 workers died and more than 14,000 workers have been infected or exposed to COVID-19 in U.S. meatpacking facilities.[9] In Canada, the numbers are between 1,500 and 2,200 for workplace infections, and 5 workplace fatalities have been reported.[10] The site of the largest single outbreak of the coronavirus in North America is a processing plant in High River, Alberta, where 949 employees tested positive for COVID-19 and 2 employees died.[11]

Working Hard or Hardly Working: Supply and Demand Disruptions for Migrant Workers

Moving up the supply chain, from grocery store clerks to employees at processing plants, the next place where COVID-19 is disrupting labour in the agri-food sector is on the field. Due to mobility restrictions on temporary foreign workers, there are concerns that crops will not be

---

8. See e.g. Joel Dryden & Sarah Rieger, "Inside the Slaughterhouse", *CBC News* (6 May 2020), online: <newsinteractives.cbc.ca/longform/cargill-covid19-outbreak>; Peter Waldman et al, "Cold, Crowded, Deadly: How U.S. Meat Plants Became a Virus Breeding Ground", *Bloomberg Businessweek* (7 May 2020), online: <bloomberg.com/news/features/2020-05-07/coronavirus-closes-meat-plants-threatens-food-supply?srnd=premium&sref=O7tM50w9>.
9. Leah Douglas, "Mapping Covid-19 in Meat and Food Processing Plants" (22 April 2020, updated 18 May 2020), online: *Food and Environment Reporting Network* <https://thefern.org/2020/04/mapping-covid-19-in-meat-and-food-processing-plants/>. See also "Trump Order to Re-Open 14 Meatpacking Plants Fails to Increase Coronavirus Testing and Safety Measures Needed to Protect Food Supply & Workers" (8 May 2020), online: *United Food and Commercial Workers Union* <ufcw.org/press/>.
10. Estimates from the United Food and Commercial Workers Union are more conservative than the numbers tracked by Factory Farm Collective, a civil society organization advocating for the elimination of animal agriculture. See "Help Protect Food Processing Workers! ACT NOW!" (8 May 2020), online: *United Food and Commercial Workers Canada* <ufcw.ca/index.php?option=com_content&view=article&id=32649:help-protect-food-processing-workers-act-now&catid=10162:directions-20-036&Itemid=2468&lang=en>; "COVID-19 Cases in Canadian Slaughterhouses and Meat Packing Plants" (9 May 2020, updated 14 May 2020), online: *Factory Farm Collective* <factoryfarmcollective.ca/covid-19/>.
11. See e.g. Kathryn Blaze Baum, Carrie Tait & Tavia Grant, "How Cargill Became the Site of Canada's Largest Single Outbreak of COVID-19", *The Globe and Mail* (2 May 2020), online: <theglobeandmail.com/business/article-how-cargill-became-the-site-of-canadas-largest-single-outbreak-of/>; Dryden & Rieger, *supra* note 8.

harvested. As with meat processing, picking fruits and vegetables is labour-intensive and farmers depend on migrant workers to do the work that locals will not. For example, Germany relies on 300,000 seasonal workers to harvest its white asparagus crops, many of whom are Romanian and were prevented from travelling abroad when Romania declared a state of emergency and implemented highly militarized lockdown measures.[12] The need for these seasonal workers was so great that Germany lobbied the Romanian government to temporarily lift lockdown measures so that farm workers could board chartered flights to pick their vegetables. Other countries have copied Germany's arrangement with Romania, including the U.K., which needed as many as 90,000 workers to harvest fruits and vegetables and was unable to recruit enough British workers despite a nation-wide appeal.[13]

Reliance on temporary foreign workers raises ethical questions. Migrant workers are frequently forced to live and work in unhygienic conditions that lack proper sanitation facilities; some have their passports taken away by employers, or are moved around at the whim of temporary employment agencies to remote locations with limited information about where they are going or what they are expected to do.[14] In the midst of the coronavirus pandemic, existing vulnerabilities may be heightened. For instance, the Jamaican government has been requiring migrant workers bound for Canadian farms to sign a liability release for any injuries or losses due to COVID-19.[15] Moreover,

12. Costi Rogozanu & Daniela Gabor, "Are Western Europe's Food Supplies Worth More than East European Workers' Health?", *The Guardian* (16 April 2020), online: <theguardian.com/world/commentisfree/2020/apr/16/western-europe-food-east-european-workers-coronavirus>.

13. Lisa O'Carroll, "Romanian Fruit Pickers Flown to UK Amid Crisis in Farming Sector", *The Guardian* (15 April 2020), online: <theguardian.com/world/2020/apr/15/romanian-fruit-pickers-flown-uk-crisis-farming-sector-coronavirus>.

14. See e.g. Sally C Moyce & Marc Schenker, "Migrant Workers and Their Occupational Health and Safety" (2018) 39 Annual Rev Public Health at 351; Gabriel Thomson, ed, *Chasing the Harvest: Migrant Workers in California Agriculture* (Brooklyn, NY: Verso, 2017); Bukola Salami, Salima Meharali & Azeez Salami, "The Health of Temporary Foreign Workers in Canada: A Scoping Review" (2016) 106:8 Can J Public Health e546; Sara Mojtehedzadeh, "A Study Urged Better Standards for Migrant Workers' Housing. Nothing Was Done. Now COVID-19 Has Struck", *The Star* (11 May 2020), online: <thestar.com/business/2020/05/11/a-study-urged-better-standards-for-migrant-workers-housing-nothing-was-done-now-covid-19-has-struck.html>.

15. Sara Mojtehedzadeh, "Migrant Farm Workers from Jamaica Are Being Forced to Sign COVID-19 Waivers", *The Star* (13 April 2020), online: <thestar.com/business/2020/04/13/migrant-farm-workers-fear-exposure-to-COVID-19.html>.

undocumented migrants may not seek medical help if they develop symptoms due to fears of deportation. In this respect, Portugal has demonstrated international leadership by setting up facilities for agricultural workers who need to be quarantined and granting temporary residence to immigrants and asylum seekers.[16]

Despite the challenges migrant workers face, they continue to seek employment abroad to support family members in low- to middle-income countries. It is troubling that one of the reasons Romania relaxed its lockdown measures for seasonal workers was due to the government's admission that there was no other income-support program available for them.[17] In 2019, estimates placed global remittances from the global migrant workforce at US$550 billion.[18] This year, however, lockdowns and border closures to non-residents mean that many temporary foreign workers have either been forced to return home or have been prevented from travelling to work. In some cases, industries that normally employ migrant workers, such as hospitality, food services, and construction, have shut down, thereby reducing demand. In the case of harvesting crops, the demand for labour is high, but travel restrictions and quarantine requirements create hurdles for getting workers to the field. The World Bank is projecting that global remittances will fall 20% in 2020.[19] In the United States, remittances will fall by US$6 billion, particularly impacting receiving households from Mexico and Central America.[20] In Nigeria, remittances, which make up 6% of the country's GDP, decreased by half in February.[21] Remittances are also expected to fall by 13% in the Philippines due to the crisis.[22]

16. European Commission, "COVID-19's Impact on Migrant Communities" (30 April 2020), online: *European Union Website on Integration* <ec.europa.eu/migrant-integration/news/covid-19s-impact-on-migrant-communities>.

17. Rogozanu & Gabor, *supra* note 12.

18. The World Bank, Press Release, 2020/175/SPJ, "World Bank Predicts Sharpest Decline of Remittances in Recent History" (22 April 2020), online: *The World Bank* <https://www.worldbank.org/en/news/press-release/2020/04/22/world-bank-predicts-sharpest-decline-of-remittances-in-recent-history>.

19. *Ibid.*

20. Manuel Orozco, "Migrants and the Impact of the COVID-19 Pandemic on Remittances" (18 March 2020), online: *Inter-American Dialogue* <https://www.thedialogue.org/wp-content/uploads/2020/03/Migration-remittances-and-the-impact-of-the-pandemic-3.pdf>.

21. "Covid Stops Many Migrants Sending Money Home", *The Economist* (16 April 2020), online: <https://www.economist.com/middle-east-and-africa/2020/04/16/covid-stops-many-migrants-sending-money-home>.

22. Phillip Inman, "World Bank Warns of Collapse in Money Sent Home by Migrant Workers", *The Guardian* (22 April 2020), online: <https://www.

For households that rely on remittances to put food on the table, a drop in income can be catastrophic. National lockdowns and physical distancing measures in the absence of government sponsored income-support programs mean that individuals have no way of seeking alternate sources of income to make up for lost wages abroad. Disruptions to the agri-food workforce are thus having multiple ripple effects across the world, including worsening a global food crisis.

A Need for Compassion in Post-Pandemic Food Systems

In April, the International Panel of Experts on Sustainable Food Systems on COVID-19 (IPES-Food), released a report with a series of recommendations to respond to the current food system crisis *and* to "turn the existing seeds of change into the foundation of a new food system."[23] What should a post-pandemic food system look like? Food system governance scholars argue that a just food system must be a democratic one.[24] It must also be a compassionate one.

Our shared humanity must be at the heart of our responses to COVID-19 and efforts to rebuild post-pandemic food systems. Here, we can look to the South African concept of Ubuntu for guidance. Nobel Peace Prize Winner and Archbishop Desmond Tutu describes Ubuntu as a philosophy of interdependence: "my humanity is caught up and is inextricably bound up in yours."[25] Tutu believed that Ubuntu could be a force to facilitate reconciliation in Apartheid and post-Apartheid South Africa. His message, that we can only survive together, is equally instructive for food system governance. We are

---

theguardian.com/global-development/2020/apr/22/world-bank-warns-of-collapse-in-money-sent-home-by-migrant-workers>; "How is COVID-19 Affecting Remittances Flows into Emerging Markets?" (30 April 2020), online: *Oxford Business Group* <https://oxfordbusinessgroup.com/news/how-covid-19-affecting-remittance-flows-emerging-markets>; Karl Lester M Yap & Siegfrid Alegado, "World Bank Forecasts Philippine Remittances to Drop 13% in 2020", *Bloomberg News Wire* (24 April 2020), online: <bnnbloomberg.ca/world-bank-forecasts-philippine-remittances-to-drop-13-in-2020-1.1426277>.

23. "COVID-19 and the Crisis in Food Systems: Symptoms, Causes, and Potential Solutions" (April 2020), online (pdf): *International Panel Experts on Sustainable Food Systems*<http://www.ipes-food.org/_img/upload/files/COVID-19_CommuniqueEN.pdf>.
24. See e.g. Ludivine Petetitin, "The COVID-19 Crisis: An Opportunity to Integrate Food Democracy into Post Pandemic Food Systems" [April 2020] European J Risk Regulation, DOI: https://doi.org/10.1017/err.2020.40.
25. Desmond Tutu, "Forward" in Dana Gluckstein, ed, *Dignity: In Honor of the Rights of Indigenous Peoples* (Brooklyn, NY: PowerHouse Books, 2010).

experiencing a unique moment in history, as consumers are forced to ask questions about where our food comes from, and to think about the people who harvest, process, transport, shelve, and deliver the food we eat. Our ability to put food on our plates is inextricably bound up in their well-being. Without compassion for workers, we expose them to occupational health and safety risks. This is literally biting the hand that feeds us.

SECTION F

GLOBAL HEALTH AND GOVERNANCE

CHAPTER F-1

"Flattening the Curve" Through COVID-19 Contagion Containment

Anis Chowdhury[*] and Jomo Kwame Sundaram[**]

Abstract

Limited, uneven, and possibly "inaccurate" tests make it impossible to know the true scale of COVID-19 infections in the global South. Nevertheless, given the grossly inadequate health systems, further undermined by neoliberal reforms, catastrophic consequences for developing countries are feared. "Flattening the curve" of new infections seeks to ensure national health systems can cope by rapidly augmenting needed capacities and capabilities. The many "known and unknown" unknowns about the pandemic, and its implications, complicate the challenges posed by the complex and very varied socio-economic conditions in most developing countries. Neglecting prompt and adequate precautionary measures due to complacency for a variety of reasons, many governments have belatedly tried to check contagion by strictly imposing extended "stay-in-shelter" "lockdowns." Success for these types of measures require full public involvement, through social mobilization, public understanding, and credible leadership, enhanced by transparency, information sharing,

* Adjunct Professor of Economics, Western Sydney University and University of New South Wales (Canberra campus); former Senior United Nations official (2008-2016).

** Senior advisor at the Khazanah Research Institute and Former economics professor until 2004; and Assistant Secretary General for Economic Development in the United Nations system (2005–2015).

wide consultation, progressive relief measures, and accountability. However, by acting early to test, trace, isolate, and treat the infected, a few authorities have avoided nationwide lockdowns. Preventive measures, such as safe physical distancing, masking facial orifices, and selective targeted quarantines, enjoy greater public acceptance and voluntary compliance with minimal draconian measures.

Résumé
COVID-19 : contrôler la contagion pour aplatir la courbe

Des tests limités, disparates et parfois inexacts nous empêchent de connaître l'ampleur réelle de la contamination à la COVID-19 dans les pays du Sud. Néanmoins, étant donné les systèmes de santé nettement inadéquats, encore minés par les réformes néolibérales, on redoute des conséquences catastrophiques pour les pays en développement. L'aplatissement de la courbe des nouvelles infections vise à faire en sorte que les systèmes de santé nationaux puissent tenir le coup en augmentant rapidement leurs capacités et leurs moyens. Les nombreuses variables, connues et inconnues, concernant la pandémie et ses répercussions s'ajoutent aux défis que posent les conditions socioéconomiques déjà complexes et très variées dans la plupart des pays en développement. De nombreux gouvernements, qui ont omis de prendre des mesures de précaution rapides et adéquates en raison d'une certaine complaisance due à divers facteurs, ont tenté, tardivement, d'enrayer la contagion en imposant un confinement strict prolongé. Pour que ce type de mesure soit couronné de succès, il faut que la population soit activement impliquée, par la mobilisation sociale, en s'assurant qu'elle comprend la situation et en lui offrant un leadership crédible, le tout renforcé par la transparence, le partage des informations, une vaste consultation, des mesures d'aide progressives et un système de responsabilisation. D'autres gouvernements, en intervenant rapidement pour tester, localiser, isoler et traiter les personnes infectées, ont su éviter un confinement à l'échelle nationale. Les mesures préventives, comme la distanciation physique, le port du masque et la mise en quarantaine sélective ciblée, sont mieux acceptées par le public et sont appliquées de façon volontaire, avec un minimum de mesures draconiennes.

Barely a month after China reported a novel coronavirus outbreak in the city of Wuhan at the end of 2019,[1] on January 30, the World Health Organization (WHO) designated the COVID-19 outbreak a "public health emergency of international concern" (PHEIC), raising the global risk of the outbreak to "very high," its highest alert level.[2] By declaring the outbreak a PHEIC as per International Health Regulations (IHR, 2005),[3] WHO thus emphasized the urgent need to coordinate international efforts to better investigate and understand COVID-19, to "minimize the threat in affected countries" and to reduce the risk of further international spread. WHO declared a "very high" risk assessment for China, and a "high" level globally. All countries were advised to "be ready to contain any introduction of the virus and its spread through active surveillance, early detection, isolation and case management, contact tracing, and prevention."

Early precautionary measures in much of the rest of China and East Asia, and in places such as Kerala state in Southwestern India, were largely successful in containing the spread of the epidemic, at least thus far. But most national authorities outside of East Asia did not take adequate early precautionary measures to contain the spread of the outbreak, typically by promoting safe "physical distancing," use of masks in public areas, and other measures to reduce the likelihood of infection.

1. On 31 Dec 2019, the Wuhan Municipal Health Commission reported a cluster of cases of pneumonia in Wuhan in Hubei Province. The next day, the WHO set up an Incident Management Support Team, putting the organization on an emergency footing to deal with the outbreak. On 12 January, China publicly shared the genetic sequence of COVID-19.
2. When a PHEIC is declared, the WHO Director-General issues temporary recommendations under the 2005 IHR, including obligations for countries to provide sufficient public health rationale and justification to WHO about any additional measures beyond what WHO recommends. This is critical to ensure the international response is evidence-based, measured, and balanced, so that unnecessary interference with travel and trade is avoided. The WHO also recommended that the global community should provide support to low- and middle-income countries to respond to the threat, and to facilitate their access to diagnostics, potential vaccines, and therapeutics. "2019-nCoV Outbreak is an Emergency of International Concern" (31 January 2020), online: *World Health Organization* <http://www.euro.who.int/en/health-topics/health-emergencies/international-health-regulations/news/news/2020/2/2019-ncov-outbreak-is-an-emergency-of-international-concern>.
3. "International Health Regulations" (2005), online (pdf): *World Health Organization* <https://apps.who.int/iris/bitstream/handle/10665/43883/9789241580410_eng.pdf?sequence=1>.

This review of developing country governance and responses tries to draw pragmatic lessons to address the COVID-19 pandemic. It notes the higher costs of not acting quickly, and the causes and implications of public health capacity vulnerabilities in developing countries. Some implications of the different policy responses in China, South Korea, Vietnam, Kerala, Argentina, and Brazil are highlighted.

Failure to Act Quickly

On January 30, there were 7,818 confirmed cases of human-to-human transmission, with the vast majority in China, and 82 cases in 18 countries outside China. But when the WHO declared COVID-19 a "pandemic" on March 11, there were more than 118,000 confirmed cases and 4,291 deaths in 114 countries.[4] More than 90% were in four countries (China, Iran, Italy, and South Korea), with new infections declining significantly in China and South Korea, 81 countries reporting no cases, and 57 reporting 10 cases or less.

The WHO Director-General expressed the hope that countries could still check the pandemic by mobilizing people to detect, test, isolate, trace, and treat those infected, quarantining them while they remained infectious. Only a handful of East Asian economies and Kerala acted early, and thus avoided highly disruptive total lockdowns and associated human and economic costs. They also secured greater community support for containment, while minimizing draconian enforcement measures.

Had far more countries done so, while requiring safe physical distancing, mask wearing, and other precautionary measures, the contagion could have been contained.[5] And where communities or large clusters had significant infection rates, targeted measures could have helped "turn the tide" on COVID-19, as in China, Korea, and Vietnam, with decisive early actions without requiring nationwide "stay-in-shelter" "lockdowns," or restrictions on movements of people within

4. "WHO Director-General's Opening Remarks at the Media Briefing on COVID-19" (11 March 2020), online: *World Health Organization* <https://www.who.int/dg/speeches/detail/who-director-general-s-opening-remarks-at-the-media-briefing-on-covid-19---11-march-2020>.
5. The WHO's initial advice was to prioritize the use of face masks only by people with COVID-19 symptoms, or by those looking after someone who may have the virus, owing to the critical shortage of medical masks.

its borders. These terms are often used differently in various contexts, even changing over time.

But most others have been slow, often lacking resolve, perhaps hoping that the virus would bypass them or that "herd immunity" would protect most of the populations exposed to the virus. A few headstrong, but very influential government leaders simply refused to acknowledge the severity of the COVID-19 threat, subsequently distracting many with conspiracy theories instead of quickly learning from and correcting the policy errors that had been made.

Thus, new infections and deaths quickly rose exponentially as the virus rapidly spread to other countries, especially to advanced countries in the West, better connected by passenger air travel. As developing countries struggled with the lack of vitally needed resources, many developed countries have been jingoistic by restricting exports of vital medical supplies, in contravention of the International Health Regulations (IHR) and WHO recommendations.

Understanding the COVID-19 Crisis

The COVID-19 pandemic is now widely considered more threatening than other viral epidemics in recent decades, since the Asian flu of the late 1950s and the Hong Kong flu of 1968. Although the fatality rate of those infected may be lower than for SARS (severe acute respiratory syndrome) in 2002–2003,[6] and COVID-19 may not be more infectious than the H1N1 virus, its particular combination of transmissibility and mortality risks has generated unprecedented fear and apprehension. SARS, by contrast, was more deadly, going deeper into the lungs, but less infectious than COVID-19, despite having similar symptoms.

The virus is considered especially dangerous as infection, via mucous in the mouth, nose, and eyes, starts in the upper respiratory tract (throat, upper airways). Those infected are also infectious very soon after being infected, when they are still asymptomatic. They may still remain without symptoms or only have mild symptoms when

6. According to the WHO, a total of 8,098 people in 26 countries had SARS; 774 died between November 2002 and July 2003, i.e., a death rate of 9.6%, whereas the COVID-19 death rate was 3.6% when it was declared a pandemic. Matt Woodley, "How Does Coronavirus Compare with Previous Global Outbreaks?" (19 February 2020), online: *The Royal Australian College of General Practitioners* <https://www1.racgp.org.au/newsgp/clinical/how-does-coronavirus-compare-with-previous-global>.

testing positive for antigens, on average about five days after being infected. They may remain asymptomatic or only mildly symptomatic later, when testing positive for antibodies.

Thus, they pose a major challenge for detection, tracing, and testing, especially for developing countries, as currently "internationally approved" tests tend to be much more expensive the earlier they can yield positive results, that is, not yield "false negatives." The vastly disparate costs of various tests effective for detection at different stages of infection, and the limited means and capacities for testing in developing countries imply that the true extent of infection is not only unknown, but may never be known.

WHO estimated a monthly global need for tens of millions of medical masks, gloves, and goggles as personal protective equipment (PPE) required for adequate COVID-19 responses. It has urged easing restrictions on the export and distribution of PPE, ventilators or respirators, and other medical supplies.[7] It has also called on PPE manufacturers to boost production by 40% and urged governments to offer incentives to accelerate production.

Although the first COVID-19 outbreak was in China, it initially seemed to bypass much of the global South, perhaps reflecting the role of passenger air travel in its uneven global spread. Nevertheless, months after China reported the outbreak to the WHO on December 31, 2019, and the first related death on January 11, predictions of catastrophic consequences, especially for developing countries, continue to grow.[8]

On March 31, the United Nations (UN) Secretary-General described the COVID-19 crisis as the greatest collective test for the "international community" since the UN's formation.[9] He urged

7. "Shortage of Personal Protective Equipment Endangering Health Workers Worldwide" (3 March 2020), online: *World Health Organization* <https://www.who.int/news-room/detail/03-03-2020-shortage-of-personal-protective-equipment-endangering-health-workers-worldwide>.
8. Anthony Faiola et al, "Public Health Experts: Coronavirus Could Overwhelm the Developing World", *The Washington Post* (1 April 2020), online: <https://www.washingtonpost.com/world/the_americas/coronavirus-developing-world-brazil-egypt-india-kenya-venezuela/2020/03/31/d52fe238-6d4f-11ea-a156-0048b62cdb51_story.html>; Robert Malley & Richard Malley, "When the Pandemic Hits the Most Vulnerable: Developing Countries Are Hurtling Toward Coronavirus Catastrophe", *Foreign Affairs* (31 March 2020), <https://www.foreignaffairs.com/articles/africa/2020-03-31/when-pandemic-hits-most-vulnerable>.
9. "Transcript of the UN Secretary-General's Virtual Press Encounter to Launch the Report on the Socio-Economic Impacts of COVID-19" (31 March 2020),

developed countries to immediately help less developed countries to bolster their health systems and capacity to check disease, especially COVID-19 transmission. Failure to do so, he warned, would contribute to "the nightmare of the disease spreading like wildfire in the global South with millions of deaths and the prospect of the disease re-emerging where it was previously suppressed."

Weak Health Systems

Health systems in most developing countries are unevenly inadequate, even in normal times. Despite several pandemics in recent years, most countries remained poorly prepared, let alone for the specific challenges posed by COVID-19. Even most health systems in Europe and North America faced major shortages of doctors, respirators, basic infection prevention (BIP) gear, PPE, and testing kits.[10]

A recent survey of the availability of four BIP and four PPE items in seven poor countries (Afghanistan, Bangladesh, Democratic Republic of Congo [DRC], Haiti, Nepal, Senegal and Tanzania) found less than a third of clinics and health centres in Bangladesh, the DRC, Nepal, and Tanzania had any face masks.[11] In all seven countries, clinics, and health centres, often the first point of public contact with the health system, had, on average, just 2.3 (of four) BIP items and two (of four) PPE items. Most countries surveyed scored poorly on health workers' preparedness in terms of the 2005 IHR to prevent the spread of diseases.

---

online: *United Nations* <https://www.un.org/sg/en/content/sg/press-encounter/2020-03-31/transcript-of-un-secretary-general%E2%80%99s-virtual-press-encounter-launch-the-report-the-socio-economic-impacts-of-covid-19>.

10. The WHO's shortened list includes (a) guidelines for infection prevention; (b) pourable water and soap or hand disinfectant; (c) surface disinfectant; and (d) a waste bin. WHO's guidance on PPE for those in direct contact with patients includes: (a) gloves; (b) face masks; (c) gowns or aprons; and (d) eye protection. See "Service Availability and Readiness Assessment (SARA)" (2015), online (pdf): *World Health Organization* <https://www.who.int/healthinfo/systems/SARA_Reference_Manual_Chapter3.pdf?ua=1>; and "Rational Use of Personal Protective Equipment (PPE) for Coronavirus Disease (COVID-19)" (19 March 2020), online (pdf): *World Health Organization* <https://apps.who.int/iris/bitstream/handle/10665/331498/WHO-2019-nCoV-IPCPPE_use-2020.2-eng.pdf>.

11. Anna Gage & Sebastian Bauhoff, "Health Systems in Low-Income Countries Will Struggle to Protect Health Workers from Covid-19" (2020), online: *Center for Global Development* <https://www.cgdev.org/blog/health-systems-low-income-countries-will-struggle-protect-health-workers-covid-19>.

While the U.S. has about 33 intensive care unit (ICU) beds per 100,000 population, the ratio is around 2 per 100,000 in India, Pakistan, and Bangladesh in South Asia. In sub-Saharan Africa, the situation is even more dire: Zambia has 0.6 ICU beds per 100,000, Gambia 0.4, and Uganda 0.1.[12] Total ICU beds in 43 of Africa's 55 countries are less than 5,000, or about 5 beds per million, compared with about 4,000 per million in Europe. There are also serious respirator shortages in Africa, with 10 countries having none.[13] The average low-income country has 0.2 physicians and 1.0 nurse per thousand people, compared to 3.0 and 8.8 respectively in high-income countries.[14]

As high-income countries scramble to secure crucial supplies such as face masks, with increasingly strident calls to ban their export, nationalize equipment producers, and invest in this sector, low-income countries face much tougher choices. Their budgets are far more limited, and they typically lack local producers for most equipment, relying on donors and multilateral organizations for procurement in the face of unreliable supply chains.

The looming COVID-19 threat to frontline health workers in low-income countries has been largely ignored. Only a fraction of needed PPE has gone to them. The WHO has dispatched 0.5 million PPE sets, while UNICEF has dispatched 100,000 N95 masks, 4.3 million gloves, and other PPE. Billionaire philanthropist Jack Ma has donated 100,000 masks and 1,000 protective suits each to every country in Africa as well as 1.8 million masks to 10 Asian countries.[15]

In recent decades, developed economies, through the International Monetary Fund (IMF) and World Bank, used aid conditionalities to demand funding cuts and neoliberal health sector reforms, for example, by imposing user fees in developing countries.[16] Instead of improving efficiency, quality, and coverage, these reforms had deleterious implications for public health, besides exacerbating

12. Malley & Malley, *supra* note 8.
13. Ruth Maclean & Simon Marks, "10 African Countries Have No Ventilators", *The New York Times* (20 April 2020), online: <https://www.nytimes.com/2020/04/18/world/africa/africa-coronavirus-ventilators.html>.
14. Gage & Bauhoff, *supra* 11.
15. *Ibid.*
16. John Lister & Ronald Labonté, "Globalization and Health System Change" in Ronald Labonté et al, eds, *Globalization and Health: Pathways, Evidence and Policy* (New York: Routledge, 2009) at 181.

inequalities in access to health care.[17] Their structural adjustment programs in developing countries, particularly in Africa, resulted in underinvestment in health care systems, rendering them poorly prepared to respond to the Ebola epidemic.[18] Besides IMF and World Bank programs, such underinvestment was also due to compromised fiscal capacities and regressive fiscal priorities.[19]

Developing Country Responses

As it is likely to take some time before an effective and affordable vaccine is available to all, it will be impossible to completely eradicate the COVID-19 threat in the near future. With no known effective treatment for the infection, as the deadly nature of the virus became clear, even in the world's most advanced and richest countries, many countries have adopted total lockdowns, often in panic and ignorance of other options. In some circumstances, as in Wuhan, and elsewhere, following earlier inaction, a lockdown is believed by many to be needed to abruptly slow the virus spread if it has reached potentially catastrophic proportions.

Accustomed to adopting supposed "best practices" prescribed by the rich and powerful, all too many governments are implementing borrowed measures without sufficiently taking into account country-specific circumstances and challenges. Besides obvious differences between developed and developing countries, especially in terms of resources, demography, and institutions, there are significant differences among developing countries themselves.

17. Timon Forstera et al, "Globalization and Health Equity: The Impact of Structural Adjustment Programs on Developing Countries" [2019] Soc Science & Medicine, online: *Science Direct* <https://www.sciencedirect.com/science/article/pii/S0277953619304897>; Saeed Sobhani, "From Privatization to Health System Strengthening: How Different International Monetary Fund (IMF) and World Bank Policies Impact Health in Developing Countries" (2019) 94:10 J Egyptian Public Health Assoc 1; Thomas Stubbs & Alexander Kentikelenis, "International Financial Institutions and Human Rights: Implications for Public Health" (2017) 38:27 Public Health Rev 1.
18. Waiswa Nkwanga, "The Ebola Crisis in West Africa and the Enduring Legacy of the Structural Adjustment Policies" (2015), online (blog): *London School of Economics* <https://blogs.lse.ac.uk/africaatlse/2015/01/26/the-ebola-crisis-in-west-africa-and-the-enduring-legacy-of-the-structural-adjustment-policies/>.
19. David Sanders, Amit Sengupta & Vera Scott, "Ebola Epidemic Exposes the Pathology of the Global Economic and Political System" (2015) 45:4 International Journal of Health Services 643; Vera Scott, Sarah Crawford-Brown & David Sanders, "Critiquing the Response to the Ebola Epidemic Through a Primary Health Care Approach" (2016) 16: 410 BMC Public Health 1.

In most slums and villages, many people often live together in one or two rooms, sharing common utensils, towels, and much else, perhaps including a toilet nearby. Safe physical distancing is virtually impossible in these circumstances. Even basic hygiene and other prescribed sanitary measures, such as washing hands with lather for at least a certain amount of time, is not easy when clean running water is scarce.

Transmission patterns are determined by social factors that are both local and intimate, which international and even national public health decision makers are often oblivious to, but which community members know all too well. Therefore, joint learning, involving both experts and affected communities, can be vital for effective responses.

Lessons learned from previous epidemics may be useful. Governments need to consider the specific nature of the COVID-19 pandemic and its unique, but nonetheless varied, implications in various contexts. After all, an effective vaccine is believed by many to be at least 18 months away. A standardized set of interventions, even ostensible best practices, is unlikely to be universally applicable, as the COVID-19 pandemic has different ramifications in various circumstances over time.

As an economy cannot be locked down for too long, authorities have to choose between lives and livelihoods rather than between life and the economy, as is often said. The bulk of the population in many developing countries is in the informal sector, earning meagre, typically daily incomes and having paltry savings. All too many developing countries do not have enough fiscal space to provide sufficient relief for vulnerable populations and small businesses for long. Hence, extending strict lockdown measures is likely to lose broad public support, even if such support is high at the beginning.

Countries can have less disruptive and less costly, yet very effective, containment strategies, especially if they act early and quickly, as timing is critical. The ability to trace and test as many suspected cases as possible, for example, those who have come into close recent contact with an infected person, is also crucial. Effective containment depends heavily on voluntary compliance, and hence, community acceptance and trust, helped by transparency and shared understanding of what needs to be done. All these require state capabilities working together ("all of government"), as well as credible and inclusive leadership to mobilize and co-ordinate the "whole of society" for effective containment of contagion, as was done in the Southwestern Indian state of Kerala, in Vietnam, and in Argentina.

Flattening the Curve?

The principal strategy adopted by most governments is to "flatten the curve," so that countries' health systems can cope with new infections by tracing, testing, isolating, and treating those infected until an approved vaccine or cure is available to all. But this is easier said than done.

Vulnerability to infection and capacity to respond depend on many factors, including health care system preparedness, leadership experience, and ability to manage specific challenges posed. Government capacity to respond depends crucially on system capacity and capabilities—for example, authorities' ability to speedily trace, isolate, and treat the infected—and available fiscal resources—for example, to quickly enhance testing capacity and secure PPE. Funding cuts, privatization, and other abuses of recent decades—in the face of rising costs, not least for medicines—have further constrained and undermined most public health systems, albeit on various pretexts.

Physical distancing, mask use, and other precautionary measures, besides mass testing, tracing, isolation, and treatment, have been able to check contagion without resorting to draconian lockdowns. Such measures have been quite successful so far in much of East Asia, Vietnam, and Kerala. Precautionary measures must be appropriate and affordable. To minimize the risk of infection, authorities can encourage and enable, if not require, changes in social interactions, including work and other public space arrangements, including for offices, factories, shops, public transportation, and classrooms.

Lockdowns can have many effects, depending on context. Good planning, implementation, and enforcement of movement restrictions, and adequate provisioning for those adversely affected, are crucial, not only for efficacy, but also for transitions before, during, and after the lockdowns. Nonetheless, lockdowns typically incur huge economic costs, distributed unevenly in economies and societies. Governments must therefore be mindful of costs, including of disruptions, and also of how policies affect various people differently. Hence, the effectiveness of a lockdown has to be judged primarily by its ability to quickly "flatten the curve" and to ensure no resurgence of infections. Success should not be measured by duration, enforcement stringency, or even unsustainable declines in new cases.

Lockdowns cannot have the effect of setting back progress and people's welfare irreversibly, that is, of delivering "economic knockouts" to the vulnerable. Most casual labourers, petty businesses reliant on daily cash turnover, and others in the "informal" economy find it especially difficult to survive extended lockdowns. Although they need more relief support than others, they are often difficult for governments to reach. Those living in crammed conditions, for example in urban slums, cannot realistically be expected to consistently practise safe distancing, but can nonetheless be enabled to sustainably take other precautionary measures within their modest means, for example, by using washable masks in public areas.

Country Policy Response Lessons

China

Many countries have restricted freedom of movement through lockdowns, citing China's response in Wuhan.[20] However, Bruce Aylward, leader of the WHO fact-finding mission to China, clarified,

> The majority of the response in China, in 30 provinces, was about case finding, contact tracing, and suspension of public gatherings—all common measures used anywhere in the world to manage [infectious] diseases... The lockdown people are referring to ... was concentrated in Wuhan and two or three other cities ... that got out of control in the beginning ... the key learning from China is ... all about the speed. The faster you can find the cases, isolate the cases, and track their close contacts, the more successful you're going to be.[21]

Therefore, the varied Chinese experiences suggest that resources should be concentrated on rapid and early detection, isolation and contact tracing, protecting the most vulnerable, and treating the infected, regardless of means, instead of mainly relying on strict, but typically "blunt" lockdown measures due to failure to act earlier.

20. "Lockdowns and Entry Bans Imposed Around the World to Fight Coronavirus" (15 March 2020), online: *Reuters* <https://www.reuters.com/article/us-health-coronavirus/lockdowns-and-entry-bans-imposed-around-the-world-to-fight-coronavirus-idUSKBN21208S>.
21. Julia Belluz, "China's Cases of Covid-19 are Finally Declining. A WHO Expert Explains Why", *Vox* (3 March 2020), online: <https://www.vox.com/2020/3/2/21161067/coronavirus-covid19-china>.

South Korea[22]

Like China, South Korea recovered rapidly from having the second highest rate of infection globally. The country is one of several, mainly East Asian, economies that have dramatically reduced or kept low the number of COVID-19 cases and related deaths without resorting to draconian lockdowns. It has thus slowed the spread of COVID-19, even in Daegu, its most infected city. The Korean authorities continue to urge physical distancing and personal hygiene. Mass gatherings are discouraged, and employers are encouraged to allow employees to work remotely.

Mass testing has been key, with South Korea doing more COVID-19 tests by country until April. Much of East Asia built up its testing capabilities following earlier epidemics in recent decades, and their authorities were thus prepared with test kits and facilities for rapid development, approval, and deployment. In South Korea, the tests have been free for those whom medical professionals recommend for testing. Others who wish to be tested are charged about US$130, but reimbursed if the result is positive, with treatment needed paid for by the government.

Another legacy of earlier epidemic experiences is governmental legal authority to collect data from those who test positive for contact tracing efforts. Artificial intelligence and big data have also been deployed for contact tracing. Such pro-active testing and contact tracing have been lauded by the WHO, which is encouraging other countries to apply lessons learned in East Asia.

Kerala[23]

The first COVID-19 case in India was detected in the southwestern Indian state of Kerala on January 30, 2020. But with precautionary measures in place even before that, with a population of 35 million, Kerala has become "a model state in the fight against COVID-19." The state health department went into action early, setting up a coordination centre on January 26 to identify, test, isolate, and treat those

22. Nazihah Muhamad Noor & Jomo Kwame Sundaram, "East Asian Lessons for Controlling Covid-19", *Inter Press Service* (26 March 2020), online: <https://www.ipsnews.net/2020/03/east-asian-lessons-controlling-covid-19/>.

23. Anis Chowdhury & Jomo Kwame Sundaram, "Kerala Covid-19 Response Model for Emulation", *Inter Press Service* (9 April 2020), online: <https://www.ipsnews.net/2020/04/kerala-covid-19-response-model-emulation/>.

infected. Through appropriate and effective early actions, it successfully slowed infections in the state, largely by promoting precautionary measures, and providing better protection for health staff well before the hugely disruptive and draconian lockdown imposed in India from late March.

The Left Front-led Kerala state government invited religious leaders, local bodies, and civil society organizations to participate in policy design and implementation, considering its specific socio-economic conditions. It has communicated effectively in different languages to educate all, and acted to prevent stigmatization of those infected, opposing the term "social distancing," with its caste connotations, insisting on "physical distancing and social solidarity."

With Kerala's long-standing achievements in education, highly educated Keralans tend to migrate to work out of state, if not abroad, seeking more lucrative employment. With the nationwide lockdown, non-residents, about 5% of Kerala's population, have returned, causing many new infections. The state has handled the migration issue well, especially compared to other state governments and the central government.

To make things worse, Kerala has been discriminated against by the central government's disaster relief fund on specious grounds. The largely agricultural state has modest fiscal resources of its own, as state governments in India have limited fiscal rights and resources. Hence, Kerala's response, by a government with very limited fiscal resources, is especially instructive to others considering early precautionary action.

Vietnam[24]

Vietnam, a poor, populous country with 97 million people, bordering China, has successfully kept down infections, with no deaths (as of May 7), by acting early to trace and test contacts, and to quarantine and treat the infected. Key features of Vietnam's response are similar to those of other much-lauded East Asian responses, with infection rates significantly lower than even Taiwan's. Vietnam has been much lauded as a low-cost COVID-19 success story to be emulated by poor countries with limited resources.

24. Anis Chowdhury & Jomo Kwame Sundaram, "Vietnam Winning New War Against Invisible Enemy", *Inter Press Service* (14 April 2020), online: <https://www.ipsnews.net/2020/04/vietnam-winning-new-war-invisible-enemy/>.

Having experienced several recent epidemics, Vietnam acted early and proactively. When China officially confirmed the first death due to the novel coronavirus on January 11, Vietnam quickly tightened health checks at all borders and airports. Other measures included closing schools, rationing surgical masks, cancelling some flights, and restricting entry to most foreigners. The measures have been imposed unevenly, as needed, rather than as blanket, across-the-board measures.

Vietnam was the first country after China to seal off a large residential area. Within a month, the government mobilized a large group of scientists to develop a fast, efficient, and affordable test kit using a WHO-approved technique. The government has also asked all citizens to make online health declarations, and regularly texts updates nationwide. Different ministries have jointly developed an "easy-to-use app" to get tested, and update information regarding infection hotspots and best practices.

A successful fund-raising campaign purchased medical and protective equipment for doctors, nurses, and others in close contact with patients, and for those quarantined. Rather than mass testing, key to wealthier South Korea's response, Vietnam has tracked down the primary (direct) and secondary (next-level indirect) contacts of those infected to trace and test those more likely to be infected.

As in Kerala, the government keeps the public fully informed, while keeping identities private to avoid stigmatization. And when Vietnamese businesses were reportedly ostracizing foreigners, the prime minister spoke out against such discrimination.

Vietnam's response has earned a high level of trust among its citizens. About 62% of Vietnamese surveyed, in the single largest global public opinion survey on COVID-19, think the Government is doing "right," compared to the global average of around 40%. Vietnam is also following in the steps of Cuba and China by donating protective suits for health care professionals, medical masks, testing equipment, and kits to other countries: the U.S., five European countries, Cambodia, Laos, and Indonesia.

Brazil[25]

Brazil's President Jair Bolsonaro has sought to resume business as usual regardless of its potentially lethal consequences, even firing his previous health minister for public remarks on the need for lockdowns and physical distancing. Official figures likely greatly understate the gravity of the situation, as there is no standardized testing method, and it is the hospitalized who are mainly being tested. The death toll is expected to be high due to late and inadequate action. Meanwhile, Brazil is digging graves around the clock in anticipation of continuing deaths due to the COVID-19 epidemic.

Despite the life-threatening risks, Bolsonaro has dismissed the threat as a media-hyped "fantasy" and preventive measures as "hysterical." He has disregarded physical distancing recommendations, urging others to also defy them, while demanding that Brazil's 27 state governors withdraw their safe distancing orders, which have been closing shops and schools to slow the pandemic that threatens to overwhelm its health care system. An executive order tried unsuccessfully to strip states of the authority to restrict people's movements. Not unlike other leaders, Bolsonaro has not hesitated to mislead the public while accusing his opponents of doing so.

As he loses support from the Brazilian elite over his handling of the crisis, he has tried to centralize authority by various means, with apparent Army support, even calling for a military coup to enhance federal executive powers to prevent and, if necessary, repress an increasingly anticipated social explosion.

Argentina[26]

Like much of the West, Argentina did not take many early precautionary actions, but became the first Latin American country to act decisively,[27] with a March 12 public health emergency presidential

25. Anis Chowdhury & Jomo Kwame Sundaram, "Covid-19: Brazil's Bolsonaro Trumps Trump", *Inter Press Service* (21 April 2020), online: <http://www.ipsnews.net/2020/04/covid-19-brazils-bolsonaro-trumps-trump/>.
26. Anis Chowdhury & Jomo Kwame Sundaram, "Argentina Responds Boldly to Coronavirus Crisis", *Inter Press Service* (5 May 2020), online: <https://www.ipsnews.net/2020/05/argentina-responds-boldly-coronavirus-crisis/>.
27. Peru was the second Latin American country to act. President Martín Vizcarra announced coronavirus lockdowns on March 16 effective from March 17. Argentina's lockdown was effective from March 19.

decree a day after the WHO declared a global pandemic, over a week after Argentina's first case was confirmed on March 3. The measures include a mandatory "stay in shelter" lockdown, with those violating the order facing harsh penalties and other "social, preventive isolation" measures. The mandatory lockdown has been extended to June 28 in Buenos Aires and some other parts of the country, with nation-wide "mandatory and preventive social distancing" remaining in place.

All arrivals from COVID-19 hot spots have to be quarantined for 14 days, regardless of nationality. All direct flights between Argentina and the U.S., as well as Europe, were suspended for 30 days from March 17, now extended indefinitely. As infections surge in neighbouring Brazil, the government has set up secure corridors in border provinces, allowing Brazilian drivers to access bathrooms, get food, and unload products, with minimal contact with Argentines.

A patchwork of regional and national laws without much coherence has resulted in very inequitable and fragmented health care coverage in Argentina. The new government, from December 2019, of left-populist President Alberto Fernandez reversed the previous Macri government's severe austerity measures under an IMF program, and the demotion of the Health Minister to a non-cabinet position, which had further undermined its already debilitated health "non-system".

The new government inherited an economy already deep in recession, with gross public debt around 93.3% of the 2019 GDP, annual inflation over 50%, poverty above 40%, unemployment at almost 10%, and the Argentine peso having lost 68% of its value in 2019.

Thus, having to lock down an economy in recession, Argentina's policy choice captures the cruel dilemma COVID-19 has posed for people and governments to choose between lives and livelihoods. After taking office, Fernandez initially increased progressive taxation to balance the budget to restore growth, rather than to pay foreign creditors. Instead of reducing social expenditure, he has cut spending benefiting the wealthy.

Argentina initially committed around 2% of GDP to an economic and social relief package, ensuring that essential services for retirees, social welfare recipients, and households earning less than about US$520 are not cut due to non-payment. As the lockdown continues, Argentina's economic relief package had grown to 3.5% of GDP by April's end.

The administration has made every employer eligible for emergency aid, postponed or reduced taxes on small businesses by up to 95%, and is paying employees half to all the monthly minimum wage. The government has required banks to extend loans at reduced interest rates to keep the economy afloat. The administration has also suspended evictions, frozen all rent increases, and forgiven penalties imposed for not paying taxes due on those in the lowest tax bracket.

Despite Argentina's divided politics, the new President stood with leaders from across the political spectrum in a display of unity to announce the March 19 lockdown. The central government is working closely with state governors and all health providers, securing private sector cooperation without nationalization. Meanwhile, the armed forces are building triage centres in case of a surge in infections. Argentina's infection and mortality rates are low, but its testing rate is well behind Chile's, although it is improving fast.

Meanwhile social, religious, and business groups deliver food to more than two million in the greater Buenos Aires area alone. Despite these relief measures, much hardship remains, especially for those relying on daily incomes. Yet, government measures have 94.7% approval, with the President's popularity soaring to 81%.

Governance, Mobilization, Leadership

In order to plan and effectively implement needed measures, enhance efficacy, and minimize disruption, an "all of government" approach would significantly improve design and implementation of needed measures. In all too many situations, public health and police authorities manage lockdowns with little meaningful consultation with the rest of government. Human resource, social protection, transport, education, media, industry, fiscal, and other relevant authorities need to be appropriately engaged to plan, design, and implement various measures, as well as post-lockdown and post-COVID-19 transitions to varying notions of "new normal."

Another condition for success is "whole of society" mobilization to secure popular participation and support for undoubtedly difficult transitions. Government transparency and explanation of evolving situations and justification of various measures undertaken are important for public understanding, cooperation, support, and legitimacy.

Flexibility is important, as well as the willingness and ability to change strategy and policies in response to new developments and realizations, especially in dealing with a fast unfolding situation with so much that is unfamiliar, or worse, misleadingly familiar. Singapore's apparent early success, for example, was not what it seemed, as it had overlooked official disincentives for possibly infected migrant workers to come forward to cooperate with authorities. One can expect the problem to be compounded when sections of a population feel particularly vulnerable, especially in dealing with state authorities, for example, those in the "grey economy" or undocumented foreign labour. Special incentives, such as full amnesties and the promise of free treatment, can be important to overcome such disincentives.

Diverse, culturally appropriate, enhanced public health and other relevant education and communications will need to be quickly developed to effectively mobilize full public engagement. The efficacy and consequences of lockdowns and other such measures are contingent on public appreciation of the challenges, and on the ability of societies to respond appropriately with socio-economic, cultural, and behavioural changes.

While the COVID-19 crisis challenges are undoubtedly unique, they are not exceptional insofar as such challenges all have unique characteristics. But perhaps the differences are far greater than with other recent epidemics, challenging earlier tested modes of response. Full social mobilization is undoubtedly needed, but such exceptional "wartime" measures must not be abused, for example, by the temptation to skew implementation for political or pecuniary advantage. Hence, success can be greatly enabled by legitimate, credible, and exemplary leadership, in government and civil society.

CHAPTER F-2

The Plausibility and Resolvability of Legal Claims Against China and WHO under the International Health Regulations (2005)

Sam Halabi[*] and Dr. Kumanan Wilson[**]

Abstract

Since the declaration of a public health emergency of international concern by the World Health Organization on January 30, 2020, accusations have been levelled against both the World Health Organization (WHO) and the People's Republic of China (PRC) for failures to adequately and effectively notify the world about the COVID-19 threat. These accusations have been followed by calls for international sanctions, withdrawal of contributions to WHO's work, and multilateral calls for investigations into the pandemic's origins. Against a backdrop of increasingly bellicose rhetoric from governments, this chapter sets forth the most straightforward legal framework for resolving disputes about PRC and WHO actions: the International Health Regulations (2005). All disputing parties are members of the agreement, which provides specific mechanisms for dispute resolution. The chapter carefully assembles the known timeline from the outbreak of the novel coronavirus in Wuhan, PRC, to the PRC's notification to WHO, to actions taken thereafter. It identifies the possible

* Manley O. Hudson Professor of Law at the University of Missouri as well as a scholar at the O'Neill Institute for National and Global Health Law at Georgetown University.

** Specialist in general internal medicine, and senior scientist at The Ottawa Hospital, innovation advisor at Bruyère Research Institute, and Professor of Medicine at the University of Ottawa.

grounds for legal complaints, and analyzes the legal alternatives for resolution.

Résumé

Vraisemblance et possibilité de résoudre les actions en justice contre la Chine et l'OMS dans le cadre du *Règlement sanitaire international* (2005)

Depuis que l'Organisation mondiale de la santé (OMS) a déclaré l'état d'urgence sanitaire mondial le 30 janvier 2020, des accusations ont été portées contre elle et contre la République populaire de Chine (RPC) pour avoir omis d'informer le monde de manière adéquate et efficace de la menace que représentait la COVID-19. Ces accusations ont été suivies d'appels à des sanctions internationales et au retrait des contributions aux travaux de l'OMS, et d'appels multilatéraux à enquêter sur les origines de la pandémie. Dans un contexte de rhétorique de plus en plus belliqueuse de la part des gouvernements, ce chapitre présente le cadre juridique le plus simple pour résoudre les différends au sujet des actions de la RPC et de l'OMS : le *Règlement sanitaire international* (2005). Toutes les parties en cause sont membres de l'accord, qui prévoit des mécanismes précis de règlement des différends. Ce chapitre présente soigneusement la chronologie connue des événements, depuis l'apparition du nouveau coronavirus à Wuhan, en RPC, jusqu'à la déclaration de la maladie à l'OMS et aux mesures prises par la suite. Il précise les motifs éventuels de plaintes et analyse les solutions envisageables sur le plan juridique.

The global response to COVID-19 should be governed by the International Health Regulations (2005), the World Health Organization (WHO)-administered agreement to which all UN member states belong.[1] Instead, the response is haphazard, and the authority of WHO and the UN Security Council are hobbled by disagreements between the United States, the People's Republic of China, and WHO. This chapter presents the legal arguments underpinning these disagreements, that doing so may facilitate solutions

1. Wilson K et al, "Strategies for Implementing the New International Health Regulations in Federal Countries" (2008) 86:3 *Bull World Health Organization* 215, DOI: <10.2471/blt.07.042838>.

drawn from law, rather than the less efficient tit-for-tats that characterize feuds between antagonistic great powers and, less frequently, international organizations. The factual and legal analysis provided herein is dependent upon facts still being reported and revised. Nevertheless, the chapter is a roadmap to reconsideration of some of the IHR (2005)'s functions and a guide to the legality of actions and measures taken by major actors over the course of a rapidly unfolding pandemic.

The process leading to the International Health Regulations (2005) was facilitated by recognition at the highest national and international organizational levels that infectious diseases posed a threat to global security, a threat of sufficient magnitude to implicate the United Nations Security Council's authority under the UN Charter. The 1980s witnessed the emergence and increase in the incidence of viral hemorrhagic fevers and HIV. By 1995, the number of people in Africa living with HIV/AIDS rose dramatically, accounting for the vast majority of people living with HIV/AIDS globally.[2]

In response, the World Health Assembly adopted resolutions charging the WHO Director-General with identifying new responses to new and re-emerging infectious diseases, because the existing International Health Regulations did not address novel infectious agents and failed to provide for an adequate response to those that were covered.[3] In 2000, the UN Security Council recognized infectious disease as an international peace and security issue.[4] Between 2000 and 2002, negotiations for a revised IHR languished at WHO.

In late 2002, an epidemic of atypical pneumonia erupted in China's Guangdong Province. China failed to disclose to WHO the emergence of the disease that would later become known as SARS until a doctor who had treated patients in Guangdong developed symptoms while in Hong Kong. The pathogen infected hotel guests, patients, and contacts in Hong Kong, Vietnam, Singapore, and Canada. Because SARS was not a notifiable disease under the IHR as they then existed, China had no legal obligation to report

2. Jonathan M Mann & Daniel JM Tarantola, eds, *AIDS in the World II: Global Dimensions, Social Roots, and Reponses* (New York: Oxford University Press, 1996).
3. World Health Organization, "Strengthening Health Security by Implementing the International Health Regulations (2005)" (2005), online: *World Health Organization* <http://www.who.int/ihr/revisionprocess/revision/en/index.html>.
4. Alex de Waal, "HIV/AIDS and the Challenges of Security and Conflict" (2010) 375:9708 The Lancet 22.

cases to WHO. WHO had no legal authority to request information from China. The outbreak of SARS facilitated the 2005 revisions of the IHR.[5]

The IHR (2005) were expanded to encompass the detection and prevention of all infectious diseases.[6] Reflecting the importance of communication for early detection and response, States Parties must inform WHO within 24 hours of any event that could be considered a "public health risk to other States requiring a coordinated international response."[7]

From public health and epidemiological perspectives, the IHR (2005) reflect disease control priorities applicable at local, regional, and national levels: rapid detection of threats through surveillance and reporting, identification of pathogens, and control measures to contain the threat and reduce transmission. Therefore, the IHR (2005) prioritizes the development of surveillance and response infrastructure (Annex 1), provides a guide to reporting (Annex 2 – providing a yes-or-no flow chart), and imposes strict timelines for detection and assessment. Early on, there is often uncertainty about a threat that could provide an obligation to report—particularly if there are likely to be negative economic consequences of reporting. Annex 2 guidance attempts to address this, but ambiguity remains. The backdrop to the PRC's and WHO's early actions regarding COVID-19 is a significant measure of scientific uncertainty.

Methodologically, this chapter analyzes the obligations imposed under Articles 6 through 17 of the IHR (2005) to the content of international disputes by reviewing the existing literature for timelines, statements, declarations, and chronology. Articles 8 and 12 through 14 are not separately analyzed, either because they are irrelevant or because their relevance is addressed within analysis of an Article with overlapping content.

5. David P Fidler, "Revision of the World Health Organization's International Health Regulations" (16 April 2004), online: *American Society of International Law* <https://www.asil.org/insights/volume/8/issue/8/revision-world-health-organizations-international-health-regulations>.
6. Sam Halabi, "The Origins and Future of Global Health Law: Regulation, Security, and Pluralism" (2020) 108:6 Georgetown LJ 1608.
7. World Health Organization, "International Health Regulations" (2005) at arts 4-5, online: *World Health Organization* <https://www.who.int/ihr/publications/9789241580496/en/>.

Claim 1: The People's Republic of China Failed to Promptly Report

IHR **Article 6** governing notification requires that:

> Each State Party shall notify WHO ... within 24 hours of assessment of public health information, of all events which may constitute a public health emergency of international concern ... as well as any health measure implemented in response...

Article 7 provides that:

> If a State Party has evidence of an ... unusual public health event within its territory, irrespective of origin or source, which may constitute a public health emergency of international concern, it shall provide to WHO all relevant public health information...

Several states accuse the PRC of violating Articles 6 and 7. The known timeline is that on December 10, 2019, one of the earliest coronavirus patients became ill. On December 16, the patient was admitted to Wuhan Central Hospital with a treatment-resistant lung infection. Between December 16 and December 27, cases multiplied. On December 27, health officials in Wuhan were told that an unclear cause was behind atypical pneumonia cases, and asked that information about those cases be compiled and transmitted. On Dec. 31, the PRC informed WHO's China office of the pneumonia cases. WHO officials responded with questions and offers of assistance. China notified the U.S. Centers for Disease Control and Prevention on January 3, 2020.

There is some question as to whether "all events" were notified either to WHO, as the IHR require, or to other States Parties. For example, PRC national authorities (as opposed to local or provincial authorities) were investigating the novel coronavirus by December 30, and perhaps earlier. If a violation of the notification provisions occurred, the question would then arise whether that violation was "material."

Claim 2: The People's Republic of China Failed to Provide WHO Timely, Accurate, and Sufficiently Detailed Public Health Information

IHR **Article 6** further governs notification of relevant public health events and requires that:

> a State Party shall … communicate to WHO timely, accurate and sufficiently detailed public health information available to it on the notified event … including case definitions, laboratory results … number of cases and deaths, conditions affecting the spread of the disease and the health measures employed; and report … the difficulties faced and support needed in responding…[8]

Between December 31 and January 15, there appear to be measures taken at municipal, provincial, and national levels in China to both share and suppress information. Researchers mapped the coronavirus's genetic information by January 2, 2020, and posted that information on a public genetic data repository on January 9, 2020. On January 14, WHO tweeted that Chinese authorities had seen "no clear evidence of human-to-human transmission of the novel coronavirus."

Epidemiologists and clinicians need to know much about new diseases to effectively respond. This includes when people get sick, their symptoms, and other characteristics, such as age, gender, and underlying medical conditions, that increase risk. During this period, the first case was confirmed in Thailand. On January 20, the first case was announced in South Korea. Zhong Nanshan, a Chinese doctor coordinating response, announced the virus could pass between people.

A *New England Journal of Medicine* study revealed that the first 425 patients in Wuhan, between December 10 and January 4, experienced long delays before admission to hospitals.[9] Person-to-person spread occurred as early as mid-December, and cases were doubling every seven days from January 11 to January 17, 2020. As early as December 30, 2019, physicians treating (what is now known as) COVID-19 patients were censured or arrested for attempting to report

8. *Ibid* at art 5.
9. Li Q et al, "Early Transmission Dynamics in Wuhan, China, of Novel Coronavirus-Infected Pneumonia" (2020) 382:13 N Engl J Med 1199, DOI: <10.1056/NEJMoa2001316>.

novel aspects of the infections. During that time, the Wuhan Health Commission claimed there were no new infections or deaths.

The case for a material breach having occurred with respect to "timely, accurate and sufficiently detailed public health information" appears stronger than the relatively short delay that accompanied China's December 31 report to WHO.

Claim 3: WHO Failed to Take into Account Reports from other Sources and Verify Reports from the PRC

Articles 9 through 11 of the IHR (2005) allow WHO to consider reports other than notifications from the notifying State Party.

> **Article 9 – Other Reports**
> WHO may take into account reports from [other] sources ... and shall assess these reports according to established epidemiological principles and then communicate information on the event to the State Party... Before taking any action based on such reports, WHO shall consult with and attempt to obtain verification from the State Party...
>
> **Article 10 – Verification**
> WHO may, when justified by ... the public health risk, share with other States Parties the information available to it ... taking into account the views of the State Party concerned...
> When WHO receives information of an event that may constitute a public health emergency ..., it shall offer to collaborate with the State Party concerned in assessing the potential for international disease spread ... and the adequacy of control measures...

On December 31, 2019, Republic of China (Taiwan) officials reported to WHO and PRC health authorities that its doctors had received reports from mainland colleagues that medical staff were becoming ill after treating patients diagnosed with atypical cases of pneumonia, indicating human-to-human transmission.

Articles 9 and 10 are deferential to the State Party's interest about how "other reports" may affect that State's interests. Although the IHR (2005) endeavour to balance public health protection with commerce and liberty interests, reporting events that may lead to the declaration of a public health emergency of international concern inevitably carries adverse economic effects for the State Party making those reports.

Claim 4: WHO Failed to Inform Other Parties to the IHR (2005)

Article 11 – Provision of Information by WHO

Subject to Paragraph 2... WHO shall send to States Parties ... as soon as possible and by the most efficient means available, in confidence, such public health information which it has received ... which is necessary to enable States Parties to respond to a public health risk...

2. WHO shall use information received ... for verification, assessment and assistance purposes under these Regulations and, unless otherwise agreed with the States Parties referred to in those provisions, shall not make this information generally available to other States Parties, until such time as:

(a) the event is determined to constitute a public health emergency ...; or

(b) information evidencing the international spread of the infection or contamination has been confirmed ...; or

(c) there is evidence that:

(i) control measures against the international spread are unlikely to succeed ...; or

(d) the nature and scope of the international movement of travellers ... that may be affected by the infection ... requires the immediate application of international control measures.

3. WHO shall consult with the State Party in whose territory the event is occurring as to its intent to make information available under this Article...

WHO declared a public health emergency of international concern (PHEIC) on January 30, 2020. The criteria for doing so under the IHR (2005) are vague. Based on the existing record, there is little evidence than any party had effectively assessed the controllability of SARS-CoV-2. The legal question, then, is whether WHO had an obligation to alert State Parties earlier than it did.

Claim 5: Temporary and Standing Measures Recommended by the WHO Director-General Did Not Comply with the Criteria Set Forth in the IHR (2005)

Article 17 – Criteria for Recommendations

When issuing ... recommendations, the Director-General shall consider:

> (a) the views of the States Parties directly concerned;
> (b) the advice of the Emergency Committee ...;
> (c) scientific principles as well as available scientific evidence ...;
> (d) health measures that ... are not more restrictive of international traffic and trade and are not more intrusive to persons than reasonably available alternatives that would achieve the appropriate level of health protection...

When it announced the PHEIC, WHO leaders did not recommend travel or trade restrictions, a decision criticized as overweighing criterion (a) over countervailing concerns. The WHO delegation that visited PRC between January 20 and 21 noted that PRC officials carefully negotiated the terminology and details of the delegation's findings. But Article 17 criteria suggest that such views are to be considered, and there remains agreement that there was (and remains) uncertainty over the uniqueness of the novel SARS coronavirus and what its differences with other coronaviruses meant for response.

Dispute Resolution Under the IHR (2005)

Whatever the determination as to material breaches committed either by the PRC or by WHO, the IHR (2005) provide the mechanisms by which those breaches may be addressed.

> **Article 56 - Settlement of Disputes**
> 1. In the event of a dispute ..., the States Parties concerned shall seek ... to settle the dispute through negotiation or any other peaceful means... Failure to reach agreement shall not absolve the parties to the dispute from the responsibility of continuing to seek to resolve it.
> 2. In the event that the dispute is not settled ... the States Parties concerned may ... refer the dispute to the Director-General, who shall make every effort to settle it.
> 3. A State Party may ... declare ... to the Director-General that it accepts arbitration as compulsory ... concerning the interpretation or application of these Regulations... The States Parties that have agreed to accept arbitration as compulsory shall accept the arbitral award as binding and final...

> 5. In the event of a dispute between WHO and … States Parties concerning the … Regulations, the matter shall be submitted to the Health Assembly.

Article 56 of the IHR (2005) provides the channel through which matters fundamental to how the treaty operates may be reviewed and ultimately incorporated into a revised instrument.

Conclusion

The IHR (2005) are the agreed governing legal framework for the global response to COVID-19. They are the law. The law addresses disputes of the type raised as to the PRC's candour in reporting to WHO, WHO's failure or not to share information with others, and WHO's assessment of PHEIC criteria. The law may have failed in the response to COVID-19 and, as we suggest, PRC's communication of timely information to the WHO. The lawful course of action is to negotiate a peaceful resolution to any disputes, including, perhaps, composition of an independent investigatory body, submission of the dispute to the WHO Director-General, consideration of binding arbitration, and, finally, resolution through the World Health Assembly.

CHAPTER F-3

COVID-19 and Africa: Does "One Size Fit All" in Public Health Intervention?

Chidi Oguamanam*

Abstract

Taking into account the socio-economic, cultural, and political dynamics of Africa, and drawing from a universe of publicly available information, this chapter explores Africa's experiences with selected aspects of COVID-19 public health and associated response measures. It aims, in part, to identify facets of the contextual dynamics of the continent that warrant creative and fit-for-context public health responses outside of a one-size-fits-all milieu. Also, the chapter identifies and reflects on some real and potential lessons and opportunities from the COVID-19 experience on the African continent that could reposition the continent and enhance its resilience in the face of the first global pandemic in a globalized and technology-driven world order.

* Full Professor in the Faculty of Law (Common Law Section), University of Ottawa, where he is affiliated with the Centre for Law, Technology and Society, the Centre for Environmental Law and Global Sustainability and the Centre for Health Law, Policy and Ethics.

Résumé
La COVID-19 et l'Afrique : peut-on adopter une approche unique en matière d'intervention en santé publique ?

En tenant compte de la dynamique socioéconomique, culturelle et politique de l'Afrique, et en s'appuyant sur un univers d'informations largement accessibles, ce chapitre explore les expériences de l'Afrique relativement à certains aspects de la santé publique et aux mesures d'intervention associées dans le contexte de la COVID-19. Il vise, en partie, à cerner les facettes de la dynamique contextuelle du continent qui justifient des réponses créatives et adaptées au contexte, dans un milieu distinct. En outre, le chapitre suscite une réflexion et identifie certaines leçons et certaines occasions, réelles et éventuelles, qui découlent de l'expérience de la COVID-19 sur le continent africain et qui pourraient repositionner ce continent et accroître sa résilience face à la première pandémie planétaire dans un ordre mondial axé sur la technologie.

Public health reifies the penetrating interface of health with virtually all aspects of socio-economic reality. For example, access to basic necessities such as food, housing, electricity, water, recreational facilities, and other critical public infrastructure are important determinants of public health. Those all face times of reckoning during public health emergencies. Since the advent of COVID-19, many countries have adopted public health response measures aimed, primarily, at stemming its spread while, at the same time, the global race to scientifically understand its pathology and develop a viable vaccine intensifies. The earliest suspicion of the outbreak of SARS-CoV-2 in Wuhan, China, was in December 2019.[1] Compared to other regions, the virus was slower in spreading to Africa, the world's poorest and most politically susceptible continent.

Egypt confirmed the continent's first index case on February 14, 2020. On February 27, Nigeria announced the arrival of COVID-19 in Sub-Saharan Africa. Shortly after, on March 11, the World Health

1. China made official report of the virus at WHO Regional Office in Wuhan, Hubei Province, on December 31, 2019. See "Novel Coronavirus (2019-nCoV) Situation Report 1" (21 January 2020), online: *World Health Organization* <https://bit.ly/2LjofHB>.

Organization (WHO) declared COVID-19 a global pandemic. Before and within this period, as COVID-19 began to spread on the continent, African countries had—but mostly missed—the opportunity to take early preventive action.[2] Taking into account the socio-economic, cultural, and political dynamics of Africa, and drawing from publicly available information, this chapter explores Africa's experiences with selected aspects of COVID-19 public health responses. It aims, in part, to identify facets of the contextual dynamics of the continent that warrant creative and fit-for-context public health responses, outside of a one-size-fits-all milieu. Also, it identifies and reflects on some lessons and opportunities from the COVID-19 experience on the African continent that could reposition the continent and enhance its resilience in the face of the first global pandemic in a globalized world order.

Africa's Existential Socio-Economic Challenges

Africa is a heterogeneous continent of 1.2 billion people and 55 countries at different levels of development and with diverse economic and human development indicators.[3] As such, it is inaccurate to make generalizations about the continent, save to indicate that all African countries are located in the category of least developed or developing countries.[4] These countries' interconnected yet diverse historical, cultural, linguistic, religious, and colonial affinities are highly complex.[5] The majority of Africans navigate developmental aspirations within fraught and fragile socio-economic structures. In its centrality to, and interconnectedness with, socio-economic realities, public health constitutes a core dimension of the existential vulnerabilities experienced by ordinary Africans. Those tensions are now heightened by the COVID-19 pandemic.[6]

2. See Mike Onyiego, "How the Spread of the Corona Virus is Testing Africa", *BBC News* (11 April 2020), online: <https://bbc.in/2WcVBoU>.
3. "Human Development Report 2019" (2019), online (pdf): *United Nations Development Programme* <https://bit.ly/3cpyEgT>.
4. But the IMF provides a classification of Sub-Saharan African countries on basis of COVID-19 impact. See International Monetary Fund, "Regional Economic Outlook: Sub-Saharan Africa – COVID-19: An Unprecedented Threat to Development" (April 2020), online: *IMF Regional Economic Outlook* <https://bit.ly/3fGC7ti>.
5. See Daniel Chigudu, "Strength in Diversity: An Opportunity for Africa's Development" (2018) 4:1 Cogent Social Sciences 1.
6. See Tracy Bach, "A Quiet Public Health Crisis in West Africa" (21 February 2016) Vermont Law School Working Paper No 2-16.

COVID-19 Public Health Response and Related Measures[7]

For ease of analysis, and not rigour, we can classify roughly four complementary sets of anti-COVID-19 public health and economic responses. The first are measures to *regulate social and behavioural conduct*. The second are measures targeting *institutional capacity and therapeutic strategy*. The third are measures in *support of R&D efforts* aimed at development of a COVID-19 vaccine, production of pandemic necessities, and scenario management—and associated policy interventions. Fourth are mostly *financial and in-kind reliefs* targeted at members of the public and businesses to cushion them, and the broader economy, against the disruptive effects of COVID-19.

Regulation of Social and Behavioural Conduct

A strain related to SARS-CoV-1, SARS-CoV-2 is a novel virus in the Corona family of viruses. It is the cause of the COVID-19 disease. Human-to-human transmission of COVID-19 happens through transmission from an infected person's respiratory droplets and through contact with fomites infected with viable COVID-19 RNA.[8] Airborne transmission is possible in treatment settings where the COVID-19 RNA particles are captured in aerosol-generating procedures or other pressurized devices.[9] Outside of these settings, the detection of COVID-19 virus in air samples, and its viability for airborne transmission for the purposes of its classification as an airborne disease, remains, at the moment, an urgent matter of public health curiosity[10] and part of COVID-19's unclear transmission dynamic.[11]

Given the literal and figurative fluidity in the transmission of the disease, governments have implemented social and behavioural control measures. They include human movement restrictions of intra- and international scope, the latter via total or partial closures of land, air, and sea borders. Some jurisdictions have implemented curfews,

7. The online encyclopedia, Wikipedia, has a country-by-country list of measures. See "National Responses to the COVID-19 Pandemic" (last modified 11 May 2020), online: *Wikipedia* <https://bit.ly/2SXz1HF>.
8. See "Modes of Transmissions of Virus Containing COVID-19: Implications for IPC Precaution Recommendations" (29 March 2020), online: *World Health Organization* <https://bit.ly/2YVsv86>.
9. *Ibid.*
10. *Ibid.*
11. See Tao Liu et al, "Transmission Dynamics of 2019 Novel Coronavirus (2019-nCoV)" [forthcoming 2020].

or total or partial lockdowns of cities, territories, and sub-national regions. These measures are designed to slow the degree and rapidity of spread in order to minimize morbidity and mortality and to avert overwhelming fragile health infrastructures.

Because humans are super spreaders of COVID-19, self-isolation and quarantine of suspected carriers and infected persons, respectively, have also been mandated. Other measures include contact tracing of infected persons, physical or social distancing[12] in public spaces, and promotion of time-tested basic hygiene through hand-washing, other forms of hand sanitization, and disinfecting of surfaces in homes and workplaces.

These measures are part of received public health wisdom for infectious disease control.[13] However, the underlying assumptions for their viability are often taken for granted, and their implementation in African settings poses significant challenges. Among the core assumptions: that average citizens have access to credible information from public health authorities, and access to basic amenities like running water, electricity, functional accommodation, public transportation, and personal identification details. However, Sub-Saharan Africa is largely deficient in three core dimensions of the multidimensional poverty index (MPI)—health, education, and standard of living—and is also deficient in other specific MPI elements: nutrition, sanitation, drinking water, electricity, housing, and assets.[14]

Effective implementation of COVID-19 pandemic awareness, physical distancing, hand sanitation, and disinfection of surfaces are implausible in the absence of the conditions that are basic assumptions underlying infectious disease control.[15] In a multitude of African contexts, the majority of people do not have reliable access to running water, live in crowded spaces (especially the vulnerable urban and suburban slum populations), and are served by decrepit, overcrowded, and poorly regulated public transportation. Buying and selling of goods is typically conducted in open-air community markets

12. Some jurisdictions prefer "physical distancing" to "social distancing" because of the nuances in meaning of the latter and unintended connotations. For the most part, the terms are used interchangeably.
13. See Dale Weston, Katherina Hauck & Richard Amlôt, "Infection Prevention Behaviour and Infectious Disease Modelling: A Review of the Literature and Recommendations for the Future" (2018) 18:1 BMC Public Health 336.
14. *Ibid.*
15. See Chidi Oguamanam, "Africa and COVID-19" (30 March 2020), online (blog): *OpenAIR* <https://bit.ly/2xSXd6J>.

characterized by intense human traffic, close physical contact, and payments in cash. Crowding is a central feature of the daily lives of the majority of Africans.[16] Add to those, meagre housing resources and paucity of vital personal identification data. Despite expanded mobile phone penetration and internet connectivity in Africa, more than half of mobile phones have non-smart features, without internet connectivity.[17] As such, dissemination of pandemic-related information will do well to rely on non-internet-dependent devices or apps, as well as traditional media such as radio and television, notwithstanding the limited supply of electricity to power TVs.

The above examples suffice to make the point that, to be effective, COVID-19 emergency public health measures in Africa need to be tailored to specific contexts. Self-isolation is largely unviable, as is mandatory self-quarantine, and contact tracing. In this situation where physical distancing is close to impossible, wearing of face masks must be non-negotiable. But as with all behavioural prescriptions, proper use of face masks requires proactive public education, particularly for less-educated populations—another example of the necessity of context-specific approaches.

Institutional Capacity and Therapeutic Strategy; Supporting R&D

As reflected by their low rankings in both the MPI and the Human Development Index (HDI),[18] many African nations' institutional capacities in the health sector are weak. Dismal physician-patient ratios[19] persist, alongside a dearth of local specialist personnel.[20] Additionally, these nations lack the resources necessary to effectively engage in the worldwide scramble for, or domestic production of,

16. See Munyaradzi Makoni, "Keeping COVID-19 at Bay in Africa" (29 April 2020), online (pdf): The *Lancet Respiratory Medicine* <https://bit.ly/3bnkStF>.
17. See Laura Silver & Courtney Johnson, "Internet Connectivity Seen as Having a Positive Impact on Life in Sub-Saharan Africa" (2018) at 12, online (pdf): *Pew Research Centre* <https://pewrsr.ch/3bm1v4q>.
18. See United Nations Development Programme, "Human Development Index (HDI)" (last visited 11 May 2020), online: *Human Development Reports* <https://bit.ly/2WlY61j>.
19. 0.25 doctors and 1.4 hospital beds per 1000 people. See Kartik Jayram et al, "Tackling COVID-19 in Africa: An Unfolding Health and Economic Crisis That Demands Bold Action" (April 2020) at 10, online (pdf): *McKinsey & Company* <https://mck.co/2STYOAE>.
20. Such as RTI specialists, ER physicians, human virologists, environmental microbiologists, etc.

COVID-19 supplies such as test kits, ventilators, and professional-grade personal protective equipment (PPE). Accordingly, global public health analysts worry that Africa may be overrun by COVID-19.[21] In a headline-catching remark, Melinda Gates stated in April 2020 that "[t]he disease is going to bite hard on the continent. I see some dead bodies in the streets of Africa."[22]

With the world's lowest levels of per capita health expenditure, and with underdeveloped health sectors, most African nations' path of least resistance in fighting the pandemic lies in early preventive action more than in therapeutic or management measures. However, the opportunity for early action has, in many countries, been missed—at least in respect of the first wave. Working in the continent's favour, however, are its past experiences with infectious diseases and public health emergencies.[23] Also, necessity is the time-tested incubator of innovation. Thus, the prognosis for Africa does not necessarily have to be bleak.[24] Africans are capitalizing on new technologies, such as 3D printing and drones, to localize and scale responses to COVID-19. South African innovators have invented the intubox (intubation box), which provides an additional layer of protection for ICU medical personnel conducting and monitoring intubation procedures.[25] Nigeria's military R&D has been brought to bear on production of ventilators and PPE, using local materials.[26] South African and Ugandan military and law enforcement personnel have been deployed to deliver relief supplies to the vulnerable.[27]

21. See International Monetary Fund, *supra* note 4; McKinsey & Company, *supra* note 19.
22. See Africa Check, "Melinda Gates Said She Feared Coronavirus in Africa Would Lead to Dead Being Put Out in Street, as in Ecuador" (20 April 2020), online: *Africa Check* <https://bit.ly/2YSCMBT>.
23. See Esther Yie Mokuwa et al, "Covid-19: What Africa Can Learn from Africa – Community Care Centres" (17 April 2020), online: *African Arguments* <https://bit.ly/3c92c2o>.
24. *Ibid.*
25. See "S. African Doctors Design Virus 'Box' to Prevent Infection", *France24* (16 April 2020), online: <https://bit.ly/3ca6IgF>.
26. See "Nigerian Military Begins Mass Production of Ventilators, PPE Kits" (21 April 2020), online: *Nigerian Investment Promotion Commission* <https://bit.ly/2xCNkdc>.
27. See South African Government, Media Statement, "Defence on Reserve Force Call Up to Combat Coronavirus COVID-19" (23 April 2020), online: *South African Government Newsroom* <https://bit.ly/2SF4jCU>; Shi Yinglun "Uganda Starts Food Relief Distribution Amid COVID-19 Lockdown", *Xinhuanet* (4 April 2020), online: <https://bit.ly/2Ww6SbQ>.

In several nations, including Ghana, Nigeria, and Kenya, local fabric and garment industries have been repurposed to mass produce face masks.[28] Ghana is using drones to transport test samples from hinterland areas to the main cities for analysis.[29] Drawing from experience in fighting Dengue fever and Ebola, a Senegalese laboratory is producing a COVID-19 diagnostic testing kit at the cost of approximately US$1,[30] giving the country the capacity to test every citizen and to support other countries. Senegalese innovators are also using 3D printing to produce ventilators at cost of US$60, while imported ventilators cost roughly US$16,000.[31] As of early May 2020, Senegal was believed to have the highest rate of recovery of COVID-19 patients in Africa, and to have the third-best rate globally.[32] While Madagascar's Artemisia-based tea, being hastily marketed as a "cure" by the government under the name Covid-Organics, is the subject of scientific skepticism[33] and requiring prudence, it nonetheless draws attention to the potential role of Africa's genetic resources and traditional knowledge in COVID-19-related R&D.[34] Many African countries are demonstrating commitment to the search for credible and affordable solutions via both traditional knowledge and cutting-edge R&D.[35] Africans are striving to take their destinies into their own hands in attacking COVID-19. But time is in short supply.

Social and Economic Reliefs for Individuals and Businesses

Governments the world over have implemented an extensive range of COVID-19 social and economic palliative measures. In developed

28. See Oluwadamilare Akinpelu "COVID-19: Entrepreneurs in Nigeria, Ghana, Kenya Begin Mass Surgical Mask Production", *Technext* (9 April 2020), online: <https://bit.ly/2yCjlm6>.
29. Alex Davies "Drones Take Flight to Carry Covid-19 Tests to Labs in Africa", *Wired* (22 April 2020), online <https://bit.ly/2SX9zlB>.
30. Nigel Roberts "Senegalese Lab Uses Expertise to Develop $1 Coronavirus Testing Kit", *BET* (4 April 2020), online: <https://bet.us/35EHnZZ>.
31. *Ibid.*
32. *Ibid.*
33. See "Coronavirus: Caution Urged over Madagascar's 'Herbal Cure'", *BBC News* (22 April 2020), online: <https://bbc.in/2SHaJS1>.
34. After initial reluctance, the WHO has endorsed a clinical trial of Covid-Organic with a promise to collaborate. See Felix Thi "WHO Calls for Clinic Trial of Madagascar's Virus Cure", *Anadolu Agency* (7 May 2020), online: <https://bit.ly/2ywcdIe>.
35. See "Ewu Monastery Develops CVD Plus for the Treatment of COVID-19", *RealNews Magazine* (30 April 2020), online: <https://bit.ly/3ftIO1J>.

countries, such measures have been aimed at cushioning the pandemic's wide-ranging disruptive effects on citizens rendered unemployed and/or constrained by lockdowns and other restrictive ordinances; and on various categories of enterprises, including large corporations, which have direct negative exposure to the impacts of the virus. These largely ad hoc measures have severely tested the policymaking ingenuity, administrative flexibility, bureaucratic efficiency, and fiscal stability of developed-world governments. Central to these governments' capacities has been the availability of reliable data necessary to identify, and deliver palliatives to, qualifying demographics. Most African nations, even in ordinary times, have precarious public finances,[36] with limited fiscal space to absorb shocks. COVID-19 disruptions have hit African mono-product economies extremely hard; for example, severe oil price drops have fiscally destabilized Nigeria, Africa's largest economy.[37] Elaborate social and economic palliatives are beyond the reach of most African countries' fiscal capacity. Even the negligible palliatives some countries are able to administer[38] are bogged down in controversy and bureaucracy.[39] In the majority of countries, there is limited socio-economic data for public administration necessary to identify those in dire straits and in need of reliefs. About 85% of Sub-Saharan Africans are informal economic operators who must go out on a daily basis to earn cash, or harvest food, needed to feed their households.[40] There is a dearth of the credible data needed to identify and reach vulnerable individuals and households in a targeted, meaningful fashion. Of the estimated 89 million Nigerians living in chronic poverty, only 3.6 million (according to the government) are targeted in the "social register" of people eligible for COVID-19 palliatives.[41]

---

36. See International Monetary Fund, *supra* note 4; McKinsey & Company, *supra* note 19; "Trade Policies for Africa to Tackle Covid-19" (27 March 2020), online (pdf): *United Nations Economic Commission for Africa* <https://bit.ly/2STpu4m>.
37. *Ibid.*
38. See International Monetary Fund, *supra* note 4 at 9.
39. See Obinna Onwujekwe, "Coronavirus: Corruption in Health Care Could Get in the Way of Nigeria's Response", *The Conversation* (4 May 2020), online: <https://bit.ly/2W7Ox5U>.
40. See Faure Essozimna Gnassingbe "Mobile Cash is the Best Way to Help Africa Fight Covid-19", *Financial Times* (12 April 2020), online: <https://on.ft.com/3c6gDE5>.
41. See "Buhari Expands Social Register from 2.6m Households to 3.6m", *The Guardian Nigeria News* (13 April 2020), online: <https://bit.ly/35NgP91>.

COVID-19 Ordinances, Law Enforcement, and Civil Liberty

Most African countries have historical legacies of dictatorship. Even in the best of times, civil liberties in Africa are fraught. Since the 1990s, most of these nations have transitioned to fledgling, fragile democracies.[42] COVID-19 emergency ordinances have resulted in many citizens across the continent being subjected to overzealous law enforcement personnel undermining the rule of law.[43] In some cases, citizens have been murdered.[44] Draconian law enforcement and legislative power grabs of various guises have crept into the polity on the back of COVID-19.[45] Details of rapidly rolled out emergency ordinances have been foggy, as they are not broadly disseminated at the time of enforcement. And access to legal services has been truncated.[46] The result is that, in many cases, the most vulnerable are victimized several times over—a dynamic that needs to be fully documented and exposed in order to eliminate impunity, whereby civil liberties are violated in the name of public health in a pandemic.[47]

Lessons, Opportunities in the Gloom of COVID-19

COVID-19 has shaken the foundation of global public health, exposed both the fragility of industrialized countries' pandemic preparedness and a moment of vacuum in global leadership, caused chiefly by the palpable abdication of the U.S. and its ongoing blame game with China. Among other considerations, those have undermined the institutional effectiveness of the WHO and related organizations. One

---

42. See Landry Signe, "The Tortuous Trajectories of Democracy and the Persistence of Authoritarianism in Africa" (2013) Stanford Center on Democracy, Development and the Rule of Law Working Paper 147, online: *SSRN* <https://ssrn.com/abstract=2237354>.
43. See "UN Raises Alarm About Police Brutality in COVID-19 Lockdowns", *Al Jazeera* (28 April 2020), online: <https://bit.ly/3bp63Xs>.
44. *Ibid.*
45. See Dima Samaro & Emna Sayadi, "Tunisia's Parliament on COVID-19; an Initiative to Fight Disinformation or an Opportunity to Violate Fundamental Rights?", *Access Now* (1 April 2020), online: <https://bit.ly/2SDXfq7>; Adamu Abuh et al, "Pressure Mounts on Reps to Suspend Infectious Disease Bill", *The Guardian Nigeria News* (5 May 2020), online: <https://bit.ly/2SGapTO>.
46. See "Lockdown: Lawyers Sue FG, Demand Categorization of Legal Practice as Essential Service", *Vanguard News Nigeria* (5 May 2020), online: <https://bit.ly/2YAjVLY>.
47. See Oluchi Aniaka, "Law and Ethics of Ebola Outbreak in Nigeria" (2014), online (pdf): *SSRN* <https://bit.ly/2AdM15q>.

result has been to delay focus on a global approach to COVID-19. The absence of concerted international solidarity to contain COVID-19 in Africa will render the entire world vulnerable. However, several lessons and opportunities for Africa can be sketched from the current realities and experiences.

First, reliance on external intervention will not optimally tap the continent's potential for resilience. African nations collectively need to leverage their variegated capacities, and experiences with infectious disease control, and to regionally scale the national response successes in Senegal and elsewhere referenced above.

Second, a copy-and-paste adoption of emergency responses crafted outside the continent will not effectively serve African realities. Adaptive approaches to emergency response measures, including extra vigilance on matters of civil liberties and rule of law, are important.

Third, COVID-19 demonstrates the core need for credible data as a governance tool in order to identify and support vulnerable demographics.

Fourth, pending improved governance over the use of data, Africa's endowment in community mobilization through religious and cultural networks, including increasingly important diaspora outreach, have demonstrable capacity to fill the gaps in government's failure to reach the most vulnerable.[48] These actors need to be more creatively integrated into African nations' fledgling social safety nets and protocols.[49]

Fifth, further growth in use of mobile money and mobile payment systems needs to be fostered, since electronic transactions do not carry the virus-spreading risks posed by physical handling of cash.[50]

Sixth, despite the current weakening of global institutional public health interventionist bodies and the tenuousness of international comity, Africa needs to strengthen its own regional health bodies as important pathways to scaling and dispersal of R&D efforts.

48. The African union recognizes the diaspora as Africa's 6th regional category, an evidence of the role and potential of that demographic in development. See Carine K Nantulya & Dewa Mavhinga, "Africa's Covid-19 Response Should Focus on People's Needs, Rights" (16 April 2020), online: *Human Rights Watch* <https://bit.ly/2xHYU6S>.

49. See Gift Dafuleya "Explainer, Why COVID-19 Provides a Lesson for Africa to Fund Social Assistance", *The Conversation* (3 May 2020), online: <https://bit.ly/2yrqLc6>.

50. See Gnassingbe, *supra* note 40.

Seventh, as a related matter, a harmonization of regional and national institutional health capacities is necessary to prepare the continent to participate in the local production of a COVID-19 vaccine under, hopefully, a global public good model.[51]

Such strengthened internal capacity will also leave African nations better positioned to negotiate the strategic fiscal relief from international creditors that will be necessary to cushion African national economies against COVID-19's devastating toll.

---

51. See Maci Kennedy McDade et al, "Aligning Multilateral Support for Global Public Goods for Health Under Global Action Plan" (2019) Duke Global Working Paper Series No 2019/15, online: *SSRN* <https://papers.ssrn.com/sol3/papers.cfm?abstract_id=3448704>.

CHAPTER F-4

Border Closures: A Pandemic of Symbolic Acts in the Time of COVID-19

Steven J. Hoffman* and Patrick Fafard**

Abstract

COVID-19 provoked unprecedented national border closures. Some countries stopped travel from particular regions, despite evidence that such closures are ineffective and illegal under the International Health Regulations (IHRs). Even more countries banned all incoming travel by non-citizens. It has been suggested that these more restrictive total border closures are theoretically effective and arguably permissible under international law. Yet a closer analysis reveals that total border closures are probably still illegal given the IHRs require countries to adopt less restrictive alternatives when possible, such as a 14-day quarantine order for incoming travellers. If border closures are largely ineffective and illegal, then why have at least 142 countries implemented them? The answer lies in the realities of politics. Even if governments know the science and law of border closures, they still feel compelled to enact them because of intense domestic pressure

* Dahdaleh Distinguished Chair in Global Governance and Legal Epidemiology, and Professor of Global Health, Law, and Political Science at York University, the Director of the Global Strategy Lab, the Director of the World Health Organization Collaborating Centre on Global Governance of Antimicrobial Resistance, and the Scientific Director of the CIHR Institute of Population and Public Health at the Canadian Institutes of Health Research.

** Full Professor in the Graduate School of Public and International Affairs at the University of Ottawa.

and to avoid blame for not acting. Therefore, border closures are best regarded as powerful symbolic acts that help governments show they are acting forcefully, even if these actions are not epidemiologically helpful and even if they breach international law. As a result, citizens should be critical of border closures when these symbolic acts are motivated by political advantage without regard to immense collateral damage.

Résumé

Fermetures des frontières : une pandémie d'actes symboliques en temps de COVID-19

La COVID-19 a provoqué des fermetures de frontières nationales sans précédent. Des pays ont interdit les entrées en provenance de certaines régions, bien qu'il soit prouvé que de telles restrictions sont inefficaces et illégales en vertu du Règlement sanitaire international. Un nombre encore plus élevé de pays ont suspendu toute arrivée sur leur territoire des non-citoyens. Ces fermetures totales des frontières, plus restrictives, sont théoriquement efficaces et vraisemblablement autorisées par le droit international. Pourtant, une analyse plus approfondie révèle qu'elles sont probablement illégales puisque le Règlement sanitaire international exige des pays qu'ils adoptent des solutions moins contraignantes lorsque cela est possible, comme une ordonnance de quarantaine de 14 jours pour les voyageurs entrants. Si la fermeture des frontières est largement inefficace et illégale, alors pourquoi est-ce qu'au moins 142 pays y ont eu recours ? La réponse se trouve dans les réalités du monde politique. Même si les gouvernements sont au fait des données scientifiques et des lois en matière de fermeture des frontières, ils se sentent obligés de la décréter en raison d'une pression intérieure intense et pour éviter d'être blâmés pour leur inaction. Par conséquent, une telle fermeture doit être considérée comme un geste symbolique puissant qui permet aux gouvernements de démontrer qu'ils agissent avec force, même si ces actions ne sont pas utiles sur le plan épidémiologique et même si elles contreviennent au droit international. Les citoyens devraient donc se montrer critiques à l'égard de la fermeture des frontières lorsqu'un tel acte symbolique est dicté par un intérêt politique, sans égard aux nombreux dommages collatéraux.

With global infectious disease outbreaks comes pressure on national governments to close their borders to citizens or residents of affected countries. Too many governments give way to this pressure. Border closures against high-risk regions, implemented by dozens of countries within the first two months of the COVID-19 outbreak (see Figure F4.1), isolate vulnerable communities, devastate fragile economies, and disincentivize affected governments from reporting new cases of disease. Targeted border closures also violate the International Health Regulations (IHR)—the legally binding instrument that governs how 196 countries respond to pandemics like COVID-19—and that in turn undermines our global public health system and the rules-based world order on which we depend.[1]

This chapter takes a critical look at national border closures in the time of COVID-19. After explaining why targeted border closures do not work and how they violate international law, we examine the more complicated case of total border closures and present the quarantining of incoming travellers as a reasonably available less restrictive alternative that is likely to be equally effective. We end by asking why nearly every government has implemented some form of border closure, if most are not supported by science or law. We conclude that border closures represent an irresistible opportunity for political leaders to show they are doing something and to redirect blame outside their jurisdiction. Such political theatre of symbolic acts means that citizens must contest and challenge border closures as they would any other questionable government action. Citizens must not unduly defer to scientists or lawyers on COVID-19 border closures because these are primarily political—not scientific or legal—decisions.

Targeted Border Closures Are Ineffective

In theory, targeted border closures are intended to prevent all incoming travel by people who might have been exposed to a pathogen, who might be carrying it, and who might transmit that pathogen to others. If people from affected areas cannot leave their country, then

1. Roojin Habibi et al, "Do Not Violate the International Health Regulations During the COVID-19 Outbreak" (2020) 395:10225 The Lancet 664 [Habibi]; Steven J Hoffman & Roojin Habibi, "Opinion: Canada Should Not Join Other Countries in Instituting Travel Restrictions – Or in Breaking International Law", *The Globe and Mail* (11 March 2020), online: <https://www.theglobeandmail.com/opinion/article-canada-should-not-join-other-countries-in-instituting-travel/>.

it is reasoned that other countries will be safe from the pathogen, as there is no human vector through which the pathogen can travel.

Border closures, unfortunately, are not so simple. The reality is that people will find a way to travel to their destination if they really need or want to do so, either by first travelling to a third country, or by travelling through unofficial channels. The former increases the global risk by increasing the distance and segments of travel. The latter makes it more difficult to identify individuals infected by the pathogen and trace those with whom they came into contact. There is also usually a gap between the time when governments announce border closures and when they can be implemented, provoking an immediate surge in travel that increases the risk of infectious disease transmission, alongside the chaos that comes with sudden stampedes of travellers.[2]

The best available empirical research evidence also supports the view that targeted border closures are likely to be ineffective.[3] For example: temporary flight bans in the United States after the September 11, 2001 terrorist attacks did not stop or diminish that season's influenza outbreak;[4] travel restrictions imposed by several countries against Mexico during the 2009 H1N1 influenza outbreak reduced travel by 40% but only delayed the virus's arrival in other countries by less than three days;[5] and epidemiologic simulations of H5N1 avian influenza found that even a 90% reduction in travel through border closures would merely slow that virus's spread by a few days to weeks in the implementing country.[6]

Case data from the first four months of the COVID-19 outbreak show that countries with targeted border closures against high-risk regions have fared no better than countries without targeted border

---

2. Doug Saunders, "Why Travel Bans Fail to Stop Pandemics", *Foreign Affairs* (15 May 2020), online: <https://www.foreignaffairs.com/articles/canada/2020-05-15/why-travel-bans-fail-stop-pandemics>.
3. Nicole A Errett, Lauren M Sauer & Lainie Rutkow, "An Integrative Review of the Limited Evidence on International Travel Bans as an Emerging Infectious Disease Disaster Control Measure" (2020) 18:1 Journal of Emergency Management 7; Ali Tejpar & Steven J Hoffman, "Canada's Violation of International Law during the 2014-16 Ebola Outbreak" (2017) 54 Canadian Yearbook of International Law 366.
4. John S Brownstein, Cecily J Wolfe & Kenneth D Mandl, "Empirical Evidence for the Effect of Airline Travel on Inter-Regional Influenza Spread in the United States" (2006) 3:10 PLoS Med 1826 at 1832.
5. Paolo Bajardi et al, "Human Mobility Networks, Travel Restrictions, and the Global Spread of 2009 H1N1 Pandemic" (2011) 6:1 PLoS ONE 1.
6. Timothy C Germann et al, "Mitigation Strategies for Pandemic Influenza in the United States" (2006) 103:15 Proceedings of the National Academy of Sciences 5935 at 5938.

closures (see Figures F4.2 and F4.3). A simple fixed-effects regression confirms that enacting targeted border closures at any period during the outbreak is not statistically associated with fewer cases of COVID-19 ($F(1,160) = 1.23$, $p = 0.268$, within $R^2 = 0.0077$) or fewer deaths ($F(1,160) = 1.49$, $p = 0.223$, within $R^2 = 0.0054$).[7]

Targeted Border Closures Are Illegal

In addition to their likely ineffectiveness, targeted border closures are also illegal. According to Article 43 of the International Health Regulations (see Box F4.1), countries are only permitted to enact "additional health measures" limiting travel during pandemics if such measures are 1) supported by science, 2) proportionate to the risks involved, and 3) respectful of human rights.[8] These three conditions are intended to protect people and economies from needless harm and to avoid disincentivizing governments from alerting the World Health Organization (WHO) to new public health risks when first identified.[9]

The targeted COVID-19 border closures do not fulfil these three requirements.[10] As described above, the science around targeted travel restrictions points against their effectiveness; research on previous outbreaks of similar viruses suggests that these restrictions typically delay their spread by only a few days. Second, targeted border closures are not proportionate to the risks involved, especially given that there are better strategies for addressing the COVID-19 outbreak, such as screening at airports, community surveillance, and public communication. Third, targeted border closures may violate human

7. In the fixed-effects regression model, each country is treated as an individual subject with repeated measures. A dummy variable was included to reflect whether a country had implemented a targeted border closure on any given day. Two statistical analyses were conducted, one with COVID-19 cases as the dependent variable of interest and a second with COVID-19-attributed deaths as the dependent variable. The F-statistic indicates model fit; neither model's results are statistically significant. The very low within R^2 value indicates that little variation in the dependent variables was explained by the enactment of targeted border closures across countries. All data were from: Max Roser et al, "Coronavirus Pandemic (COVID-19)" (last updated 26 May 2020), online: *Our World in Data* <https://ourworldindata.org/coronavirus-data-explorer> [Roser].
8. World Health Organization, "International Health Regulations (2005)" (2005), online (pdf): *World Health Organization* <http://www.who.int/ihr/publications/9789241580496/en/>.
9. Habibi, *supra* note 1.
10. *Ibid.*

rights obligations when they unfairly discriminate against those who appear to be from the most affected countries. As described by Jamie Liew in Chapter D-7 of this book, these travel restrictions may be more about pacifying fears of racialized persons, reinforcing racism and xenophobia, than anything else.

Total Border Closures Are Possibly Legal But Probably Illegal

While it is clear that targeted border closures are illegal under the International Health Regulations, more uncertain is the international legal status of total border closures that have been enacted by at least 113 countries, including Brazil, Canada, France, Germany, Russia, and South Africa.[11] Whereas targeted border closures limit travel from particular countries perceived as high-risk, total border closures ban inbound travellers from all countries.

At first glance, many people might understand total border closures to be even more restrictive than targeted border closures and as such assume that they would be just as illegal under Article 43 of the International Health Regulations. Yet the purpose of the Article 43 limitations on travel restrictions was to avoid unnecessarily amplifying the economic and social consequences of public health risks in affected countries, and to avoid disincentivizing all countries from reporting risks when they appear. Indeed, countries are naturally less likely to report a new infectious disease outbreak in their jurisdiction if they are worried about facing targeted border closures that do not typically work anyway. But total border closures do not primarily or only punish specific affected countries; rather, most costs from total border closures are endured by the citizens and economies of the country that enacts them. Because of that dynamic, total border closures were neither anticipated nor specified by the International Health Regulations. Indeed, the 196 countries that are parties to the instrument may not have intended to prevent total border closures if a time came when such closures were desired.

Even if this purposive interpretive argument does not pass muster, countries enacting total border closures could still point to the absence of opposing scientific evidence as a rationale in defence. Thereby, they can skirt the first condition on additional health measures imposed by

11. Our World in Data, "International Travel Controls During the COVID-19 Pandemic" (last visited 25 May 2020), online: *Our World in Data* <https://ourworldindata.org/grapher/international-travel-covid>.

Article 43 of the International Health Regulations. Specifically, countries could argue that there is no scientific evidence either way on the effectiveness of total border closures. Previous studies have evaluated targeted border closures, not total border closures. And this COVID-19 outbreak is additionally unique in how much of the world's international travel stopped in such a short period of time. Indeed, even if there were studies showing that total border closures did not work, there is still a possibility that they would work in these extraordinary times. A country could potentially argue that the constrained travel environment during the COVID-19 outbreak may make total border closures effective by reducing the viability of incoming travel via third countries and unofficial channels.

Besides, while it makes good sense for an instrument like the International Health Regulations to prevent countries from punishing others with unjustifiable targeted border closures, the international legal principle of sovereignty protects the ability of countries to close their borders.[12] The Article 43 limitation on additional health measures in the International Health Regulations must then be read more narrowly to only prevent countries from enacting border closures when they have discriminatory effects on other countries. This means that non-discriminatory total border closures could be legal under international law, even when the less restrictive but discriminatory targeted border closures are clearly illegal.

All of that being said, if total border closures are enacted for public health reasons, then, according to Article 43.1 of the International Health Regulations, countries must still ensure that "such measures shall not be more restrictive of international traffic and not more invasive or intrusive to persons than reasonably available alternatives that would achieve the appropriate level of health protection."[13] This provision means that countries are obliged to deploy less restrictive border measures if they are available and if they would attain comparable health protection in a non-discriminatory way. Those countries that do not deploy less restrictive measures when they are able to effectively do so would be violating international law.

12. Samantha Besson, "Sovereignty" (last updated April 2011), online: *Oxford Public International Law* <https://opil.ouplaw.com/view/10.1093/law:epil/9780199231690/law-9780199231690-e1472>; Steven J Hoffman, "The Evolution, Etiology and Eventualities of the Global Health Security Regime" (2010) 25:6 Health Policy Plan 510.

13. World Health Organization, *supra* note 8.

Mandatory Quarantine Is a Less Restrictive Alternative

For many countries, a reasonably available alternative to total border closures would be to temporarily quarantine all people entering a country. This policy option compels all incoming travellers to isolate for the maximum incubation period of COVID-19 (for example, 14 days)[14] so that potentially asymptomatic and pre-symptomatic cases can safely be identified without the risk of spreading the SARS-CoV-2 virus to others. This option builds on a proven intervention—quarantine[15]—and is non-discriminatory in terms of race, ethnicity, sex, gender, citizenship, residency, and other factors (although, of course, the downstream consequences of quarantine disproportionately affect people facing conditions of marginalization, including poverty, homelessness, disability, racism, and xenophobia). This means that temporarily quarantining all travellers coming into a country would likely meet the Article 43 conditions, in that this measure is supported by science, proportionate to the risks involved, and respectful of human rights.

Would temporarily quarantining all incoming travellers for 14 days be equally as effective as completely closing the border? Probably, at least so long as quarantine measures were fully implemented and enforced. Indeed, previous studies highlight that the vast majority of citizens in democratic societies comply with public health orders when they make logical sense, when their value is properly explained, and when they have the means to safely do so.[16] Governments can additionally promote compliance by requiring travellers to have credible quarantine plans, sequestering travellers without credible plans to government-run quarantine sites, randomly auditing compliance, zealously prosecuting violators, bringing public attention to prosecutions, and advertising steep punishments for violating quarantine orders.

Not every government has the bureaucratic capacity to implement this more nuanced border measure. But most wealthier countries should have the needed capacity, and all countries can attempt

14. Stephen A Lauer et al, "The Incubation Period of Coronavirus Disease 2019 (COVID-19) from Publicly Reported Confirmed Cases: Estimation and Application" (2020) 172:9 Annals of Internal Medicine 577.
15. Barbara Nussbaumer-Streit et al, "Quarantine Alone or in Combination With Other Public Health Measures to Control COVID-19: A Rapid Review" (2020) 4 Cochrane Database of Systematic Reviews.
16. R K Webster et al, "How to Improve Adherence with Quarantine: Rapid Review of the Evidence" (2020) 182 Public Health 163.

this approach either before or simultaneous to total border closures, the latter of which can later be lifted if the quarantining of all incoming travellers proves effective and feasible. Assuming so, this approach represents a reasonably available alternative that would achieve the appropriate level of health protection in a less restrictive and non-discriminatory manner—meaning that Article 43.1 of the International Health Regulations would legally require national governments to make use of this alternative instead of total border closures, if it is feasible to do so.

Border Closures Are Symbolic Acts to Avoid Blame

If targeted border closures are ineffective and illegal, and if total border closures are only theoretically effective and probably illegal, then why have at least 142 countries implemented one of these border control measures?

The answer lies in the realities of politics. Even if governments know the science and international law of border closures, they will still feel compelled to enact them because of intense pressure from powerful domestic political actors who might otherwise blame them for not taking every possible action. Such criticism could come from opposition parties, sub-national governments, civil society organizations, academics, and/or journalists, depending on the political institutions of a society and how they give voice to and structure criticism. For example, political pressure to enact border closures may be particularly intense in those countries with federal structures, wherein sub-national governments may look for opportunities to assign blame to the national government, as it controls national borders. The same logic is true for countries with multi-party systems and freedom of the press. The ruling party may feel pressure to implement border closures to deny their political adversaries and the media the opportunity to criticize them, particularly during an election year. Even more pressure would be faced by national leaders with all three political institutions—a federal structure, multi-party system, and press freedoms—like Canada, which was indeed one of the earlier countries to enact a total border closure, on March 18, 2020 (see Figure F4-1).[17]

17. Justin Trudeau, News Release, "Prime Minister Announces New Actions Under Canada's COVID-19 Response" (March 16 2020), online: *Justin Trudeau, Prime Minister of Canada* <https://pm.gc.ca/en/news/news-releases/2020/03/16/prime-minister-announces-new-actions-under-canadas-covid-19-response>.

Therefore, in the context of a pandemic as significant and unprecedented as COVID-19, border closures are best regarded as powerful symbolic acts that help governments show they are acting forcefully, even if these actions are not epidemiologically helpful and even if they breach international law. Broad dramatic gestures like border closures can garner political support independent of whether they are effective or legal. Such symbolic acts become ever more instrumentally important—and politically valuable—the more a government feels it has insufficient knowledge, tools, or options to address the actual problem it faces in a way that will satisfy the demands of its citizens and critics.

Furthermore, border closures have the additional political advantage of implicitly assigning blame for the health emergency to people or governments outside of one's own country. They discourage citizens from reflecting on the frailty of their own country's public health system or the consequences of past policy choices, like insufficient public health investment, that have led to their vulnerability.

The reality of border closures as blame-avoiding symbolic acts means that these decisions must be subject to the usual political contestation that comes with political decisions in democratic societies. To avoid such political contestation is to deny the accountability of political leaders. The challenge we have seen in the current COVID-19 pandemic is that governments have justified their border closures by citing expert advice apparently received from epidemiologists and legal counsel. Essentially, political leaders have sought public support for their border closures by asking citizens to defer to government scientists and lawyers. But, of course, these decisions are not based only on science or law. They are political. And as a result, citizens must not acquiesce uncritically. Deferring to government leaders and other authorities on border closures, even in a pandemic emergency, undermines the systems of political accountability on which democracies depend. Citizens owe it to themselves to be critical of governments when they take symbolic action for political advantage without regard to immense collateral damage.

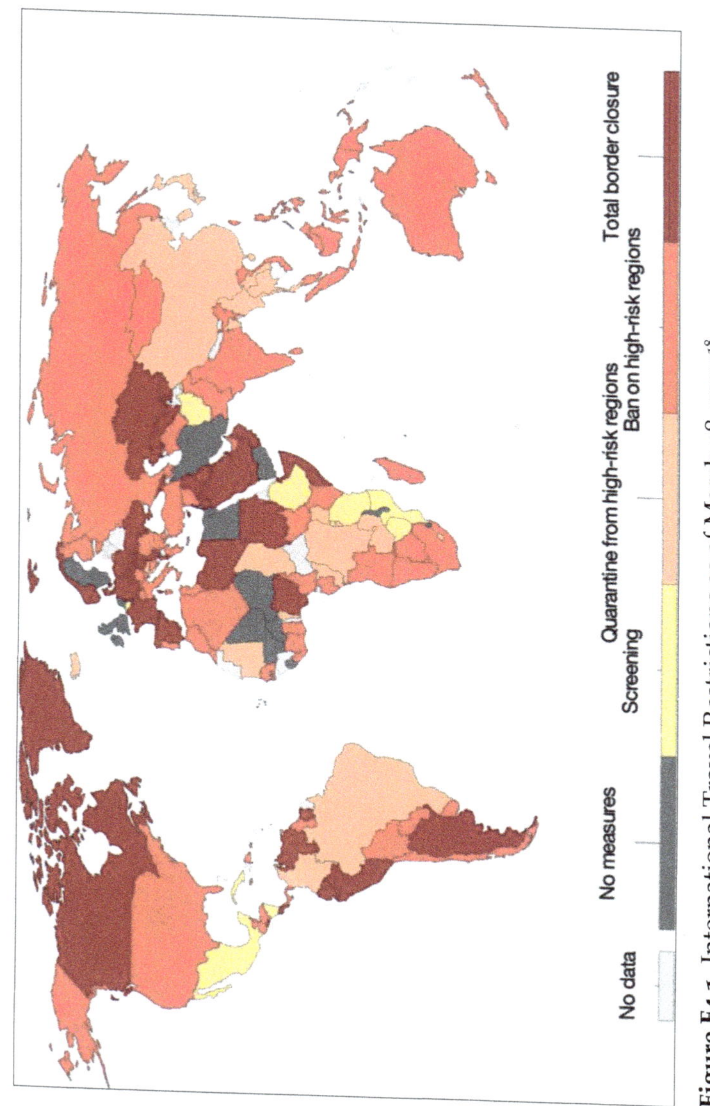

Figure F4.1 International Travel Restrictions as of March 18, 2020[18]

Source: Max Roser et al, "Coronavirus Pandemic (COVID-19)" (last updated 26 May 2020), online: Our World in Data <https://ourworldindata.org/coronavirus-data-explorer> [Roser].

18. Roser, *supra* note 7.

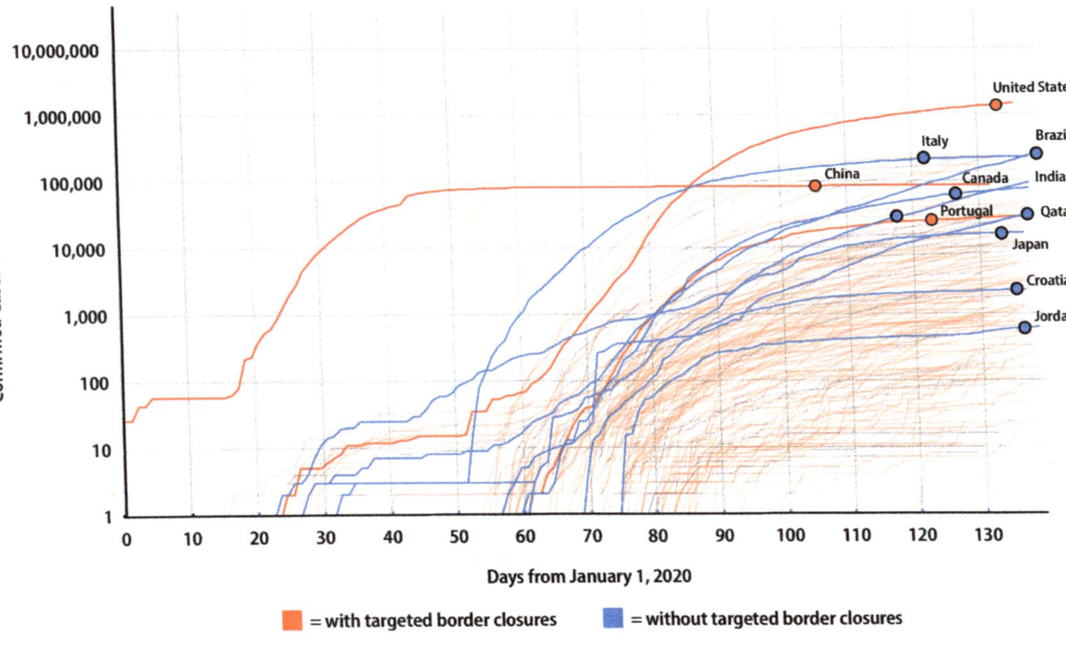

Figure F4.2 COVID-19 Cases in Countries With and Without Targeted Border Closures Against High-Risk Regions[19]

Source: Max Roser et al, "Coronavirus Pandemic (COVID-19)" (last updated 26 May 2020), online: Our World in Data <https://ourworldindata.org/coronavirus-data-explorer> [Roser].

19. *Ibid.*

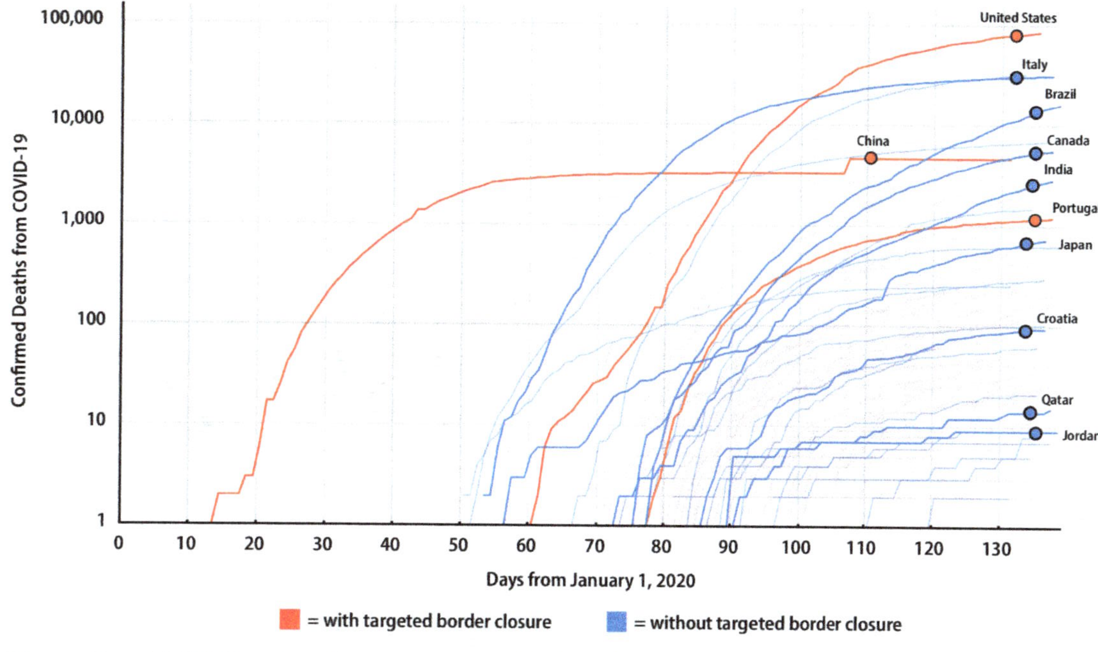

Figure F4.3 COVID-19 Deaths in Countries With and Without Targeted Border Closures Against High-Risk Regions[20]

Source: Max Roser et al, "Coronavirus Pandemic (COVID-19)" (last updated 26 May 2020), online: Our World in Data <https://ourworldindata.org/coronavirus-data-explorer> [Roser].

20. *Ibid.*

Explanation for Figure F4.1: As early as March 18, 2020, 18 countries had mandated quarantines for incoming travellers from high-risk regions like China, 55 countries had imposed bans against travel from high-risk regions, and 37 countries had enacted total border closures. March 18, 2020, was chosen as the map's date of reference because several countries enacted total border closures on that day, including Canada, Georgia, Oman, Venezuela, and Somalia. Two months later, on May 18, 2020, 14 countries had quarantines for travellers from high-risk regions, 29 countries had bans against travel from these regions, and 113 countries had total border closures.

Explanation for Figures F4.2 and F4.3: Countries with targeted border closures against incoming travellers from high-risk regions (red) have fared no better than countries without targeted border closures (blue).

Box F4.1 International Health Regulations (2005)

Article 43 on Additional Health Measures[21]

43.1. These Regulations shall not preclude States Parties from implementing health measures, in accordance with their relevant national law and obligations under international law, in response to specific public health risks or public health emergencies of international concern, which:

a. achieve the same or greater level of health protection than WHO recommendations; or

b. are otherwise prohibited under Article 25, Article 26, paragraphs 1 and 2 of Article 28, Article 30, paragraph 1(c) of Article 31 and Article 33, provided such measures are otherwise consistent with these Regulations.

Such measures shall not be more restrictive of international traffic and not more invasive or intrusive to persons than reasonably available alternatives that would achieve the appropriate level of health protection.

43.2. In determining whether to implement the health measures referred to in paragraph 1 of this Article or additional health measures under paragraph 2 of Article 23, paragraph 1 of Article 27, paragraph 2 of Article 28 and paragraph 2(c) of Article 31, States Parties shall base their determinations upon:

21. World Health Organization, *supra* note 8.

a. scientific principles;
b. available scientific evidence of a risk to human health, or where such evidence is insufficient, the available information including from WHO and other relevant intergovernmental organizations and international bodies; and
c. any available specific guidance or advice from WHO.

43.3. A State Party implementing additional health measures referred to in paragraph 1 of this Article which significantly interfere with international traffic shall provide to WHO the public health rationale and relevant scientific information for it. WHO shall share this information with other States Parties and shall share information regarding the health measures implemented. For the purpose of this Article, significant interference generally means refusal of entry or departure of international travellers, baggage, cargo, containers, conveyances, goods, and the like, or their delay, for more than 24 hours.

43.4. After assessing information provided pursuant to paragraphs 3 and 5 of this Article and other relevant information, WHO may request that the State Party concerned reconsider the application of the measures.

43.5. A State Party implementing additional health measures referred to in paragraphs 1 and 2 of this Article that significantly interfere with international traffic shall inform WHO, within 48 hours of implementation, of such measures and their health rationale unless these are covered by a temporary or standing recommendation.

CHAPTER F-5

COVID-19 and Accountable Artificial Intelligence in a Global Context

Céline Castets-Renard* and Eleonore Fournier-Tombs**

Abstract

This chapter identifies two of the key elements in accountable artificial intelligence infrastructure globally—ethical modelling and responsible data. The chapter takes a global perspective and highlights issues of particular relevance to countries that were already in humanitarian crises, such as food insecurity and conflict, explaining how these play into the way that epidemiological models should be constructed. Furthermore, it examines vulnerability from the perspective of aid recipients and migrants, to evoke the type of guidelines and laws that should be taken into account for data protection and privacy.

Résumé

La COVID-19 et l'intelligence artificielle responsable dans un contexte mondial

Ce chapitre aborde deux des principaux éléments d'une infrastructure d'intelligence artificielle responsable à l'échelle mondiale : la

* Full Professor of Law at the Faculty Law (Civil Law Section) of the University of Ottawa, and member of the Center of Law, Technology and Society.

** Senior data scientist focusing on anticipatory financing of humanitarian crisis, on joint appointment at UNOCHA's Centre for Humanitarian Data and the World Bank's Disaster Risk Financing Unit.

modélisation éthique et les données responsables. Dans une perspective mondiale, il met en lumière des questions particulièrement pertinentes pour les pays qui étaient déjà en situation de crise humanitaire (insécurité alimentaire, conflits, etc.), en expliquant comment ces questions influent sur la manière dont les modèles épidémiologiques devraient être construits. En outre, ce chapitre se penche sur la vulnérabilité du point de vue des bénéficiaires de l'aide et des migrants, pour évoquer le type de lignes directrices et de lois qui devraient être prises en compte pour assurer la protection des données et de la vie privée.

The COVID-19 pandemic has brought to light vulnerabilities in all domains, while also showing the promise of strong, thoughtful solutions. Artificial intelligence, one of the most impactful research areas of the last decade, is no exception. The COVID-19 crisis is being called a "data-driven pandemic."[1] As countries seek to understand, confine, find cures, develop vaccines, protect the vulnerable, and deconfine the population, the use of artificial intelligence-based solutions has been very appealing, and in some cases, disturbing.

Fundamentally an analytical tool, what we call artificial intelligence in this context, is actually a hybrid of computer science and statistics that allows for rapidly evolving models that learn and adapt over time. In large part due to stronger computational power and massive data storage capacities, a series of powerful techniques have emerged that allow for fast and more accurate predictions in many domains. It should therefore come as no surprise that, at a time where uncertainty and doubt has been universal, computational modelling has gone mainstream.

For instance, artificial intelligence models are being used in three medical research fields—testing, treatment, and vaccinations.[2] As early as January 2020, BenevolentAI's algorithms[3] were combing

1. Roberto Rocha, "The Data-Driven Pandemic: Information Sharing with COVID-19 is 'Unprecedented'", *CBC News* (17 March 2020), online: <https://www.cbc.ca/news/canada/coronavirus-date-information-sharing-1.5500709>.
2. Swati Bhonde, Jayashree Prasad & Madhulika Bhati, "Predictive Analytics to Combat with COVID-19 Using Genome Sequencing" (April 15, 2020), online: *SSRN* <https://ssrn.com/abstract=3580692>.
3. "Benevolent AI Website" (May 2020), online: *Benevolent AI* <https://benevolent.ai>.

through thousands of research papers in order to identify the drugs that might be used to treat the disease. Google's DeepMind[4] used its AI algorithms to understand the proteins that might make up the virus. While there is no doubt that the use of artificial intelligence has been successfully accelerating medical advances, there is a concern that the use of these techniques might be seen as a panacea, and that the results produced may be used without proper testing.[5]

Furthermore, in the last few months, mobile applications have been developed, notably based on contact tracing tools to identify "contact" subjects and anticipate the risks of contamination[6] (such as *StopCovid* in France, or *Covi* in Canada). While the effectiveness of these applications remains uncertain,[7] the potential for violations of civil rights and freedoms is clear. The issues relating to privacy and the protection of sensitive health and geolocation data have been widely highlighted by protection authorities, especially under the *Personal Information Protection and Electronic Documents Act* (PIPEDA) in Canada. Federal, provincial, and territorial privacy guardians issued a joint statement calling on governments to ensure that COVID-19 contact tracing applications respect key privacy principles.[8] Beyond that, the most vulnerable parts of our population—the poor, the historically socially excluded—are naturally the ones most affected by the virus, as mentioned by the Ontario Human Rights Commission.[9]

4. R Tiernan, "Google DeepMind's Effort on COVID-19 Coronavirus Rests on the Shoulders of Giants" (March 6, 2020), online: *ZD Net* <https://www.zdnet.com/article/google-deepminds-effort-on-covid-19-coronavirus-rests-on-the-shoulders-of-giants>.
5. "Doctors are Using AI to Triage COVID-19 Patients. The Tools May Be Here to Stay" (23 April 2020), online: *MIT Technology Review* <https://www.technologyreview.com/2020/04/23/1000410/ai-triage-covid-19-patients-health-care/>.
6. Mirjam Kretzschmar, Ganna Rozhnova & Michiel van Boven, "Effectiveness of Isolation and Contact Tracing for Containment and Slowing Down a COVID-19 Epidemic: A Modelling Study" (6 March 2020), online: *SSRN* <https://ssrn.com/abstract=3551343>.
7. "Show Evidence that Apps for COVID-19 Contact Tracing Are Secure and Effective" (29 April 2020), online: *Nature Editorial* <https://www.nature.com/articles/d41586-020-01264>.
8. Office of the Privacy Commissioner of Canada, News Release, "Privacy Guardians Issue Joint Statement on COVID-19 Contact Tracing Applications" (7 May 2020), online: *Office of the Privacy Commissioner of Canada* <https://www.priv.gc.ca/en/opc-news/news-and-announcements/2020/nr-c_200507>.
9. "Actions Consistent with a Human Rights-Based Approach to Managing the COVID-19 Pandemic" (May 2020), online: *Ontario Human Rights Commission* <http://www.ohrc.on.ca/en/actions-consistent-human-rights-based-approach-managing-covid-19-pandemic>.

Discrimination against them could be reinforced by the use of technology that can lead to the accessing of certain government services being refused. Finally, the use of this type of technology will contribute to greater acceptance by our society of generalized technological surveillance.[10] In the past, the declaration of a state of emergency to combat terrorism has led to the incorporation of special measures into law that allow greater surveillance.[11]

Beyond these important concerns, much of the relevant research has focused on the wealthier nations of China, Western Europe, and North America—the first to be hit by the pandemic. However, as the virus continues to spread, poorer countries are not being spared. In this chapter, we explore the impact of artificial intelligence solutions to the COVID-19 pandemic in a global context and we focus in particular on countries with middle to low human development levels.[12] These populations are bound to be more vulnerable, not only to the pandemic impacts, but also to inappropriate uses of artificial intelligence. We consider predictive analysis and modelling and, then, the governance of data. We conclude by proposing a path forward for ensuring the accountable use of artificial intelligence globally.

Machine Learning and Impact Modelling

BlueDot,[13] a Canadian start-up, was among the first organizations in the world to identify the emerging risk from COVID-19 in Hubei province, and to sound the alarm before the U.S. Centers for Disease Control and Prevention did, on January 6, and before the World Health Organization followed suit three days later.[14] The start-up combines

10. Federica Lucivero et al, "Covid-19 and Contact Tracing Apps: Technological Fix or Social Experiment? (April 10, 2020), online: *SSRN* <https://ssrn.com/abstract=3590788>.
11. See for instance in France: Céline Castets-Renard, "Online Surveillance in the Fight Against Terrorism in France" in T-E Synodinou et al, eds, *EU Internet Law Regulation and Enforcement* (Switzerland: Springer, 2017). In Canada, see Kent Roach, "Canada's Response to Terrorism" in Victor V Ramraj et al, eds, *Global Anti-Terrorism Law and Policy* (Cambridge, UK: Cambridge University Press, 2005).
12. "The Human Development Index" (last visited 28 May 2020), online: *United Nations Development Programme* <http://hdr.undp.org/en/content/human-development-index-hdi>.
13. "BlueDot" (last visited 28 May 2020), online: *BlueDot* <https://bluedot.global>.
14. Geoffrey Vendeville, "U of T Infectious Diseases Expert AI Firm Now a Part of Canada's AI Arsenal" (27 March 2020), online: *U of T News* <https://www.utoronto.ca/news/u-t-infectious-disease-expert-s-ai-firm-now-part-canada-s-covid-19-arsenal>.

natural language processing and machine learning to gather insights on the emergence and spread of infectious diseases around the globe.

Research organizations have used modelling techniques to predict the timing and severity of the crisis and to compare the impacts of different possible intervention scenarios. These epidemiological models typically have a compartmental structure, where the model is divided into four broad categories—susceptibility, exposure, infectivity, and recovery (or death). The researchers thus calculate the percentage of the population at each stage, over time. However, the infectivity levels partly depend on the vulnerability of a person, particularly in terms of respiratory weakness. The elderly, but also those with chronic respiratory illness such as asthma, HIV/AIDS, and tuberculosis, are also more likely to have severe symptoms requiring hospitalization. As there is no cure (at the time of writing this), the recovery of those who require and receive intensive care is anywhere between 30% and 70%.[15] This depends on the quality of care received, as well as on the person's own immune system.

There have been many objectives of impact modelling. Firstly, having a sense of the number of people requiring critical care, as well as the timing of the peak number of cases, has allowed governments to allocate hospital resources appropriately. Secondly, the modelling has allowed the theoretical testing of different intervention strategies, in order to "flatten the curve," meaning to slow the infection rate and reduce the overall number of cases at the peak. These intervention strategies, in turn, have been implemented, often based solely on the model results.

One of the most impactful modelling initiatives in the COVID-19 crisis was spearheaded by Imperial College in London.[16] It showed a significant improvement of the crisis by implementing strong measures—physical distancing for the entire population, school closures, and contact tracing. However, there are many countries where the social and economic costs of such interventions in the models threatened to exceed the epidemic itself. In these cases, cultural and ethical impact modelling would take these other costs into account by including appropriate scenarios and population segmentation. An initiative by the London School of Hygiene and Tropical Medicine, for example,

15. Pavan K Bhatraju et al, "Covid-19 in Critically-Ill Patients in the Seattle Area: A Case Series" [2020] New England J Medicine.
16. Robert Verity et al, "Estimates of the Severity of Coronavirus 2019: A Model-Based Analysis" (2020) 20 Lancet 669.

detailed other intervention measures, primarily related to reduction of vulnerability to acute infection and shielding of the high-risk populations without complete lockdowns.

For instance, according to the Food and Agriculture Organisation of the UN (FAO),[17] more than one third of the population of Afghanistan is considered severely food insecure, a condition that, according to available literature, would make them more vulnerable to acute infection than their better-nourished counterparts. Consequently, given the feedback loop between food insecurity, COVID-19, and intervention scenarios, an ethical and accountable modelling methodology would take a very different approach than the original Imperial College model. Rather than focusing on an age parameterization, which would show increased vulnerability to severe infection as a person ages, a model for younger, but more food insecure, countries would include a breakdown of the level of malnutrition and food insecurity. This example reveals that ethical modelling in the pandemic is not only a technical problem, but one that must take into account a contextual understanding of the realities in each country, as well as the impact of computing and disseminating model results. Furthermore, the accuracy and diversity of the data are also important issues. The most vulnerable communities could be under- or over-represented in a dataset, a common error that could lead to a wrong interpretation and an inappropriate decision.

While age is not a vulnerability that can be reversed, food insecurity most certainly is, and so are certain treatable co-infections. Models that include these and other kinds of contextual parameters will provide realistic and attainable options for governments trying to mitigate the crisis.

Responsible Governance of Data

The responsible use of data is an important component of accountable AI in the COVID-19 pandemic. This is of particular relevance in situations of vulnerability, where individuals do not feel they are able to consent to breaches in their privacy and personal data use. As highlighted by the Office of the Privacy Commissioner of Canada, during a public health crisis, emergency legislation may

17. "Integrated Food Security Phase Classification: Afghanistan" (May 2020), online: *The Integrated Food Security Phase Classification* <http://www.ipcinfo.org/ipc-country-analysis/details-map/en/c/1152636/>.

supersede privacy laws.[18] Even worse, people already in positions of vulnerability as aid recipients or refugee claimants have very little to control over their own data protection and very few have the actual capacity to consent.

Importantly, data used to fight COVID-19 can be subverted for other, more nefarious, purposes. The security firm FireEye has reported that personal data was used in Syria to monitor and target dissidents.[19] In the past, data used by humanitarian organizations to distribute aid has been hacked and diverted in this way in a number of other conflict-ridden areas, including Yemen.[20] The information collected during a pandemic includes health information of populations that are marginalized or even oppressed. Humanitarian organizations are having to prevent the nefarious use and misappropriation of the personal data of the most vulnerable and impoverished persons in the world by actors ranging from militaries to authoritarian regimes to amorphous hacker armies.[21] Moreover, the collection and use of population data can also generate risks of racial discrimination based on data concerning vulnerable communities. It is therefore essential to protect sensitive information that concerns not only individual information but also group-level information.

The Centre for Humanitarian Data, a part of the United Nations Centre for the Coordination of Humanitarian Affairs, has published responsible data guidelines, with a focus on countries experiencing humanitarian crisis.[22] These guidelines include precautions for anonymization, understanding sensitive data, and techniques, such as Statistical Disclosure Control, which may ensure that data is safe to publish. The Centre has also developed a Peer Review Framework, which aims to provide ethical oversight of analytical models

18. "Privacy and the Covid-19 Outbreak" (March 2020), online: *Office of the Privacy Commissioner of Canada* <https://www.priv.gc.ca/en/privacy-topics/health-genetic-and-other-body-information/health-emergencies/gd_covid_202003/>.
19. FireEye, "Behind the Syrian Conflict's Digital Frontlines" (February 2015), online (pdf): *FireEye* <https://www.fireeye.com/content/dam/fireeye-www/global/en/current-threats/pdfs/rpt-behind-the-syria-conflict.pdf>.
20. "In Search of Better Data Protection for Those Caught in Conflict" (1 February 2019), online: *Open Canada* <https://www.opencanada.org/features/search-better-data-protection-those-caught-conflict/>.
21. *Ibid.*
22. Centre for Humanitarian Data, "FAQ on Data Responsibility for Covid-19" (11 May 2020), online: *Humanitarian Data Exchange* <https://data.humdata.org/faq-data-responsibility-covid-19>.

developed for humanitarian purposes. The objective of this effort is to sensitize technical specialists who may not be familiar with the ethical dimensions and impact of their work.

As we have seen, data used in artificial intelligence, whether for medical purposes or for epidemiological modelling, can be extremely sensitive, with implications for the personal privacy and security of individuals and groups. Given the pre-existing tendency to overlook the privacy needs and rights of residents of developing countries and the current de-prioritization of privacy legislation in the face of the pandemic response, this problem is likely to get worse.

Conclusion

There is no one-size-fits-all solution to the COVID-19 pandemic. However, thanks to the recent advances in artificial intelligence, we will be able to deal more quickly and effectively with this crisis. But the use of artificial intelligence has risks. This is most certainly the case for privacy protection, which already is lacking in humanitarian emergency contexts.

The societal and democratic impacts of artificial intelligence, used as a decision-support tool for governments at all levels, will need to be considered from the start. This kind of application is even more critical for developing countries, which have fewer resources to address the crisis and have less resilience to its compound effects. More than ever, therefore, we need to highlight and mitigate the adverse effects of these technologies, particularly when they impact vulnerable populations.

CHAPTER F-6

International Trade, Intellectual Property, and Innovation Policy: Lessons from a Pandemic

Jeremy de Beer* and E. Richard Gold**

Abstract

This chapter addresses intersections among international trade law, intellectual property rights, and domestic innovation policies to prevent, detect, and treat pandemics. Structural issues with Canada's innovation system affected preparedness for this pandemic and, unless remedied, will impede responses to future crises. In this chapter, we suggest aligning domestic and international policy measures to nuance Canada's approach to intellectual property and accelerate Canada's global contributions through open science.

Résumé

Commerce international, propriété intellectuelle et politique d'innovation : les leçons d'une pandémie

Ce chapitre traite des recoupements entre le droit commercial international, les droits de propriété intellectuelle et les politiques nationales d'innovation pour prévenir, détecter et traiter les pandémies. Les problèmes structurels du système d'innovation canadien ont affecté la préparation à cette pandémie et, s'ils ne sont pas corrigés,

*. Full Professor at the University of Ottawa's Faculty of Law.

** James McGill Professor with McGill University's Faculty of Law and a senior fellow at the Centre for International Governance Innovation (CIGI).

ils entraveront les réponses aux crises futures. Dans ce chapitre, nous suggérons d'harmoniser les mesures politiques nationales et internationales afin de nuancer l'approche du Canada en matière de propriété intellectuelle et d'accélérer les contributions du pays sur la scène mondiale grâce à la science ouverte.

In the early stages of the COVID-19 pandemic caused by SARS-CoV-2, policy attention around international trade law, intellectual property rights, and domestic innovation policies focused mostly on patents and compulsory licensing. There was also some discussion, but less action, regarding other intellectual property rights, such as copyrights or trade secrets. One reason is that the global system governing trade in scientific and technical knowledge leaves governments little room to manoeuvre with domestic intellectual property policy in the short term.[1] Therefore, while Canada and other countries should exploit flexibilities immediately, we argue that long-term policy opportunities are more important.

Canada's policy frameworks are poorly aligned with the country's characteristics. Canada has succeeded, and can succeed again, in aspects of the drug (or vaccine or diagnostic) development process.[2] But Canadians are unlikely to do so alone, given the conditions of our pharmaceutical industry.[3] For example, an Ebola vaccine was discovered in a Canadian laboratory supported by significant public investments, but a misguided proprietary strategy of patenting and exclusive licensing stalled clinical trials and eventually left most of the credit and profit to foreign firms.[4] Canada's plans for a national immunization strategy after SARS was underfunded and unsuccessful.[5] After years of criticism, it remains questionable whether Canada

1. Jeremy de Beer, "Introduction to Intellectual Property Law", in Oonagh E Fitzgerald, Valerie Hughes & Mark Jewett, eds, *Reflections on Canada's Past, Present and Future in International Law* (Waterloo: CIGI Press, 2018).
2. See Jason W Nickerson and Matthew Herder, this volume.
3. See Industry Canada, *Canada's Pharmaceutical Industry and Prospects* (Discussion Paper) (Kirkland: IMS Brogan, 2014).
4. Matthew Herder, Janice E Graham & Richard Gold, "From Discovery to Delivery: Public Sector Development of the rVSV-ZEBOV Ebola Vaccine" (2020) JL & Biosciences 1.
5. Public Health Agency of Canada, *Learning from SARS: Renewal of Public Health in Canada* (Executive Summary) (Ottawa: Public Health Agency of Canada, 8 November 2004).

has the capacity to do independent clinical trials.[6] And questions have been raised about Canada's biomanufacturing capacity.[7]

It is plausible that Canada can overcome some of these challenges with its current approaches to innovation policy. But we argue, instead, that the experience of addressing COVID-19 offers an opportunity to jump-start structural transformations in Canada's innovation system that would otherwise take decades to achieve. Canada's most realistic route to develop and ensure access to vaccines, diagnostics, and therapeutics is via international cooperation in open science. To accomplish this, Canada should rethink rather than abandon intellectual property as one tool of innovation policy.[8] We recommend aligning domestic and international intellectual property strategy with a broader array of innovation policy levers to adjust the conditions underlying Canada's biomedical innovation system.

Access under Current International Trade and Intellectual Property Rules

Researchers around the world have begun questioning the role of intellectual property in light of SARS-CoV-2 and COVID-19. Analyses cover general intellectual property and public health developments in the first months of the pandemic;[9] the coronavirus patent landscape and challenges related to "crisis-critical products";[10] intellectual property aspects of vaccines in the context of innovation law and policy;[11]

6. Standing Senate Committee on Social Affairs, Science and Technology, *Prescription Pharmaceuticals in Canada: Final Report* (March 2015) (Chair: Kelvin K Ogilvie) at 7; "Strategic Planning Report: A Pan-Canadian Clinical Trial Strategy" (2018) at 12, online (pdf): *Canadian Clinical Trials Coordinating Centre* <www.cctcc.ca/wp-content/uploads/2018/03/CCTCC-Report_Final.pdf>.
7. Nathaniel Lipkus, "Canadian Access to Coronavirus Treatment is Threatened by Weak Manufacturing Capacity", *The Globe and Mail* (10 April 2020), online: <https://www.theglobeandmail.com/business/commentary/article-canadian-access-to-coronavirus-treatment-is-threatened-by-weak/>.
8. Jeremy de Beer, Richard Gold & Mauricio Guaranga, "Intellectual Property Management: Policy Issues and Options" (2011), online (pdf): *Genome Canada* <www.genomecanada.ca/sites/default/files/pdf/en/Research_Policy-Directions-Brief.pdf>.
9. Ellen 't Hoen, "Protect Against Market Exclusivity in the Fight Against COVID-19" [2020] Nature Medicine.
10. Frank Tietze et al, "Crisis-Critical Intellectual Property: Findings from the COVID-19 Pandemic" (2020) Centre for Technology Management Working Paper No 2.
11. Ana Santos Rutschman, "The Intellectual Property of Vaccines: Takeaways From Recent Infectious Disease Outbreaks" (2020) 118 Mich L Rev Online 170.

transnational issues with copyright and related rights;[12] compulsory licensing and other patent issues for developing countries;[13] and more.

Canada was among the world's first movers to address patent issues before problems arose by making changes to its compulsory licensing law through its *COVID-19 Emergency Response Act*.[14] The government and anyone it authorizes can obtain a one-year licence to make, sell, or use patented technologies necessary to address the pandemic on a simple application to the patent office. While the patent owner must still be paid adequate remuneration, the emergency approach avoids any need for negotiations over reasonable terms prior to getting the licence.[15] The approach is not perfect, however. Among other things, the *Act* establishes a September 30, 2020, sunset clause that will inevitably be too soon for the most promising technology. Further, the one-year duration of licences is overly restrictive, rendering it uneconomical to start production on generics. Canada's emergency licensing powers, in our view, ought to last as long as the pandemic.

Canada's compulsory licensing provisions are likely more useful for existing devices or repurposed drugs than for new vaccines or antivirals. That is because, for new inventions, it takes years for patents to issue and liability for infringement only begins 18 months after filing—after, we hope, the emergency ends. Even if there is some liability for use of those inventions, this will likely represent only the reasonable cost of a licence.

Nonetheless, giving government the power to issue compulsory licences without protracted negotiations over the terms of access to vaccines, therapeutics, or other technologies was a necessary measure.[16] It reassures Canadians that patents will not impede a rapid response to the pandemic, and it encourages innovators to be

12. Marketa Trimble, "COVID-19 and Transnational Issues in Copyright and Related Rights" [4 May 2020] Intl Rev Intellectual Property & Competition L.
13. Krishna Ravi Srinivas, "Intellectual Property Rights and Innovation in the Times of Corona Epidemic" (April 2020), online (pdf): *Research and Information System for Developing Countries* <infojustice.org/wp-content/uploads/2020/04/RaviSrinivas.pdf>.
14. Bill C-13, *An Act respecting certain measures in response to COVID-19*, 1st Sess, 43 Parl, 2020, cl 51 (as passed by the House of Commons 24 March 2020).
15. *Patent Act*, RSC 1985, c P-4, s 66.
16. Christian Clavette & Jeremy de Beer, "Patents Cannot Impede Canada's Response to COVID-19 Crisis" (6 April 2020), online: *Centre for International Governance Innovation* <www.cigionline.org/articles/patents-cannot-impede-canadas-response-covid-19-crisis>.

proactive and reasonable about ensuring access to intellectual property protected technologies.[17]

Documents compiled by Knowledge Ecology International, a non-governmental organization monitoring global developments on this topic, show that Canada's actions are in line with or even leading other countries in exploring options to mitigate adverse impacts of patents on solutions to the pandemic.[18] But there remains a major cross-border issue that Canada's domestic patent law amendment does not solve: the ability to export patented technologies to other countries, especially developing countries, and to import drugs manufactured elsewhere.

In 2003, Canada handcuffed itself by declaring to the World Trade Organization that it would not avail itself of the ability to import patented medicines made under compulsory licence elsewhere. Member States of the WTO agreed to amend the Agreement on Trade-Related Aspects of Intellectual Property Rights (TRIPS) to allow this importation, but developed countries declined, *en masse*, to allow themselves to use this provision.[19] This misstep can and should be undone with a simple notice to the WTO, if Canada has the political will to do so.

Beyond patents, there remain other intellectual property issues relevant to the COVID-19 crisis. These include, for example, limits on Canadians' ability to access scientific publications, research, and test data, epidemiological models, algorithms, and artificial intelligence related to SARS-CoV-2 and COVID-19 due to copyrights and contracts.[20] Copyright may also constrain online teaching in the

17. *Ibid.*
18. "KEI Blogs and Research Notes on COVID-19/Coronavirus" (2020), online: *Knowledge Ecology International* <www.keionline.org/coronavirus>.
19. The HIV/AIDS crisis in Africa and elsewhere led to the 2001 Doha Declaration that TRIPS should not prevent countries from taking measures to protect public health and subsequent amendments to the TRIPS Agreement itself. World Trade Organization, *Declaration on the Trips Agreement and Public Health*, WTO Doc WT/MIN(01)/DEC/2. 4th Sess. The amendments, while complex, basically allow countries with manufacturing capacity to export patented medicines to other countries with no manufacturing capacity. TRIPS, Art 31*bis*. Somewhat ironically, given its own weak capacity, Canada became the first country worldwide to reform its domestic law (*An Act to Amend the Patent Act and the Food and Drugs Act [The Jean Chrétien Pledge to Africa Act]*, SC 2004, c 23) and then export patented medicines when it sent generic HIV/AIDS medicines to Rwanda. And somewhat short-sightedly, Canada had opted itself out of the chance to benefit from similar measures by other countries.
20. The Wellcome Trust was among the first to call on researchers, journals, and funds to ensure that research findings and data relevant to the pandemic are

COVID-19 era by rendering certain digital learning materials inaccessible.[21] There are even media reports of firms attempting to obtain trademarks on terms such as COVID-19.[22]

The province of Ontario is encouraging publicly funded researchers, research institutions, and/or private companies to seek intellectual property rights, believing that patenting will ensure that economic outcomes from a COVID-19 Rapid Research Fund will benefit Ontario.[23] It is plausible that, based on this approach, Canadians can try to bargain for access to the intellectual property of other firms across the globe. However, the costs of implementing this short-term strategy—including the cash, time, and opportunity costs to acquire and license out rights—is unlikely to be a wise investment. Another possible, but in the end poor, policy would be to embrace high prices on drugs, vaccines, and equipment in Canada on the mistaken belief that this will attract investment.[24] But firms make rational decisions as to where to conduct research based on capacity and resources, not on the basis of the rents they can extract in that particular jurisdiction. So a winner-take-all patent bonanza—which, by the way, other countries are better positioned to win—results in runners-up receiving nothing for competing instead of collaborating.

---

shared rapidly and openly. David Carr, "Sharing Research Data and Findings Relevant to the Novel Coronavirus (COVID-19) Outbreak" (31 January 2020), online: *Wellcome* <wellcome.ac.uk/coronavirus-covid-19/open-data>.

21. See, for example Eoin O'Dell, "Coronavirus and Copyright—or, the Copyright Concerns of the Widespread Move to Online Instruction—Updated" (15 March 2020), online (blog): *Cearta.ie* <www.cearta.ie/2020/03/coronavirus-and-copyright-or-the-copyright-concerns-of-the-widespread-move-to-online-instruction/>; Marketa Trimble, "COVID-19 and Transnational Issues in Copyright and Related Rights" [4 May 2020] Intl Rev Intellectual Property & Competition L; Samuel Trosow & Lisa Macklem, "Fair-Dealing and Emergency Remote Teaching in Canada" (21 March 2020), online (blog): *Sam Trosow* <samtrosow.wordpress.com/2020/03/21/fair-dealing-and-emergency-remote-teaching-in-canada/>; Michael Geist, "David Porter on the Benefits of Open Educational Resources as Millions Shift to Online Learning" (30 March 2020), online (podcast): *Law Bytes* <www.michaelgeist.ca/2020/03/lawbytes-podcast-episode-45/>.

22. Liam Casey, "Two Montreal Lawyers File Application to Trademark the Term COVID-19", *The Globe and Mail* (17 April 2020), online: <https://www.theglobeandmail.com/canada/article-two-montreal-lawyers-file-application-to-trademark-the-term-covid-19-2/>.

23. Office of the Premier, News Release, "Ontario Leading COVID-19 Research in Canada" (21 May 2020), online: *News Ontario* <https://news.ontario.ca/opo/en/2020/05/ontario-leading-covid-19-research-in-canada.html>.

24. Richard C Owens, "Our Drug Discovery System Seems Broken", *Financial Post* (5 May 2020), online: <https://business.financialpost.com/opinion/our-drug-discovery-system-seems-broken>.

The most significant problem with recommendations based on increasing patent rights or engaging in strategic patent bargaining is that it ignores who actually does pandemic research. Unfortunately, there is little incentive for firms, acting alone, to invest in pandemic research; they only do so when publicly funded or when working in collaboration with publicly funded institutions.[25] Canada has faced an unfortunate example of this when it licensed and paid for the rVSV-ZEBOV Ebola vaccine, only to have all the financial benefits accrue to a foreign firm.[26] Similarly, drugs such as remdesivir, that show some limited advantage in some studies, were publicly funded yet privately controlled.[27] For better or worse, governments and philanthropies will remain the major funders of research into pandemic as well as neglected and rare diseases.

While overhauling the whole of intellectual property law is neither necessary nor appropriate, this pandemic should inspire new strategic thinking about the role of intellectual property and other policy levers.

Strategic Policy Principles for Post-COVID-19 Innovation Policy Alignment

Sometimes we need to pay attention to what our actions tell us. Immediately following the start of the COVID-19 outbreak, scientists, government laboratories, and firms around the world drastically altered their behaviour. They engaged in radical sharing of data, materials, and ideas to fight the virus. In a matter of weeks, scientists openly shared samples, sequenced the SARS-CoV-2 virus, and shared proteins associated with it. Because of this sharing, researchers, government labs, and firms quickly developed diagnostics, put vaccines

25. Ana Santos Rutschman, "The Intellectual Property of Vaccines: Takeaways From Recent Infectious Disease Outbreaks" (2020) 118 Mich L Rev Online 170.

26. Matthew Herder, Janice E Graham & Richard Gold, "From Discovery to Delivery: Public Sector Development of the rVSV-ZEBOV Ebola Vaccine" (2020) JL & Biosciences 1.

27. Kathryn Ardizzone, "Role of the U.S. Federal Government in the Development of GS-5734/Remdesivir" (25 March 2020), online (pdf): *Knowledge Ecology International* <www.keionline.org/wp-content/uploads/KEI-Briefing-Note-2020_1GS-5734-Remdesivir.pdf>; E Richard Gold et al, "Canada Needs a Proactive Pandemic Innovation Strategy", *The Hill Times* (11 May 2020), online: <https://www.hilltimes.com/2020/05/11/open-science-anti-viral-drug-development-critical-to-canadas-pandemic-response/247148>.

into clinical trials, and began work repurposing old drugs to fight the disease.[28]

This COVID-19 stimulated move away from proprietary science—in which we patent everything and keep it secret until we do—to open science—where we do not clog up the system and do share research outcomes, data, materials, and tools —reflects a longer-term dissatisfaction over drug and vaccine development generally: drugs are increasingly expensive to develop, and our investments are producing less and less.[29] This is a global problem; one that Canada can only address in coordination with the international community.

If Canadians are to have access to the vaccines and antivirals to end or manage the COVID-19 crisis, Canada will need to cooperate globally. In this moment of heightened nationalism, Canada will need to be at the table—funding and supporting global efforts—to ensure it has a say in how those vaccines and antivirals are distributed. This implies an all-of-government approach in which Canada aligns domestic and trade policy to maximize its ability to exercise soft power.

More specifically, Canada's all-of-government approach needs to achieve the following. First, Canada needs to develop a drug discovery ecosystem that addresses Canadian strengths and weaknesses, and is not simply an ill-fitting adaptation of foreign innovation models. Second, Canada needs to invest in research and development not only because of the (relatively small) chance that a Canadian will develop the key vaccine or drug, but to be in the circle of experts and nations working together to find a cure. This will likely provide Canada with early access to an eventual vaccine or drug. Third, because it is not possible to control the virus in Canada without also doing so internationally, Canada needs to ensure that other countries, particular developing and least developed countries, have the ability to implement similar policies without restrictions. That is, solving the problem in Canada would be useless if the rest of the world were not able to do the same.

Because innovation and drug policy cross many federal (not to mention provincial[30]) ministries, Canada has a large number of

28. "Coronavirus: Everyone Wins When Patents Are Pooled", *Nature* (20 May 2020), online: <https://www.nature.com/articles/d41586-020-01441-2>.
29. E Richard Gold, "The Coronavirus Pandemic Has Shattered the Status Quo on Drug Development. We Should Build on That", *Fortune* (26 March 2020), online: <fortune.com/2020/03/26/coronavirus-vaccine-drug-development-open-science-covid-19-treatment/>.
30. Jeremy de Beer & Craig Brusnyk, "Intellectual Property and Biomedical Innovation in the Context of Canadian Federalism" (2011) 19 Health LJ 45.

domestic levers with which to achieve its goal. While there are a number of ways the country can configure these levers, what is critical is that these be aligned with each other and with foreign and trade policy. First, we discuss the domestic policy levers and then turn to those available to Canada internationally.

Domestic Levers

Because the majority of the science that addresses pandemics involves university and public laboratories, Canada needs to develop a strategy that accelerates science, moves it into clinical trials and, eventually, into the clinic. Currently, however, Canada is saddled with a strategy in which universities and public laboratories seek patents, and then license those patents out to industry partners. Not only has this strategy failed to produce any sustainably successful global firms, it has caused delays.[31] Canada needs to develop a university and public laboratory strategy that aims at broad dissemination and collaboration, especially with international partners, rather than just trying to generate more patents. As we noted earlier, this involves a recalibration, not a rejection, of intellectual property. There are other forms of intellectual property—such as data protection and trademarks, as two examples—that are fully compatible with open collaboration, allow follow-on research, and give Canadian firms an advantage in accessing the tacit knowledge emerging from our institutions. In fact, the largest Canadian preclinical drug deal was based on open sharing and access to tacit knowledge.[32]

While most Canadian institutions struggle to break even with outdated intellectual property acquisition strategies, other Canadian institutions are becoming world leaders in open science partnerships among academic, industry, and government researchers. This made-in-Canada model has not only advanced research but has led to drugs that are going through clinical trials today. Canada needs to build on this experience and expertise by targeting pandemic drug and vaccine funding to open science partnerships. Funding calls could be limited to

31. E Richard Gold, "Should Universities Get Out of the Patent Business?" (3 April 2019), online: *Centre for International Governance Innovation* <www.cigionline.org/articles/should-universities-get-out-patent-business>.

32. "Ontario Teams Collaborate to Discover First-in-Class Drug for Blood Cancers" (2019), online: *Ontario Institute for Cancer Research* <ar.oicr.on.ca/en/translating.html>.

those collaborations in which members fully accept open science principles and agree to transparently report on progress. Existing measures specifically designed for open science exist and ought to be used.[33]

In addition to funding open science, Canada can amend its drug approval regulations to provide longer periods of data protection for drugs approved by regulators by an additional two or more years with conditions that innovators promise to claim no patent rights, agree to publish all data openly, and accept price caps on drugs sold.[34] Canada can also ease tax rules regarding activities in which charities can and cannot participate. Canada's current rules are among the most restrictive in the world. In particular, they limit the ability of charities to invest in projects, such as vaccine and drug development that may result in commercial benefit for certain partners. As the philanthropic sector is a major funder, worldwide, of drug research and given that pharmaceutical firms are important partners in these efforts, tax rules need to be relaxed in a way that will ensure the public benefit of the work of charities but permit other partners to profit.

International Levers

Enhancing Canadian capacity to carry on drug and vaccine development will only achieve scale if we work with international partners. Further, the course of a pandemic will be determined by its weakest link. Thus, if Canada hopes to combat COVID-19 and future pandemics, it will need to ensure that all countries participate in the research effort or, at the least, have equal access to the drugs and vaccines that are eventually developed.

There are a few critical international and trade policy levers that align with this goal and build on Canada's domestic drug development policy. The first such lever is to fund international consortia, such as the Structural Genomics Consortium, that conduct open science. Canada ought to encourage domestic universities and firms to lead or at least participate in these consortia. Global open science partnerships are Canada's best guarantee of ensuring access to pandemic drugs and vaccines at home and combatting the virus abroad.

Given Canada's pre-eminence in open science partnerships (despite these being the minority form of partnership), it should

33. E Richard Gold et al, "An Open Toolkit for Tracking Open Science Partnership Implementation and Impact" (2019) 3 Gates Open Research 1442.
34. *Food and Drug Regulations*, CRC, c 870, s C.08.004.1.

actively bring the open science model to international governmental bodies, such as the Organisation for Economic Co-operation and Development (OECD) and the World Intellectual Property Organization. Canada has historically used the OECD to exercise soft power by convincing other countries to adopt solutions and policies made in Canada. The COVID-19 and post-COVID-19 world is an opportunity for Canada to return to these fora in an active way.

Finally, Canada needs to support developing countries that are calling for greater access to existing drugs and devices and for access to the tools necessary to both participate in research and access the fruits of that research. This means supporting the use by countries of compulsory licences to access patented technology and pooling to access tools and other pandemic-related technology. During a previous public health crisis involving HIV/AIDS, Canada became the first country worldwide to reform its domestic law to enhance developing countries' access to patented medicines[35] and then used the new powers to export generic antiretrovirals to Rwanda.[36] While that experience was far from perfect, it set a precedent for global leadership. Now is the time for Canada to step up as an international role model for open science.

Conclusion

The COVID-19 crisis presents an opportunity to improve Canada's approach to biomedical innovation at home and abroad. Canada should seize this chance to rethink the role of intellectual property acquisition vis-à-vis other domestic and international policy levers. With a more nuanced approach to intellectual property and greater emphasis on open science, Canada can emerge from this pandemic with a healthier biomedical innovation ecosystem to fight or, better, prevent the next one.

35. *An Act to amend the Patent Act and the Food and Drugs Act (The Jean Chrétien Pledge to Africa Act)*, SC 2004, c 23.

36. See Tania Bubela & Jean-Frédéric Morin, "Lost in Translation: The Canadian Access to Medicines Regime From Transnational Activism to Domestic Implementation" (2010) 18 Health LJ 113; Jean-Frédéric Morin & E Richard Gold, "Consensus-Seeking, Distrust and Rhetorical Entrapment: The WTO Decision on Access to Medicines" (2010) 16:4 European J Intl Relations 562; E Richard Gold & Jean-Frédéric Morin, "Promising Trends in Access to Medicines" (2012) 3:2 Global Policy 231.

CHAPTER F-7

COVID-19 Vaccines as Global Public Goods

Jason W. Nickerson* and Matthew Herder**

Abstract

There is growing awareness that the only end to the COVID-19 pandemic, without causing an unacceptably large number of deaths, will be with one or more vaccines mass-produced and readily available to meet the world's needs. A flurry of research and development activities are underway; however, the way the vaccine research and development system is currently constructed is not optimized to develop, manufacture, and equitably distribute vaccines on a global scale. In this chapter, we propose that resolving the tension between these realities requires a different approach to health innovation, one that operationalizes the concept of global public goods throughout the phases of vaccine development, manufacturing, and distribution. We argue that such an approach is not only the morally correct thing to do, given the scale of needs and the risk that the public has accepted by financing the development of various experimental vaccines, but it is also the only possible way of ensuring sufficient global manufacturing capacity and equitable distribution of any vaccines

* Clinical Scientist at the Bruyère Research Institute, and Adjunct Professor of Common Law in the Centre for Health Law, Policy and Ethics at the University of Ottawa.

** Director of the Health Law Institute at Dalhousie University in Halifax, Nova Scotia, and Associate Professor at Dalhousie University's Faculties of Medicine and Law.

that prove effective against COVID-19. We detail what adopting a global public goods approach to vaccine production would require in Canada, in an effort to encourage other jurisdictions to follow the same approach.

Résumé
Les vaccins contre la COVID-19 comme biens publics mondiaux

Nous sommes de plus en plus conscients du fait que la seule issue à la pandémie de COVID-19, sans occasionner un nombre inacceptable de décès, sera la production en masse d'un ou de plusieurs vaccins facilement accessibles pour répondre aux besoins du monde entier. Une multitude d'activités de recherche et de développement sont en cours à cet effet. Cependant, la façon dont le système de recherche et de développement des vaccins est actuellement construit n'est pas optimale pour les développer, les fabriquer et les distribuer équitablement à l'échelle mondiale. Dans ce chapitre, nous suggérons que pour dissiper la tension entre ces réalités, il faut adopter une approche différente de l'innovation en matière de santé, une approche qui concrétise le concept de biens publics mondiaux tout au long des phases de développement, de fabrication et de distribution des vaccins. Nous soutenons qu'une telle approche est non seulement correcte du point de vue moral, étant donné l'ampleur des besoins et le risque que le public a accepté de prendre en finançant le développement de divers vaccins expérimentaux, mais qu'il s'agit de la seule façon possible de garantir une capacité de production mondiale suffisante et une distribution équitable de tout vaccin qui s'avérerait efficace contre la COVID-19. Enfin, nous exposons en détail ce qu'exigerait l'adoption d'une approche des biens publics mondiaux pour la production de vaccins au Canada, afin d'encourager d'autres pays à suivre la même démarche.

There is growing awareness that the only end to the COVID-19 pandemic, without causing an unacceptably large number of deaths, will be with one or more vaccines, mass-produced and readily available to meet the world's needs.[1] Yet, no vaccine for any coronavirus

1. Gavin Yamey, "To End this Pandemic We'll Need a Free Vaccine Worldwide", *Time* (15 April 2020), online: <https://time.com/5820963/end-pandemic-free-vaccine-worldwide/>.

in humans, let alone the specific coronavirus at the heart of the present pandemic—known as SARS-CoV-2—exists at this point in time. Further, the way the global vaccine research and development system is currently constructed and operated is not optimized to develop, manufacture, and equitably distribute vaccines. Given these conflicting realities, a new approach to health innovation is required.

Specifically, we argue that any COVID-19 vaccines must be re-conceptualized as global public goods rather than publicly subsidized, privately controlled commodities. By "public good" we mean that COVID-19 vaccines—while material in form—are, at bottom, information-based products. That is, once knowledge about a given vaccine's safety and effectiveness against SARS-CoV-2 is in hand, only resources (for example, manufacturing facilities) and law (for example, patent law) can limit its consumption; the underlying knowledge about how to make and use them, absent these limitations, is both non-rivalrous and non-exclusive. Because of the demand for such vaccines, and their central importance to securing adequate public health within and across countries, no one nation, or private manufacturer, alone can guarantee their provision; rather, their development and production will, of necessity, be a global endeavour, thus the term "global" public goods.[2] We argue that this conceptualization of COVID-19 vaccines as global public goods must be carried through the entire process of producing, testing, manufacturing, and distributing any resulting COVID-19 vaccines. To make it concrete, we outline how this global public goods approach might be achieved in the Canadian setting, while also recognizing that the approach must be adopted elsewhere as well if global needs are to be met.

Public Financing of COVID-19 Research and the Public Sector's Capacity to Do More

Like many other knowledge-based goods in the health domain, vaccines are not usually treated as public goods, on the strength of the argument that without the promise of exclusivity, private companies would not undertake the lengthy, costly process of developing them for human use. Patent rights and other legal protections from

2. Inge Kaul, Isabelle Grunberg & Marc Stern, *Global Public Goods: International Cooperation in the 21st Century* (Oxford: Oxford University Press, 1999).

potential competitors are used to motivate, coordinate, and sustain vaccine R&D, from discovery and preclinical stages of research (often performed by publicly funded institutions) through to clinical trials involving human participants, manufacturing, and regulatory approval (usually run by the private sector). Most vaccines and drug therapies that reach the market follow this pattern.[3]

There are several limitations associated with this publicly subsidized, privately appropriated approach. Principal among them are that health conditions or diseases which afflict the world's poor[4] or carry less predictable financial returns typically command very little interest. Prior to COVID-19, coronaviruses were an example of this lack of interest: only six interventions reached the clinical trial phase of development, all of which relied heavily on public funding.[5]

Governments around the world have made massive amounts of funding available to support R&D of COVID-19 vaccines, drugs, and other technologies. Canada has contributed more than C$1 billion toward COVID-19 R&D, at least C$850 million of which is for vaccine and therapeutics-related research[6,]; the U.S. has provided roughly the same amount to two companies with vaccines in development,[7] on top of many more billions being devoted to coronavirus R&D. A recent pledging conference raised €7.5 billion for COVID-19 vaccine

3. For example, every drug approved in the United States in 2016 emerged from public sector science. Ekaterina Galkina Cleary et al, "Contribution of NIH Funding to New Drug Approvals 2010-2016" (2018) 115:10 Proc Natl Acad Sci 2329. See also Ashley J Stevens et al, "The Role of Public-Sector Research in the Discovery of Drugs and Vaccines" (2011) 364:6 N Engl J Med 535.
4. Patrice Trouiller et al, "Drugs for Neglected Diseases: A Failure of the Market and a Public Health Failure?" (2001) 6:11 Trop Med Int Health 945.
5. Zain Rivzi, "Government Funds Coronavirus Research While Pharma Sits By", *Public Citizen* (19 February 2020), online: <https://www.citizen.org/article/blind-spot/>.
6. Justin Trudeau, News Release, "Canada and international partners launch the Coronavirus Global Response" (4 May 2020), online: *Justin Trudeau, Prime Minister of Canada* <https://pm.gc.ca/en/news/news-releases/2020/05/04/canada-and-international-partners-launch-coronavirus-global-response>. Canadian Institute of Health Research, "Government of Canada invests $27M in Coronavirus Research — Details of the Funded Projects" (2020), online: *Government of Canada* <https://www.canada.ca/en/institutes-health-research/news/2020/03/government-of-canada-invests-27m-in-coronavirus-research--details-of-the-funded-projects.html>.
7. Julie Steenhuysen, "J&J, Moderna Sign Deals with U.S. to Produce Huge Quantity of Possible Coronavirus Vaccines" (30 March 2020), online: *Reuters* <https://www.reuters.com/article/us-health-coronavirus-johnson-johnson-idUSKBN21H1OY>.

development, eliciting pledges from 46 countries, philanthropic organizations, and private companies.[8]

Despite these unprecedented injections of funding, the approach to R&D appears fundamentally unchanged. Apart from a joint statement in favour of data openness, which many national health research funders as well as private sector players have signed,[9] there is little indication that a global public goods approach will be pursued. On the contrary, efforts to move away from a proprietary approach, for example, by creating a global clearinghouse of intellectual property rights, have been thwarted.[10]

The good news is that the capacity of public sector science is under-realized. Contrary to the standard view that the public sector's role is limited to discovery and preclinical research, Canada's National Microbiology Laboratory, combined with other publicly funded institutions and civil society organizations, demonstrated their ability to problem solve many technical challenges of manufacturing a clinical grade vaccine and establishing its safety and effectiveness against Ebola. While this eventually culminated in the approval of "*r*VSV-ZEBOV" by the U.S. Food and Drug Administration in 2019,[11] the government lab's decision to patent and license the vaccine to a small biotechnology company in 2010 failed to advance the vaccine toward clinical trials prior to the 2014-2015 Ebola epidemic.[12] Only as the outbreak escalated, and governments mobilized more resources, did Merck, which now controls *r*VSV-ZEBOV, become motivated to

8. European Union, "Funds Raised" (2020) online: *European Union* <https://global-response.europa.eu/pledge_en>.
9. Wellcome, "Sharing research data and findings relevant to the novel coronavirus (COVID-19) outbreak" (31 January 2020), online: *Wellcome Trust – Open Data* <https://wellcome.ac.uk/coronavirus-covid-19/open-data>.
10. Notably, entities such as the Coalition for Epidemic Preparedness Innovations (CEPI), which have both a mandate and formal policies to facilitate equitable access, have opposed such initiatives. See James Love, "WHO Member States Poised to Adopt Weaker than Needed COVID-19 Resolution After Tortuous Negotiations" (13 May 2020), online: *Knowl Ecol Int* <https://www.keionline.org/33044>. For background on CEPI, see Brenda Huneycutt et al, "Finding Equipoise: CEPI Revises its Equitable Access Policy" (2020) 38:9 Vaccine 2144-2148."
11. Matthew Herder, Janice E Graham & Richard Gold, "From Discovery to Delivery: Public Sector Development of the rVSV-ZEBOV Ebola Vaccine" [16 January 2020] J Law Biosci, online: <https://academic.oup.com/jlb/advance-article/doi/10.1093/jlb/lsz019/5706941>.
12. *Ibid.*

get involved.[13] To help realize a global public goods vision of vaccine production against COVID-19, a different approach is required.[14]

Producing a COVID-19 Vaccine in Canada as a Global Public Good

Discovery and Development

Researchers in publicly-funded institutions have been at the forefront of infectious disease research, including for coronaviruses, even though industry interest in infectious diseases has waned. Many, if not all, of the interventions that the world is now scrambling to develop—antiviral treatments, diagnostics, and vaccines—have their origins in platforms or technologies developed by researchers in public institutions.[15,16] Despite this massive public investment, it appears that few if any strings have been attached to the funding to ensure access and affordability of any resulting technologies. One company that has received Canadian funding for a COVID-19 vaccine testified before Parliament that no such requirements exist, though the company noted that part of their overall strategy was to ensure global availability.[17]

Unlike other jurisdictions, where federal research funding carries "march-in rights," which the government can theoretically invoke to improve access to a federally funded technology,[18] in Canada, outside of federal laboratories,[19] no analogous legal power exists with respect

13. *Ibid.*
14. Mariana Mazzucato, Henry Lishi Li & Ara Darzi, "Is It Time to Nationalise the Pharmaceutical Industry?" (2020) 368 BMJ, online: <http://www.bmj.com/content/368/bmj.m769>.
15. Justin Hughes & Arti K Rai, "The Public Role in Drug Development: Lessons from Remdesivir" (8 May 2020), online: *STAT* <https://www.statnews.com/2020/05/08/acknowledging-public-role-drug-development-lessons-remdesivir/>.
16. Nathan Vanderklippe, "National Research Council Strikes Deal with China to Develop COVID-19 Vaccine in Canada", *The Globe and Mail* (May 12, 2020), online: <https://www.theglobeandmail.com/world/article-national-research-council-strikes-deal-with-china-to-develop-test/>.
17. House of Commons, Standing Committee on Health, 43-1, No 16 (30 April 2020), online: *Our Commons* <https://www.ourcommons.ca/DocumentViewer/en/43-1/HESA/meeting-16/evidence>.
18. Carolyn L Treasure, Jerry Avorn & Aaron S Kesselheim, "Do March-In Rights Ensure Access to Medical Products Arising From Federally Funded Research? A Qualitative Study" (2015) 93:4 Milbank Q 761.
19. Pursuant to the *Public Servants Inventions Act*, RSC 1985, c P-32, inventions generated in a federal lab are the property of the Crown. In theory, this could allow for a different approach; however, recent cases, such as the rVSV-ZEBOV Ebola

to publicly funded research. Moving forward, all funding agreements should contain explicit clauses on affordable pricing and equitable access, in addition to the data sharing commitments that appear to be included already. While such clauses have seldom been used in the past, precedents do exist. The government of France recently included a specification in a licensing agreement for the drug Onasemnogene abeparvovec (Zolgensma®), that French patients should have access at a price that "would not constitute an obstacle for patients to have access to the therapy."[20] Model equitable access clauses, or benefit-sharing commitments,[21] are also available.[22]

For the funding that has already been distributed, Canadian governments must secure commitments by other means if any resulting vaccine is to become a global public good. Negotiation may work; if not, and assuming the intervention in question is the subject of a patent, the federal government could threaten to invoke its new compulsory licensing authority, added as part of the COVID-19 emergency response legislation,[23] in order to encourage the patent holder to make the intervention affordably and broadly available.

Human Clinical Trials

On May 12, the National Research Council of Canada (NRCC) announced a collaboration with CanSino Biologics Inc. (CanSinoBIO) to conduct bioprocessing and clinical development of a COVID-19 candidate vaccine.[24] The vaccine uses the NRCC's HEK293 cell line, which was previously licensed to CanSinoBIO, and is the first candidate vaccine to enter Phase II trials; the Canadian Center for

vaccine, indicate that the government tends to adhere to the standard proprietary approach to commercializing discoveries. See Herder et al, supra note 12.

20. James Love, "'Reasonable' Pricing Could Limit the Cost for Zolgensma in France – STAT", *Stat News* (18 September 2019), online: <https://www.statnews.com/2019/09/18/zolgensma-reasonable-pricing-france/>.
21. Amy Kapczynski, "Order without Intellectual Property Law: Open Science in Influenza" (2017) 102:6 Cornell Law Rev 1539.
22. David Branigan, "UAEM: In 'Historic' Shift, Universities in Canada Adopt Licensing Promoting Access to Medicines" (1 November 2018), online: *Intellect Prop Watch* <https://www.ip-watch.org/2018/11/01/uaem-historic-shift-universities-canada-adopt-licensing-promoting-access-medicines/>.
23. *Patent Act*, RSC, c P-4, s 19.4.
24. Nathan Vanderklippe, "National Research Council Strikes Deal with China to develop COVID-19 Vaccine in Canada", *Globe Mail* (12 May 2020), online: <https://www.theglobeandmail.com/world/article-national-research-council-strikes-deal-with-china-to-develop-test/>.

Vaccinology, will lead clinical trials in Canada—yet another instance of clinical research being financed and led by the public sector.

Provided that appropriate access and affordability safeguards are contained in the agreement between CanSinoBIO and the Government of Canada, this model may be on the right track for leveraging the collective benefits and strengths of both the public and private sectors: a technology developed in collaboration between public and private actors, being evaluated by publicly funded researchers, could allow for data transparency, open sharing of manufacturing know-how, flexible intellectual property provisions, and access and pricing guarantees.

None of those details are in the public domain at present, although the intellectual property associated with the vaccine candidate reportedly remains under CanSinoBIO's control.[25] In return for making the vaccine available in Canada, the company is getting the benefit of Canada paying for and running clinical trials, the results of which the company will presumably include in any future submissions to regulatory agencies. To ensure that the knowledge that is generated through these trials is rigorously evaluated, it is essential that Canadian researchers retain control over the data and in turn make it openly available for independent scrutiny in a timely fashion.

Manufacturing and Distribution

Canada cannot manufacture the world's COVID-19 vaccine supply—production capacity simply will not allow for it, though investments have been made to increase Canada's public vaccine manufacturing capacity.[26] A strategy for transferring vaccine technology and manufacturing know-how to a network of other vaccine producers is necessary, not only for pragmatic reasons of supply, but also to avert a parallel pandemic of poorly manufactured or outright falsified vaccines that often emerge when demand outstrips supply.[27] Discovering a vaccine that works is the initial challenge; next is determining a

25. *Ibid*.
26. Justin Trudeau, News Release, "Prime Minister Announces New Support for COVID-19 Medical Research and Vaccine Development" (23 April 2020), online: *Justin Trudeau, Prime Minister of Canada* <https://pm.gc.ca/en/news/news-releases/2020/04/23/prime-minister-announces-new-support-covid-19-medical-research-and>.
27. Paul N Newton, "COVID-19 and Risks to the Supply and Quality of Tests, Drugs, and Vaccines" (1 June 2020) 8:6 The Lancet E754.

manufacturing strategy capable of meeting quality-assured, equitable global demand. If, for example, the CanSinoBIO vaccine candidate proves effective against SARS-CoV-2 in trials, it may be necessary for the NRCC to transfer its know-how to other manufacturing sites and/or ramp up its own production beyond domestic needs, whether or not CanSinoBIO grants permission to do so.[28]

If COVID-19 vaccine technologies are to become global public goods, governments need to act to ensure that information, data, and manufacturing know-how are shared globally, and that systems are in place to ensure manufacturing processes, access strategies, and quality control monitoring of diversified manufacturing and supply chains. These measures are necessary to avert a crisis of equity and to avoid the perpetuation of the pandemic by having the vaccine made available to only some people. The scientific work to develop a vaccine has been characterized as a global act of scientific solidarity; so too should the work of manufacturing and distributing it; thus, governments can and should take steps to ensure intellectual property is not a barrier to globalized sharing of know-how and vaccine production.

Conclusion

Without a plan for how to ensure equitable worldwide distribution of a Canadian (or any) vaccine, the status quo is inequitable distribution both within and among countries. There is precedent for this concern: during the 2009 influenza A(H1N1) pandemic, wealthy countries purchased nearly all doses of the vaccine.[29] More recently, the United States may have attempted to secure exclusive access to a German COVID-19 vaccine.[30] If nationalizing vaccine production is to help realize a globally accessible COVID-19 vaccine, then it cannot devolve into vaccine nationalism.

28. As noted above, Canada has added a "public health emergency" compulsory licensing provision to its *Patent Act*, which can be used to override CanSinoBIO's patent rights, without negotiation, if necessary to address the emergency.
29. David P Fidler, "Negotiating Equitable Access to Influenza Vaccines: Global Health Diplomacy and the Controversies Surrounding Avian Influenza H5N1 and Pandemic Influenza H1N1" (4 May 2010) 7:5 PLoS Med e1000247.
30. Aitor Hernández-Morales, "Germany Confirms that Trump Tried to Buy Firm Working on Coronavirus Vaccine" (15 March 2020), online: *Politico* <https://www.politico.eu/article/germany-confirms-that-donald-trump-tried-to-buy-firm-working-on-coronavirus-vaccine/>.

The bare minimum that the Canadian government ought to do is to ensure that pricing and access strategies are applied to any vaccine that benefited from Canadian public funds. A practical, legally enforceable commitment from Canada and other countries to treat a COVID-19 vaccine as a global public good, accessible to everyone who needs it, is not only the morally right thing to do to facilitate access, it also reflects the financial and intellectual investments made by the public. It may be the only way of ensuring that the pandemic ends, not just for some, but for all.

Biographies

Editors

Colleen M. Flood is the University of Ottawa Research Chair in Health Law and Policy and inaugural Director of the Ottawa Centre for Health Law, Policy and Ethics. From 2017 to 2018, she served as Associate Vice-President Research at the University of Ottawa. From 2000 to 2015, she was Professor and Canada Research Chair in the Faculty of Law, University of Toronto. From 2006 to 2011, she served as a Scientific Director of the Institute for Health Services and Policy Research, one of the Canadian Institutes of Health Research. Her research interests are focused on the role of law in shaping health and health care systems and the appropriate roles for the public and private sectors. She is the author/editor of twelve books (two of which are in multiple editions) and editor of *Halsbury's Laws of Canada: Public Health* (2019 Reissue) and teaches a course called the Law of Modern-Day Plagues.

Vanessa MacDonnell is Associate Professor at the University of Ottawa Faculty of Law and Co-Director of the uOttawa Public Law Centre. She researches in the areas of Canadian constitutional law, constitutional theory, comparative constitutional law, and criminal law and procedure. In 2019, she spent six months as Scholar-in-Residence in the Constitutional, Administrative and International Law Section of the

Department of Justice Canada and was a Kathleen Fitzpatrick Visiting Fellow in the Laureate Program in Comparative Constitutional Law at Melbourne Law School. Vanessa is currently completing a three-year research project on quasi-constitutional legislation funded by the Social Sciences and Humanities Research Council of Canada (SSHRC). Other recent projects focus on global constitutionalism and on examining the civil servant's role in the implementation of constitutional rights. She is a member of the Global Young Academy.

The Honourable **Jane Philpott** is Professor of Family Medicine, Dean of the Faculty of Health Sciences, and Director of the School of Medicine at Queen's University in Kingston, Ontario. She is a medical doctor, educator, and former Member of Parliament. She received her Doctor of Medicine degree from the University of Western Ontario. She completed a Family Medicine residency at the University of Ottawa, then both a Tropical Medicine fellowship and a Master of Public Health from the University of Toronto. Dr. Philpott spent the first decade of her medical career in Niger, West Africa. In 1998, she moved to Stouffville, Ontario, where she served as a family physician for 17 years. She was Chief of Family Medicine at Markham Stouffville Hospital and an Associate Professor in the Faculty of Medicine at the University of Toronto. In 2015, Dr. Philpott was elected as the Member of Parliament for Markham-Stouffville. She served in numerous federal cabinet positions from 2015 to 2019, including Minister of Health, Minister of Indigenous Services, President of the Treasury Board, and Minister of Digital Government. Her research interests include medical education, primary care, and the Indigenous health workforce.

Sophie Thériault is Full Professor and Vice-Dean (Academic) in the Faculty of Law (Civil Law Section) at the University of Ottawa. From 2015 to 2017, she served as the Vice-Dean of Graduate Studies in Law at the University of Ottawa. Professor Thériault's research focuses on Indigenous Peoples' rights in the context of natural resources extraction; Indigenous environmental governance; environmental justice and environmental rights; and food security and sovereignty for Indigenous Peoples. Her work examines the myriad ways in which state law dispossesses, subjugates, and marginalizes Indigenous Peoples, especially in relation to the extraction of natural resources from their traditional lands. It also focuses on the role of law in creating, reproducing, and potentially remediating environmental injustices for Indigenous Peoples and other marginalized groups. Professor Thériault is a member of the Executive Committee of the Alumni Network of the Pierre Elliott Trudeau Foundation and of the Global Young Academy.

Sridhar Venkatapuram is an academic practitioner in global health ethics and justice. He is Associate Professor at King's College London, and Director of Global Health Education and Training at the King's Global Health Institute. His interdisciplinary training includes international relations (Brown), history (SOAS), global public health (Harvard), sociology, and political philosophy (Cambridge). He has worked with organizations including Human Rights Watch, Doctors of the World, the Population Council, Open Societies Institute, Welcome Trust, Health Foundation, U.K. Parliament of Science & Technology, and recently, the World Health Organization. He is a member of the Independent Panel on Global Governance for Health, a trustee of Medact, and a fellow of the Salzburg Global Seminar, Human Development & Capabilities Association, the RSA (Royal Society for the encouragement of Arts, Manufactures and Commerce), and U.K. Faculty of Public Health, among others. His PhD was an argument for every human being's moral right to health, examined and passed without corrections by Nobel Laureate Amartya Sen. It was the basis of his first book, titled *Health Justice: An Argument From the Capability Approach* (Polity Press). He publishes in diverse scholarly journals on public and global health ethics, social determinants of health, the capabilities approach, health equity, and global governance for health. His Twitter handle is @sridhartweet.

Contributors

Hugh Armstrong is Distinguished Research Professor and Professor Emeritus of Social Work, Political Economy, and Sociology at Carleton University. He has served as a Co-Investigator on the "Re-imagining Long-Term Residential Care: An International Study of Promising Practices" project and on several related research projects.

Pat Armstrong is Distinguished Research Professor in Sociology at Toronto's York University and a Fellow of the Royal Society of Canada. She held a Canadian Health Services Research Foundation/Canadian Institutes of Health Research (CHSRF/CIHR) Chair in Health Services and Nursing Research and chaired Women and Health Care Reform, a group funded for over a decade by Health Canada. She has served as both Chair of the Department of Sociology at York and Director of the School of Canadian Studies at Carleton University. She is also a board member of the Canadian Health Coalition and, until recently, the Canadian Centre for Policy Alternatives. She is Principal Investigator of "Reimagining Long-term Residential Care: An International Study of Promising Practices." Focusing on the fields of social policy, women, work, and health and social services, she has published widely, authoring or co-authoring such books as *Critical to Care: The Invisible Women in Health Services* (University of Toronto Press); *Wasting Away: The Undermining of Canadian Health Care* (Oxford University Press); *The Double Ghetto: Canadian Women and Their Segregated Work* (Oxford University Press); and *Wash, Wear, and Care: Clothes and Laundry in Long-Term Residential Care* (McGill-Queen's University Press). Much of this work makes the relationship between paid and unpaid work central to the analysis.

Amir Attaran is by training an immunologist and lawyer, and he has been active in efforts against infectious disease in Canada and globally for over two decades, particularly on malaria, HIV/AIDS, and now COVID-19. He is a professor in both the Faculty of Law and the School of Epidemiology and Public Health at the University of Ottawa. He is also an active litigator, of the Bar of Ontario.

Louise Bélanger-Hardy est professeure titulaire à la Faculté de droit, Section de common law, de l'Université d'Ottawa où elle a été vice-doyenne (1996-1999, 2013-2014 et 2020). Ses domaines d'enseignement sont le droit des délits et de la responsabilité extracontractuelle, ainsi que le droit de la santé. Elle est membre de l'Institut de recherche LIFE et du Centre de droit, éthique et politique de la santé, tous deux à l'Université d'Ottawa. Pendant plus de 10 ans, elle a été membre de tribunaux administratifs spécialisés en matière de réglementation des professions et des services de santé en Ontario. Elle a été membre de comités d'éthique de la recherche à l'Université d'Ottawa, à la Société canadienne du sang et à Santé Canada. Dans sa recherche, elle s'intéresse à la responsabilité civile des professionnels de la santé, à la réglementation des professions de la santé, à la santé mentale, au consentement aux soins et à la recherche ainsi qu'aux enjeux de sécurité dans le contexte des soins à domicile.

Louise Bélanger-Hardy is Full Professor in the Faculty of Law, University of Ottawa, where she has been Vice-Dean (1996–1999, 2013–2014, and 2020). She teaches Tort Law (common law and Québec civil law) and Health Law. She is a member of the Life Research Institute and the Centre for Health Law, Policy and Ethics, both at the University of Ottawa. For over ten years, she held cross-appointments to administrative tribunals dealing with health professions and health services in Ontario. She has been a member of the Research Ethics Board at the University of Ottawa, Canadian Blood Services, and Health Canada. Her research interests include professional responsibility, regulation of health professions, mental health, consent in the medical and research settings, and liability issues in the context of home-based care.

Sarah Berger Richardson is Assistant Professor in the University of Ottawa's Faculty of Law (Civil Law Section), where she teaches food and agricultural law, civil liability, and administrative law. She is a member of the Law Society of Ontario and President of the Canadian Association of Food Law and Policy. Professor Berger Richardson's research focuses on the regulation of food production and farming, with a particular emphasis on the meat industry. She holds a doctorate from McGill University's Faculty of Law and her dissertation examined the ways that socio-cultural and moral perspectives on how livestock should be raised and slaughtered are considered in the design of meat inspection systems. She holds a Master of Law (LLM) from Tel Aviv University, where she was a research fellow at the Manna Center in Food Safety and Security. She previously served as a law clerk at the Supreme Court of Israel and the Canada Agricultural Review Tribunal.

Ivy Lynn Bourgeault is Professor in the School of Sociological and Anthropological Studies at the University of Ottawa, and she holds a University Research Chair in Gender, Diversity and the Professions. She leads the Canadian Health Workforce Network and the Empowering Women Leaders in Health initiative. Dr. Bourgeault has garnered an international reputation for her research on the health workforce, particularly through the lens of gender. She was inducted into the Canadian Academy of Health Sciences in 2016 and received the 2017 University of Ottawa Award for Excellence in Research. Her recent research interests include care relationships in home and long-term care and the psychological health and safety of professional workers.

Kelly Bronson is Canada Research Chair in Science and Society at the University of Ottawa. She is a social scientist studying science-society tensions that erupt around controversial technologies (GMOs, fracking, big data) and their governance. Her research aims to bring community values into conversation with technical knowledge in the production of evidence-based decision-making. She has published her work in regional (*Journal of New Brunswick Studies*), national (*Canadian Journal of Communication*), and international journals (*Journal of Responsible Innovation, Big Data and Society*).

Mel Cappe is Professor in the Munk School of Global Affairs and Public Policy, University of Toronto. From 2006 to 2011, he was President of the Institute for Research on Public Policy. Prior to that, he was High Commissioner for Canada to the United Kingdom for four years. Before that he served as Clerk of the Privy Council, Secretary to Cabinet, and Head of the Public Service. Earlier in his career he held senior economic and policy positions in the Departments of Finance and Industry. He was Deputy Secretary to the Treasury Board, Deputy Minister of the Environment, Deputy Minister of Human Resources Development, Deputy Minister of Labour, and Chairman of the Employment Insurance Commission. He was a commissioner on Canada's Ecofiscal Commission. He is also a Board Member of the Canadian Institute for Climate Choices. He is Chair of the Boards of the Health Research Foundation and Canadian Blood Services. He has graduate degrees in Economics from the Universities of Western Ontario and Toronto and honorary doctorates from both. He is an Officer of the Order of Canada and a recipient of the Queen's Diamond and Golden Jubilee Medals. His research interests are in governance and decision-making.

Céline Castets-Renard is currently Full Professor of Law at the Faculty of Law (Civil Law Section) of the University of Ottawa, and member of the Center of Law, Technology and Society. She holds the University Research Chair on Accountable AI in a Global Context. She also holds the Research Chair on Law, Accountability, Social Trust in AI granted by the French Government (ANR-3IA), within the Artificial and Natural Intelligence Toulouse Institute (ANITI). She was Full Law

Professor at Toulouse Capitole University (France) from 2002 to 2019, and Junior Member of the Institut Universitaire de France (IUF) (2015–2019). She also was Fulbright Visiting Scholar at Fordham Law School, Center of Law and Information Policy (CLIP) (2017–2019) and Visiting Scholar at Yale Law School, Internet Society Project (2018–2019). Her research on law and technology addresses issues in an American and European perspective, such as data and privacy, cybersecurity, regulation of platforms, and the law of AI. She also studies the accountability of algorithms and automated decision-making in a sectorial approach; for instance, predictive policing.

Timothy Caulfield is Canada Research Chair in Health Law and Policy, Professor in the Faculty of Law and the School of Public Health, and Research Director of the Health Law Institute at the University of Alberta. His interdisciplinary research on topics like stem cells, genetics, research ethics, the public representations of science and public health policy has resulted in over 350 academic articles. He has won numerous academic and writing awards and is a Fellow of the Royal Society of Canada and the Canadian Academy of Health Sciences. He frequently contributes to the popular press and is the author of two national bestsellers: *The Cure for Everything: Untangling the Twisted Messages About Health, Fitness and Happiness* (Penguin, 2012) and *Is Gwyneth Paltrow Wrong About Everything? When Celebrity Culture and Science Clash* (Penguin, 2015). His most recent book is *Relax, Dammit! A User's Guide to the Age of Anxiety* (Penguin Random House, 2020). Professor Caulfield is also the host and co-producer of the award-winning documentary TV show *A User's Guide to Cheating Death,* which has been shown in over 60 countries, including streaming on Netflix in North America.

Jennifer A. Chandler is Full Professor of Law and holder of the Bertram Loeb Research Chair at the University of Ottawa. She teaches mental health law and policy and neuroethics. She currently sits as a member of the Advisory Board for the Institute for Neurosciences, Mental Health and Addiction within the Canadian Institutes of Health Research (CIHR). Professor Chandler regularly contributes to Canadian governmental policy in the area of biomedical law and regulation. She was a member of the government-commissioned Expert Panel on Medical Assistance in Dying, addressing the question of access to medical assistance in dying for people with psychiatric conditions. She is currently chairing the law and ethics working group of Canadian Blood Services looking at the legal definition of brain death and criteria for determination of brain death, and she chairs the ethics committee of the Canadian Society for Transplantation. She has just completed a term as an elected member of the Board of Directors of the International Neuroethics Society and currently serves on the international editorial boards of multiple neuroethics journals and book series. Her research interests include the law and ethics of the brain sciences, mental health law and policy, and organ donation and transplantation.

Y. Y. Brandon Chen is a lawyer and a social worker by training. He is Assistant Professor in the University of Ottawa's Faculty of Law (Common Law Section). He has served as a board member of the Canadian Centre on Statelessness and as the co-chair of the Committee for Accessible AIDS Treatment. His research interests lie at the intersection between health and international migration, including such topics as migrant health care, migration and HIV/AIDS, and medical tourism.

Anis Chowdhury is Adjunct Professor of Economics, Western Sydney University and University of New South Wales (Canberra campus). He served at the United Nations Department of Economic and Social Affairs (UN-DESA, New York) as Senior Economic Affairs Officer and Chief, Financing for Development Office (Multi-stakeholder Engagement Section), and at the Economic and Social Commission for Asia and the Pacific (UN-ESCAP, Bangkok) as Director of Macroeconomic Policy and Development Division and Statistics Division. Prior to joining the United Nations in 2008, he was Professor of Economics at Western Sydney University. He was the founder and chief editor of the *Journal of the Asia Pacific Economy*, where he now serves as co-editor. He is also on the editorial board of *Economic and Labour Relations Review*. He has published widely on macroeconomic policies, sustainable development, financing for development, international political economy, labour markets, and industrial policy.

Aimée Craft is an internationally recognized leader in the area of Indigenous laws, treaties, water, and Canadian constitutional law. She prioritizes Indigenous-led and interdisciplinary research, including visual arts and film, co-leads a series of major research grants on

Decolonizing Water Governance, and works with many Indigenous nations and communities on Indigenous relationships with and responsibilities to *nibi* (water). She plays an active role in international collaborations relating to transformative memory in colonial contexts and relating to the reclamation of Indigenous birthing practices as expressions of territorial sovereignty. Professor Craft is Associate Professor at the Faculty of Common Law, University of Ottawa, and an Indigenous (Anishinaabe-Métis) lawyer from Treaty 1 territory in Manitoba. She is the former Director of Research at the National Inquiry into Missing and Murdered Indigenous Women and Girls and the founding Director of Research at the National Centre for Truth and Reconciliation. She practised at the Public Interest Law Centre for over a decade and in 2016 she was voted one of the top 25 most influential lawyers in Canada. *Breathing Life into the Stone Fort Treaty*, her award-winning book, focuses on understanding and interpreting treaties from an Anishinaabe *inaakonigewin* (legal) perspective.

Paul Daly holds the University Research Chair in Administrative Law and Governance at the University of Ottawa, to which he was recruited from the Faculty of Law, University of Cambridge. Previously, he was successively Assistant Professor, Associate Dean, and Associate Professor at the Faculté de droit, Université de Montréal and held visiting positions at Harvard Law School and Université Paris II, Panthéon-Assas. A graduate of University College Cork (BCL, LLM), the University of Pennsylvania Law School (LLM), and the University of Cambridge (PhD), his influential scholarly work on administrative law has been widely cited, including by the Supreme Court of Canada, various other Canadian courts and tribunals, the Irish Supreme Court, and the High Court of Australia. His blog, *Administrative Law Matters*, was the first blog ever cited by the Supreme Court of Canada. Since September 1, 2019, he has been a part-time Review Officer of the Environmental Protection Tribunal of Canada. His research interests span the broad field of comparative public law, especially judicial review of administrative action and complex constitutional issues.

Jeremy de Beer is Full Professor at the University of Ottawa's Faculty of Law, where he creates and shapes ideas about technology innovation, intellectual property, and global trade and development. An award-winning professor recognized for exceptional contributions to research and law teaching, Jeremy helps solve practical challenges related to innovation in the digital economy, life sciences, industries, and the clean technology sector. He is also an author or editor of 5 books and has published more than 50 peer-reviewed chapters and articles. Jeremy has a history of successfully leading international projects. He is the co-founder and director of the Open African Innovation Research Network, a Senior Fellow at the Centre for International Governance Innovation and a Senior Research Associate at the University of Cape Town's Intellectual Property Unit. As a practising lawyer and expert consultant, Jeremy has argued numerous cases before the Supreme Court of Canada, advised businesses and law firms, and consulted for agencies ranging from national governments to the United Nations. Jeremy holds a BA and LLB from the University of Saskatchewan and a BCL from the University of Oxford.

Patrick Fafard is Full Professor in the Graduate School of Public and International Affairs at the University of Ottawa. He has had a lengthy career spanning both government and academe. He has served in senior management positions with the Governments of Canada and Saskatchewan. Patrick has published extensively in a number of policy fields, including health, trade and the environment, intergovernmental relations, and Canadian federalism. His current research includes the governance of organ donation and transplantation, a comparative study of public health leadership and public health as a political project. Patrick serves as Associate Director of the Global Strategy Lab (York University and University of Ottawa) and he is a member of the University of Ottawa Centre for Health Care Law, Policy and Ethics.

Leilani Farha is the former United Nations Special Rapporteur on the Right to Housing and Global Director of The Shift, an international movement to secure the right to housing. Her work is animated by the principle that housing is a social good, not a commodity. Leilani has helped develop global human rights standards on the right to housing, including through her topical reports on homelessness, the financialization of housing, informal settlements, rights-based housing strategies, and the first UN Guidelines for the implementation of the right to housing. Leilani has worked to advance the right to housing in countries around the world, including Egypt, India, Indonesia, Nigeria, Philippines, Portugal, South Korea, Spain, Sweden, and the United States. Her research interests include the financialization of housing, the human right to housing, rights-based community engagement, and housing policy.

Katherine Fierlbeck is McCulloch Professor of Political Science at Dalhousie University. Her research interests focus on health care governance, federal health systems, and comparative health system analysis. Her recent books include *Health Law and Policy From East to West: Analytical Perspectives and Comparative Case Studies* (2020, with Joaquin Cayón de las Cuevas), *Health System Profiles: Nova Scotia* (2018), *Comparative Health Care Federalism* (2015), *Canadian Health Care Federalism* (2013, with William Lahey), and *Health Care in Canada: A Citizen's Guide to Politics and Policies* (2011).

Alexandra Flynn is Assistant Professor at the University of British Columbia's Allard School of Law. Her teaching and research focus on municipal law and governance. Professor Flynn's current project, funded by the Social Sciences and Humanities Research Council of Canada (SSHRC), focuses on the legal relationship between Indigenous communities and municipal governments. The goal of this project is to illuminate the legal obligations of municipal governments, including the duty to consult and accommodate, to create reciprocal, respectful relationships with Indigenous Peoples and First Nations. She is the author of many academic and popular media contributions and is currently working on a book entitled *Micro Legal Spaces: The Laws of Neighbourhoods and Communities,* which examines overlapping geographies and governance of city spaces, including the formal and informal bodies that represent residents. She has a long history working in law and policy and is a past TEDx speaker and a frequent media commentator.

Eleonore Fournier-Tombs is a senior data scientist focusing on anticipatory financing of humanitarian crises, on joint appointment at UNOCHA's Centre for Humanitarian Data and the World Bank's Disaster Risk Financing Unit. She has a PhD in Computational Social Science from the University of Geneva and recently completed a postdoctoral fellowship at McGill University's School of Information Science. Eleonore has worked at the United Nations since 2011 and received the Secretary General's Award in 2012 for her work at the Rio+20 Conference. She is currently a member of the International Observatory on the Societal Impacts of AI and Digital Technology

(OBVIA) in Montreal, as well as a senior researcher at the Canada Research Chair for Accountable AI in a Global Context at the University of Ottawa. Her research interests include computational political science (notably, to measure deliberative democracy), AI ethics and policy, and AI in a humanitarian context.

Marie-France Fortin is Assistant Professor in the University of Ottawa's Faculty of Law. She is a PhD graduand from the University of Cambridge, where she completed a thesis titled "A Historical Constitutional Approach to the King Can Do No Wrong: Revisiting Crown Liability." She holds an LLB from Université Laval (profil international Université de Paris II Panthéon-Assas) and a Master of Law degree in international law from the University of Cambridge and a Master of Law from Harvard Law School. Her research interests include the broad field of public law, constitutional theory, comparative constitutional law, Crown liability and legal history in public law, as well as water law and policy. Marie-France received several awards and scholarships, including The Right Honourable Paul Martin Sr. Scholarship, the Frank Knox Memorial Fellowship, and a doctoral scholarship from the Pierre Elliott Trudeau Foundation. She served as a law clerk to the Honourable Morris J. Fish at the Supreme Court of Canada from 2007 to 2008. She has practised law in prominent Canadian law firms and acted as legal counsel for various departments and governmental organizations at both the federal and provincial levels. She has been a member of the Québec Bar since 2007.

Linda Garcia est professeure à l'École interdisciplinaire des sciences de la santé et directrice de l'Institut de recherche LIFE de l'Université d'Ottawa. Avant de se joindre au corps professoral de l'Université d'Ottawa en 1993, elle a travaillé pendant plus de 10 ans dans un grand hôpital d'enseignement en tant qu'orthophoniste. Après avoir obtenu son doctorat sous la direction du professeur Yves Joanette et aidé à fonder le programme d'audiologie et d'orthophonie, elle a créé l'École interdisciplinaire des sciences de la santé et en a été la première directrice en 2010, avant de devenir vice-doyenne de la Faculté des sciences de la santé en 2014 et directrice de l'Institut de recherche LIFE en 2018. Les intérêts de recherche personnels de Linda portent sur l'impact des environnements physiques, sociaux, technologiques et cliniques sur la qualité de vie des personnes atteintes de troubles neurologiques, en particulier la démence. Elle s'intéresse au développement d'interventions qui comprennent des approches basées sur les interactions humaines, particulièrement dans les milieux de vie des soins de longue durée.

Linda Garcia is Professor in the Interdisciplinary School of Health Sciences and Director of the LIFE Research Institute at the University of Ottawa. Prior to joining the University in 1993, Professor Garcia worked for over ten years in a large teaching hospital as a speech-language pathologist and department head. After completing her PhD with Dr. Yves Joanette, she worked as a professor in the Audiology and Speech-Language Pathology Program. She then moved on to help create the Interdisciplinary School of Health Sciences and became its first director in 2010, prior to becoming Vice-Dean of the Faculty of Health Sciences in 2014 and the Director of the LIFE Research Institute in 2018. Her research interests focus on the impact of social and physical environments on the functioning of individuals with neurological disorders, especially dementia. She is interested in developing interventions that include approaches based on human interactions and improving quality of life in long-term care.

Michelle Giroux est professeure titulaire à la Faculté de droit, Section de droit civil, à l'Université d'Ottawa et membre du Barreau du Québec. Elle est également membre du Laboratoire de recherche interdisciplinaire sur les droits de l'enfant, du Centre de droit, de politique et d'éthique de la santé et de l'Institut de recherche LIFE, à l'Université d'Ottawa. Elle enseigne le droit des personnes et de la famille, le droit médical, la bioéthique et le droit de la santé publique. En 2012, la professeure Giroux a fait partie du Comité de juristes experts nommés par le gouvernement du Québec pour mettre en œuvre les recommandations de la Commission parlementaire spéciale sur la question de mourir dans la dignité. Elle est membre du Comité consultatif de la Commission du droit de l'Ontario sur le projet *Améliorer les dernières étapes de la vie*. Ses intérêts de recherche portent notamment sur les enjeux liés à la procréation médicalement assistée et aux soins de fin de vie.

Michelle Giroux is Full Professor in the Faculty of Law (Civil Law Section) at the University of Ottawa and a Member of the Québec Bar. She is also a member of the Interdisciplinary Research Laboratory on the Rights of the Child, the Centre for Health Law, Policy and Ethics and of the LIFE Research Institute, at the University of Ottawa. She teaches persons and family law, law and medical ethics, and public health law. In 2012, Professor Giroux was on the panel of legal experts appointed by the Government of Québec to implement the report of the Select Committee on Dying with Dignity. She sits on the Law Commission of Ontario's Advisory Group for the Project on Improving the Last Stages of Life. Her research interests include assisted reproduction and end of life care.

E. Richard Gold is a James McGill Professor with McGill University's Faculty of Law and a Senior Fellow at the Centre for International Governance Innovation (CIGI). As a McGill Professor, he was the founding director of the Centre for Intellectual Property Policy. Richard teaches intellectual property, international intellectual property, comparative intellectual property, and innovation policy with a research focus on the life sciences. Over the years, Richard has provided advice to Health Canada, Industry Canada, the Canadian Biotechnology Advisory Committee, the Ontario Ministry of Health and Long-Term Care, the Organisation for Economic Cooperation and Development, the World Health Organization, the World Intellectual Property Organization, and UNITAID. Richard's research has been published in high-impact journals in science, law, philosophy, and international relations. In addition, he has filed amicus briefs with the Supreme Court of the United States, the United States Court of Appeals for the Federal Circuit, the Supreme Court of Canada, and a tribunal that adjudicated an investor-state dispute under the North American Free Trade Agreement. Richard has a Bachelor of Science from McGill University, an LLB (honours) from the University of Toronto, and an SJD and LLM from the University of Michigan Law School.

Vanessa Gruben is Vice-Dean of the English Common Law Program and Associate Professor and a member of the Centre for Health Law, Policy and Ethics at the University of Ottawa. Her research interests include legal and ethical issues regarding professional self-regulation, assisted reproduction, organ donation, and harm reduction. She is co-editor of the 5th edition of Canada's leading health law text, *Canadian Health Law and Policy*, with Joanna Erdman and Erin Nelson (LexisNexis, 2017). Her most recent book is *Surrogacy in Canada: Critical Perspectives in Law and Policy*, co-edited with Alana Cattapan and Angela Cameron (Irwin Law, 2018). Her research has been funded by the Canadian Institutes of Health Research, the Social Sciences and Humanities Research Council, Canadian Blood Services, and the Foundation for Legal Research. Professor Gruben teaches graduate and undergraduate courses in Health Law and Public Health Law, as well as a seminar on Access to Health Care.

Mona Gupta is a psychiatrist at the Centre Hospitalier de l'Université de Montréal (CHUM) and Clinician-Investigator at the Centre de Recherche du CHUM. She is also Associate Clinical Professor in the Department of Psychiatry and Addictions of the Université de Montréal. The broad theme of her area of inquiry is the interface of ethics and epistemology in psychiatry. Her specific research interests include standards of evidence and conceptions of errors in psychiatry, intersubjectivity, and assisted dying for persons with mental disorders.

Sam F. Halabi is the Manley O. Hudson Professor of Law at the University of Missouri, as well as a scholar at the O'Neill Institute for National and Global Health Law at Georgetown University. He served as the 2017-18 Fulbright Canada Research Chair in Health Law, Policy, and Ethics at the University of Ottawa. Prof. Halabi is the author of *Intellectual Property and the New International Economic Order* (Cambridge University Press, 2018) and he has edited (with Lawrence O. Gostin and Jeffrey S. Crowley) *Global Management of Infectious Disease After Ebola* (Oxford University Press, 2017). He has authored or co-authored more than 30 articles and book chapters in legal and medical publications, including the *Georgetown Law Journal*, the *Journal of the American Medical Association* (JAMA), and the *Lancet*. Prof. Halabi advises or has advised domestic and international organizations including the World Health Organization, the National Foundation for the Centers for Disease Control and Prevention, and the Global Virome Project. His research interests include global health law, intellectual property aspects of access to health care and medicines, and health care financing.

Lorian Hardcastle is Assistant Professor in the Faculty of Law and Cumming School of Medicine at the University of Calgary, where she is also a member of the AMR One Health Consortium and the O'Brien Institute for Public Health. Lorian obtained her JD with Health Law and Policy Specialization from Dalhousie University and her LLM and SJD from the University of Toronto. She also completed a fellowship at the O'Neill Institute for National and Global Health Law at Georgetown University. Lorian's work has been published in numerous legal and health policy journals, including the *Canadian Medical Association Journal, University of Pennsylvania Law Review, Healthcare Policy, Alberta Law Review, Queen's Law Journal,* and *Journal of Law, Medicine & Ethics.* She is the author of *Introduction to Health Law in Canada*. Lorian is a frequent contributor to health policy debates in the media. She has appeared numerous times on CBC, Global, and CTV, and her writing has been published in several Canadian newspapers, including the *Globe and Mail, Toronto Star, Calgary Herald, Edmonton Journal,* and *Ottawa Citizen*. Lorian's research interests include public health law, liability and governance of health facilities and health professionals, and governmental liability in the health sector.

Simon Hatcher is Full Professor of Psychiatry at the University of Ottawa. He moved to Ottawa from Auckland, New Zealand, in 2012. He trained in psychiatry in the U.K. and then worked in New Zealand in the Department of Psychological Medicine at the University of Auckland. His main research interests include suicide, self-harm, psychotherapies, clinical trials and e-therapies. His research lab *Hatching Ideas Hub* focuses on clinical trials in underserved populations. He works in a First Responder Clinic, the homeless shelters, and at The Ottawa Hospital.

Matthew Herder is Director of the Health Law Institute at Dalhousie University in Halifax, Nova Scotia, and is also Associate Professor at Dalhousie University's Faculties of Medicine and Law. Matthew's research focuses on biomedical innovation policy, with a particular emphasis on intellectual property rights and the regulation of medical interventions, including pharmaceuticals, biologics, and medical devices. In 2018, he was appointed a member of the Patented Medicine Prices Review Board, Canada's national drug price regulator, and he became a member of the Royal Society of Canada's College of New Scholars, Artists and Scientists in 2019. He has published extensively and engaged in various forms of policy advocacy in an effort to help reform how knowledge about the safety and effectiveness of medical interventions is generated and governed.

Jeffery G. Hewitt joined Osgoode Hall Law School in 2019 as an Assistant Professor. He holds an LLB and an LLM from Osgoode and was called to the Bar of Ontario in 1998. His research and teaching interests include Indigenous legal orders and governance, constitutional law, human right, and business law, as well as art and law and visual legal studies. Professor Hewitt has presented his research work nationally and internationally to a range of audiences. He is mixed-descent Cree and works with Rama First Nation as well as other Indigenous Elders and leaders in the promotion of Indigenous legal orders. He is a past president of the Indigenous Bar Association of Canada and is currently director of the National Theatre School.

Steven J. Hoffman is the Dahdaleh Distinguished Chair in Global Governance and Legal Epidemiology and Professor of Global Health, Law, and Political Science at York University, the Director of the Global Strategy Lab, the Director of the World Health Organization Collaborating Centre on Global Governance of Antimicrobial Resistance, and the Scientific Director of the CIHR Institute of Population and Public Health at the Canadian Institutes of Health Research. He holds courtesy appointments as Professor of Clinical Epidemiology and Biostatistics (Part-Time) at McMaster University and Adjunct Professor of Global Health and Population at Harvard University. He is an international lawyer licensed in both Ontario and New York who specializes in global health law, global governance and institutional design. His research leverages various methodological approaches to craft global strategies that better address transnational health threats and social inequalities. Past studies have focused on access to medicines, antimicrobial resistance, health misinformation, pandemics, and tobacco control. Steven previously worked as a Project Manager for the World Health Organization in Geneva, Switzerland, and as a Fellow in the Executive Office of the United Nations Secretary-General Ban Ki-moon in New York City, where he offered strategic and technical input on a range of global health issues.

Adam R. Houston is a PhD candidate (Law) at the University of Ottawa, working at the intersection of global health and human rights. He holds a JD from the University of Victoria and an MA in Global Development Studies from Queen's University (where his award-nominated thesis focused upon reconciling disparate approaches to HIV and tuberculosis in South Africa's first integrated National Strategic Plan). He won the Outstanding Student Award in his LLM (Health Law, Global Health & Justice) from the University of Washington. He has worked all across Canada and around the world with such organizations as Avocats sans frontières Canada (ASFC), the Pacific Islands AIDS Foundation (PIAF), and the Institute for Justice & Democracy in Haiti (IJDH), the latter as part of their groundbreaking advocacy around United Nations accountability for the Haitian cholera epidemic. He has also taught courses on topics related to health, human rights, and justice at multiple Canadian universities. His current research focuses on access to off-patent essential medicines and on human rights considerations in the response to tuberculosis and other infectious diseases.

Adelina Iftene is Assistant Professor at Schulich School of Law, Dalhousie University and the incoming Associate Director of the Health Law Institute at Dalhousie. Adelina teaches criminal law, evidence and imprisonment, and prison policy. Her major research work explores issues related to prison health and access to justice for prisoners, and her book *Punished for Aging: Vulnerabilities, Rights, and Access to Justice in Canadian Penitentiaries* was published by University of Toronto Press in 2019. Adelina's current research interests include end of life and incarceration, compassionate release mechanisms, sentencing of old and sick individuals, and evidentiary issues related to undercover investigations.

Martha Jackman is Professor of constitutional law in the Faculty of Law, University of Ottawa, where she has taught in the French Common Law Program since 1988. She was a consultant to the Auditor General of Canada (Federal Support of Health Care Delivery Audit), the Canadian Bar Association Health Care Task Force, the Royal Commission on New Reproductive Technologies, and the Commission on the Future of Health Care in Canada. She is the Co-Chair of the National Association of Women and the Law, a past board member of the Canadian Health Coalition, and has acted as legal counsel in Charter test cases, including before the Supreme Court of Canada in *Eldridge v British Columbia* (1997) and *Chaoulli v Québec* (2005). In 2007, she was awarded the Law Society of Ontario Medal; in 2015, she was the recipient of the Canadian Bar Association's Touchstone Award; and in 2017, she was elected to the Royal Society of Canada. Her research interests include socio-economic rights, federalism, the Canadian Charter, equality, and health.

Jomo Kwame Sundaram was an economics professor until 2004 and Assistant Secretary General for Economic Development in the United Nations system (2005–2015). He is senior advisor, Khazanah Research Institute, and was an occasional advisor to the last Malaysian government (2018–2020) and Founder/Chair, International Development Economics Associates. He received the Wassily Leontief Prize for Advancing the Frontiers of Economic Thought in 2007.

Yasmin Khaliq is currently studying in the Programme de common law en français at the University of Ottawa. Dr. Khaliq comes from a health care background with both a Bachelor of Science in Pharmacy and a Doctorate in Pharmacy. She has extensive hospital experience in patient care, teaching, drug information, and research. Specifically, she has worked in the areas of critical care, infectious diseases, hematology/bone marrow transplantation, gynecology-oncology, and geriatrics. In more recent years, Dr. Khaliq has focused on the specialty of mental health and, in particular, mental health and the law. She has been a member of both the Consent and Capacity Board and the Ontario Review Board in Ontario. Her research interests include access to care for the mentally ill, as well as the forensic mental health system.

Martine Lagacé est professeure au Département de communication et membre de l'Institut de recherche LIFE à l'Université d'Ottawa. Ses intérêts de recherche portent sur la communication intergénérationnelle, l'âgisme, l'identité et les relations intergroupes. Les travaux de la professeure Lagacé ont grandement contribué à l'avancement des connaissances sur les aspects psychosociaux du vieillissement, particulièrement quant aux tenants et aboutissants de la discrimination basée sur l'âge. Elle a mené plusieurs enquêtes de terrain au Canada et à l'échelle internationale, auprès des travailleurs comme des patients âgés, afin de mieux comprendre les manifestations et les répercussions de l'âgisme. Dans le monde francophone, ses travaux universitaires sur l'âgisme font figure de pionniers. Elle a d'ailleurs dirigé deux ouvrages sur l'âgisme : *Comprendre et changer le regard sur le vieillissement* (2010) et *Représentations et discours sur le vieillissement* (2015), publiés aux Presses de l'Université Laval.

Martine Lagacé is Professor in the Department of Communication and a member of the LIFE Research Institute at the University of Ottawa.

Her research interests are in intergenerational communication, ageism, identity, and intergroup relations. Dr. Lagacé has contributed greatly to the advancement of knowledge on the psychosocial aspects of aging, particularly as they relate to discrimination based on age. She has led several field surveys in Canada and abroad, with workers as well as older patients to better understand the manifestations and impacts of ageism. Her academic work on ageism has been innovative, particularly in the francophone community. She has edited two books on the topic of ageism: *Comprendre et changer le regard sur le vieillissement* (2010) and *Représentations et discours sur le vieillissement* (2015), published by les Presses de l'Université Laval.

Yves Le Bouthillier is Professor in the Faculty of Law at the University of Ottawa (Common Law Section, French Common Law Program). He teaches in the areas of public law, including citizenship, immigration and refugee law, and in public international law. He is the co-author, with Delphine Nakache, of a forthcoming book on citizenship law in Canada, and he has previously published with her a volume on this topic in French. He has held various positions within the Faculty (Vice-Dean of the French Common Law Program, Co-director of the IUCN Academy of Environmental Law) and outside (President of the Law Commission of Canada, Scholar-In-Residence at the Department of Global Affairs).

Olivia Lee is is a resident physician at the University of Ottawa, Department of Psychiatry. Before committing to medicine, she was a law student at the University of Ottawa and obtained her law degree prior to starting residency. She has assisted in research on genetic discrimination, privacy policy, health outcomes of people who use drugs, neuroethics, and the intersection between mental illness and the legal system. She has also led health advocacy projects at both the provincial and federal levels and will sit as the Resident Doctors of Canada representative on the Canadian Medical Association Ethics Committee for the 2020–2021 term. Her research interests include the interaction between mental illness and the legal system, medical assistance in dying, neuroethics, and the mental health of vulnerable populations.

Anne Levesque is Assistant Professor in the French Common Law Program in the Faculty of Law at the University of Ottawa. She obtained her Master's in International Human Rights from Oxford

University, where she studied with a full scholarship from the Baxter & Alma Ricard Foundation. Anne was admitted to the Bar in Ontario in 2008 and practised human rights law in private practice and also in a community legal clinic. She has appeared before several administrative tribunals, Canadian courts of all levels, including the Supreme Court of Canada, and regional and international human rights bodies. She is one of the lawyers who represented the First Nations Child and Family Caring Society in its human rights case leading to a historic victory in 2016 which affirmed the right to equality for more than 165,000 First Nations children in Canada. Her research and publications focus on human rights and public interest litigation.

Jamie Chai Yun Liew is an immigration and refugee lawyer and Associate Professor in the Faculty of Law, University of Ottawa. She has appeared before the Immigration and Refugee Board, the Federal Court of Canada, and the Supreme Court of Canada. She is the co-author (with Donald Galloway) of *Immigration Law*, published by Irwin Law. Jamie is a member of the litigation committee of the Canadian Council for Refugees and engages in advocacy work with the Canadian Association of Refugee Lawyers and Amnesty International. Her research focuses on how law and public policy marginalizes immigrants, migrants, refugees, refugee claimants, and stateless persons. Her writing has looked at legal barriers in making gender-based refugee claims, as well as the challenges LGBTQ refugees and migrants with mental illness face in the immigration system. Jamie's socio-legal work examines barriers to family reunification that immigrants face and how immigration policy has constructed the irregular border crossers at the Canada-U.S. border as "illegal." Her current research examines how law constructs stateless persons in Canada and Malaysia and how the legal concept of "alternative remedies" has prevented migrants and stateless persons from fully accessing protections in the *Charter of Rights and Freedoms*.

Katherine Lippel is Full Professor of Law in the Faculty of Law (Civil Law Section) at the University of Ottawa and has held the Distinguished Research Chair in Occupational Health and Safety Law since March 2020. Between 2006 and 2020, she held the Canada Research Chair in Occupational Health and Safety Law (http://www.droitcivil.uottawa.ca/chairohslaw). She is also a member of the Québec Bar and of the CINBIOSE research centre. She specializes in legal issues related to occupational health and safety, workers' compensation, and return to work after work injury. She currently leads a research partnership funded by Social Sciences and Humanities Research Council of Canada (SSHRC) and Canadian Institutes of Health Research (CIHR) entitled "Policy and Practice in Return to Work After Work Injury: Challenging Circumstances and Innovative Solutions". In 2017, she was awarded the SSHRC Gold Medal, the Council's highest award. Her research interests include the role of law in the prevention of occupational illness and disease, workers' compensation, the prevention of disability, and return to work after work injury.

Deborah McGregor is Canada Research Chair in Indigenous Environmental Justice, cross-appointed with Osgoode Hall Law School and the Faculty of Environmental Studies, York University. Professor McGregor has been at the forefront of Indigenous environmental justice and Indigenous research theory and practice. Over the years, she has achieved international recognition through her creative and innovative approach, using digital and social media to reach Indigenous communities and the general public. Her work has been shared through the Indigenous Environmental Justice (IEJ) project website (https://iejproject.info.yorku.ca/) and the UKRI International Collaboration on Indigenous research website (https://www.indigenous.ncrm.ac.uk).

Ravi Malhotra is Full Professor in the Faculty of Law (Common Law Section), cross-appointed to the School of Rehabilitation Sciences, University of Ottawa. A graduate of Harvard Law School, he has published widely in numerous journals, including the *McGill Journal of Law and Health*, the *Ottawa Law Review*, and the *Windsor Yearbook on Access to Justice*. He has also published numerous books, including the anthologies *Disability Politics in a Global Economy: Essays in Honour of Marta Russell* (Routledge) and *Disabling Barriers: Social Movements, Disability History and the Law* (with Benjamin Isitt). He is currently completing a biography (under contract with UBC Press) on a double amputee and socialist militant, E. T. Kingsley (with Benjamin Isitt). From 2017 to 2019, he served as Vice-Dean (Graduate Studies). His research interests include labour law, disability rights law, and human rights law.

Carissima Mathen is Professor of Law at the University of Ottawa. A leading constitutional scholar, she is the author of *Courts Without*

Cases: The Law and Politics of Advisory Opinions (Hart, 2019) and *The Tenth Justice: Judicial Appointments, Marc Nadon, and the Supreme Court Act Reference* (UBC Press, 2020) (with Michael Plaxton). She is a former Director of Litigation for the Women's Legal Education and Action Fund (LEAF), where she undertook path-breaking equality rights litigation. An award-winning media commentator, Professor Mathen has given hundreds of interviews in all media formats and published numerous op-eds. She pioneered the practice of "live tweeting" from the Supreme Court of Canada and is committed to public education and legal literacy. Professor Mathen is a recipient of the Law Society Medal, one of the highest honours bestowed by the Law Society of Ontario. In addition to her two books, Professor Mathen has published on all aspects of constitutional law, as well as in criminal law, legal theory, and law and technology. Her current research interests include a reconceptualization of the doctrine of arbitrariness in constitutional and criminal law and how to balance social media regulation with freedom of expression.

Kwame McKenzie is the CEO of Wellesley Institute and is an international expert on the social causes of mental illness and suicide, and the development of effective, equitable health systems. Kwame is also Director of Health Equity at the Centre for Addiction and Mental Health (CAMH), and Professor in the Department of Psychiatry at the University of Toronto. As a policy advisor, clinician, and academic with over 200 papers and 5 books, Kwame has worked across a broad spectrum to improve population health and health services for over two decades. He is currently a member of the National Advisory Council on Poverty and previously was an advisor to Ontario's basic income pilot project. He sits on the board of United Way Toronto and the Ontario Hospitals Association. In addition to his academic, policy, and clinical work, Kwame is a columnist for the *Guardian*, *Times-online*, and *Toronto Star*, and is a past BBC Radio presenter.

Jason Millar holds the Canada Research Chair in the Ethical Engineering of Robotics and AI and is Assistant Professor at the University of Ottawa's School of Electrical Engineering and Computer Science, with a cross-appointment in the Department of Philosophy. He has authored book chapters, policy reports, and articles on the ethics and governance of robotics and AI. Jason consults internationally on policy and ethical engineering issues in emerging autonomous vehicle technology. His work is regularly featured in the media, including articles in such publications as WIRED and *The Guardian*, and in interviews with the BBC, CBC, and NPR. He recently authored a chapter titled "Social Failure Modes in Technology and the Ethics of AI: An Engineering Perspective," for the forthcoming *Oxford Handbook of Ethics of AI* (OUP). He also authored a chapter on ethics settings for autonomous vehicles in *Robot Ethics 2.0* (OUP), and co-authored a chapter on metaphors in technology governance for the *Oxford Handbook on the Law and Regulation of Technology* (OUP). His research interests include developing tools and methodologies engineers can use to integrate ethical thinking into their daily engineering workflow, and focusing on applications in automated vehicles, artificial intelligence, health care robotics, and social and military robotics.

Delphine Nakache is Associate Professor in the Faculty of Law at the University of Ottawa (Common Law Section, French Common Law Program). She teaches courses in the areas of public international law, humanitarian law, and immigration and refugee law. As an investigator in several funded projects, she has researched and published on issues related to the human rights and security-based implications of migration, citizenship, and refugee laws and policies, both in Europe and in Canada. Her main focus is on issues surrounding the protection of migrant workers, asylum seekers, and non-status migrants, and on barriers to citizenship for disadvantaged immigrants. She also regularly provides consultancy work for the United Nations or the Government of Canada. Delphine is the author (with Yves Le Bouthillier) of a forthcoming book on *Citizenship Law in Canada* (to be published by Thomson Reuters/Carswell in 2021).

Jason W. Nickerson is a Clinical Scientist at the Bruyère Research Institute, an Adjunct Professor in the Centre for Health Law, Policy and Ethics at the University of Ottawa, and a Humanitarian Affairs advisor for Doctors Without Borders/Médecins Sans Frontières (MSF). As a respiratory therapist, he has worked in adult critical care and anesthesia in hospitals throughout Canada and has worked extensively in global public health response internationally during emergencies, including armed conflicts, disease epidemics, and sudden onset disasters. He currently works on intersecting issues of humanitarian diplomacy and response, health policy, and medical research and development, with a focus on ensuring access to the highest quality of medical care for people affected by crises. His research focuses on health policies that improve and hinder access to medicines and other health technologies, particularly controlled medicines for pain relief, anesthesia, and palliative care.

Chidi Oguamanam is Full Professor in the Faculty of Law (Common Law Section), University of Ottawa, where he is affiliated with the Centre for Law, Technology and Society, the Centre for Environmental Law and Global Sustainability and the Centre for Health Law, Policy and Ethics. He holds numerous research fellowships and affiliations with leading global organizations. Dr. Oguamanam leads, and is associated with, many research consortia, including the ABS Canada project and the Open African Innovation Research Partnership network (Open AIR). He is the author of several books and publications that reflect a wide range of interdisciplinary research interests spanning intellectual property's interface with Indigenous knowledge systems, global knowledge governance dynamics, biodiversity conservation, equitable access to and use of data, genetic and health resources, and the new and emerging innovation landscape for development. He was named to the Royal Society of Canada College of New Scholars, Artists and Scientists. Dr. Oguamanam is the editor of *Genetic Resources, Justice and Reconciliation: Canada and Global Access and Benefit Sharing*.

Jennifer A. Quaid is Vice-Dean Research and Communications in the Faculty of Law (Civil Law Section) at the University of Ottawa, where she teaches criminal law, competition law, and corporate law. Professor Quaid is a leading legal expert and scholar in organizational criminal liability, nationally and internationally. Her scholarship, policy work, and extensive public engagement focus on when and how law can be used to stimulate good governance and ethical business practices, particularly in the prevention of serious harm flowing from the materialization of foreseeable operational risks, such as corruption, fraud, and failure to take appropriate measures to protect public safety and the environment. Among her current funded projects, Professor Quaid is leading a four-year comparative study of the use of non-trial resolution mechanisms in corruption matters that brings together researchers in Canada, France, and Switzerland. A member of the Bars of Québec, Ontario, and New York, Prof. Quaid practised law before joining the academy, first with the Department of Justice Canada (Competition Law Division) and then with Sullivan

& Cromwell LLP in New York and Melbourne. She clerked for the Honourable Frank Iacobucci of the Supreme Court of Canada. Her research interests include Corporate Criminal Liability, Criminal Law, Competition Law, Anti-Corruption Law, Corporate Law, Corporate Governance, and Organization Studies.

Vardit Ravitsky is Full Professor in the Bioethics Program, School of Public Health, Université de Montréal. She is President of the International Association of Bioethics and Director of Ethics and Health at the Centre for Research on Ethics. She is a 2020 Trudeau Foundation Fellow and Chair of the Foundation's COVID-19 Impact Committee. She is also a member of the Standing Committee on Ethics of the Canadian Institutes of Health Research (CIHR), the Advisory Board of CIHR's Institute of Genetics, and the Genomics and Society Working Group of the National Human Genome Research Institute (NHGRI). Previously, she was faculty at the Department of Medical Ethics at the University of Pennsylvania. Her research is funded by Canada's leading funding agencies. She has published over 160 articles and commentaries on bioethical issues. Her research interests include the intersection between bioethics and public policy, and the way cultural perspectives frame bioethical reflection. Much of her research touches on the ethics of genomics and reproduction, and covers topics such as the ethical, social, and legal aspects of public funding of in vitro fertilization; the use of surplus frozen embryos; posthumous reproduction; pre-implantation genetic diagnosis; gamete donation; epigenetics; non-invasive prenatal testing; germline and somatic gene editing; and mitochondrial replacement.

David Robitaille est professeur titulaire à la Section de droit civil et codirecteur du Centre de droit public de l'Université d'Ottawa. Ses travaux de recherche et publications ont remporté de nombreux prix et subventions, dont la Médaille d'or de la gouverneure générale du Canada attribuée à la meilleure thèse de doctorat en sciences humaines à l'Université d'Ottawa en 2008. Le professeur Robitaille a été directeur de la *Revue générale de droit* de 2012 à 2014, obtenant au passage une subvention du CRSH pour l'Aide aux revues savantes. Il est aussi avocat-conseil auprès du Centre québécois du droit de l'environnement (CQDE) et du cabinet de droit municipal DHC Avocats de Montréal. Au cours des dernières années, il a plaidé devant la Cour d'appel du Québec, la Cour d'appel de l'Ontario et la Cour d'appel fédérale dans des litiges de droit constitutionnel et d'environnement d'intérêt public. Il agit aussi comme avocat du CQDE et d'Équiterre dans le dossier de la constitutionnalité de la tarification fédérale du carbone devant la Cour suprême du Canada. Il contribue régulièrement à la vulgarisation scientifique par de nombreuses entrevues avec les médias et la publication d'articles d'opinion dans les journaux. Il a été clerc de l'honorable juge François Pelletier à la Cour d'appel du Québec en 2002-2003. Ses recherches et publications récentes, subventionnées par le CRSH, portent notamment sur le fédéralisme et les interactions entre les compétences provinciales et fédérales en matière de transport interprovincial, de droits et libertés et d'environnement.

David Robitaille is Full Professor in the Faculty of Law (Civil Law Section) and Co-Director of the Public Law Centre, University of Ottawa. He has earned numerous awards and grants for his research projects and publications, including the Governor General's Gold Medal, awarded to the best thesis in the humanities at the University of Ottawa in 2008. He was the Director of the *Revue générale de droit*, the peer-reviewed journal of the Civil Law Section, from 2012 to 2014, for which he earned a Social Sciences and Humanities Research Council of Canada (SSHRC) Aid to Scholarly Journals grant. He is also legal counsel to the Québec Environmental Law Centre (CQDE) and at DHC Avocats, a municipal law firm in Montreal. In recent years, he has appeared before the Québec Court of Appeal, the Ontario Court of Appeal, and the Federal Court of Appeal in public interest constitutional and environmental law cases. He is also the legal counsel for the CQDE and Équiterre in the case on the constitutionality of the federal carbon pricing scheme before the Supreme Court of Canada. He regularly contributes to the popularization of science through numerous interviews with the media and the publication of op-eds in newspapers. He served as a law clerk to the Honourable Justice François Pelletier at the Québec Court of Appeal in 2002–2003. His recent research and publications, funded by Social Sciences and Humanities Research Council of Canada (SSHRC), have focused on federalism and the interaction between provincial and federal jurisdictions in the areas of interprovincial transportation, rights and freedoms, and the environment.

Teresa Scassa is Canada Research Chair in Information Law and Policy in the Faculty of Law, University of Ottawa. She is Chair of the Canadian Statistics Advisory Council, member of the Digital Strategy

Advisory Panel for Waterfront Toronto, and member of the Canadian Advisory Council on Artificial Intelligence. Teresa is also a Senior Fellow with CIGI's International Law Research Program. She is the author of *Canadian Trademark Law*, and co-author of *Digital Commerce in Canada*, and *Canadian Intellectual Property Law*. She is a co-editor of the books *Law and the Sharing Economy* and *Interdisciplinary Approaches to Intellectual Property Law*. Her research interests include privacy law, data governance, intellectual property law, law and technology, law and artificial intelligence, and smart cities.

Tess Sheldon is Assistant Professor in the Faculty of Law at the University of Windsor. She writes, presents, and teaches extensively on a variety of mental health, access to justice, disability, and human rights topics. She explores law's possibilities (and perils) to confront the regimes that reflect and reinforce economic and social exclusion, including of persons with disabilities and consumers/survivors of the psychiatric system.

Kaitlin Schwan is Director of Research at The Shift, an international movement to secure the right to housing. She is also a Senior Researcher at the Canadian Observatory on Homelessness (York University), and she teaches social policy at the University of Toronto's Faculty of Social Work, where she is appointed Assistant Professor, Status Only. Since completing her PhD in Social Work at the University of Toronto, Kaitlin's research has focused on homelessness prevention in Canada and beyond, particularly for women and youth. Across her work, Kaitlin uses research to build bridges between evidence, advocacy, policy, and lived expertise in order to advance housing justice for all. Her research interests include homelessness prevention, the human right to housing, community-based participatory research, and women's homelessness and housing issues.

Jeffrey Simpson is the author of seven books, including one on the Canadian health care system, which won the Donner Prize for the best book on Canadian public policy. He was the *Globe and Mail*'s national affairs columnist for 32 years and is now a Senior Fellow at the Graduate School of Policy and International Affairs at the University of Ottawa. He has received eight honorary degrees from universities across Canada and has won many awards for his book, magazine, and newspaper writing. He retired in 2016.

Terry Skolnik is Assistant Professor in the Faculty of Law (Civil Law Section) at the University of Ottawa. Prior to joining the Faculty, he was an affiliated scholar and a Scholar-in-Residence at NYU's Center for Human Rights and Global Justice (CHRGJ). He served as a law clerk for the Honourable Justice Russell Brown at the Supreme Court of Canada. Before entering academia, he worked as a police officer with the Montreal Police Service. His primary research interests are criminal law, legal philosophy, constitutional law, criminal evidence and procedure, poverty law, and the intersections between those fields.

Bryan Thomas is a Senior Research Fellow at the Centre for Health Law, Policy and Ethics and Adjunct Professor with the Faculty of Law, University of Ottawa. His research spans a wide range of topics, including Canadian and comparative health law and policy, health rights litigation, long-term care, global health law, and the role of religious arguments in legal and political discourse. Dr. Thomas holds an SJD from the University of Toronto and a Master's degree in philosophy from Dalhousie University.

Grégoire Webber is Canada Research Chair in Public Law and Philosophy of Law at Queen's University, Visiting Fellow at the London School of Economics and Political Science, and Executive Director of the Supreme Court Advocacy Institute. He was formerly Legal Affairs Advisor to the Minister of Justice and Attorney General of Canada and senior policy advisor with the Privy Council Office. His research areas are in jurisprudence, human rights, and public law.

Daniel M. Weinstock holds the Katharine A. Pearson Chair in Civil Society in the Faculties of Law and Arts at McGill University. Since 2013, he has been the director of McGill's Institute for Health and Social Policy. For 20 years, between 1992 and 2012, he was Professor in the Faculty of Law at the Université de Montréal and the Founding Director of that university's Centre de recherche en éthique. His research interests have focused on democracy and on the challenges posed by the ethnocultural and religious diversity of modern liberal democracies. He is presently leading a project on harm reduction as a key ingredient of public policy across a wide range of policy domains.

Kumanan Wilson is a specialist in general internal medicine and senior scientist at The Ottawa Hospital, innovation advisor at Bruyère

Research Institute and Professor of Medicine at the University of Ottawa. He is the CEO of CANImmunize, a pan-Canadian digital immunization application. His research interests include public health policy with a focus on blood safety, public health security, and immunizations. He also has expertise in big data and digital health.

www.ingramcontent.com/pod-product-compliance
Lightning Source LLC
Chambersburg PA
CBHW050327270326
41926CB00016B/3342
9780776636405